HANDBOOK OF SURGERY

Edited by

THEODORE R. SCHROCK, M.D.

Professor of Surgery
University of California
School of Medicine
San Francisco, California

with 95 illustrations

TENTH EDITION

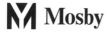 **Mosby**

St. Louis Baltimore Boston Chicago London Madrid
Philadelphia Sydney Toronto

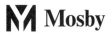
M Mosby

Dedicated to Publishing Excellence

Publisher: George Stamathis
Editor: Susie Baxter
Developmental Editor: Anne Gunter
Project Manager: Linda Clarke
Production Editor: Vicki Hoenigke
Senior Book Designer: Gail Morey Hudson

Tenth Edition

Printed in the United States of America
Composition by Clarinda Company
Printing/binding by Malloy Lithography, Inc.

Mosby–Year Book, Inc.
11830 Westline Industrial Drive, St. Louis, Missouri 63146

International Standard Book Number ISBN 0-8016-7637-1

94 95 96 97 98 CL/MA 9 8 7 6 5 4 3 2 1

Contributors

Except where noted, the contributors are affiliated with the School of Medicine, University of California, San Francisco.

F. William Blaisdell, M.D.
Professor and Chairman, Department of Surgery, University of California, Davis, California

Martin S. Bogetz, M.D.
Associate Professor of Clinical Anesthesia

Orlo H. Clark, M.D.
Professor of Surgery

Alfred A. deLorimier, M.D.
Professor of Surgery

Paul A. Fitzgerald, M.D.
Clinical Professor of Medicine

Dennis J. Flora, M.D.
Valley Medical Center, Fresno, California

Chris E. Freise, M.D.
Post-Doctoral fellow, Liver Transplantation Division

Barbara S. Gold, M.D.
Assistant Professor
Department of Anesthesiology, University of Minnesota, Minneapolis

William H. Goodson III, M.D.
Professor of Surgery

Michael R. Harrison, M.D.
Professor of Surgery

Edward C. Hill, M.D.
Emeritus Professor of Obstetrics, Gynecology, and Reproductive Sciences

John C. Hutchinson, M.D.
Clinical Professor of Medicine and Surgery

Ernest Jawetz, M.D., Ph.D.
Emeritus Professor of Microbiology and Medicine

Harry E. Jergesen, M.D.
Associate Clinical Professor of Orthopedic Surgery

Fraser Keith, M.D.
Assistant Professor of Surgery

Suzanne M. Kerley, M.D.
Assistant Professor of Plastic and Reconstructive Surgery

Eugene S. Kilgore, M.D.
Clinical Professor of Surgery

Frank R. Lewis, Jr., M.D.
Professor of Surgery, Case-Western Reserve University,
Cleveland, Ohio

Stephen J. Mathes, M.D.
Professor of Surgery

Scot H. Merrick, M.D.
Assistant Professor of Cardiothoracic Surgery

Anne E. Missavage, M.D.
Assistant Professor of Surgery, University of California,
Davis, California

William L. Newmeyer III, M.D.
Associate Clinical Professor of Surgery

Cornelius Olcott IV, M.D.
Bay Area Cardiovascular Medical Group

Lawrence H. Pitts, M.D.
Professor of Neurological Surgery

John P. Roberts, M.D.
Assistant Professor of Surgery

Hope S. Rugo, M.D.
Assistant Clinical Professor of Medicine

William P. Schecter, M.D.
Associate Clinical Professor of Surgery

Theodore R. Schrock, M.D.
Professor of Surgery

George F. Sheldon, M.D.
Professor and Chairman, Department of Surgery, University
of North Carolina, Chapel Hill

Patrick S. Swift
Assistant Professor, Department of Radiation Oncology

Thomas A. Tami, M.D.
Assistant Professor of Otolaryngology

Emil A. Tanagho, M.D.
Professor and Chairman, Department of Urology

Donald D. Trunkey, M.D.
Professor and Chairman, Department of Surgery, Oregon
Health Sciences University, Portland

Alan P. Venook
Assistant Professor, Department of Medicine,
Hematology/Oncology

Flavio Vincenti, M.D.
Professor of Clinical Medicine

To-Nao Wang, M.D.
Assistant Clinical Professor of Surgery

Robert S. Warren
Assistant Professor of Surgery

Preface

Handbook of Surgery is a concise, portable first reference for student, resident, and general physician. It is intended for use "on the scene" to give the readers some idea what questions to ask when taking a history, what physical signs to elicit, what tests to order, what other diagnostic possibilities to consider, and what treatment to institute immediately.

The tenth edition of *Handbook of Surgery* has been substantially revised to incorporate current knowledge and practice. New chapters have been added on Oncology and Organ Transplantation to reflect the continuing diversification of surgery. New authors have extensively revised the chapters on Pulmonary System, Surgical Infections, Head and Neck Surgery, Heart and Great Vessels, and Orthopedics.

My previous publisher, Richard C. M. Jones, has retired, and this tenth edition is published by Mosby–Year Book, Inc. I look forward to continuing success with this *Handbook of Surgery*.

Theodore R. Schrock

Contents

1

Shock and Trauma

Donald D. Trunkey

I. SHOCK

Shock is defined as peripheral circulatory failure causing tissue perfusion to be inadequate to meet the nutritional requirements of the cells and remove the waste products of metabolism. In the simplest terms, therefore shock is **inadequate tissue perfusion.**

Shock may be classified as hypovolemic, traumatic, septic, cardiogenic, neurogenic, or miscellaneous (e.g., anaphylactic reactions and insulin shock).

A. HYPOVOLEMIC SHOCK is the result of decreased blood volume due to acute and severe loss of blood, plasma, or body water and electrolytes. Hypovolemia accounts for nearly all shock seen within the first 24 hours of injury. Clinically, the patients have cool, mottled extremities. Hemorrhage, burns, bowel obstruction, peritonitis, and crush injuries are some of the common causes. A fall in venous pressure, a rise in peripheral vascular resistance, and tachycardia are characteristic of hypovolemic shock.

Factors that make a patient especially susceptible to hypovolemic shock include: **age** (the very young and the elderly tolerate loss of body water or plasma poorly); **chronic illness** (such patients often have a reduced blood volume and relatively small acute losses may precipitate shock); **anesthesia** (paralysis of vasomotor tone may cause shock in a patient who has compensated for a reduced blood volume); **adrenal insufficiency** (profound hypotension may be induced by minimal stress if corticosteroids are not supplied during and after trauma, operation, or illness).

1. Pathophysiology. Events in the microcirculation progress in phases.

a. Compensation phase. The first response of the circulation to hypovolemia is contraction of precapillary arterial sphincters; this causes the filtration pressure in the capillaries to fall. Because osmotic pressure remains the same, fluid moves into the vascular space with a corresponding increase in blood volume. If this compensatory mechanism is adequate to return blood volume to normal, the capillary sphincters relax and microcirculatory flow returns to normal. If shock is prolonged and profound, the next phase is entered.

b. Cell distress phase. If vascular volume has not been restored, the precapillary sphincters remain closed, and arteriovenous shunts open up to divert arterial blood directly back into the venous system, thus maintaining circulation to more important organs such as heart and brain. Cells in the bypassed segment of the microcirculation must rely on anaerobic metabolism for energy. The amount of glucose and oxygen available for the cell decreases, and metabolic waste products such as lactate accumulate. Histamine is released, resulting in closure of the postcapillary sphincters, and this mechanism serves to slow the remaining capillary flow and hold the red blood cells and nutrients in the capillaries longer. The empty capillary bed constricts almost completely; very few capillaries remain open.

c. Decompensation phase. Just before cell death, local reflexes (probably initiated by acidosis and accumulated metabolites) reopen the precapillary sphincters while the postcapillary sphincters stay closed. Prolonged vasoconstriction of the capillary bed damages endothelial cells and results in increased capillary permeability. When capillaries finally reopen, fluid and protein are leaked into the interstitial space; capillaries distend with RBCs, and sludging occurs. Cells become swollen, are unable to utilize oxygen, and die.

d. Recovery phase. If blood volume is restored at some point in the decompensation phase, effects on the microcirculation may still be reversible. Badly damaged cells may recover, and capillary integrity may be regained. The "sludge" in the microcirculation is swept into the venous circulation and eventually into the lungs, where these platelet and white cell aggregates are filtered out and produce postshock pulmonary failure (see Chapter 2). Other capillaries may be so badly damaged and filled with sludge that they remain permanently closed; cells dependent upon these capillaries die.

2. Diagnosis. Clinical assessment permits classification of hypovolemic shock as mild, moderate, or severe (Table 1-1). The compensatory mechanisms act to preserve blood flow to the heart and brain at the expense of all others; thus, in severe shock, there is marked constriction of all other vascular beds.

Table 1-1. Clinical classification of hypovolemic shock

Mild shock (up to 20% blood volume loss)

Definition: Decreased perfusion of nonvital organs and tissues (skin, fat, skeletal muscle, and bone).

Manifestations: Pale, cool skin. Patient complains of feeling cold.

Moderate shock (20%-40% blood volume loss)

Definition: Decreased perfusion of vital organs (liver, gut, kidneys).

Manifestations: Oliguria to anuria and slight to significant drop in blood pressure, mottling in extremities (especially legs).

Severe shock (40% or more blood volume loss)

Definition: Decreased perfusion of heart and brain.

Manifestations: Restlessness, agitation, coma, cardiac irregularities, ECG abnormalities, and cardiac arrest.

From Dunphy JE, Way LW, editors: *Current Surgical Diagnosis & Treatment,* ed 3, Lange.

3. Treatment. Shock is an acute emergency: **act promptly!**

a. Keep the patient recumbent—do not move the patient unnecessarily.

b. Establish and maintain an airway.

c. Place one or more large IV catheters.

(1) Do a cutdown in the long saphenous vein at the ankle; this method is rapid and safe.

(2) Do a cutdown on the basilic vein in the antecubital space so that central venous pressure can be monitored.

(3) Percutaneous insertion of subclavian or jugular catheters is not recommended because the veins are collapsed in hypovolemic shock. Femoral vein catheters may be placed percutaneously in unusual circumstances, e.g., when a single physician is available for resuscitation.

d. Parenteral fluids. Begin **immediately** to restore blood volume. In mild or moderate shock, the choice of fluid is important because endothelial permeability may be increased or microvascular forces altered, resulting in "capillary leak" which compounds the problems if colloid is given (Table 1-2).

(1) *Crystalloids* are preferred in the initial treatment of shock. They are readily available and effectively restore vascular volume for brief periods. Crystalloids also lower blood viscosity and enhance resuscitation of the microcir-

Table 1-2. Fluid resuscitation of shock

I. Crystalloids

    A. Isotonic sodium chloride

    B. Hypertonic sodium chloride

    C. Balanced salt solution: (1) Ringer's lactate; (2) *Ringer's acetate;* (3) Normosol, Plasmolyte, etc.

II. Colloid

    A. Blood: (1) Low-titer O negative blood; (2) *Type-specific;* (3) Typed and crossed; (4) Washed red cells; (5) Fresh red cells

    B. Plasma and its components: (1) Plasma—fresh frozen; (2) Albumin; (3) Plasmanate

    C. Plasma substitutes: (1) Clinical dextran (MW 70,000); (2) Low molecular weight dextran (MW 40,000)

---

culation. Resuscitation and restoration of perfusion with balanced salt solution correct the acidosis. Occasionally, some sodium bicarbonate may be required, and serial blood pH measurements are a guide. Overcorrection of acidosis is more harmful than the opposite.

(2) *Colloids*

(a) *Blood* is available in emergencies as low-titer O negative or type-specific. O negative blood has the theoretical disadvantage of isoimmunization or difficulty with typing and cross-matching later; this is probably not a major consideration. Type-specific blood can be used until cross-matched blood becomes available (45 minutes).

If shock persists after 2 liters of crystalloid have been infused, or if shock recurs after the patient initially responds, whole blood should be transfused immediately.

(b) *Plasma* and albumin solutions are detrimental in prolonged severe shock. They leak through capillary membranes, taking water with them and thus exacerbating the interstitial edema. Plasma and its components should be withheld until capillaries regain their integrity (about 24 hours).

(c) *Plasma substitutes* (dextrans) interfere with function of the reticuloendothelial system and depress the already impaired immune mechanisms in shock patients. Clinical dextran coats red cells, making typing and cross-matching difficult; low molecular weight dextran coats platelets and may contribute to bleeding.

Table 1-3. Variables frequently monitored in shock

Measurement	Typical normal values	Typical values in severe shock
Arterial blood pressure	120/180	<90 mm Hg systolic
Pulse rate	80/minute	>100/minute
Central venous pressure	4-8 cm saline	<3 cm
Hematocrit	35%-45%	<35%
Arterial blood:		
pH	7.4	7.3
PO_2	95 mm Hg	85 mm Hg
PCO_2	40 mm Hg	<30 mm Hg
—HCO_3	23-25 mEq/L	<23 mEq/L
Lactic acid	12 mg/dl	>20 mg/dl
Urine:		
Volume	50 ml/hour	<20 ml/hr
Specific gravity	1.015-1.025	>1.025
Osmolality	300-400 mOsm/kg water	>700 mOsm/kg water

   e. The underlying cause of shock should be investigated and treated while resuscitation is underway. Failure of resuscitation almost always reflects persistent massive hemorrhage, and definitive operative treatment offers the only chance for survival. Ineffective resuscitation should not be continued at the expense of delaying surgery to control hemorrhage.

   f. Evaluation of treatment. The amount of fluid a patient should receive is governed by the patient's response; there is no rigid formula. Constant close monitoring is essential (see Table 1-3). Urine output is the most useful sign.
   (1) *Left atrial filling pressure* is rarely measured directly, but the pulmonary artery wedge pressure is a useful approximation, and it should be monitored in critical patients. Central venous pressure is sufficiently accurate in the great majority of patients. In mild or moderate shock, resuscitation may be permitted to raise atrial filling pressure as high as 20 torr without risk. In severe shock, however, atrial filling pressure must be kept at or near normal

(3-8 torr) because higher pressures aggravate interstitial edema. Pressures up to 12-14 torr can be tolerated if the patient is receiving positive-pressure ventilation, particularly PEEP. It is important to remember that filling pressure measurements are not indicated in acute resuscitation of injured patients except when primary myocardial dysfunction is likely or apparent.

(2) *Urine output* should be monitored. If a patient is in shock, a urinary catheter should be placed during resuscitation if not contraindicated by urethral trauma. Urine output >0.5 ml/kg/hour is a good index of visceral blood flow, specifically renal blood flow.

(3) Additional signs of successful resuscitation include an alert, oriented patient and adequate peripheral perfusion as judged by clinical criteria.

(4) Blood pressure, pulse rate, and respiratory rate should be recorded every 15-30 minutes.

(5) *Hematocrit* should be measured every few hours if continued bleeding is suspected. The hematocrit usually falls gradually over a period of 24-48 hours because of hemodilution even if bleeding has stopped, but can equilibrate in 3-4 hours if balanced salt solution is being administered.

(6) *Blood gases* should be determined repeatedly (see Table 1-3).

(7) Other measurements obtained in certain circumstances include cardiac output, oxygen delivery, oxygen consumption, and pulse oximetry.

g. Failures of resuscitation

(1) If both atrial filling pressure and urine output are increased, too much fluid is being given, and the infusion rate should be slowed immediately.

(2) If both atrial filling pressure and urine output are below normal, more volume is required. Additional intravenous (IV) access can be obtained. If perfusion cannot be improved, immediate surgical control of bleeding is necessary.

(3) When atrial filling pressure is elevated and urine output is low, measurement of cardiac output is useful.

(a) High atrial filling pressure, low urine output, and high or normal cardiac output indicate deficient renal function. This may be documented by urine/plasma ratios of creatinine, sodium, and osmolarity. Give mannitol (12.5-25 g IV) followed by infusion of mannitol 50 g in 500-1000 ml of balanced salt solution. No more than 75-100 g of mannitol should be given.

(b) High atrial filling pressure, low urine output, and low cardiac output suggest that an inotropic agent is needed (Table 1-4). (i) **Dopamine hydrochloride,** 200 mg in 500 ml of sodium injection USP (400 μg/ml), is given initially at a rate of 2.5 μg/kg/minute. These doses stimulate both dopaminergic receptors, which increase the renal blood flow and urine output, and the β-adrenergic cardiac receptors, which increase the cardiac output. Higher levels stimulate alpha receptors to cause systemic vasoconstriction, and doses above 20 μg/kg/minute reverse the vasodilatation of the renal vessels achieved at lower levels. (ii) **Isoproterenol,** a β-adrenergic stimulator, increases cardiac output by its action on the myocardial contraction mechanism, and it also produces peripheral vasodilatation. Give 1-2 mg in 500 ml of 5% dextrose in water IV. Isoproterenol should not be used if the heart rate is >100-120 minute lest cardiac arrhythmias develop.

(4) There is no convincing evidence that corticosteroids or ganglionic blocking agents are of value in hypovolemic shock.

B. TRAUMATIC SHOCK is considered separately from hypovolemic shock because it is a combination of hypovolemic shock and tissue injury. Traumatic shock is markedly worse than pure hypovolemic shock (bleeding duodenal ulcer) because tissue injury is a potent activator of the inflammatory cascade.

C. SEPTIC SHOCK is most often due to gram-negative septicemia, although infection by gram-positive bacteria can also cause shock. Trauma, diabetes mellitus, hematologic diseases, corticosteroid therapy, immunosuppressive drugs, and radiation therapy increase susceptibility to infection and thus predispose to septic shock.

1. Pathophysiology

a. Gram-negative septicemia causes a generalized increase in capillary permeability, loss of fluid from the vascular space, and pooling of blood in the microcirculation. All of these mechanisms contribute to hypovolemia. There may also be a direct toxic effect on the heart, with depression of myocardial function. In many cases there is a rise in pulmonary vascular resistance; this may produce right heart dilatation which can impair left ventricle function. Peripheral vascular resistance usually is lowered.

Table 1-4. Adrenergic drugs used in hypotensive states (Effects graded on a scale of 0-5)

| Drug | Vasomotor effect | | Cardiac stimulant (inotropic effect) | Cardiac output | Renal and splanchnic blood flow |
	Vaso-constriction	Vaso-dilatation			
α-adrenergic					
Phenylephrine (Neo-Synephrine)	5	0	0	Reduced	Reduced
Mixed α- & β-adrenergic					
Norepinephrine (Levophed)	4	0	2	Reduced	Reduced
Metaraminol (Aramine)	3	2	1	Reduced	Reduced
Epinephrine (Adrenalin)	4	3	4	Increased	Reduced
Dopamine (Inotropin)	2	2	2	Usually increased	Increased
β-adrenergic					
Isoproterenol (many trade names)	0	5	4	Increased	Usually reduced

b. Gram-positive septicemia occasionally produces hypovolemia, but loss of fluid from the vascular space usually is limited to the area of infection. Exotoxemia, which can occur with gram-positive septicemia, can be as devastating as endotoxemia.

c. Disseminated intravascular coagulation (DIC) may develop in septic shock (see later in this chapter).

2. Diagnosis

a. Symptoms and signs. (1) The inciting infection may be obscure. (2) Confusion and restlessness are early indications. (3) The skin is warm and the pulses full initially; vasoconstriction develops later if adequate fluid volumes are not given. (4) Pulmonary hypertension and hyperventilation. (5) Urine output is normal at first, then it slows rapidly.

b. Laboratory tests. (1) Inability to metabolize glucose (glycosuria, hyperglycemia) is an early finding. (2) Respiratory alkalosis. (3) Hemoconcentration is common. (4) Early leukopenia followed by leukocytosis; usually the leukocyte count is 15,000 or more with a shift to the left. (5) Identification of the responsible organism(s) is urgent. Obtain cultures on samples of blood, sputum, urine, drainage fluid, and any other suspicious site. A Gram-stained smear of infected fluid may suggest the origin of the problem and guide emergency therapy.

3. Treatment. As in other forms of shock, the objective of treatment is to improve tissue perfusion. In addition, the underlying infection must be treated.

a. Volume replacement. The initial fluid should be balanced salt solution; colloids are particularly prone to leak from capillaries and aggravate interstitial edema in septic shock. Blood pressure may remain low despite adequate perfusion. It is important to monitor other parameters, such as urine output, to assess perfusion.

b. Antibiotic therapy. Large doses of specific antibiotics should be given if the organism is known; if not, a "best guess" should be made as to the responsible bacteria, and antibiotics are given accordingly (see Table 4-1). It is better to treat with broad-spectrum coverage early and then choose more specific antibiotics when identity and sensitivity are known.

c. Surgical drainage. If an abscess or other accessible focus of infection is identified, it should be drained, debrided, or decompressed promptly. Antibiotics and fluid resuscitation do not salvage the patient if the source of infection is not found and drained.

d. Supportive measures. Close attention should be paid to maintenance of ventilation. Accompanying disorders must be treated. If the patient continues to deteriorate, cardiovascular support with inotropic agents may be required as in hypovolemic shock. Hypotension with adequate perfusion is not an indication for cardiotonics or vasoactive drugs.

e. Corticosteroids have both beneficial and deleterious effects in septic shock (Tables 1-5, 1-6). Because the disadvantages outweigh the advantages, the use of corticosteroids in septic shock cannot be recommended.

D. CARDIOGENIC SHOCK. Some degree of cardiac failure, usually left ventricular, can be detected in 20-50% of patients with acute myocardial infarction.

1. Diagnosis. Clinical findings are often absent or minimal. Dyspnea, pulmonary rales, diastolic gallop, accentuated pulmonary second sound, pulsus alternans, and pulmonary venous congestion on chest radiographs may or may not be present. The radiographic changes take time to develop and are

Table 1-5. Biochemical and metabolic effects of corticosteroids

Increased hepatic glucose	Hyperaminoacidemia
Increased secretion of glucagon	Inhibition of lipogenesis—selective
Induces negative calcium balance	Blocks increased capillary endothelial permeability
Markedly inhibits exudation of inflammatory cells	May maintain plasma membrane integrity
Suppresses T-helper cell	Stabilizes lysosome membrane
Depresses myocardial inotropism	

Table 1-6. Acute complications of corticosteroid therapy in the shock patient

Peptic ulceration	Intestinal perforation
Pancreatitis	Sodium and water retention
Impaired wound healing	Suppression of the immune response

slow to resolve, so they are not very helpful acutely. Hypotension is often the first sign that cardiac failure is more severe than suggested by other parameters.

2. Treatment

a. Treatment of **moderate left ventricular failure** consists of diuretics (e.g., furosemide, 20-200 mg IV), oxygen, and limitation of sodium intake.

b. More aggressive treatment is required for severe LV failure. Such patients should have monitoring of arterial pressure, pulmonary artery wedge pressure, and cardiac output. The stroke work index can be computed, and rational therapy is based on the specific hemodynamic abnormality found.

(1) Low LV filling pressure (<12 torr), normal cardiac output, and low arterial pressure indicate hypovolemia. Replace volume, beginning with 1 dl of saline or balanced salt solution. If cardiac output does not increase as LV filling pressure rises to 15-20 torr, stop volume replacement to avoid pulmonary edema which may occur abruptly.

(2) Elevated LV filling pressure, normal cardiac output, and normal blood pressure suggest that vigorous diuresis should be attempted with large doses of furosemide. Avoid volume depletion from excessive diuresis.

(3) Normal LV filling pressure, normal cardiac output and low arterial pressure reflect a failure of compensatory peripheral vasoconstriction which is generally not seen with cardiogenic shock. The goal is to maintain blood pressure but not increase the stroke work index. As long as perfusion remains adequate, treatment is seldom needed.

(4) Elevated LV filling pressure (>20 torr), low cardiac output, and arterial blood pressure at or >90 torr is a pattern for which vasodilator therapy can be given. Drugs such as sodium nitroprusside, phentolamine, or nitroglycerine infused slowly IV, decrease the impedance to LV ejection. Reduced LV volume and filling pressure may improve the LV stroke work index, lower MVO_2, and improve perfusion to the brain, heart, and kidneys. Arterial blood pressure should be 90 torr or more before vasodilators can be given safely; if vasopressors cannot be used to raise blood pressure without elevating LV filling pressure and aggravating cardiac failure, aortic balloon counterpulsation may be useful as a temporary aid to make vasodilator therapy possible.

E. NEUROGENIC SHOCK is due to a failure of arterial resistance from nervous or psychic stimulation (e.g., sudden pain or fright), vasodilator drugs (nitrites), spinal anesthesia, or spinal trauma. Blood pools in dilated capacitance vessels, and blood pressure falls. Cardiac activity increases to fill the dilated vascular bed and preserve tissue perfusion.

Prodromal symptoms and signs are pallor, cold sweat, weakness, lightheadedness, and occasionally nausea. Fainting is accompanied by transient hypotension and bradycardia.

Neurogenic shock is self-limiting. Resting in a recumbent or head-down position with the legs elevated for a few minutes is usually sufficient. If the patient is sitting down, and reclining is not possible, have him bend forward with his head between his knees. When faintness or prostration persists, other types of shock must be considered.

High spinal anesthesia induces neurogenic shock by paralyzing the vasoconstrictor nerves. Treatment consists of placing the patient in the head-down (Trendelenburg) position and administering a vasopressor agent. Acute traumatic paraplegia or quadriplegia causes neurogenic shock. Associated injuries are common in these patients, and hypovolemia must be assumed to be responsible for shock until proved otherwise. However, if no bleeding is found and the patient is well-perfused, judicious use of α-agents such as phenylephrine maintains higher blood pressure without increasing the risk of respiratory complications in these patients.

F. ANAPHYLACTIC REACTIONS. These catastrophic allergic reactions may occur within seconds or minutes after the parenteral administration of animal sera or drugs; rarely, they develop after oral ingestion of drugs or foods. Anaphylaxis represents hypersensitivity induced by previous injection or ingestion, although occasionally no history of earlier exposure can be obtained.

1. Diagnosis. The most conspicuous clinical feature may be laryngeal edema, bronchospasm, or vascular collapse. Symptoms and signs include apprehension, generalized urticaria or edema, a choking sensation, wheezing, cough, or status asthmaticus. In severe cases, hypotension, loss of consciousness, dilatation of pupils, incontinence, convulsions, and death occur suddenly.

2. Treatment. This is a life-threatening emergency. **Act immediately!**

a. Position the patient for comfort and ease of respiration.

b. Establish an airway and maintain oxygenation. If respirations have ceased, give artificial respiration by mouth-to-mouth, mask or endotracheal tube.

c. Drug therapy. Epinephrine is the drug of choice for emergency use. It may be necessary to give IV antihistaminics, steroids, and aminophylline also.

(1) *Epinephrine hydrochloride:* give 1 ml of 1:1000 solution IM; repeat dose in 5-10 minutes and later as needed. For more rapid effect, give 0.1-0.4 ml of 1:1000 solution in 10 ml of saline slowly IV or intrathecally.

(2) *Antihistaminics:* give diphenhydramine hydrochloride (Benadryl) or tripelenamine hydrochloride (Pyribenzamine) 10-20 mg IV if the response to epinephrine is not prompt and sustained.

(3) *Steroids:* give hydrocortisone hemisuccinate (Solu-Cortef) 100-250 mg or prednisolone hemisuccinate (Meticortelone Soluble) 50-100 mg IV over 30 seconds. The dosage depends upon the severity of the patient's condition. Repeat the drug at increasing intervals (1, 3, 6, 10 hours, etc.).

(4) *Aminophylline* injection, 0.25-0.5 g in 10-20 ml of saline, is given slowly IV if bronchospasm is severe. Dose may be repeated in 3-4 hours.

3. Prophylaxis. Avoid using potentially dangerous drugs or sera if possible. Be particularly cautious when administering parenteral medications to patients with a history of allergy or previous reaction. Give injections slowly and keep individuals under close observation for an hour or more thereafter.

Always perform a sensitivity test (intradermal or conjunctival) before injecting animal sera or other agents to which a hypersensitivity reaction may occur. When sensitivity is demonstrated by a positive test or is suggested by the history, the patient must be desensitized by the administration of a series of divided doses.

II. FIRST AID

A. GENERAL PRINCIPLES

1. Determine the extent of injury quickly.

2. Treat all life-threatening conditions immediately. Assessment and treatment often must be done simultaneously. Remember the ABCs: Airway; Breathing; Circulation.

3. Control hemorrhage, splint fractures, and arrange transportation so that definitive treatment may be given promptly.

B. EVALUATION OF THE PATIENT

1. If possible, obtain a history to ascertain the degree and type of damage and any serious underlying medical problems (e.g., cardiac disease or diabetes mellitus). The family or rescue personnel may be able to provide useful information, such as amount of blood at the scene or whether a steering wheel injury occurred. Rescue personnel can also describe the condition of the patient during transportation.

2. Examine the patient thoroughly after major trauma with special attention to the following:

a. Quickly undress the patient and log-roll him or her from side to side to check for posterior wounds. Assess peripheral perfusion by examining the skin of the extremities.

b. Respiratory distress. Assess adequacy of ventilation. Stridor and suprasternal or intercostal retraction indicate airway obstruction. Cyanosis is due to poor oxygenation until proved otherwise. Shortness of breath may reflect chest injury, shock, or head injury. In respiratory arrest, begin mouth-to-mouth resuscitation immediately.

c. Cardiac arrest. Check for carotid pulses immediately; if absent, start cardiopulmonary resuscitation.

d. Shock. If peripheral perfusion is diminished, quickly examine the neck veins. If the neck veins are distended, shock is due to cardiac or preload causes. Assume that hypovolemia is the cause of shock if the neck veins are flat. Additional criteria for the assessment of shock are described in Section I.

e. External wounds and bleeding. Control bleeding promptly, using direct pressure, and apply a sterile dressing.

f. Neurologic injuries. Evaluate by repeated examination of state of consciousness, cranial nerve signs, gross skin sensation, ability to move extremities, rectal examination, and peripheral reflexes (see Chapter 17). Get brain, cervical, and spinal radiographs to rule out cervical fractures. Protect the neck with axial orientation and backboard until fractures are ruled out.

g. Fractures and dislocations. Palpate carefully from head to foot; move all joints cautiously and exert gentle pressure on the spine, chest, and pelvis. Pain, swelling, ecchymosis, deformity, and limitation of motion are classic signs of fracture and dislocation. Splint all fractures as quickly as possible to prevent further soft tissue and neurovascular damage.

h. Internal injury. Overt localizing signs are often minimal. Hypovolemic shock in the absence of external bleeding indicates internal hemorrhage. Chest films may localize blood in one or other hemithorax. Repeated abdominal examination, serial hematocrit, and serial leukocyte counts are helpful in localizing visceral injury. Peritoneal lavage may be indicated to rule out internal bleeding.

C. EMERGENCY TREATMENT
1. Respiratory distress
a. When due to airway obstruction (Figure 1-1). (1) Quickly clear the airway by suctioning secretions and removing foreign material from the mouth and pharynx. (2) Hold up the patient's chin, pull out the tongue, or force the mandible forward by pressure behind the angle of the jaw to overcome soft tissue obstruction of the hypopharynx. Oropharyngeal airways may be useful in the unconscious patient. (3) A bag and mask are often sufficient to ventilate the patient initially. Endotracheal intubation may be required in some instances. (4) Cricothyroidotomy is useful if an airway cannot be achieved by other means, or if the cervical spine injury or maxillofacial trauma prevent oral or nasotracheal intubation.

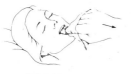

Pull out tongue

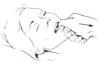

Chin Lift

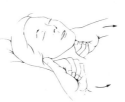

Jaw thrust

FIGURE 1-1. Relief of airway obstruction.

b. When due to other causes: Maintain a clear airway, treat the underlying cause, and increase the inspired oxygen concentration if possible.

c. Respiratory arrest. Clear the airway and institute mouth-to-mouth resuscitation.

2. Cardiac arrest. See Chapter 2.

3. Shock. Anticipate and prevent shock by the measures outlined below:

a. Control hemorrhage and such contributing causes as exposure and pain. Reduce anxiety by reassurance and explanations to the patient.

b. Keep the patient comfortable, warm, and in a recumbent position. Avoid rapid changes of position.

c. Splint all fractures and apply traction if necessary to relieve pain and reduce soft tissue injury.

d. Transport as quickly as possible to a hospital. Provide prior warning to the hospital when possible.

e. For definitive treatment see Section I.

4. External bleeding

a. Venous and minor arterial bleeding can be controlled by direct pressure on the wound with sterile gauze or a clean cloth; elevate the bleeding extremity if possible.

b. Major arterial bleeding. Compression of the major artery proximal to the wound plus direct pressure on the wound controls almost all external arterial hemorrhage. A tourniquet is rarely necessary. Traumatic amputation and uncontrolled hemorrhage when only one person is available for resuscitation may require the use of a tourniquet. **Caution:** Faulty use of a tourniquet may cause irreparable vascular or neurologic damage. Tourniquets should not be left on longer than 30 minutes.

5. Pain. Distinguish fear and excitement from real pain. Severe injuries cause surprisingly little discomfort. Immobilization of injured parts often relieves distress. When pain is severe, give morphine sulfate, 2-4 mg IV every hour. **Caution:** Narcotics are contraindicated in coma, head injuries, respiratory distress, and hypovolemia. The IV route is quick and sure. Peripheral vasoconstriction may delay absorption of a subcutaneous injection and leads to overdosage if multiple injections are later absorbed at the same time. Inform the patient that he has received morphine and record the time and dosage on a note or tag affixed to his wrist, ankle, or forehead.

6. Open wounds

a. Remove gross foreign debris. Apply sterile dressing or a clean cloth and secure firmly in place.

b. Do not place antiseptic solutions or antibacterial powders in the wound. It is not necessary to cleanse the skin around the wound with soap or antiseptic.

c. Arrange for the earliest possible cleansing, debridement, and closure under aseptic conditions.

7. Fractures. Splint all fractures as quickly as possible to prevent further soft tissue and neurovascular damage. Patients suspected of having cervical spine fractures should be maintained in an axial orientation or transported in Gardner-Wells tongs.

8. Transportation of the injured patient. Improper methods of moving patients can cause further injury. Lift severely injured patients with care, and improvise stretchers (blankets, boards, and doors) when necessary. Transport patients in the recumbent position on a stretcher, preferably in an ambulance.

The physician administering first aid is morally, and in some areas legally, responsible for the patient until care is assumed by another physician.

III. BURNS

Burns may be caused by heat, ultraviolet light, x-rays, nuclear radiation, electricity, chemicals, and mechanical abrasions. Thermal injury from fire, steam, or scalding liquids is the most common type of severe burn.

A. STRUCTURE AND FUNCTION OF THE SKIN

1. Structure. The skin is the largest organ in the body; it ranges from 0.25 m^2 to 1.8 m^2 and is divided into two layers, the epidermis and the dermis.

a. The epidermis is a very thin layer of epithelial cells. The outermost cells are cornified dead cells which provide protection against the environment.

b. The dermis is a thick layer composed of fibrous connective tissue containing blood vessels, nerves, and the epithelial appendages (hair follicles, sebaceous glands, and sweat glands).

2. Function. The skin is a physical barrier to penetration of the body by microorganisms. The small numbers of bacteria that penetrate intact skin are destroyed by immunologic cells in the dermis. The skin (especially the dermis) prevents excessive loss of body fluids by evaporation.

Sweat glands help regulate body temperature by increasing or decreasing the amount of water of evaporation. These glands also act as crude excretory organs by eliminating excess water, small amounts of sodium, chloride, and cholesterol compounds, and traces of albumin and urea.

The skin is a sensory organ; it allows a person to recognize and adapt to changes in the physical environment and thus provides important protection.

The skin serves as a person's identity (color, texture, grain, fingerprints).

The skin synthesizes vitamin D by the effects of sunlight on certain cholesterol compounds in the corium.

B. DETERMINANTS OF SEVERITY OF INJURY

1. Depth. The depth of a burn significantly affects its healing. It may be difficult to evaluate depth, especially in infants whose skin is very thin. Certain symptoms and signs are helpful, but frequently the exact depth of injury can be determined only by observation over a period of days or weeks.

a. First-degree burns involve only the epidermis and are usually caused by sunlight or brief scalding. Tissue damage is minimal. Pain is the predominant symptom. The burned skin is erythematous, and there may be very mild edema. Systemic effects are rare. Pain resolves in 48-72 hours, and healing takes place uneventfully in 5-10 days.

b. Second-degree burns involve all of the epithelium and much of the dermis. The burn is characterized by redness and blisters. **Superficial** second-degree burns usually heal with minimal scarring in 10-14 days unless they become infected. **Deep** second-degree burns extend to the depths of the dermis, and the dead covering resembles a third-degree burn except that it is usually red and may blanch when touched. Healing occurs by regeneration of epithelium from sweat glands and follicles; this process takes 25-35 days. Dense scarring is common. Deep second-degree burns may become full thickness if they become infected or they become ischemic from inadequate resuscitation. Fluid losses and metabolic effects are the same as in third-degree burns.

c. Third-degree (full-thickness) burns are characterized by a dry, tough, leathery surface that is usually brown, tan, or black, although it may even be white or red. Blisters are uncommon. These burns are anesthetic because pain receptors have been destroyed. If pressure is applied to the burn, the surface does not blanch and refill because the tissue is dead and the blood vessels are thrombosed. It is not always easy to distinguish second- from third-degree burns. If there is any question, assume they are third-degree and treat them as such.

2. Surface area. The size of a burn is usually expressed as a percentage of the total body surface area and is most accurately estimated from age-related charts (Figure 1-2). Accurate determination of the percentage of total body burn is useful because it directly relates to severity of injury, it is a good prognostic index, and it helps determine which patients should be treated in specialized burn facilities. Fluid replacement is governed by the burn size.

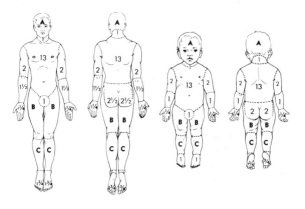

Relative Percentages of Areas Affected by Growth

Area	Age					
	0	1	5	10	15	Adult
A = half of head	9.5	8.5	6.5	5.5	4.5	3.5
B = half of one thigh	2.75	3.25	4	4.25	4.5	4.75
C = half of one leg	2.5	2.5	2.75	3	3.25	3.5

FIGURE 1-2. Table for estimating extent of burns. In adults, a reasonable system for calculating the percentage of body surface burned is the 'rule of nines': each arm equals 9%, the anterior and posterior trunk each equal 18%, and each leg equals 18%; the sum of these percentages is 99%.

3. Age. Burns of any given depth and surface area inflict higher mortality in children under 2 years and adults over age 60. The mortality in infants is attributed to immature immune competence; older adults often have associated diseases that increase mortality.

4. Associated diseases. Diabetes, congestive heart failure, pulmonary disease, and chronic treatment with immuno-suppressive drugs are among the conditions that make patients less able to tolerate burns.

5. Location of the burn is another determinant of severity. For example, burns of the hands, even if only second-degree, may result in scarring and contractures which render the hand useless unless expert treatment is started early. Further, even minor burns of both hands may make it impossible for the patient to care for himself outside the hospital. Patients with perineal burns should be hospitalized because of the high incidence of infection.

6. Associated injuries. Inhalation injury, fractures, head injuries, and other trauma contribute to the impact of a burn on the patient.

7. Type of burn. Patients with certain types of burns should always be admitted to a specialized facility. Electrical or chemical burns may appear, superficially, to be quite minor injuries, but they often involve deep structures and are difficult to manage.

8. Pediatric burns. Burned children should be admitted to the hospital when the physician doubts that the parents are able to care for what appears to be a simple wound. Neglect can result in disability from relatively minor initial injuries. If suspicion exists that the burn might have been intentional, the child must be admitted to the hospital, a fact that cannot be overemphasized.

C. OUTPATIENT CARE OF BURNS. General guidelines for admission to specialized facilities are outlined in Table 1-7. Before treating a burn victim as an outpatient, the physician should have a clear understanding of the family situation and whether or not the patient or the family can take care of the burn wound.

The best first aid for a minor burn wound at home is **immersion in cool tapwater;** no other agents are necessary, and some may be damaging. Following initial assessment, wounds should be cleansed and debrided with a cool physiologic saline solution.

Table 1-7. Classification of severity of burns

Major burn injury: Must be admitted to a specialized facility

2° burn >25% BSA* (Adults)
2° burn >20% BSA (Children)
3° burn >10% BSA

Most burns involving hands, face, eyes, ears, feet, or perineum

Most patients with:
Inhalation injury
Electrical injury
Burn injury complicated by other major trauma

Poor-risk patients with burns

Moderate uncomplicated burn injury: May need admission to the hospital

2° burn of 15-25% BSA (Adults)
2° burn of 10-20% BSA (Children)
3° burn <10% BSA

Minor burn injury: Usually treated as outpatient

2° burn <15% BSA (Adults)
2° burn <10% BSA (Children)
3° burn <2% BSA

*Body surface area

Controversy exists regarding **debridement of blisters.** Debridement leaves a cleaner wound with less chance of infection to develop in the blister fluid. The disadvantage is that the wound is more painful. All blisters that involve joint spaces on the hand should be debrided, and very large blisters in any location are best treated by debridement.

Tetanus prophylaxis (see Chapter 4).

The use of **antibiotics** immediately after a burn is controversial. Penicillin prevents the development of streptococcal wound infections, but these infections occur in only 5% of patients. If penicillin is given, it should be discontinued after 48 hours; in no case should broad-spectrum antibiotics be used. Generally, antibiotics should be reserved to treat specific infections.

The wound should be covered with a **bulky dressing.** The patient is instructed to remove the dressing, wash the wound with mild soap and tepid water, and replace the dressing at least daily. The pain caused by dressing changes is reduced by soaking the dressing with tepid water prior to removal or by using a nonadherent gauze impregnated with a bland emulsion.

Xenograft (pigskin) and plastic membranes are very useful in treating some minor wounds.

Topical antibacterial agents in the outpatient care of burns are the subject of debate. There are no well-controlled studies that demonstrate significant improvement with these compounds.

In most instances, wounds will heal in 15-20 days; grease and flame burns may require longer.

D. ACUTE RESUSCITATION. Hospitalized patients should be assessed and treated as rapidly as with any other major injury.

1. Airway maintenance. The airway takes first priority. Smoke inhalation should be suspected if fire occurred in a closed space or if there are thermal injuries to the face, nares, or upper torso. Blood gases, including carboxyhemoglobin, should be determined. Oxygen should be administered. If the patient has extreme air hunger or is in critical condition, endotracheal intubation is indicated. When in doubt intubate.

2. Fluid therapy. If the burn is >10% third-degree or >20% second-degree, a urinary catheter and a large IV line should be inserted.

Crystalloid solution is preferred during the first 24 hours. The amount of crystalloid solution administered depends upon the response of the individual; formulas are useful guidelines but should not be adhered to rigidly if circumstances dictate otherwise. The **Baxter formula** is recommended among the various ones available: **First 24 hours**—balanced salt solution (lactated Ringer's injection), 4 ml/kg/%burn; give half of this during the first 8 hours and the other half over the next 16 hours; **Second 24 hours**—5% dextrose in water (2000 ml maintenance) and plasma in sufficient amounts to restore normal plasma volume. All formulas are only approximations and should be modified for each patient based on their perfusion.

Monitoring of fluid resuscitation: Pulmonary artery and central venous monitoring lines are associated with increased complications in burn patients. Urine output remains the best means of monitoring resuscitation. 0.5 ml/kg/hour is the acceptable minimal output in adults; 1 ml/kg/hour in children. Parameters such as peripheral perfusion and sensorium should also be followed.

In patients with inhalation injury, minimal administration of fluid is prudent, but fluid should not be restricted at the expense of renal function because the combination of inhalation injury and renal failure carries a high mortality.

Children may require more free water than older patients; this can be monitored by frequent determinations of serum osmolality or serum sodium. Urine specific gravity can also be used to assess the amount of free water needed.

3. Tetanus toxoid (0.5 cc) should be administered to all patients. If the wound is >50% of the body surface area, 250 units of tetanus immune globulin (human) should also be administered.

4. Give IV narcotic (morphine 0.1 mg/kg or meperidine 1-2 mg/kg) to relieve pain. Give all medications IV.

E. CARE OF THE BURN WOUND. There are three methods of caring for the burn wound: the exposure method, occlusive dressings, and primary excision.

1. The exposure method is used on areas that are conveniently left exposed, such as the face. The burn is initially cleansed and allowed to dry. A second-degree burn forms a crust that usually brushes off after 2-3 weeks, leaving minimal scarring. The advantage of exposure treatment is that the patient is not immobilized in bulky dressings. The disadvantage is that the protection against infection afforded by sterile dressings is absent.

2. Occlusive dressings, nearly always combined with topical antibacterials, are the most common methods of burn care. The ointment or cream may be applied to the patient or to the gauze. The antibacterial agent most frequently used today is silver sulfadiazine. Other compounds are listed in Table 1-8.

3. Primary excision of the burn is gaining popularity. Methods include tangential excision, excision with special knives such as the laser or plasma scalpel, and primary excision down to fascia. In most instances, the wound is covered with autograft, homograft, or xenograft, depending on availability of these tissues.

Regardless of the method of wound care, patients are usually bathed daily when the dressings or cream are washed off. Debridement of all loose tissues is performed during the bath.

Circumferential burns of the extremity or the trunk may require *escharotomy* to prevent venous obstruction from edema beneath the constricting eschar. Longitudinal escharotomy, or incision of the burn wound, may decompress these compartments. An escharotomy on the chest may relieve tightening and restriction of ventilation.

Table 1-8. Comparison of common topical agents

	Mafenide	Silver nitrate	Silver sulfadiazine	Povidone-iodine ointment
Spectrum	Antibacterial	Antibacterial	Antibacterial	Antibacterial, antifungal
Penetration of wound	Good	Poor	Fair	Good
Effect on eschar	Results in delayed separation	Dries eschar	Softens eschar for easy debridement	Tans eschar, making it dry and tough
Allergy	Common in children	None	Rare	Relatively uncommon in children
Pain	~40% of patients	Painless	Painless	Burning sensation in ~11%
Type of dressing	Exposure or dressings	Thick occlusive dressings	Exposure or dressings	Usually dressings
Mobility	Motion of joints maintained	Impedes movement of joints	Motion of joints maintained	Impedes movement of joints
Ease of use	Easy	Difficult because of attention to dressing	Easy	Easy
Metabolic changes	Carbonic anhydrase inhibitor	Electrolyte deficiencies and methemoglobinemia	Neutropenia	Elevation of PBI

Another form of wound incision is the *grid escharotomy*. This is indicated if there is gross infection beneath the eschar; it serves to drain the wound and aid in debridement. The procedure is a series of multiple parallel incisions made diagonally across the burn with other multiple incisions made at right angles to them, dividing the wound into a grid with squares of about 2 cm^2.

The therapeutic objective in third-degree burns is to remove all dead skin and to cover the defects with autografts. Multiple operations may be required. If insufficient skin is available for autografting, xenograft or homograft is an acceptable substitute temporarily.

The maintenance of joint motion during burn care is important. Loss of motion is related to two factors: immobilization and pain. The use of splints and elevation to maintain functional position of hands and feet, followed by aggressive physical therapy, minimizes these undesirable sequelae.

F. NUTRITION IN THE BURN PATIENT. Metabolic requirements are increased 2-4 fold after thermal injury. Nutrition may be maintained by oral or tube feeding or total parenteral nutrition in descending order of preference.

Positive nitrogen balance is the goal; if it cannot be achieved with oral feedings, supplemental tube feedings or total parenteral nutrition is necessary.

A daily count of caloric intake is mandatory; daily weight should be recorded, and nitrogen balance studies are obtained as indicated.

Tube feedings are given in the form of a blenderized diet or commercial preparations. The latter may be hyperosmolar, and care must be taken to avoid hyperosmolar coma and diarrhea.

Management of total parenteral nutrition is described on page 175.

Antacids should be given to prevent stress ulcers.

Supplemental vitamins and iron are required by most patients.

G. COMPLICATIONS

1. Sepsis is the most common cause of morbidity and mortality in the burn patient, particularly pneumonia.

a. Pneumonia should be prevented, if possible, by vigorous pulmonary toilet and frequent assessment of tracheobronchial flora. If the patient has sustained an inhalation injury, get Gram stains of the sputum daily. If polymorphonuclear leukocytes or overgrowth of organisms is seen, appropriate antibiotics should be instituted and changed if necessary when results of cultures and sensitivities are available. Radiographs should be used as corroborative evidence.

b. The burn wound is also a source of infection. The wound should be cultured, preferably by quantitative methods, at least twice a week. If burn wound sepsis occurs, systemic antibiotics should be given based on cultures and sensitivities. Subeschar injections of antibiotics should also be considered. However, the definitive treatment of burn wound infection remains excision, usually to fascia.

c. Other potential sources of infection are septic thrombophlebitis, catheter sepsis, and acalculous cholecystitis.

2. Bleeding from stress ulcers is a common complication of major burns but can be prevented by routine administration of antacids. If bleeding occurs the problem is evaluated and treated like upper gastrointestinal bleeding in any patient (see Chapter 12).

3. Unique complications in children include seizures from electrolyte imbalance, hypoxemia, infection and drug administration; gastric dilatation, treated by nasogastric tube decompression; and hypertension, which occurs in approximately 30% of children and may require treatment with vasodilators.

H. RESPIRATORY FAILURE IN BURNS. Inhalation injuries are caused by three mechanisms: heat, carbon monoxide poisoning, and inhalation of noxious gases. About 60% of burn fatalities are directly or indirectly due to inhalation injury.

1. Direct inhalation of heat is not a common cause of damage below the vocal cords because of the efficient way the upper airway cools inspired gases. This may occur, however, if the victim is exposed to heat in a closed room, if steam is inhaled, or if superheated soot is inhaled.

2. Carbon monoxide poisoning should be suspected in any patient with inhalation injury. Carbon monoxide poisoning is confirmed by measurement of carboxyhemoglobin levels. Symptoms are listed in Table 1-9.

3. The kinds of noxious chemicals inhaled in smoke depend upon the type of materials that are burning (Table 1-10).

4. Treatment, in addition to the measures listed above, consists of humidifying the inspired gases, tracheobronchial toilet, bronchial dilators in some cases, and mechanical ventilation if necessary. In general, the following criteria are used for institution of mechanical ventilation:

Table 1-9. Carbon monoxide poisoning

HbCO level	Severity	Symptoms
20% HbCO	Mild	Headaches, mild dyspnea, visual changes, confusion
20-40% HbCO	Moderate	Irritability, diminished judgment, dim vision, nausea, easy fatiguability
40-60% HbCO	Severe	Hallucinations, confusion, ataxia, collapse, coma
60% HbCO	Fatal	

Table 1-10. Sources of noxious chemicals in smoke

Polyethylene Polypropylene	Clean burning Combustion to CO_2 and H_2O
Polystyrene	Copious black smoke and soot—CO_2, H_2O, some CO
Wood Cotton	Aldehydes (Acrolein)
Polyvinylchloride Acrylonitrile	Hydrochloric acid
Polyurethane Nitrogenous compounds	Hydrogen cyanide
Fire retardants may produce toxic fumes	Halogens (F_2, Cl_2, Br_2) Ammonia

a. Inability to oxygenate arterial blood as shown by arterial oxygen tension <60 mm Hg on room air or an alveolar-arterial oxygen difference of 300 on 100% inspired oxygen.

b. Inability to ventilate adequately (arterial PCO_2 >50 mm Hg)

c. Vital capacity <10 cc/kg body weight or <three times normal tidal volume.

5. The use of steroids in patients with inhalation injury is contraindicated. **Hyperbaric oxygen** has been used but has not been proven to be more effective than mechanical ventilation with 100% oxygen.

I. ELECTRICAL INJURIES are divided into three categories: true electrical current injury, electrothermal burns caused by arcing of the current, and flame burns resulting from ignition of clothing.

Tissues in the body vary in their resistance to passage of electrical current. Bone has the highest resistance. Heat is stored and dissipated into the surrounding muscle, causing myonecrosis and subsequent myoglobinuria which may lead to renal failure. Blood and nerve are the least resistant. Current passing through vessels may damage the intima and cause thrombosis; gangrene of extremities or intestine may be the consequence. Current passing through the brain may cause seizures or apnea. Ventricular fibrillation may result from electrical current passing through the chest.

Alternating current has an additional hazard compared with direct current, because it may cause tetanic contractions and severe muscle and bony injuries. The heart is very sensitive to 60-cycle AC.

Almost all patients with electrical injuries should be admitted to the hospital because the injury is often underestimated and sequelae are common.

Cutaneous burns are treated as other burns.

Myoglobinuria is treated by alkalinizing the urine and giving an osmotic diuretic (e.g., mannitol).

Late sequelae such as thrombosis of vessels are treated as they appear.

In injuries from high-tension electrical sources, the amputation rate is at least 50%.

J. REHABILITATION OF THE BURN PATIENT includes treatment of both psychological and physical problems. Patients should be informed that achievement of optimal results may require years. The physician should be realistic as to what the 'optimal' results are.

The patient must take special care of the healed skin. Direct exposure to sunlight should be avoided; screening agents are useful on areas such as the hands and face. Creams and lotions to prevent drying and cracking are required. Lanolin, A&D ointment, and Eucerin are all effective.

Hypertrophic scar and keloid formation are common; they may be minimized by pressure dressings for 6 months following the injury.

Physical therapy is essential to restore motion to joints injured by the burn or immobilized in dressings.

The family of a burn victim undergoes extreme stress.

There are often feelings of guilt. An experienced psychiatric nurse is an integral member of the burn team.

IV. MISCELLANEOUS INJURIES

A. COMMON SOFT TISSUE INJURIES

1. Abrasion. Loss of superficial epithelium caused by friction. The abraded surface bleeds from exposed capillaries. Treatment consists of cleansing the wound and application of sterile dressings; alternatively, abrasions may be left undressed.

2. Contusion (bruise). Interstitial hemorrhage and tissue damage from blunt trauma. Superficial contusions are minor, but fractures of underlying bones and injuries of internal organs must be ruled out. Application of an ice pack within the first few hours may limit the interstitial hemorrhage and subsequent ecchymosis.

3. Hematoma. Liquid or clotted blood in the subcutaneous or intramuscular spaces. Hematoma is usually associated with contusion. Most hematomas are resorbed, and surgical evacuation is seldom necessary. Clotted blood cannot be aspirated through a needle; incision, with careful aseptic technic, is the best method of evacuation.

4. Laceration. A tear or cut in soft tissues. The basic steps in management are debridement, irrigation, and wound closure, usually under local anesthesia. Always examine for damage to nerves and tendons and for the presence of foreign material. Lacerations of the hand, face, the scalp, and those associated with loss of skin require special care (see Chapters 15 to 17).

a. Wound closure. Primary closure is immediate suture of a wound. Absorbable material is used in the deeper layers and fine nonabsorbable sutures are placed in the skin. Lacerations that occur under relatively clean conditions may be closed primarily up to 24 hours after injury. Primary closure is used whenever possible for lacerations of the head and neck where blood supply is excellent and the cosmetic result is important.

Delayed primary closure is used for contaminated wounds or those seen after 24 hours. A single layer of petrolatum gauze is placed in the wound and covered with fluffed gauze. The wound is examined in 4-5 days and loosely closed with sutures or adhesive tape if it appears clean.

Secondary closure is suture closure of heavily contaminated wounds after several days. Many times it is better to allow such a wound to heal spontaneously by second intention than to attempt suture approximation of granulating surfaces.

b. Antibiotics. Most small or clean lacerations do not require antibiotic therapy. When contamination is marked or when delayed primary closure is contemplated, systemic penicillin therapy is justified.

c. Tetanus prophylaxis is recommended if contamination by soil is suspected (see Chapter 4).

5. Penetrating wound. The chief complications of penetrating wounds are perforation of a viscus, introduction of bacteria, and retained foreign body. Treatment must be individualized. Clean puncture wounds and through-and-through missile wounds that cause no serious damage may require only observation. Penetrating injuries that drive clothing or other foreign material into the wound must be explored and debrided. Tetanus prophylaxis is usually indicated.

6. Foreign body. Any open wound may contain a foreign body. Small, inert foreign bodies <1 cm beneath the skin can usually be left alone and checked by radiography several months later. A foreign body should be removed if it protrudes through the skin; if it causes pain; if it consists of or is contaminated by dirt, cloth, wood, or other material likely to cause infection or reaction; if the wound is infected or draining; or if the foreign body may migrate to or impinge upon important structures. Tetanus prophylaxis should be given as indicated in Chapter 4. Exploration of a wound to extract a foreign body should be performed only after the foreign material has been localized by (a) radiographs in two or more planes with lead markers on the skin, (b) placing identifying marks on the skin under fluoroscopy, or (c) inserting a needle down to the foreign body under fluoroscopy.

B. BITES AND STINGS

1. Human bites (see also Chapter 16). Human bites are serious because of the virulence of aerobic and anaerobic organisms in the mouth. These bacteria are already proliferating under human conditions when they are implanted in the bite wound. Deep penetrating wounds of the knuckles incurred by fighting are especially serious owing to frequent involvement of the metacarpophalangeal joint and extensor tendon. When the hand is opened, the glide of the extensor tendon carries infecting organisms proximally into anaerobic sites on the back of the hand. Cellulitis appears within 24-72 hours and may extend rapidly. Marked pain and swelling due to necrosis and abscess formation are the typical findings in the advanced case.

Emergency treatment of the fresh human bite wound consists of irrigation and debridement, extending the wound as required. Aerobic and anaerobic cultures should be taken and tests made for antibiotic sensitivity. **Do not suture the wound;** cover it with petrolatum gauze and dry dressing and splint the hand and wrist as necessary. Observe for infection, and administer full doses of penicillin pending the results of antibiotic sensitivity tests. Tetanus prophylaxis should be given.

If a human bite wound is seen late, obtain cultures, drain abscesses, place the patient at bed rest with the part elevated, apply hot moist packs, and give penicillin until the antibiotic of choice can be chosen on the basis of sensitivity.

2. Animal bites (see also Rabies in Chapter 4)

a. Dog bites. Small penetrating wounds should be thoroughly irrigated and left open. Lacerations are debrided, irrigated, and sutured according to the usual principles. Tetanus prophylaxis is usually indicated.

b. Cat bites and scratches. Cat bites are more likely to cause infection than dog bites. Cleanse the area thoroughly with soap and water, apply a dry sterile dressing, splint the part if possible, and observe for infection. Administer penicillin pending antibiotic sensitivity studies. Tetanus prophylaxis is given.

Cats may also transmit a condition known as **cat-scratch fever.** At the wound site there is localized cellulitis followed by regional lymphadenopathy; the nodes may suppurate. Encephalitis or pneumonitis occurs rarely.

3. Snake bites. Nonpoisonous snake bites may cause pain but are otherwise minor. Four types of poisonous snakes are found in the United States: rattlesnake (several species), copperhead, cottonmouth moccasin, and coral snake. The venom of poisonous snakes contains proteolytic enzymes that are neurotoxic or hemotoxic. Neurotoxins cause respiratory failure; hemotoxic venoms cause hemolysis, local hemorrhage, and bleeding from mucous membranes.

The manifestations of poisonous snake bites are severe and persistent local pain, redness, and swelling followed rapidly by nausea, vomiting, and collapse. About 15% of adults bitten by rattlesnakes die.

Treatment is outlined below:

a. Determine if the bite was made by a poisonous snake. Pit vipers have fangs that make 2 puncture wounds where they enter the skin. Nonpoisonous snakes lack fangs, and the bite leaves semicircular rows of tooth marks. However, coral snakes, which are poisonous, leave the same semi-circular imprint.

b. Immobilization and transportation. Keep the patient recumbent and quiet; muscular action tends to spread venom. Transport the patient by stretcher to a hospital at once. Give barbiturates for restlessness. **Do not give alcohol.**

c. Tourniquet. Apply a loose tourniquet proximal to the bite. The tourniquet should be left loose enough to permit insertion of a finger between it and the skin. It can be left continuously in place for 1 hour.

d. Cold pack. Application of an ice pack to the wound slows absorption of the venom and relieves pain. Packing of the entire extremity in ice is not advised.

e. Care of the wound. (1) Wash the wound thoroughly with soap and water to remove venom from the skin. (2) If appropriate facilities are available within the first half-hour (or 1.5 hours if a tourniquet has been in place), the bite wound can be elliptically excised with a 1-inch margin to the depth required to remove the venom, which may be down to the fascia or into the muscle. This may remove 90% of the venom.

f. Antivenin. Species-specific antivenin should be administered as soon as possible after testing for sensitivity to horse serum. (Follow printed instructions in the package.) Identification of the snake is important in order to choose the correct antivenin. Polyvalent pit viper antivenin and coral snake antivenin are available from Wyeth Laboratories or from the National Center for Disease Control, Atlanta, GA, and from other sources in southeastern United States.

g. Other measures. (1) Treat respiratory failure by oxygen administration and artificial ventilation (see Chapter 2). (2) Treat shock (see Section I). (3) Antibiotics have no value. (4) Corticosteroids relieve symptoms temporarily but do not lower mortality. Do not give steroids if the patient is receiving antivenin. (5) Extensive tissue necrosis requires debridement. (6) Fasciotomy may be necessary if severe edema compresses nerves or vessels in an extremity.

4. Spider bites and scorpion stings. Bites and stings of many spiders and scorpions cause only local pain, redness, and swelling. Several species are quite venomous, however. The toxin of the black widow spider *(Lactrodectus mactans)* causes severe systemic symptoms, including generalized muscular pains, abdominal cramps, nausea, vomiting, and collapse. Abdominal muscles may become rigid, resembling an acute abdominal emergency.

If symptoms are severe, give specific spider or scorpion antiserum after skin testing. For convulsions or muscle cramps, give calcium gluconate, 10 ml of 10% solution IV, and repeat as needed. Additional measures include hot baths and control of restlessness with barbiturates. Treat the local wound by application of cold compresses. If the skin becomes necrotic, excision and grafting may be indicated.

The brown recluse spider *(Loxosceles reclusa)* can cause a severe painful bite with systemic symptoms and an indolent ulcer that may take weeks to heal. The favored current treatment, provided there are no contraindications, is Dapsone (4-4' diaminodiphenylsulfone) 25 mg orally twice daily, up to 100 mg/day until there are no signs of inflammation. Most wounds require debridement and some grafting.

C. BLAST AND CRUSH INJURY

1. Blast injury. The blast force from an explosion can damage lungs and abdominal viscera. Localizing symptoms and signs frequently are delayed.

Diffuse alveolar hemorrhage with dyspnea and frothy hemoptysis is typical of blast injury to the lungs. Tracheal intubation or tracheostomy may be required to remove secretions and administer oxygen. Do not overlook pneumothorax or hemothorax.

Mild contusions of the abdominal viscera cause moderate discomfort and occasionally colicky pain that subsides in 48-96 hours. More serious injuries with impending or actual perforation produce signs of peritoneal irritation or shock. Rupture of the ear drum causes severe pain and often deafness. No local treatment is required. Packs and ear drops are contraindicated.

2. Crush injury. The crush syndrome is compression injury, shock, and acute renal insufficiency. Shock results from extravasation of blood and plasma into injured tissues after release of compression that has lasted for an hour or more. Renal failure is a consequence of prolonged shock and the nephrotoxic effect of myoglobin released from ischemic or dead muscle. Dark, brownish-red urine should make one suspicious of myoglobinuria; it must be treated promptly with an osmotic diuretic and alkalinization of the urine.

D. THERMAL INJURIES OTHER THAN BURNS

1. Heat stroke. About 4000 Americans die of heat stroke each year. The great majority of these victims are over 50 years old.

Early clinical symptoms include headache, dizziness, nausea, and visual disturbances. The skin is hot, flushed, and dry; absence of sweating is an important sign. The skin loses its vascular resistance, and cutaneous vasodilatation is prominent. Conversely, pulmonary vascular resistance is usually increased with high normal or elevated central venous pressure. A hyperdynamic state is common; heart rate and cardiac output are increased.

Renal problems result from decreased perfusion and myoglobinuria; the latter is due to rhabdomyolysis and disseminated intravascular clotting. Rectal temperatures may be as high as 42-44° C. Confusion, ataxia, seizures, and coma are common neurologic manifestations.

The objective of treatment is rapid lowering of body temperature by means of ice packs and cold water. The rectal temperature should be reduced to 39° C, after which one should proceed more slowly. Intravenous fluids and support of respiration may also be necessary, and heparin should be given for disseminated intravascular clotting.

2. Heat cramps are painful spasms of the voluntary muscles of the abdomen and extremities due to depletion of body salt by profuse sweating. Heavy manual labor in a hot environment may result in the loss of 3-4 liters of sweat (containing 0.2%-0.5% sodium chloride) per hour. Persons working in high-temperature areas should drink fluids liberally and should add 1 level teaspoon of salt to each quart of water, or they should take a sodium chloride tablet (1 g) with each 1-2 glasses of water. Commercially available drinks (e.g., Gatorade) can be used.

In addition to cramps, there may be muscle twitchings. The skin is moist and cool, and body temperature is normal or only slightly elevated. Laboratory studies show a low serum sodium.

The condition is treated by moving the victim to a cool place. Cramps frequently subside on rest alone. Give sodium chloride, 1 g, orally every hour with 1-2 glasses of water, until 15 doses have been administered. In severe cases, 1-2 liters of physiologic saline should be given IV.

3. Cold injury. The fundamental pathologic process is the same in all types of cold injury: arterial and capillary spasm, ischemia, and tissue damage. Blistering and edema due to plasma leakage through capillary epithelium are characteristic. The most serious destruction occurs in the skin and subcutaneous tissue, because cooling is greatest in these superficial structures. In the great majority of cold injuries, the tissues are not actually frozen. Freezing injury (frostbite) does not occur until the skin temperature drops to −4 to −10° C.

Likelihood of cold injury is increased by immobility, venous stasis, occlusive arterial vascular disease, previous cold injury, and a high wind-chill index.

a. Prevention. "Keep warm, keep dry, and keep moving." Wear wind-proof and water-repellant clothing, change wet garments and foot gear as quickly as possible, and maintain the circulation by frequently exercising the arms, legs, fingers, and toes. Avoid constrictive clothing and shoes and prolonged dependency of the feet. Head gear is mandatory because more body heat is lost from the head than from any other site. Protect the ears; they are the most commonly injured structures.

b. Trench foot (immersion foot) is the mildest form of cold injury. It usually results from exposure of wet feet to temperatures of 0-4° C for several hours. The first symptom is an uncomfortable coldness followed by numbness. Throbbing, aching, or burning and varying degrees of redness, cyanosis, edema, blistering, and skin necrosis occur after rewarming. The tissues may become gangrenous in severe cases of trench foot.

c. Chilblain (pernio) is the second most severe type of cold injury. It develops after prolonged exposure to temperatures below −6° C. It commonly affects the dorsum of the hand, but it may also involve the legs, particularly the anterior tibial surfaces in young women. Chilblain is characterized by a transient bluish-red caste to the skin with mild edema and pain, but blisters seldom form.

Treatment consists of rewarming the affected area promptly. Avoid trauma, massage, and excessive heat. Elevate the part if edema is present. Protect from infection by gently cleansing and placement of a sterile, dry dressing over open vesicles and ulcers. The area may be sensitive to cold and painful after it heals. Hyperhidrosis can also result.

d. Frostbite is the most severe form of cold injury and is due to actual freezing of the tissue fluid. The length of exposure necessary to produce frostbite varies from a few seconds to several hours, depending upon the temperature of the environment and the wind-chill index.

Symptoms and signs: Local sensations of coldness or stinging give way to numbness, and the skin becomes pale. Hyperemia may occur after rewarming; during this phase the skin is acutely painful, warm, and red or bluish. These changes are followed by varying degrees of edema, blistering, and skin necrosis, depending upon the depth of injury. The phase of hyperemia and local warmth gives way to cyanosis, hyperhidrosis, and coldness with persistent burning pain. Prenecrotic skin becomes dark brown and finally black. These areas of dry gangrene eventually mummify and separate in 1-2 months.

Immediate treatment: (1) Rewarm rapidly by immersion in water at 40-42° C, with body heat, or by exposure to warm air. During rewarming, maintain adequate perfusion by IV fluids; patients vasodilate during this phase. Do not expose to an open fire. Maintain general body warmth. (2) Avoid trauma. All casualties with foot involvement are stretcher cases; do not massage the affected part. (3) Prevent infection. Cleanse the part gently with bland soap. Dressings are not necessary if the skin is intact. (4) If blistering has occurred, debridement and placement of a biologic dressing such as pigskin may be helpful.

General treatment: (1) Absolute bed rest is required when the feet are involved. (2) Slight elevation of the part may control edema but marked elevation diminishes the blood flow and is contraindicated. (3) Expose closed lesions to room air at temperature of 21-23° C. (4) Rigid asepsis is mandatory in dressing open lesions. Use loosely applied sterile dry gauze or xenograft. (5) Heparin may be of some value in preventing secondary thrombosis in surrounding areas if it is begun within 24 hours after thawing and continued for 1 week. (6) Tetanus prophylaxis (see Chapter 4). (7) Regional sympathectomy performed as early as possible after a severe full thickness cold injury may conserve tissue, promote rapid demarcation and healing, diminish pain, and minimize or eliminate some late sequelae.

Surgical treatment: Debride conservatively. Amputate only when demarcation is definite. Remove superficial necrotic tissue with aseptic precautions and cover large open areas with skin grafts as early as possible. In general, the tissue loss in cold injury will be less than appears likely initially. Necrosis may be superficial, and the underlying skin may heal well.

Treatment of sequelae: (1) Neurologic measures: late sequelae such as hyperhidrosis, coldness, cyanosis, edema, chronic ulcers, and pain may be palliated by sympathectomy. (2) Orthopedic measures: pain in the feet on weight-bearing should be treated with well-fitted shoes and the use of pads, supports, and other orthopedic devices. Contractures due to fibrosis of muscles may require surgical release.

E. DROWNING. Respiratory obstruction is the primary disturbance in drowning. Spasm of the larynx usually develops, and this leads to acute oxygen deprivation and respiratory arrest. Only a small amount of water may be aspirated, but the stomach is often filled with water. The body is cold, and the face is cyanotic and congested.

1. Emergency treatment

a. Clear the airway. Remove mucus and foreign matter manually from the nose and throat, and drain water from the respiratory tract by gravity. Use suction if available. If possible, insert an endotracheal tube and inflate the lungs with oxygen, using an anesthesia bag.

b. Begin mouth-to-mouth respiration immediately and continue until spontaneous respiration returns or until death is absolutely certain.

c. If heart action fails, combine mouth-to-mouth breathing with closed chest massage. If ventricular fibrillation is suspected, attempt external defibrillation if equipment is available (see Chapter 2).

d. Loosen or remove constrictive clothing.

e. Keep the patient comfortable and warm.

f. In cases of near drowning in salt water, blood studies may indicate the need for intravenous infusions to correct hemoconcentration, electrolyte disturbances, or hypovolemia.

2

Preoperative and Postoperative Care

Evaluation and preparation of patients preoperatively and care for them postoperatively share equal importance with events in the operating room. The operation itself is but one phase in a continuum of care that begins when surgeon and patient first meet and continues long after placement of the last suture.

Diagnostic evaluation of diseases requiring operation is described in appropriate chapters elsewhere in this book. This chapter discusses subjects that pertain to all patients with major surgical problems.

PREOPERATIVE EVALUATION AND PREPARATION

Theodore R. Schrock

I. EVALUATION

The primary purpose of preoperative evaluation is to identify problems that affect surgical risk. (See also specific sections later in this chapter.) In addition, examination may detect other health problems that need attention, perhaps with greater urgency than the proposed operation. The increasing practice of same-day surgery can make the task of evaluation more difficult, but we must make every effort to be thorough.

A. HISTORY. A complete health history should be obtained, including the present illness, past illnesses, and associated diseases. Inquire about bleeding tendencies, current medications, and allergies.

B. PHYSICAL EXAMINATION. The cardiorespiratory system deserves careful attention. Do not overlook peripheral pulses, rectal examination, and pelvic examination (unless contraindicated by age, marital status, and so on).

C. LABORATORY TESTS. Studies have shown that costs and risks outweigh the benefits of most routine preoperative screening laboratory tests in adults. Tests should be selected thoughtfully and for specific reasons.

D. RADIOGRAPHY. Chest radiographs should be obtained only if indicated by history or findings.

G. OTHER STUDIES. ECG is not required routinely in adults under age 40 years undergoing uncomplicated noncardiac surgical procedures.

II. PREPARATION

A. CORRECT DISORDERS that affect surgical risk as much as possible. These problems are discussed in more detail below. Shock, hypovolemia, anemia, electrolyte imbalance, respiratory infection, cardiac decompensation, diabetic acidosis, renal insufficiency, and hyperthermia must be treated (or the operation postponed) in elective cases; in emergencies, the need for operation immediately may dictate that complete correction cannot be achieved.

B. INFORMED CONSENT. The patient and the family should be advised of alternative forms of therapy. The nature of the operation and its risks must be outlined and the signature of the patient or legal guardian obtained on the operative permit. In emergencies, with the patient unconscious and the family unavailable, operation may have to be done without a permit. The surgeon should know and follow local legal requirements. In some states, thorough discussion of transfusion alternatives is required.

C. PREOPERATIVE NOTE. The surgeon should enter a note into the record summarizing the history, findings, and indications for operation. The statement should include the fact that informed consent has been obtained.

D. PREOPERATIVE ORDERS
  1. Skin preparation. The patient should bathe thoroughly the night before operation. The umbilicus is a repository for desquamated epithelium and dirt; it should be cleansed by the patient or nursing staff. Hair should be removed from the incision site immediately before the operation. Shaving skin with a razor increases bacteria and contributes to wound infection.

Hair is better removed with an electric clipper using disposable heads.

2. Diet. No solid food should be taken for 12 hours and no liquids for 8 hours preoperatively. Infants having operation first thing in the morning should have the 4 AM feeding omitted.

3. Intravenous fluids. Consideration should be given to IV fluid administration before operation for elderly or debilitated patients, patients given vigorous bowel preparation, those having operations late in the day, or prior to major vascular reconstructions.

4. Bowel preparation. Thorough mechanical (and antibacterial) preparation is essential if colorectal surgery is planned. Other indications for preoperative bowel cleansing include chronic constipation; recent barium studies of the GI tract; ingestion of antacids containing aluminum or calcium; operations frequently followed by delayed bowel function (i.e., most abdominal operations). Partial evacuation of the colon is achieved by bisacodyl (Dulcolax) tablets (2-3) orally, or bisacodyl (10 mg) rectal suppository. (See Chapter 4.)

5. Medications. Bear in mind that the patient will be NPO for about 8 hours preoperatively. Medications during that time are given IV or IM, although in some cases it is permissible to give medications orally with a sip of water—check with the anesthesiologist. Anesthetic premedications, including sedatives at bedtime, are usually ordered by the anesthesiologist (Chapter 3).

Medications currently taken by the patient may or may not be continued up to the time of operation. No rules can be stated that cover all possibilities, and each drug should be decided upon individually. Insulin, corticosteroids, cardiac drugs, and antihypertensive mediations require special attention (see below).

Antibiotics should be started preoperatively if they are used as prophylaxis against infection (see Chapter 4).

Low-dose heparin should be given preoperatively to some (see page 131).

6. Laboratory tests. Blood should be drawn for tests in the morning before operation in certain patients. Examples include blood glucose in diabetics, serum potassium in patients with renal failure, hematocrit if large blood loss is anticipated.

7. Blood transfusion. Blood should be cross-matched with the patient if the need for transfusion is anticipated. Blood components (e.g., platelets) must be arranged for in advance if they will be needed. Autologous blood should be set aside 2-3 weeks in advance of elective operations in suitable patients. Some states require that patients be informed of all alternatives, including directed blood donations.

8. Activity. Ambulatory patients should be awakened and instructed to walk before sedation is given preoperatively.

9. Bladder. If a urinary catheter will not be used, the patient should void before anesthetic premedications are given. A Foley catheter is used in pelvic surgery, lengthy operations, operations with large blood loss, etc.; insert the catheter after the patient is anesthetized if there is no need for it earlier.

10. Respiratory. Patients with pulmonary disease should have a brief session of coughing and deep breathing with the incentive spirometer to clear secretions accumulated during the night.

11. Nasogastric tube. Unless the patient has GI obstruction, a full stomach, or some other special reason, a nasogastric tube can be inserted after induction of anesthesia if a tube is required.

12. Venous and arterial catheters. A venous line is inserted the night before operation if preoperative IV fluids are required. Large-bore venous catheters should be used if large blood loss is expected or if cardiac compensation is marginal. Arterial catheters in ill patients or in those undergoing extensive operations can be inserted in the operating room as a rule.

13. If **pneumatic compression stockings** or boots are planned for prevention of lower extremity phlebothrombosis, they should be applied and calibrated with the patient awake.

POSTOPERATIVE CARE

Theodore R. Schrock

I. POSTOPERATIVE ORDERS

An operation automatically cancels all previous orders in most institutions. Postoperative orders must be written to cover all aspects of care.

A. The **TYPE OF OPERATION** should be stated so that the nursing staff and physicians unfamiliar with the patient know what problems to look for.

B. VITAL SIGNS. The surgeon should specify acceptable limits for each vital sign; if a limit is exceeded, the surgeon should be notified (e.g., "notify surgeon if pulse rate is <60 or >100"). The limits are different for each patient.

1. Blood pressure, pulse, and respiratory rate should be recorded every 15 minutes—more often in some cases—until the patient is stable. Thereafter, vital signs should be recorded hourly for several hours, then every 4 hours. The frequency of these observations obviously depends upon the nature of the operation and the patient's condition. Temperature usually is recorded every 4 hours, but some patients become hypothermic during operation and others have fever before operation; these people are monitored more frequently.

2. Central venous pressure is measured along with the other signs. Specify the lower and upper limits that are acceptable for the individual patient.

3. Arterial pressure lines should be maintained once established. The line should be flushed with physiologic saline every 30 minutes. Arterial pressure usually is displayed continuously on a monitor.

4. Pulmonary artery pressure is measured in certain critical patients.

5. Continuous monitoring of ECG is advisable in ill patients.

6. Other monitors should be listed with changes that require notification of the surgeon.

C. ACTIVITY AND POSITION. These orders depend entirely upon the patient's condition and the operation performed. The patient should be kept at bedrest until stable. For routine cases, patients are allowed to walk with assistance the evening of operation.

Position is usually supine initially, but patients should be turned from side to side every 30 minutes while unconscious and hourly thereafter. Order active and passive motion of lower extremities if pneumatic boots are not used. Special precautions are required if the extremities are paralyzed from spinal anesthesia.

Position should be specified—e.g., supine, foot of bed elevated, sitting.

D. DIET. Nothing is permitted by mouth after most major operations; in some cases, a specific diet can be ordered immediately. Patients who are NPO initially are permitted to take liquids when intestinal function resumes, and food is allowed once liquids are known to be tolerated. "Full liquid" diet is an unnecessary step in dietary progression; sweet milkshakes and other items often are unpalatable to the postoperative patient. As a rule, solid food is permissible after clear liquids are tolerated. See page 173 for tube and IV feedings.

E. RESPIRATORY CARE. Patients on ventilators are monitored closely in intensive care settings. Patients who are breathing spontaneously should be urged to cough and hyperventilate every hour or two to prevent atelectasis. An incentive spirometer is useful to encourage deep breathing.

F. INTRAVENOUS FLUIDS. Orders are written for the type of fluids and the rate of infusion (see Fluids and Electrolytes, in this chapter). Be certain that an order is written for every venous line; unnecessary lines should be removed.

G. URINARY SYSTEM. The rate of urine flow in catheterized patients is monitored as are the vital signs, usually hourly. If no catheter is present, the surgeon should be notified if the patient does not void by a certain time, preferably 6 hours after operation.

H. INTAKE AND OUTPUT of fluids from all sources should be recorded at intervals, usually every 8 hours, and body weight is measured daily following major operations. Minor procedures do not require such close monitoring.

I. TUBES, PACKS, AND DRAINS. Care of each of these items should be specified (see below).

J. MEDICATIONS
1. Analgesics. Narcotics are required for relief of pain in most patients. Morphine and meperidine (Demerol) are used commonly. In the recovery room or ICU, where the patient is monitored closely, narcotics are best given in small doses IV (e.g., morphine sulfate 1-2 mg) every 1-2 hours. On the ward, PCA allows the patient to self-administer narcotics IV on demand but within limits set by the physician. The other option is narcotics in IM doses (e.g., morphine sulfate 5-8 mg) every 3-4 hours. Doses vary with the patient; if more is needed, give it. But remember that narcotics depress respiration and that the most common cause of preoperative restlessness is hypoxemia, not pain; **narcotics given to the restless hypoxemic patient may be fatal.** Epidural morphine requires close attention by the anesthesiologist.

2. Antibiotics should be continued if necessary.

3. Other medications. Insulin, corticosteroids, antihypertensives, and others should be prescribed as indicated. Scrutinize the list of preoperative medications and make a decision whether or not each is essential immediately postoperatively. Drugs must be given parenterally in patients who are NPO. Other medications not taken previously may be required by the nature of the disease or the operation.

K. LABORATORY TESTS AND RADIOGRAPHS. Need for these studies varies. Hematocrit, serum electrolytes, urinalysis, arterial blood gases, ECG, and chest radiographs are among those frequently ordered. Do not order laboratory tests thoughtlessly.

L. SPECIAL. Orders should be written to observe for developments that pertain to the particular operation performed (e.g., neurologic signs after a neurosurgical procedure, pulses distal to arterial reconstruction).

II. DAILY ORDERS

New orders must be written and old ones renewed. IV fluids, medications, activity, diet, laboratory tests, radiographs, removal of drains and tubes, frequency of vital signs, etc. should be changed as necessary. Orders remain in force long after they become obsolete because no one remembers to cancel them. Review orders each day and cancel those that are no longer essential. This relieves the nursing staff of unnecessary burdens and frees them for more important tasks.

III. PROGRESS NOTES

A. DAILY PROGRESS NOTES provide a record of the patient's recovery. Like all entries into the medical record, these notes should be factual, concise, and dispassionate. The following parameters should be listed daily in the immediate postoperative period:

1. General description: mental alertness, mood, tolerance to pain, etc.

2. Vital signs.

3. Activity.

4. Respiratory status.

5. Intake and output: note output of tubes and drains specifically.

6. Diet (e.g., tolerance of liquids or food).

7. Intestinal function (flatus or stool per rectum, abdominal distention).

8. Wound.

9. Laboratory tests.

10. Special observations relevant to the operation.

11. Complications not mentioned earlier.

12. Plans for changes in treatment.

B. PROBLEM-ORIENTED RECORD. The problem-oriented (Weed) system of medical records requires that a progress note be made daily for each active problem. For example, an active problem may be "cholecystectomy." Information is listed under each of four headings for each active problem: Subjective, Objective, Assessment, Plans **(SOAP).** This method helps ensure that problems are not forgotten postoperatively, and it helps the surgeon to think logically about the patient's condition.

IV. CARE OF PACKS, DRAINS, AND TUBES

A. PACKS. Certain wounds are packed with gauze of various types because they are heavily contaminated or infected, they are too large to close primarily, they are bleeding, or for other reasons. Packed wounds drain fluid and should be covered with absorbent dressings that must be changed when they become saturated. An effort is made to keep some packed wounds sterile in anticipation of delayed primary closure; others are obviously unsuited for sterile precautions. Packs should be removed as soon as possible; the timing is dependent entirely upon the circumstances in each case.

B. DRAINS are placed to permit egress of fluids that are already present or are anticipated to accumulate. Some surgeons use drains rarely, others frequently. Drains in body cavities quickly become sealed off so that they are effective in only a local area; drainage of the entire peritoneal cavity is impossible.

1. Types of drains

a. Soft rubber or plastic tubes. Hollow soft rubber tubes (e.g., Penrose drains) act as wicks; fluid does not usually flow through the collapsed lumen. Most surgeons prefer one of the newer soft plastic tubes (e.g., Jackson-Pratt) that connect to a vacuum-operated reservoir.

b. Gauze. Strips of gauze provide a wick, and fluid moves by capillary action. The gauze ceases to be effective when its interstices are saturated. Gauze drains usually are used only in superficial locations.

c. Sump drains of various designs have two or more lumens; one is for the egress of fluid and is placed on suction, and the other allows air to enter from the outside to maintain patency. Some surgeons prefer them if large volumes of drainage are expected over prolonged periods and for drainage of recesses of the body where gravity works against exit of fluid.

2. Management

a. The skin opening must be covered with sterile dressings. The dressings should be changed sterilely, unless the drainage is already infected; in this case, care should be taken to avoid spreading contamination to other patients.

b. Irrigation of drains is used in some circumstances to maintain patency or to cleanse the cavity. Irrigation carries a risk of introducing bacteria. Sump tubes can be irrigated through the air vent or the drainage lumen. Penrose drains cannot be irrigated.

c. Drains should be removed as soon as possible. Long drains should be shortened and removed stepwise over a period of days to allow the tract to close from the depths. Some drains (e.g., those placed in subphrenic abscesses) are removed very gradually to avoid leaving residual pockets of infection along the tract. Alternatively, a large drain may be replaced by successively smaller ones; the tract is obliterated as the last tube is withdrawn slowly.

3. Complications

a. Drains are foreign bodies, they incite inflammation, and fluid emerges alongside drains for this reason alone. It is unnecessary, therefore, to wait until all drainage ceases before drains are removed; essentially, drains never stop draining.

b. Infection in the tract, and within the body cavity as far as the drain extends, is a problem if drains are left in for more than a few days or if sterile precautions are not observed.

Drains placed to remove fluid and prevent infection may in fact cause infection by allowing bacteria to enter from the skin surface.

c. Drains interfere with healing of incisions if they exit through the operative wound.

d. Drains placed in proximity to intestinal anastomoses interfere with defenses of the peritoneal cavity against infection, prevent adherence of omentum to the anastomosis, and contribute to leakage of anastomoses.

e. Abdominal drains cause adhesions that may lead to intestinal obstruction.

f. Drains may erode into adjacent structures (e.g., the intestine). Rigid tubes are more likely to erode, but even soft rubber or plastic drains do so if left for a week or more.

g. Drains may recede into the body cavity. They should be fastened securely to the skin at all times. Drains sometimes break, leaving a portion of the foreign body in the wound when it is withdrawn. Persistent infection and drainage are the consequences. Examine removed drains to be sure they are intact.

h. The wound through which the drain is placed may not be large enough so that fluid accumulates inside rather than emerging to the outside.

C. TUBES

1. Nasogastric tubes are used to remove gas and fluid from the stomach. Plastic sump tubes are used almost exclusively. Size 16 Fr is sufficient for most purposes.

a. Insertion in an awake patient
(1) Inform and reassure the patient.
(2) The tube is easier to insert if it is stiffened by cooling it in ice for a few minutes.
(3) *Estimate the proper length* to be inserted as follows: hold the distal end of the tube at the xiphoid; measure with the tube to the tip of the nose, then back to the ear and around the ear once. Mark this spot on the tube.
(4) Lubricate the tube.
(5) With the patient sitting up and with head tilted slightly back, slide the tube gently through the nares into the pharynx. Remember that the floor of the nasal passage courses inferiorly; if the tube is oriented superiorly, it will injure the turbinates.
(6) Plastic tubes have a curve from being packaged in a coil; when the tip of the tube is in the pharynx, rotate it 180

degrees so that the tip points posteriorly. This helps avoid insertion into the trachea.

(7) Have the patient swallow (sips of water may help) as the tube is slowly and gently advanced through the esophagus. Coordinate gentle advancement with swallowing until the tube enters the stomach. Advance until the previously marked point in the tube is at the anterior nares.

(8) Gastric contents can be aspirated easily when the tube is properly positioned. Air can be injected through the tube and borborygmi heard over the stomach; this test is not entirely reliable. A better test is irrigation with saline; most of the irrigant should be retrieved with aspiration on the syringe if the patient is supine and the tube is well situated.

(9) Secure the tube to the nose. Take care not to wrap tape tightly around the nose lest pressure necrosis occur. The tube should emerge forward and downward from the nares in a straight line, not pressed upward against the nose as it is when taped to the forehead.

b. Management

(1) *Suction.* Intermittent low vacuum should be used for simple tubes. Sump tubes can be connected to higher suction because continual ingress of air through the vent prevents occlusion of the lumen by gastric mucosa.

(2) *Irrigation.* Simple tubes must be irrigated with 30 ml of air every hour. Sump tubes do not require irrigation as frequently, although the tips of some models of nasogastric tube can become occluded even though the sump mechanism continues to function.

(3) *Removal.* The tube is removed as soon as it is no longer needed.

c. Problems and complications

(1) *Discomfort.* Nasogastric tubes are uncomfortable nuisances, and surgeons increasingly choose not to use them in routine abdominal cases.

(2) *Respiratory.* Nasogastric tubes interfere with ventilation of the lungs and coughing to clear secretions. Removal of tube helps atelectasis to resolve.

(3) *Drying of the mouth and pharynx* results from mouth-breathing. Lubricants to the lips and mouthwashes help.

(4) *Necrosis of the nares* was mentioned above; it is preventable.

(5) *Esophagitis* results from reflux around the tube that lies across the gastroesophageal junction and breaks the barrier normally provided by the lower esophageal sphinc-

ter. Prolonged nasogastric intubation can lead to esophageal stricture for this reason, and in some cases the stricture presents a therapeutic challenge for months after operation. Swallowing of antacids around the tube or instillation of antacids through it may prevent this complication.

(6) *Vomiting* around the tube usually results from poor placement; the tube should be repositioned.

(7) *Fluid depletion* and electrolyte derangement from nasogastric suction can be significant. H^+, Cl^-, K^+, and Na^+ may be lost in large amounts and must be replaced by IV fluids. Electrolyte losses through the tube are exaggerated if the patient takes water or ice chips by mouth.

(8) Other complications include nasal bleeding, sinusitis, otitis media, parotitis, laryngitis, necrosis of the pharynx, and retropharyngeal abscess.

2. Long intestinal tubes are used to decompress the small bowel proximal to an obstruction. Nasogastric tubes do just as well if secretions and gas above an obstruction can reflux back into the stomach where the tube resides. Long tubes also are used by some surgeons to 'splint' the intestine and (it is hoped) permit adhesions to form without causing obstruction after extensive abdominal operations. Surgeons vary greatly in their fondness for long intestinal tubes; some use them regularly and others very rarely find them necessary or even helpful.

a. Types of tubes

(1) *Single-lumen tubes* have a balloon at the distal tip into which 2 ml of mercury are injected (e.g., Cantor tube), or the tip has a steel weight instead (e.g., Johnston tube). Other single-lumen tubes have no balloon or weight; they are usually intended for insertion during operation, with the surgeon guiding the tip of the tube through the upper GI tract. An example is the Leonard tube.

(2) *Double-lumen tubes.* One lumen is for aspiration of intestinal contents and the other permits inflation of the balloon at the distal end with air, saline, or mercury after the tube is inserted. A disadvantage is the small lumen for suction; it occludes easily. An example is the Miller-Abbott tube.

b. Insertion. Most long tubes are passed nasally, but sometimes a tube is placed through the mouth during an operation. Still another route is through a jejunostomy constructed at operation; this method was described by Baker. Interventional radiologists are very helpful in passing tubes beyond the stomach. If an interventional radiologist is not available, the following procedure is used for nasal insertion:

(1) Measure the distance to the stomach as described for nasogastric tubes. Inform and reassure the patient.

(2) Lubricate the tube and pass it through the nares into the pharynx.

(3) If the tube has no balloon that requires direct instillation of mercury (Cantor tube), grasp the tip of the tube in the pharynx, pull it through the mouth, and add the mercury. Make a pinhole perforation of the balloon to avoid progressive distention by gas that diffuses into the rubber bag.

(4) Replace balloon into the pharynx and advance it into the stomach.

(5) Progression of the tube into the duodenum is facilitated by placing the patient on the right side, with the head of the bed elevated 30 degrees. Fluoroscopy may be necessary to assist in this step.

(6) Once the tube enters the duodenum, the balloon of a Miller-Abbott type tube is inflated. It should not be taped to the nose or elsewhere at this point; because it advances slowly by peristaltic action, the tube should be lubricated frequently at the nares. Radiographs record the progress. When properly positioned, the tube is taped to the nose.

c. Management. Low vacuum suction is used. All long tubes, including the double-lumen types, must be irrigated frequently.

d. Removal. Long intestinal tubes are withdrawn slowly, a few inches at a time, at intervals of a few minutes. Tape the tube to the nose after each withdrawal so that this length of tube cannot move distally again. When the balloon reaches the pharynx, withdraw it through the mouth and cut it off; remove the tube through the nose. If the tube cannot be withdrawn from above, sever the tube at the nose and allow it to pass per rectum; this method should be needed rarely.

e. Problems and complications

(1) Distention of the balloon by gases diffusing into the balloon is prevented by making a pinhole opening as described above.

(2) Rupture of the balloon, even containing mercury, is usually not serious.

(3) With double-lumen tubes, irrigating fluid can be instilled inadvertently into the balloon instead of the lumen. This can overdistend and rupture the balloon; very rarely, the

balloon distends so greatly that intestinal wall is perforated. Be certain to mark the two channels before inserting the tube.

(4) Reverse intussusception during removal is avoided by slow stepwise withdrawal as described.

(5) Because long tubes decompress obstructed intestine and thus relieve pain, obstructions can proceed to strangulation without the surgeon's awareness of this development until too late — the result of misuse of long tubes.

3. Bile duct tubes. Straight or T-shaped, rubber or plastic tubes are placed into the extrahepatic bile ducts for external drainage, for decompression, for subsequent cholangiography and stone extraction, and sometimes as an internal stent through a bile duct anastomosis.

T-tubes are the most common bile duct tubes. Long-armed T-tubes have one limb that passes through the ampulla into the duodenum; these tubes may obstruct the pancreatic duct and should not be used.

a. Management

(1) The skin around the tube should be cleansed daily and covered with a sterile dressing at all times.

(2) The tube is sutured to the skin at operation; in addition, it should be securely taped to the skin to avoid accidental withdrawal.

(3) The tube is connected to gravity drainage.

(4) Irrigation of the tube with saline or antibiotic solution is advocated by some surgeons; others believe that irrigation may introduce bacteria, raise the pressure in the biliary tree, and cause cholangitis.

(5) Tubes are removed at varying intervals after operation, depending on the indication for placement of the tube. Tubes used for decompression after routine bile duct exploration are usually removed about 2 weeks later, after a T-tube cholangiogram shows that the duct is normal. Tubes placed for other reasons are left for weeks, months, or even permanently. Tubes are removed by gentle steady traction.

b. Problems and complications

(1) The tube may be accidentally withdrawn, partially or completely. If the tube is partially removed and bile still drains through or around it, leave the tube in and obtain a tube-cholangiogram immediately. If the tube is completely withdrawn, try to pass a straight catheter through the tract; this must be done immediately, and even then it

may be impossible to reinsert the tube in the first few days after operation because a firm tract has not yet formed. An interventional radiologist has the best chance for success. Watch these patients closely for bile peritonitis or subhepatic collection.

(2) Tubes may become occluded by blood clot or sludge. Irrigation may be attempted to dislodge the occluding material. If left for long periods, all bile ducts become occluded by debris.

(3) Cholangitis is a risk if high pressure develops in ducts contaminated by bacteria. Such pressure may result from forceful irrigation or occlusion of the tube.

4. Other tubes. Chest tubes are discussed in Chapter 9. Tubes for esophageal tamponade are discussed in Chapter 12.

GENERAL CONDITIONS AFFECTING SURGICAL RISK

Theodore R. Schrock

Specific nonsurgical diseases affecting surgical risk are discussed in the next section. General conditions affecting risk are considered here.

A. AGE. Patients at the extreme ages of life have a greater risk of complications or death from operation because they have a narrow margin of safety; small problems that might be well-tolerated by a young adult are quickly compounded in children or geriatric patients, sometimes with catastrophic consequences.

1. Infants. Special problems in pediatric surgical patients are discussed in more detail in Chapter 19.

a. Infants become severely *hypovolemic* from small losses of blood or fluid.

b. Vitamin K deficiency in neonates may result in bleeding from hypoprothrombinemia; give water-soluble vitamin K, 2 mg IM, one dose only.

c. Fever may cause convulsions or cardiovascular collapse; temperature should be lowered preoperatively by sponging with water and alcohol or application of ice packs. Elective operation should be postponed if child is febrile.

2. The elderly

a. Operative risk should be judged on the basis of *physiologic* rather than chronologic age. Do not deny the elderly patient a needed operation because of age alone. The hazard of the average major operation for the patient over 60 years of age is increased only slightly provided there is no serious cardiovascular, renal, or other systemic disease.

b. Assume that every patient over 60 years of age, even in the absence of symptoms and physical signs, has generalized arteriosclerosis and potential limitation of myocardial and renal reserve. Accordingly, the preoperative evaluation should be comprehensive.

c. Occult cancer is not infrequent in this age group; investigate suggestive GI and other complaints.

d. The elderly patient is apt to develop cardiac failure if the circulation is overloaded with excessive fluids. Monitor intake, output, body weight, vital signs, and serum electrolytes closely.

e. Elderly people generally require smaller doses of narcotics, sedatives, and anesthetics than younger patients. Respiratory depression may result from narcotics; several drugs can cause mental confusion.

B. OBESITY. Obese surgical patients have a greater than normal tendency to serious concomitant disease and a higher incidence of postoperative wound and thromboembolic complications. Obesity also increases the technical difficulty of anesthesia and surgery. It may at times be advisable to delay elective surgery until the patient loses weight by appropriate dietary measures.

C. COMPROMISED OR ALTERED HOST. A patient is a "compromised or altered host" if capacity to respond normally to infection and trauma has been significantly reduced by some disease or agent. Obviously, preoperative recognition and special evaluation of these patients are important. Increased susceptibility to infection and delayed wound healing are major postoperative problems.

Increased susceptibility to infection may arise from:

1. Drugs, such as corticosteroids, immunosuppressive agents, cytotoxic drugs, and prolonged antibiotic therapy. Infections in these patients may be caused by common bacteria, but sometimes fungi and other organisms that are rarely pathogenic are responsible.

2. Malnutrition.

3. Renal failure.

4. Granulocytopenia and diseases which produce immunologic deficiency, including lymphomas, leukemias, hypogammaglobulinemias, and AIDS.

5. Uncontrolled diabetes mellitus.

D. ALLERGIES AND SENSITIVITIES. A history of untoward reaction or sickness after injection, oral administration, or other use of any of the following substances should be noted so that these materials may be avoided:

1. Penicillin and other antibiotics.

2. Narcotics.

3. Aspirin or other analgesics.

4. Local anesthetics.

5. Tetanus antitoxin or other sera.

6. Iodine or other antiseptic.

7. Any other medications.

8. Food (e.g., chocolate, milk, eggs).

9. Adhesive tape.

E. CURRENT DRUGS. Drugs currently taken by the patient should be considered for continuation, discontinuation, or dosage adjustment. Medications such as insulin and corticosteroids must usually be maintained and their dosage carefully regulated during the operative and postoperative periods. Anticoagulants are an example of medications to be strictly monitored or eliminated preoperatively.

The anesthesiologist is concerned with the long-term preoperative use of CNS depressants (e.g., barbiturates, opiates, alcohol), which may be associated with increased tolerance for anesthetic drugs, and with tranquilizers (e.g., phenothiazine derivatives) and antihypertensive agents, which may be associated with hypotension in response to anesthesia.

NONSURGICAL DISEASES AFFECTING SURGICAL RISK

I. CARDIAC DISEASE

John C. Hutchinson

Cardiac conditions severe enough to impair the capacity of the heart to respond to stress can increase operative risk.

Myocardial failure, ischemia, or serious arrhythmia may be precipitated by operation or its complications in patients who have minimal or absent cardiac symptoms under normal conditions. Cardiovascular function may be adversely affected by such common sequelae of surgery as apprehension, severe pain, fluid and electrolyte imbalance, infection, hypoxemia, hypercapnia, hypovolemia, altered peripheral resistance, hypotension, tachycardia, bradycardia, and arrhythmia. The cardiac patient, therefore, requires careful preoperative evaluation and close observation during and after operation. A cardiologist should be consulted if a significant cardiac condition is present preoperatively or if it develops in the postoperative period.

Cardiac conditions most commonly associated with increased surgical risk are as follows: cardiac failure or limited myocardial reserve; coronary heart disease with a history of myocardial infarction or angina pectoris; major arrhythmia; hypertension associated with coronary artery disease; valvular heart disease; and congenital heart disease.

A. PREOPERATIVE EVALUATION

1. History and physical examination. The most common symptoms of heart disease are dyspnea, fatigue, chest pain, and palpitation. Signs include cardiac enlargement, murmurs, hypertension, arrhythmias, and such evidence of cardiac failure as distention of neck veins, dependent edema, rales, liver enlargement, and ascites. A past history of angina pectoris, myocardial infarction, Stokes-Adams attacks, stroke, cerebral ischemic attacks, intermittent claudication, or previous treatment for heart disease or hypertension should alert the surgeon to the possibility of a cardiac abnormality requiring special study.

Conditions that contraindicate elective surgery because of increased risk are new angina pectoris, crescendo angina pectoris, preinfarction angina, acute myocardial infarction, severe aortic stenosis, a high degree of AV block, and congestive failure.

2. Special examinations. If symptoms, signs, or past history is suggestive of heart disease, the following examinations may further clarify the diagnosis and the functional state of the heart.

a. Electrocardiography is useful diagnostically and as a baseline for evaluating subsequent changes. It may provide evidence of arrhythmia, myocardial hypertrophy or strain, coronary artery disease, digitalis effect, or electrolyte disturbance.

A normal ECG does not exclude important coronary artery disease.

In general, a stable abnormality in the ECG, in the absence of cardiac failure or angina pectoris, indicates that the operative risk is probably only slightly increased. A patient with a healed myocardial infarction has an added mortality factor of 3%-5% or greater if the infarction occurred in the preceding 6 months. Assessment of the stability of the current ECG pattern requires comparison with past tracings, if at all possible.

b. Chest radiographs should be checked for abnormalities in the size and shape of cardiac and vascular contours and for evidence of valvular calcifications and pulmonary vascular congestion. Serial films are helpful for comparison.

c. Central venous pressure. Elevations >10 cm H_2O demonstrate right ventricular failure. Normal CVP does not exclude left ventricular failure.

d. Cardiac catheterization and angiography are rarely required except in preparation for cardiac surgery. However, if a patient with serious congenital or coronary heart disease is under consideration for elective surgery, it may be necessary to complete one or both of these studies in order to decide whether corrective cardiac surgery should take precedence.

e. Determination of pulmonary arterial wedge pressure is possible by use of the Swan-Ganz flow-directed catheter, and indicates left ventricular filling pressure. Serial values <10 mm Hg may be associated with shock; >25 mm Hg, with pulmonary edema.

f. Exercise tolerance tests may be warranted if coronary heart disease is a possibility. An exercise thallium scan greatly increases the specificity of the exercise test, especially in the presence of preexisting ECG abnormalities. A simple rough exercise tolerance test is to have the patient walk up three flights of stairs. If this can be accomplished without precipitating angina and without stopping because of dyspnea, there probably is no significant deficit in cardiopulmonary function.

g. Echocardiography. Totally without risk, this non-invasive method of studying heart anatomy and function has become a powerful tool. The origin of murmurs, the severity of valvar lesions, the contractility of the ventricles, the size of the atria and hence their inferred pressures, and the presence of focal contractile abnormalities signifying old myocardial infarction are important examples of information that can be reliably derived by skillful echocardiographic study. Transesophageal intraoperative echocardiographic monitoring of heart function can provide a sensitive sign of cardiac ischemia and is thus useful in patients who must be operated upon despite known coronary disease.

h. Nuclear medicine studies. The cardiac wall motion, especially of the left ventricle, can be imaged by comparing the size and shape of the radioactively-labeled blood pool in systole and diastole. The intramyocardial distribution of thallium is an indication of coronary blood flow: a defect at rest identifies a myocardial infarction, and a reversible defect during exercise or pharmacologic stress signifies ischemia. Technetium pyrophosphate labels recent myocardial infarction. These tests are particularly useful in the diagnosis of coronary artery disease, which presents such a common preoperative problem and such a variable operative risk depending upon the stability of the pathophysiologic process.

B. PREOPERATIVE PREPARATION. The cardiac patient should achieve the best possible cardiac status before surgery. Special attention should be paid to correction of electrolyte imbalance, fluid excess, and anemia. Alert all those concerned with the patient's care during and after the operation to the importance of avoiding hypotension, hypoxia, excessive sodium, fluid, and blood administration, and undue pain or excitement. These stresses may precipitate major cardiac complications.

1. Cardiac failure should be treated before surgery. Patients with mild cardiac failure whose symptoms and signs are controlled with digitalis and diuretics have only a slightly increased surgical risk, provided that they are able to perform ordinary activities without symptoms.

2. Coronary artery disease. Many surgical patients, mostly in the older age group, have either occult or symptomatic coronary artery disease. A history of previous myocardial infarction or angina is frequently obtained, and its implication must be assessed. Important danger signals, indicating markedly increased surgical risk, are crescendo in the character of the anginal pain at rest, and the possibility of preinfarction angina or actual recent myocardial infarction. Under these circumstances, elective surgery should be deferred.

When emergency surgery must be done in spite of recent myocardial infarction, the mortality rate has been 30%-50%. Surgery that is important but not urgent should be delayed at least 3 weeks if possible following myocardial infarction. Elective surgery should be postponed 6 months. If at least 6 months have elapsed following a myocardial infarction, if the coronary artery disease is stable as evidenced by no change in pattern of pain or in the serial ECG, if there are no signs of cardiac failure, and if the indications for surgery are definite, operation can be undertaken.

3. Arrhythmias. Atrial premature beats occur more frequently in diseased hearts and may forebode supraventricular arrhythmias, for which monitoring is indicated. Occasional ventricular premature beats generally have no definite significance. When ventricular premature beats are frequent and arise from multiple foci, when they occur with rapid ventricular rates or in runs, or when they appear during digitalis administration, they may be an indication of severe myocardial disease or digitalis toxicity and thus may require preoperative study and treatment. Partial (second degree) or complete (third degree) heart block indicates organic heart disease. The patient should be monitored; prior to a surgical procedure, it may be advisable to insert a transvenous electrode catheter into the right ventricle and have a pacemaker available in case ventricular standstill occurs. These patients may be candidates for permanent pacemakers.

4. Hypertension. Moderate hypertension alone does not affect the surgical risk significantly unless renal or cardiac complications are present. Patients with uncomplicated chronic hypertension, even with left ventricular hypertrophy and an abnormal ECG, tolerate surgery well if there is no evidence of coronary heart disease or cardiac failure and if renal function is normal. Operative risk is minimized by controlling the blood pressure into the range 140-160/85-95. This control may require the continuation of antihypertensive drugs through the entire operative period. If thiazides have been used, be certain that the body potassium level is normal. Catechol depletion following reserpine, methyldopa, and guanethidine can be managed satisfactorily if the anesthesiologist is forewarned and is prepared to give vasopressors if hypotension occurs. If the blood pressure rises out of control in the operative period, sodium nitroprusside, by carefully regulated IV infusion (0.5-10 μg/kg/min) is a useful and powerful temporary measure. Other agents for the acute control of hypertension are sublingual nifedipine, IV nitroglycerin (5-100 μg/min), hydralazine (10-25 mg), or labetolol (20-80 mg every 10 minutes or 2 mg/min infusion).

5. Valvular heart disease. Acquired valvular conditions that affect operative risk adversely are severe aortic stenosis and tight mitral stenosis. An aortic systolic murmur without significant valvular disease or important left ventricular hypertrophy does not increase the mortality rate. Mitral insufficiency is usually well-tolerated, but tight mitral stenosis may result in pulmonary edema, especially if the patient has the abrupt onset of atrial fibrillation. Assessment of the severity of valvular heart disease by echocardiography is currently widely available.

6. Congenital heart disease. Uncomplicated ventricular or atrial septal defect does not usually increase surgical risk. Coarctation of the aorta and patent ductus arteriosus should usually be repaired before other kinds of elective surgery. Cyanosis indicates right-to-left intracardiac shunting, which increases during vasodilatory anesthesia. Vasoconstrictor drugs may be necessary to avoid profound desaturation. In all cyanotic heart conditions the danger of emboli, such as clots or bubbles, crossing to the arterial circulation is very high. Extreme caution should be exercised with all IV injections.

C. PROGNOSIS. Generalizations about the cardiac patient's prognosis for survival of surgery are difficult. Large series of cardiac patients have shown an average mortality of only 3% after major abdominal and thoracic surgery. Certain cardiac conditions, however, are associated with an inherently greater surgical risk. Coronary heart disease is the commonest of these encountered in practice. In general, surgical mortality for major procedures is doubled by congestive heart failure or angina with mild exertion. Risk is further increased in the presence of serious arrhythmia or a history of myocardial infarction within 6 months. Angina at rest quadruples the risk, and recent myocardial infarction raises the risk to a practically prohibitive level.

II. PULMONARY DISEASE

Frank R. Lewis, Jr.

Operative morbidity and mortality are adversely affected by acute and chronic diseases of the respiratory tract. The extent of preoperative assessment required depends upon the patient's age, evidence of preexisting disease, and the type of operation to be performed. Operations under local anesthesia generally require minimal respiratory evaluation. Any procedure involving general anesthesia requires more attention to pulmonary risk. Patients over age 60 years and patients with chronic pulmonary disease should have brief mechanical pulmonary function testing (vital capacity and forced expiration volume) and preoperative arterial blood gas determination. Patients in the highest risk groups and those who are to undergo thoracotomy, particularly if pulmonary resection is contemplated, should have extensive testing of pulmonary function.

Acute respiratory conditions affecting operative risk are mainly infections. Any respiratory infection (e.g., pharyngitis, bronchitis, or pneumonitis) is a contraindication to elective surgery and should be resolved for 1-2 weeks before operation is done. If emergency operation is required in the presence of acute respiratory infection, inhalation anesthetics should be avoided if possible, and antibiotic therapy should be administered if a bacterial cause is evident.

Most pulmonary conditions that present a significant risk are chronic and involve some degree of airway obstruction. Chronic bronchitis, bronchiectasis, emphysema, and asthma are the usual conditions. Smoking is a common accompaniment of these disorders and is a significant risk factor in itself. Assessment of chronic pulmonary disease requires evaluation of airway obstruction and vital capacity (see in the following section). A history of sputum production should be obtained, and if present, sputum should be studied by smear and culture. Purulent sputum is an indication for specific antibiotic treatment preoperatively, usually for a period of 1-2 weeks until the sputum is no longer purulent and the amount of sputum decreases. Copious production of sputum should raise the possibility of bronchiectasis or lung abscess. Smokers should abstain for 2 weeks before elective operations.

A. PREOPERATIVE EVALUATION. Initial assessment of the patient for pulmonary disease is based on information obtained from the history, physical examination, and any exercise testing carried out. In patients who will undergo minor surgical procedures, and in those who are at minimal risk even if major procedures are planned, the assessment may stop at this point. If a question is raised, or if obvious pulmonary problems exist, clinical evaluation is not enough, and specific laboratory tests must be done to categorize the pulmonary dysfunction and its severity.

1. History. The essential features to be elicited are a history of known pulmonary disease or symptoms, positional or exercise limitations that produce shortness of breath, respiratory difficulties with previous operations, smoking, sputum production, and hemoptysis. Any positive items in the history must be followed up in detail and the cause specifically determined.

2. Physical examination. Physical findings to be noted are the rate and character of respirations, thoracic anatomy, presence or absence of respiratory distress, use of accessory muscles of respiration, and evidence of restriction of rib cage motion on one or both sides.

a. Patients with chronic bronchitis and emphysema often have an increased anterior-posterior thoracic diameter and a noticeably prolonged expiratory phase to their breathing. In severe cases, the use of accessory muscles of respiration may be marked with the patient laboring, even at rest, to exchange adequate amounts of air.

b. Tachypnea is an often overlooked symptom of respiratory problems, especially acute ones. If the patient is unable to breathe deeply enough, he compensates by breathing more rapidly.

A second cause of tachypnea is increased stiffness of the lungs; this usually occurs with acute conditions. When the lungs become stiff (decreased compliance), the elastic work of breathing is accentuated, and less energy is expended if the tidal volume is small and the rate is high.

A third reason for tachypnea is a marked increase in physiologic dead space which results in an increased fraction of wasted ventilation with each breath. In order to achieve a given amount of alveolar ventilation, the rate or depth must be increased.

All of these problems represent significant pulmonary disease and increased surgical risk. Tachypnea (>25 respirations/minute) in any patient signals the need for intensive investigation of the cause.

3. Simple **exercise testing** is a rough indication of the patient's functional reserve. The ability to walk vigorously on the level for about 100 meters and to climb two flights of stairs without pausing are commonly used exercise tests. If the patient is about to undergo thoracic or major abdominal surgery and is unable to do these tests, further pulmonary function studies must be obtained.

B. PULMONARY FUNCTION TESTS

1. Physiology. Transport of oxygen from the external environment to the intracellular organelles that utilize it in metabolism may be analyzed in five steps: (1) Physical exchange of air in the environment with gas in the alveoli of the lung.

(2) Diffusion of oxygen from alveoli into the pulmonary capillaries. (3) Transport of oxygenated blood from pulmonary capillaries to peripheral tissue beds. (4) Diffusion through peripheral capillary walls and the interstitial space into oxygen-consuming cells. (5) Intracellular utilization by mitochondria.

The first two steps in this cycle are ordinarily evaluated with pulmonary function tests. The third step is evaluated by studies of cardiac function and oxygen-carrying capacity of the blood. The last two steps cannot be assessed by usual clinical methods, but they may be investigated by certain research procedures which measure tissue PO_2 tensions.

2. Ventilation

a. Physical exchange of gas from the environment to the alveolar space is defined as ventilation. Total volume of gas exchanged per minute is termed the **minute ventilation.** A portion of this goes to ventilate the physiologic dead space and is termed the wasted or dead space ventilation, and the remainder goes to ventilate alveolar spaces which are perfused with blood and is defined as **alveolar ventilation.** Only the latter is effective in gas exchange.

b. Mechanical breathing function relates generally to three factors: the relative stiffness of the lungs; the muscle power which is available to overcome this resistance and move gas in and out of the lungs; and the resistance of the airways through which the air moves.

c. Vital capacity is the maximal amount of air that a patient can move from full inspiration to full expiration; it provides a measure of the first two factors. If the lungs are excessively stiff (low compliance), or if the intercostal muscles and diaphragm are weak, vital capacity is reduced. Normal vital capacity is 65-70 ml/kg of body weight. A vital capacity of at least 10-15 ml/kg (approximately 15%-20% of normal) is needed to maintain spontaneous ventilation.

d. In patients who are intubated, the relative stiffness of the lungs may be assessed directly by measuring the volume of gas that can be exchanged with a given pressure change. This is defined as **compliance** (the inverse of stiffness) and is expressed as ml/cm H_2O pressure.

e. Airway resistance is determined by measuring the volume of gas that can be exhaled forcibly in 1 second (FEV_1). Normally, >80% of vital capacity can be exhaled in 1 second. If <70% is exhaled, some degree of obstruction is present. If <60% can be exhaled in 1 second, the obstructive disease is severe. If the FEV_1 is reduced, more sophisticated tests of pulmonary function are indicated, including measurement of maximal expiratory flow rates, flow volume curves, airway resistance, and changes in these measurements after the use of bronchodilators.

f. The arterial carbon dioxide tension (Pco_2) provides an index of the adequacy of alveolar ventilation. Normal values are 38-42 mm Hg. Elevation of the Pco_2 under resting conditions reflects compromised pulmonary function, usually obstructive in nature, and must be evaluated.

3. Alveolar-capillary diffusion. The second phase of oxygen transport is the diffusion of oxygen from the alveoli into the blood in the pulmonary capillaries. Diffusion is evaluated by measuring arterial oxygen tension (PO_2). Under normal conditions of breathing room air, the arterial oxygen tension will be >95 mm Hg in patients <40 years of age. Normal values decline approximately 5 mm Hg for each decade of additional age. Pulmonary parenchymal diseases (e.g., atelectasis, pneumonia, aspiration, fat embolism, or pulmonary embolism) can cause marked hemoglobin desaturation, and the arterial PO_2 while breathing room air may be as low as 40 or 50 mm Hg. Any reduction <70 mm Hg while breathing room air is an indication of significant parenchymal disease. Maintain arterial PO_2 >60 mm Hg by increasing the concentration of inspired oxygen, either by mask or, if necessary, by endotracheal intubation.

C. PREOPERATIVE PREPARATION. After the extent of pulmonary disease has been defined, a decision must be made about the risk it poses for the patient. In certain cases, the risk may be sufficiently great to contraindicate the proposed operation, e.g., when a pneumonectomy might make it impossible for the patient to ventilate adequately with the remaining lung. In most circumstances, however, preoperative preparation improves respiratory function to the point that the patient can tolerate the operation. If emergency surgery is necessary for a life-threatening condition, whatever risk is present must be accepted and an attempt must be made to treat the pulmonary disease in the postoperative period.

1. Acute respiratory conditions. When respiratory problems are due to acute infections, the patient should be treated with antibiotics and the operation postponed. Emergency operations must be done despite respiratory infection. Specific antibiotics are chosen initially on the basis of a gram stain of the sputum or pharyngeal swab and changed if necessary when results of culture and sensitivity tests become available.

2. Chronic respiratory conditions. Patients who have chronic lung disease cannot be returned to a normal state, and some compromise must be reached which represents the best achievable pulmonary function. They should be hospitalized for 1-2 weeks and treated with antibiotics, nebulized bronchodilators, intermittent positive pressure ventilation, postural drainage, and respiratory exercises. With significant pulmonary impairment, planned postoperative endotracheal intubation and mechanical ventilation may be necessary.

III. RENAL DISEASE

Flavio Vincenti

A. CAUSES OF CHRONIC RENAL FAILURE include the following:

1. Primary glomerular diseases (e.g., glomerulonephritis).

2. Renovascular diseases, including nephrosclerosis from hypertension. Hypertension plays a dual role in chronic renal disease. It may be the primary problem leading to renal failure, or it may occur in the course of other renal diseases and accelerate the progression to renal failure.

3. Metabolic diseases with renal involvement (diabetes and amyloidosis).

4. Interstitial nephritides, including nephrotoxic diseases.

5. Obstructive uropathy.

6. Chronic nonobstructive pyelonephritis (a rare cause of renal failure).

7. Polycystic kidney disease.

8. Hereditary nephritis.

B. MANIFESTATIONS OF CHRONIC RENAL FAILURE. Symptoms and signs of renal disease frequently reflect the degree of renal failure; on the other hand, it is not uncommon for patients with marked impairment of renal function to be essentially asymptomatic.

1. Diminished renal reserve. Although renal reserve is diminished, the excretory and regulatory functions of the kidney are still adequate.

a. Creatinine clearance is >30 ml/min.

b. The BUN rises, but the value may still be within the normal range.

c. Symptoms are usually absent except for nocturia, which is an early manifestation of the loss of concentrating ability.

2. Renal failure

a. Creatinine clearance is <30 ml/min and the BUN is distinctly elevated (azotemia).

b. A variety of symptoms (fatigue, poor appetite, pruritus) may occur.

c. Anemia, acidosis, hyperphosphatemia, hypocalcemia, and hyponatremia can develop.

d. Significant hyperkalemia is absent unless the intake of potassium is greatly exaggerated.

3. Uremia is the terminal phase of renal failure and is present when the creatinine clearance is <10 ml/min; the BUN is usually well above 100 mg/dl. Symptoms and their severity vary greatly.

a. CNS dysfunction may be manifested by the loss of higher integrative functions, memory loss, personality changes, and alteration in consciousness.

b. Peripheral nervous system disease includes sensory and motor neuropathy, the restless leg syndrome, fasciculations, and asterixis.

c. Hypertension, congestive heart failure, and edema are frequently present.

d. Pericarditis and pericardial effusion may occur in the terminal stages of uremia; these signs were ominous in the predialysis era.

e. GI symptoms include nausea, vomiting, anorexia, weight loss, metallic taste, and enterocolitis.

f. Hematologic disorders. Anemia, bleeding tendency due to platelet dysfunction, and impaired immunologic function.

g. Endocrine-metabolic. Impaired carbohydrate tolerance, hyperlipidemia, abnormal TFTs, hyperuricemia, infertility, and sexual dysfunction.

h. Musculoskeletal. Bone pain, pathologic fractures, hypocalcemia, hyperphosphatemia, hyperparathyroidism, osteomalacia, and metastatic soft tissue calcification.

C. PREOPERATIVE EVALUATION
1. Laboratory tests

a. Determination of BUN, serum creatinine, and routine urinalysis are adequate screening tests for renal disease.

b. A freshly voided urine sample may yield much information about the renal disease. Hematuria may be secondary to glomerular disease or to a lesion in the collecting system. Different types of casts are found in the urine of advancing renal disease. Red-cell casts are very strongly suggestive of an inflammatory glomerular lesion (glomerulonephritis), and white-cell casts, especially in the presence of bacteria, are indicative of acute pyelonephritis.

c. In patients with reduced muscle mass, serum creatinine can remain within the range of normal even though creatinine clearance is no more than 20% of normal.

d. A BUN:creatinine ratio well above 10:1 may reflect prerenal azotemia, GI bleeding, enhanced catabolic states, or the catabolic effect of drugs (e.g., tetracycline, steroids).

2. Radiography. Chest radiographs in patients with chronic renal disease frequently show an enlarged cardiac silhouette, prominent pulmonary vasculature, and, in later stages, pleural or pericardial effusions. Ultrasonography is a simple noninvasive study that can be used to determine renal size and the presence of obstruction with hydronephrosis. Renal scans are not very helpful in chronic renal disease. Antegrade or retrograde pyelography is required to establish the diagnosis in chronic obstruction.

D. PREOPERATIVE PREPARATION

1. Evaluate renal function carefully.

2. Correct electrolyte imbalance. In severe renal failure, hemodialysis may be advisable.

3. Anemia is a frequent finding. Hemodialysis patients adapt to hematocrits in the range of 20% and do not need transfusions unless significant losses occur. Give blood transfusions cautiously to avoid cardiac decompensation.

4. Patients with severe renal failure may have bleeding because of platelet dysfunction. Elective surgery should be delayed until platelet dysfunction has been reversed by hemodialysis and/or the use of desmopressin acetate (or DAVP), conjugated estrogen, and cryoprecipitate plasma.

5. Continue all antihypertensive medications, including beta-blockers and catecholamine-depleting drugs, until the night before surgery. Discontinuation of clonidine may result in paroxysmal hypertension; abrupt withdrawal of propranolol may precipitate cardiac arrhythmias. Patients likely to be NPO postoperatively may benefit from having a clonidine patch placed prior to surgery.

6. Patients on diuretic therapy may require correction of volume contraction and hypokalemia.

7. Avoid nephrotoxic drugs whenever possible and be alert to medication that may accumulate because of decreased renal excretion (Table 2-1).

8. Radiographic studies requiring contrast media should be done sparingly, because these substances are potentially nephrotoxic.

E. POSTOPERATIVE CARE

1. Record daily weights, input, and output.

2. Determine BUN, creatinine, and electrolytes daily.

3. Maintain fluid and electrolyte balance. If in doubt, measure urinary electrolytes. Severe hyperkalemia may occur within hours after operation in previously normokalemic patients. Use care with potassium supplementation.

4. Acidosis should be corrected gradually and carefully. Rapid correction of acidosis may lead to respiratory alkalosis, CNS depression, and decreased oxygen delivery.

5. Postoperative hypertension frequently is related to excessive fluid replacement. Antihypertensive therapy should be initiated with a diuretic agent. In renal failure, furosemide is more effective than thiazides and can be used in doses ranging from 40-200 mg, orally or IV. Episodes of acute hypertension can be treated with clonidine 0.1 mg every hour (total 0.6 mg) or nifedipine 10-20 mg every 2-4 hours. Refractory hypertensive crises should be treated with IV diazoxide 100-300 mg, IV labetolol 20 mg, or nitroprusside by constant IV infusion.

6. Diet. Restrict proteins to 0.75-1 g/kg/day in moderately azotemic patients. The diet should include adequate calories. Most patients with chronic renal failure can ingest a diet containing normal amounts of sodium and potassium. Patients with salt-wasting diseases, such as medullary cystic disease, may need to be supplemented with additional sodium chloride. Those with nephrotic syndrome or hypertension may need salt restriction.

Table 2-1. Dosage reduction of antibiotics in renal failure

None or minor	Moderate	Major	Avoid
Cefadroxil	Amdinocillin	Cefamandole	Methenamine
Cefaclor	Imipenem	Cefonicid	Nalidixic acid
Cefoperazone	Cilastatin	Ceforanide	Nitrofurantoin
Cefotaxime	Aztreonam	Cefoxitin	Sulfonamides
Chloramphenicol	Cephalexin	Ceftazidime	Tetracycline
Clindamycin	Cephalothin	Cefsulodin	Aminosalicylic acid
Carmdacilin	Cefazolin	Clavulanic acid	
Doxycycline	Cefuroxime	Aminoglycosides	
Erythromycin	Cefotetan	Carbenicillin	
Ethionamide	Moxalactam	5-Fluorocytosine	
Isoniazid	Amphotericin B	Ticarcillin	
Isoxazolylpenicillins	Ampicillin	Norfloxacin	
(dicloxacillin, nafcillin)	Ethambutol	Ciprofloxacin	
Lincomycin	Methicillin	Ceftizoxime	
Rifampin	Metronidazole		
Sulbactam	Penicillin G		
	Trimethoprim/		
	sulfamethoxazole		
	Mezlocillin		
	Azlocillin		
	Piperacillin		

IV. DISORDERS OF HEMOSTASIS

Hope S. Rugo

Patients with hemostatic defects may require surgical or other invasive procedures. The goal of preoperative screening is to identify patients at increased risk for intraoperative or postoperative bleeding in order to take preventive action. Because specific replacement therapy is often available, it is essential to identify the exact defect preoperatively whenever possible. When the appropriate history and laboratory screening tests are obtained before surgery in patients with preexisting bleeding disorders, both excessive intraoperative bleeding and unnecessary blood transfusions may be avoided.

A. SCREENING. Screening procedures must test all components responsible for hemostasis (see below). Regardless of the reason for preoperative screening, remember that screening tests are seldom useful except in the context of a careful personal and family history as well as a focused physical examination and general laboratory assessment. The overall assessment made on the basis of this evaluation guides the selection of tests for hemostasis. Routine undirected preoperative screening to detect bleeding risk using the PT and PTT is not useful unless risk groups are established, and laboratory tests alone may be misleading.

1. History and physical examination. A careful and detailed history is the best way to detect mild to moderate bleeding disorders. These patients may have normal preoperative screening tests. The history should cover common hemostatic stresses including menses, labor and delivery, dental work and extractions, tonsillectomy, and lacerations as well as major surgery. It is very important to determine whether or not the patient has ever withstood a hemostatic stress and to what degree in order to determine the contribution of the history to the evaluation. Consultation with a hematologist is advised before undertaking major surgery on a patient with a known hemostatic defect. An outline including the essential details of an appropriate history is listed below:

A. Have you ever had surgery, including tooth extractions?
  1. Did you have prolonged bleeding after the surgery? Did you have to stay in the hospital longer than you expected owing to excessive bleeding?
  2. If you have had a tooth extracted, how long did it take for the bleeding to stop? Did the bleeding stop and then start up again after a day or two?

3. Have you ever required a blood transfusion? If so, what for? Did you receive transfusions during or after surgery?

B. Do you develop frequent bruises? Are the bruises larger than a quarter? Do you bruise without remembering a specific injury?

C. Do you have frequent nose bleeds? Did you have frequent, severe, or prolonged nose bleeds as a child? Have you ever been hospitalized for nose bleeding?

D. Do you bleed for more than 5 minutes when you cut yourself or bite your cheek?

E. Have you had prolonged or heavy menstrual periods requiring medical therapy? If you have had children, did you have any bleeding problems when you delivered your children? Did you require a transfusion?

F. Do you have any blood relatives who have had problems with bleeding or bruising? With surgery?

G. Are you taking any medications now? Have you taken aspirin, headache, cold, or pain medicines in the last week? Which medicines?

A detailed past and present medical history including use of alcohol should also be included. The physical examination should include examining the skin for petechiae (usually seen in dependent areas), ecchymoses, and telangiectasias, the abdomen for hepatomegaly or splenomegaly, and the joints for evidence of old hemarthroses.

2. Laboratory tests. Hemostatic tests fall into two major groups; general screening tests and specific tests that measure coagulation factors or platelet function. Essential screening tests include tests of primary hemostasis (platelet-vascular problems), the platelet count, and bleeding time, and tests of secondary hemostasis (clotting factor problems)—the PTT (intrinsic pathway) and PT (extrinsic pathway).

The platelet count detects quantitative platelet abnormalities, and the bleeding time detects qualitative platelet defects. Remember that platelet clumping may lead to falsely low platelet counts. The bleeding time is affected by many other factors, including capillary integrity, hormonal status, medications, hematocrit, and technic in performing the procedure. In addition, the bleeding time is abnormal if the platelet count is below 80,000. For these reasons, the bleeding time may vary considerably in the same individual. In general, abnormalities in the bleeding time do not appear to correlate with bleeding risk during surgery. The test is used primarily to diagnose congenital bleeding disorders and to assess the response to treatment of qualitative platelet disorders. *The PT and PTT detect only severe deficiencies of clotting factors—generally less than 25% to 30% of normal levels.* Examples of abnormalities detected by these screening tests and several other common tests of hemostasis are shown in Table 2–2.

3. Risk categories. The history obtained above and the nature and urgency of the surgical procedure direct the necessary hemostatic work-up. A schema is presented for risk assessment and screening tests below:

a. Level 1. Negative bleeding history and low-risk procedure. The patient has given a negative bleeding history. The procedure planned is minor, such as a skin or soft tissue biopsy or a dental extraction. This includes procedures in which local pressure can easily be applied and the site is easily visible. No laboratory evaluation is necessary to screen for a coagulation abnormality.

b. Level 2. Positive bleeding history and low-risk procedure. The patient has given a significant history for bleeding. The following tests are indicated: PT, PTT, platelet count, and bleeding time (depending on the platelet count and specific history). If any of the above tests are abnormal, further work-up may be indicated. See the specific abnormality below for guidelines.

c. Level 3. Negative bleeding history and high-risk procedure*: PT, PTT, and platelet count.

d. Level 4. Positive bleeding history and high-risk procedure*: PT, PTT, platelet count, and bleeding time, if needed.

B. EVALUATION OF SCREENING TESTS

1. Isolated prolonged PT. A prolonged PT suggests either vitamin K deficiency, oral anticoagulant therapy with warfarin (Coumadin), liver disease, or, in the correct clinical setting, acute or chronic DIC. Vitamin K deficiency occurs in patients with malabsorption, or biliary tract disease, in patients who are not eating or have a poor diet, and in patients taking broad-spectrum antibiotics. In all of the above disorders, the

---

*A high-risk procedure is one that impairs hemostasis, such as cardiac surgery (platelets are damaged by the bypass pump) and prostatectomy (urokinase release), and one in which even the most minimal postoperative bleeding is hazardous, such as surgery of the central nervous system.

Table 2-2. Common tests of hemostasis

Test	Component measured	Pathologic states
PT	Extrinsic and common pathway	Liver failure, DIC, vitamin K deficiency, factor VII deficiency, hypofibrinogenemia or dysfibrinogenemia
PTT	Intrinsic and common pathway	DIC, lupus anticoagulant, deficiency or inhibitors of factors VIII, XI, XII
Platelets	Quantitative platelets	Immune destruction, decreased production, splenic sequestration
Bleeding time	Platelets (quantitative) Platelets (qualitative) Capillary integrity	Thrombocytopenia, aspirin use, von Willebrand's disease, uremia, platelet storage pool defects
Fibrinogen	Fibrinogen (functional)	DIC, fibrinolytic states
Russell's viper venom time	Common pathway (activates factor X)	**Lupus anticoagulant,** deficiency or inhibitor of factors X or V, prothrombin, or fibrinogen
Factor inhibitor assay	PT or PTT of test plasma mixed Normal plasma	**Inhibitors** to specific factors (acquired antibodies)

PTT may also be prolonged if the condition is more advanced or excessive warfarin is consumed.

The easiest and most efficient diagnostic tool is a trial of vitamin K administration. In the absence of recent warfarin therapy, the PT should correct to normal within 24 hours. If the procedure is urgent, the degree of prolongation of the PT helps in risk assessment. Generally, a PT of 15 seconds or less is considered safe for most surgical procedures and is not associated with a specific increase in bleeding. This recommendation depends on the underlying cause of the prolonged PT. Patients with vitamin K deficiency or liver disease with an isolated mild prolongation of the PT have an otherwise normal hemostatic mechanism. In contrast, patients with DIC have a severe hemostatic deficiency, usually also associated with circulating fibrin split products resulting from increased fibrinogen turnover. These split products interfere with platelet aggregation and worsen the hemostatic defect. Undetected chronic mild DIC can be a source of considerable intraoperative and postoperative bleeding. Clearly, these patients need additional evaluation and postponement, if possible, of surgery.

If the PT is prolonged to greater than 15 seconds, the risk of bleeding during surgery increases significantly. This degree of prolongation indicates a more serious deficiency of clotting factors. Again, the cause of the prolonged PT is important. If the patient has liver disease, other hemostatic abnormalities are likely present and require evaluation before major surgery is performed. For major procedures, the hemostatic defect must be corrected (see medical management). For minor procedures or those involving noncritical and not highly vascular organs in which bleeding can be directly visualized, a PT of up to 18 seconds is acceptable.

2. Isolated prolonged PTT. A prolonged PTT may be due to several problems that have a very different significance for the surgical patient. A patient with a clear history of bleeding and a prolonged PTT probably has a defect of a coagulation factor in the intrinsic pathway. By far the most common abnormality involves factor VIII or the antihemophilic factor (factor VIII$_{AHF}$, hemophilia A). Less commonly, there may be an abnormality of factor IX (hemophilia B) or XI. In this situation, specific factor levels must be measured to adequately assess the degree of risk and to direct management.

If the patient is deficient in factor VIII, it must then be determined whether the patient has hemophilia A or von Willebrand's disease. The hemophilias occur only in males and are characterized by deep tissue bleeding (hemarthroses, muscle hematomas, retroperitoneal bleeding) spontaneously or after minimal trauma. Patients with von Willebrand's disease have a deficiency in factor VIII as well as a platelet defect. It occurs in both sexes and is characterized primarily by mucocutaneous bleeding and purpura. Even if the patient has a normal bleeding time, von Willebrand's disease cannot be excluded. Mild hemophilia A and mild von Willebrand's disease may be indistinguishable from the history and mildly prolonged PTT alone. Hematology consultation should be obtained for further diagnostic work-up.

A patient with recent onset of bleeding and a prolonged PTT may have an acquired inhibitor of factor VIII. This disorder is most commonly seen in elderly patients, postoperatively, and postpartum and can result in serious bleeding complications. The diagnosis of a factor inhibitor is made by obtaining a factor inhibitor screen, most commonly referred to as a mixing study. This test is performed by mixing patient plasma with normal plasma. The PTT is usually normal at time 0 but then prolongs over a period of 1 to 4 hours after the initial mix. If the mixing test is positive, specific factor levels must be measured to determine which factor is affected. An acquired inhibitor to factor VIII is the most common. Management of patients with acquired inhibitors is complicated and requires hematology consultation.

If the patient has a normal bleeding history and an isolated prolongation of the PTT, the most likely diagnosis is a lupus anticoagulant. The lupus anticoagulant is seen in a variety of diseases, including SLE and liver disease, in older age, in otherwise normal patients, and in patients taking various drugs including phenothiazines and antiarrhythmics. Unlike patients with a factor inhibitor (see above), patients with the lupus anticoagulant *are not at risk* for excessive bleeding and can safely undergo surgical procedures. The diagnosis is made by performing a mixing test and a Russell's viper venom test. The mixing test should result in a prolonged PTT at time 0; in other words, the PTT does not correct with the mixing test. The Russell's viper venom time is prolonged if the patient has a lupus anticoagulant and is normal if the patient has a clotting factor deficiency. Patients with a lupus anticoagulant may have an increased risk for thrombosis, especially in the postoperative period.

If the patient has no bleeding history, the mixing test is negative, and factors VIII, IX, and XI are normal, it is unlikely that the patient has an underlying bleeding disorder. Potential causes of a prolonged PTT in such a patient include laboratory artifact and traces of heparin in the blood sample. Heparin can be removed from the blood sample by a simple laboratory procedure and the PTT rechecked.

3. Isolated thrombocytopenia. Isolated thrombocytopenia in adult patients is usually an acquired disorder caused by increased platelet destruction or decreased platelet production. Congenital abnormalities are rare and usually are associated with severe bleeding. Platelet disorders are associated with mucocutaneous bleeding (petechiae, purpura, nose bleeds) rather than the deep tissue bleeding seen in clotting disorders.

Increased platelet destruction occurs in ITP, secondary (e.g., vasculitis, SLE) and drug-induced thrombocytopenias, TTP, hemolytic-uremic syndrome, and DIC. Decreased platelet production is responsible for thrombocytopenia in aplastic anemia, leukemias, other bone marrow failure states, and bone marrow suppression due to drugs or chemotherapy. Splenic pooling may occur in patients with splenomegaly.

The cause of the thrombocytopenia should be determined, as it may be an indication of a serious underlying disorder and helps to determine the potential usefulness of platelet transfusions before or after surgery. Platelet survival in ITP and related disorders may be markedly shortened, with transfused platelets circulating for less than 1 hour in some patients. Platelet survival may be normal in patients with decreased platelet production, and bleeding can usually be prevented with platelet transfusions. Patients with splenomegaly have an enlarged splenic platelet pool so that transfused platelets pool in the spleen rather than circulating in the peripheral blood. The platelet count in these patients may be improved with multiple transfusions.

4. Isolated prolonged bleeding time. The two most common causes of an acquired prolonged bleeding time are thrombocytopenia and ingestion of antiplatelet drugs. A platelet count should always be obtained before a bleeding time is ordered, although, as noted above, the bleeding time may be normal in immune thrombocytopenia.

Aspirin is the most common medication that prolongs the bleeding time. In normal individuals, the bleeding time is prolonged by 2 to 4 minutes past the normal range. This is not usually associated with excessive intraoperative or postoperative bleeding. In high-risk procedures, the safest policy is to delay surgery for 5 to 7 days after the last ingestion of aspirin. The effects of other drugs, including nonsteroidal antiinflammatory agents, are usually rapidly reversible over 2 to 3 days. This is also true of the β-lactam antibiotics, including synthetic penicillins and cephalosporins. High doses of these drugs can cause a significant abnormality in platelet function which takes several days to return to normal after discontinuing the antibiotic.

Other causes of a prolonged bleeding time include von Willebrand's disease, uremia, myeloproliferative disorders, hyperglobulinemic states (multiple myeloma, Waldenstrom's macroglobulinemia), amyloidosis, and congenital qualitative platelet defects. Controversy exists over the use of the bleeding time as a screening test before surgical procedures. It is clear that the degree of prolongation correlates imperfectly with the risk of bleeding at the time of surgery. The bleeding time varies with a number of factors, one of which is the nature of the underlying disease. For this reason, it is a useful test only when it is indicated by the patient's history and is evaluated with that history in mind. Generally, a bleeding time of greater than 20 minutes (with the normal range at less than 9 minutes) might be expected to result in a significant increase in bleeding at the time of surgery. However, a patient with von Willebrand's disease and a modestly prolonged bleeding time at 12 to 15 minutes may have moderately severe operative bleeding, whereas a patient with a myeloproliferative disorder may have a bleeding time of 20 minutes with no increased bleeding at all. Special consideration is given to the treatment of uremia and von Willebrand's disease below.

5. Combined defects involving the PT and PTT. Prolonged PT and PTT are usually indications of an underlying disorder causing multiple factor deficiencies. The most common causes are DIC and liver disease. A patient with DIC should be further evaluated by measuring fibrin split products and a functional fibrinogen level to further assess bleeding risk, which may be considerable.

Other causes of a prolonged PT and PTT include warfarin therapy and occasionally the presence of a lupus anticoagulant. Although the lupus anticoagulant prolongs primarily the PTT, the PT may be prolonged by 2 to 3 seconds as well. Congenital deficiency of a factor in the common pathway of coagulation (factors V or X or prothrombin) is a rare cause of a combined defect that is usually diagnosed in childhood.

6. Negative screening tests but a significant bleeding history. Various disorders that result in an increased bleeding risk are not picked up on the standard screening tests covered above. The following disorders must be considered and an appropriate work-up should be done under these circumstances:

a. Mild hemophilia. The PTT is prolonged only if factor levels are below 25% to 30%. Therefore, patients with factor VIII$_{AHF}$ or factor IX deficiency who have levels of 25% to 30% or higher have a normal PTT despite a high risk of excessive bleeding with major surgery or major trauma. These patients usually tolerate minor surgery well without need for treatment. Most patients give a history of bleeding with trauma or previous surgery. The PTT is normal, but specific factor assays confirm the diagnosis of mild hemophilia.

b. von Willebrand's disease or mild qualitative platelet disorders. Patients with von Willebrand's disease or a mild qualitative platelet disorder may have normal screening tests but give a personal history of excessive bleeding. Usually, these patients are not at high risk for bleeding with minor surgery. If the procedure is elective, an aspirin screening test may be useful to make the diagnosis. A 625-mg dose of aspirin is given to the patient, and bleeding time is measured in 2 hours. The likelihood of a patient having von Willebrand's disease or a qualitative platelet disorder is higher if the bleeding time is prolonged beyond the range specified for normal patients taking aspirin. About 90% of patients with von Willebrand's disease have an abnormal response to aspirin. If von Willebrand's disease is suspected on the basis of this test, hematology consultation should be obtained for further diagnostic studies.

C. MEDICAL MANAGEMENT OF PATIENTS WITH HEMOSTATIC DEFECTS UNDERGOING SURGERY

1. Acquired bleeding disorders

a. Vitamin K deficiency. Patients with a PT prolonged up to 1.5 times normal tolerate minor procedures such as liver biopsy, paracentesis, and thoracentesis without excessive bleeding. Replacement is necessary for longer prothrombin times or prior to major surgery. The urgency of the planned surgery dictates the type of replacement given. For elective surgery, 5 to 10 mg of vitamin K administered intramuscularly completely corrects the PT and PTT within 24 to 48 hours. Partial correction is seen as early as 6 hours.

Emergency surgery that cannot be postponed for vitamin K requires factor replacement. Fresh frozen plasma or factor IX concentrates are used to correct the PT. Ten to 15 cc/kg of fresh frozen plasma should correct the PT to a safe range. If the PT is greater than 20 seconds, it may be difficult to completely correct the PT and PTT with plasma alone owing to volume limitations (each unit of plasma is 250 to 300 cc).

b. Anticoagulants. Most patients receiving chronic anticoagulation therapy are treated with sodium warfarin. This drug inhibits the vitamin K–dependent clotting factors II, VII, IX, and X.

For elective surgery, warfarin should be discontinued 3 to 4 days before the operation to allow the PT to gradually return to 15 seconds or less. Warfarin can then be resumed 2 to 3 days after surgery. When the PT returns to normal or close to normal, the patient requiring chronic anticoagulation is at high risk for thrombotic complications. The degree of risk depends on the reason for anticoagulation. For this reason, subcutaneous or intravenous heparin is used to bridge the gap between stopping warfarin and achieving adequate anticoagulation again postoperatively. It is important that anticoagulation be maintained, especially in the postoperative period when patients are generally hypercoagulable.

For emergency surgery, vitamin K or fresh frozen plasma should be given. Vitamin K corrects the PT to a safe level within hours; fresh frozen plasma acts immediately but may take considerable time to infuse owing to volume limitations (see above). If vitamin K is used, the patient may be relatively refractory to re-anticoagulation with warfarin for as long as 1 week. However, it is the preferred therapy if time permits, as it avoids the use of a pooled blood product such as fresh frozen plasma and its inherent infectious risks. Heparin may be used for anticoagulation during this period.

c. Liver disease. As discussed above, many hemostatic abnormalities associated with liver disease may be very difficult or impossible to correct. The abnormalities include factor deficiency due to decreased synthesis, excessive fibrinolysis with increased fibrin split products (which interfere with platelet aggregation), and thrombocytopenia due to splenic sequestration. Factor deficiency can be corrected with fresh frozen plasma and cryoprecipitate (to correct fibrinogen). Thrombocytopenia may be difficult to correct even with platelet transfusions owing to splenic sequestration. Fibrinolysis is difficult to manage, and no specific treatment is available to clear circulating fibrin split products. Hence, defects beyond specific deficiencies of factors are often impossible to correct.

Elective surgery in patients with severe liver disease can be quite dangerous and should be performed only when absolutely necessary. Occasionally, plasmapheresis is used to remove circulating split products and enhance hemostasis (patients receive a large transfusion of normal plasma as replacement) in patients with acute liver failure who are scheduled for urgent liver transplantation. Patients may also receive a continuous infusion of fresh frozen plasma intraoperatively and postoperatively in this setting.

d. DIC. DIC is usually acute or subacute but can be chronic in the setting of underlying malignancy or chronic liver disease. Patients with chronic DIC may be at high risk for bleeding or thrombosis. The PT and PTT are usually normal, but the platelets and fibrinogen are low, and the fibrin split products are elevated. If surgery is necessary (and often as chronic therapy to control chronic DIC), low- to moderate-dose heparin is used to reverse the hemostatic defect and prevent complications resulting from the consumption of coagulation factors and the presence of circulating fibrin split products. The heparin is maintained as a low-dose continuous infusion or as an intermittent small dose given subcutaneously. The level of fibrinogen (and often the platelet count) is used to monitor therapy.

e. Thrombocytopenia. What level of thrombocytopenia is acceptable before a surgical procedure? For low-risk procedures, a platelet count of at least 50,000/μl is recommended, but certain procedures may be performed without complication at lower counts. For example, simple skin biopsies are well tolerated when the platelet count is as low as 30,000/μl. High-risk procedures should generally be done when the platelet count is above 80,000 to 90,000/μl. Patients with immune thrombocytopenic purpura (peripheral destruction) may have a normal bleeding time and often tolerate procedures at lower platelet counts without significant bleeding. The patient's individual bleeding history is very useful in this situation. Severe bleeding is likely if the platelet count is below 20,000/μl.

Patients with immune thrombocytopenia require special management preoperatively. Prophylactic platelet transfusion should not be given unless there is life-threatening bleeding. Corticosteroids often raise the platelet count within about 1 week so that elective operations can safely be performed, and steroids can usually be rapidly tapered postoperatively. If urgent or emergent surgery is required, intravenous gammaglobulin can be used both to rapidly (but temporarily—usually lasts about 3 weeks) raise the platelet count and to increase the patient's responsiveness to transfused platelets. Often splenectomy is required for the long-term management of patients with idiopathic immune thrombocytopenia.

Nonimmune thrombocytopenia can often be managed by platelet transfusion alone. A posttransfusion platelet count should be obtained prior to beginning surgery to ensure an adequate rise in platelets.

The above recommendations must be used only if platelet function is normal. Additional qualitative platelet defects are found in uremia and in patients taking aspirin-like (antiplatelet) drugs. These patients have bleeding in excess of that expected from the absolute platelet count. The management of uremic bleeding is discussed below.

f. Thrombocytosis. Platelet counts greater than 600,000/μl may be seen transiently after splenectomy or other major operations or in patients with chronic inflammatory and neoplastic diseases. This reactive thrombocytosis does not cause bleeding or thrombosis and does not require treatment.

Clinically significant thrombocytosis occurs in myeloproliferative diseases such as polycythemia vera, chronic myelogenous leukemia, and others. These patients may have an increased risk for bleeding or thrombosis during and after surgery owing to qualitative platelet defects and the increase in red cell mass seen in polycythemia vera. It is essential that the platelet count and red cell mass be controlled before elective surgery to avoid significant morbidity and mortality. Hematology consultation should be obtained.

g. Uremia. Uremia causes a qualitative defect in platelet function that can result in a high risk of bleeding with even minor surgical procedures. The risk of bleeding is usually monitored by the bleeding time, although again, it correlates poorly with the patient's own risk of bleeding. The treatment of choice for elective procedures is rigorous dialysis as close to the planned surgery as possible (less than 24 hours). If the patient still has a high risk of bleeding assessed either by the bleeding time or by past history during hemostatic stress, DDAVP or cryoprecipitate can be used.

DDAVP may result in short-term return to normal hemostasis in patients with uremic bleeding. The maximum effect on bleeding time after infusion is seen in 1 hour, with little effect remaining after 8 hours. A dose of 0.3 μg/kg is given intravenously in advance to test the response with bleeding times. Unfortunately, DDAVP is not effective in repeated doses unless at least 1 day is allowed to pass between doses. Cryoprecipitate also may be used when DDAVP and dialysis are not effective at stopping bleeding. Conjugated estrogens have been used for persistent bleeding on a chronic basis and may be moderately effective.

2. Congenital bleeding disorders. Surgery on patients with congenital bleeding disorders should be performed only in coordination with a hematologist. Severe deficiencies must be replaced before, during, and after operation. If emergency surgery is necessary on a patient with congenital hemostatic defect but the exact nature of the defect is unknown, the patient should be given fresh frozen plasma, which provides all the clotting factors (but not platelets).

a. Hemophilia. Treatment of hemophilia is based on the degree of factor deficiency and the planned procedure. Patients with severe hemophilia usually have a factor level of less than 1% of normal, whereas patients with very mild hemophilia may have a level of 25% of normal. The calculated dose of factor to be replaced is based on the desired level for the surgical procedure and the distribution of the factor in plasma.

Patients with hemophilia A are given factor VIII concentrates, and patients with hemophilia B are given factor IX complex. Factor VIII concentrates currently on the market are considered safe in terms of HIV and hepatitis risk. In addition, recombinant factor VIII is now available. A factor IX complex has been recently produced which is much safer in terms of infectious risk. Factor IX complex contains factors II, VII, IX, and X, and prolonged administration results in an increased risk of DIC. A new product containing only pure factor IX is now available for prolonged administration, which should eliminate thrombotic complications. Cryoprecipitate (factor VIII) and fresh frozen plasma (factor IX) should not be used unless emergency factor replacement is required and specific concentrates are not available.

Very minor procedures (e.g., a biopsy) are treated with a limited number of infusions of factor intended to raise the patient's level to about 50%. Factor is given immediately prior to and for 1 to 2 days after the procedure. Major procedures, especially orthopedic surgery, require maintaining factor levels at greater than 50% for 7 to 10 days following surgery. Prior to surgery, levels are usually raised to 100%. Factor levels must be obtained to assess the adequacy of replacement.

b. von Willebrand's disease. von Willebrand's disease is actually a heterogeneous group of diseases that vary in severity and response to treatment. Cryoprecipitate has been used to treat patients prior to surgery, but the infectious risk of products such as cryoprecipitate and fresh frozen plasma is considerable over a lifetime of therapy. Purified factor VIII products and DDAVP are now available and have essentially no infectious risk.

Factor VIII products have not been used to treat von Willebrand's disease in the past because the method of purification markedly reduced the amount of von Willebrand factor in the preparation. Newer technics for purifying factor VIII concentrates have resulted in products with high von Willebrand factor activity.

DDAVP stimulates the release of endogenous factor VIII and von Willebrand factor. The bleeding time is usually measured before and after administration of DDAVP as a trial to assess response before recommending this therapy. If major surgery is planned, DDAVP may be given on alternating days with factor replacement, as the beneficial effect of DDAVP decreases or is eliminated with repeated consecutive doses.

c. Congenital qualitative platelet disorders. Patients with qualitative platelet defects who have an unacceptably prolonged bleeding time or significant bleeding history should be treated with random donor platelet transfusions preoperatively and postoperatively. One unit of platelets usually raises the platelet count by $10,000/\mu l$ in a 70-kg individual. Many patients have been previously transfused and may be alloimmunized and therefore relatively refractory to platelet transfusions. In this situation, cross-matched or HLA-compatible platelets are obtained in advance of the planned procedure. Some patients may be refractory even to matched platelets, so a posttransfusion count prior to surgery should always be obtained.

V. ENDOCRINE DISORDERS

Paul A. Fitzgerald

A. DIABETES MELLITUS. Patients should be screened for unsuspected diabetes with a urinalysis and serum glucose; glycosuria or a serum glucose >140 mg/dl should cause suspicion for diabetes.

About 15% of diabetics have severe insulin deficiency and are classified as type I insulin-dependent because they are dependent upon insulin to avoid ketoacidosis; they are usually juveniles when diabetes first occurs. The rest have partial insulin deficiency or insulin resistance and are classified type II non–insulin-dependent because they are not ordinarily dependent upon insulin to avoid ketoacidosis; they are usually adults when diabetes first occurs. NIDDM patients may require insulin for hyperglycemia if diet and oral medications are ineffective or in times of illness or surgical stress.

The diagnosis of diabetes requires either (1) *fasting* glucose over 140 mg/dl on two occasions or (2) a diagnostic 2-hour OGTT: a venous plasma glucose over 200 mg/dl at 2 hr and some other time (30, 60, 90 minutes) after 100 g of liquid glucose. (Note: Postprandial capillary and arterial plasma glucose can be about 30% higher than venous plasma glucose owing to tissue glucose utilization.)

1. Complications

a. Hyperglycemia can produce a solute diuresis that may result in hypovolemia if fluid intake is inadequate. Severe hyperglycemia with dehydration may produce hyperosmolar coma or ketoacidosis.

b. Hypoglycemia caused by insulin or oral hypoglycemics may produce brain injury and intraoperative hemorrhage.

IV access should be maintained longer than in nondiabetics, so 50% dextrose (10-25 ml) can be administered quickly for serious hypoglycemia. Keep glucagon, 1 mg, available to be given IM for serious hypoglycemia when venous access is difficult. Oral dextrose or fruit juice should be within the patient's reach.

c. Atherosclerosis is accelerated in the presence of smoking, hypertension, hyperlipidemia, or nephropathy. Such patients have an increased risk for ischemic stroke, myocardial infarct, and lower extremity ischemia. They often do not tolerate hypotension, severe anemia, or hypoxia as well as otherwise healthy patients of the same age.

d. Nephropathy most frequently occurs in diabetes of >10 years' duration. Proteinuria is usually a first sign of renal disease and should evoke caution in the use of large volumes of IV saline which may produce severe edema. Hyperosmolar IV contrast may cause acute tubular necrosis, especially in diabetics with a serum creatinine of >2 mg/dl. Nonionic contrast agents offer less risk for renal damage. Nephrotoxic drugs should be avoided when possible.

e. Retinopathy most frequently occurs in diabetes of

>10 years' duration. Visual impairment most often occurs from macular edema, neovascular glaucoma (rubeosis iridis), and/or proliferative retinopathy with vitreous hemorrhage. Retinopathy may require laser treatment. In the presence of proliferative retinopathy, excessive increases in venous pressure may induce a vitreous hemorrhage (avoid Valsalva maneuvers, heavy lifting, straining due to constipation, spirometry, or mechanical ventilation, especially with positive end-expiratory pressure).

f. Neuropathy may present as numbness or paresthesias in the extremities, especially the feet. Patients with severe neuropathy must have the feet examined daily during prolonged hospitalization because bed pressure may produce serious unsensed ulcerations. Heel ulcerations may be prevented with heel pads. Casts must be well padded and molded. Neuropathy may also acutely affect major nerves (cranial nerves III, VI, VII) or major nerve trunks.

Neuropathy may affect visceral organs such as the stomach (**diabetic gastroparesis**). Patients should receive nothing by mouth for at least 12 hours preoperatively in order to reduce the possibility of postoperative emesis and aspiration. Diarrhea and/or constipation and male impotence are also common. Impaired bladder innervation may cause urinary retention, especially after intraabdominal or pelvic surgery. This may require bladder catheterization but may also respond acutely to urecholine. Cystitis is common, especially after instrumentation, owing to postvoiding residual urine in the bladder, and may progress to pyelonephritis.

g. Microvascular disease and impaired wound healing. Diffuse microvascular disease makes diabetics more prone to pressure ulcerations. Decubitus ulcers may form with bedrest and heal poorly in diabetics. Patients should have vigorous decubitus precautions including heel, elbow, or sacral padding and frequent turning. Alternating pressure mattresses are useful. Good blood glucose control must be maintained in the first postoperative week.

Wounds often heal poorly in diabetics and wound infections are more common. Healing in ischemic tissues may be promoted with nasal oxygen administration. Ischemic foot lesions may be healed by improving blood flow by angioplasty or bypass surgery where feasible.

2. Controlling blood sugar: methods

a. Blood and urine glucose monitoring. Measure the

blood glucose 4 times daily (before meals and at bedtime), more frequently on the day of surgery, and hourly during general anesthesia.

Blood for testing may be obtained from the fingertip using lances. During surgery, obtain a drop of blood from the fingertip, earlobe, or an arterial line; glucose determinations on blood obtained from a running IV infusion are often inaccurate.

Glucose determination may be done at the bedside. A **large** drop of blood is placed on a glucose oxidase test strip which is then read with the aid of a portable device. Visually read strips may underestimate hyperglycemia; monitoring devices are preferable but their accuracy must be checked.

Urine testing for glucose and acetone may be done four times daily on hospitalized diabetics. Certain drugs affect urine glucose oxidase tests and may cause false-negative results (ascorbic acid, L-dopa, methyldopa, salicylates, ketones).

b. Diet should be "diabetic" so that foods are not given which have excess sugar or fat. Obese diabetics need caloric restriction.

Nasogastric tube feedings should be used judiciously in diabetics. Total parenteral nutrition (TPN) can cause severe hyperglycemia; regular insulin should be added to the TPN formulation as required, usually starting with about 10 units/L.

Obese patients do not require nasogastric feeding or TPN as long as blood glucose is controlled, proper hydration is maintained, and potassium, calcium, phosphorus, and necessary vitamins are supplemented as indicated. Insulin or sulfonylurea requirements may decrease as calories are restricted and weight falls. Starvation ketosis and ketonuria may occur in calorie-restricted obese diabetics and is a natural consequence of fat catabolism; it should not be confused with ketoacidosis.

    (1) *For diet-controlled NIDDM patients,* caloric restriction is indicated if the patient is obese. Diets as low as 800-1200 calories may be safely prescribed for obese adult patients and do not impair wound healing because such patients have adequate energy stores. Diabetics not taking oral hypoglycemic drugs or insulin should receive no dextrose in the IV fluids. Nevertheless, stress of illness, surgery, or hyperalimentation may cause significant hyperglycemia (blood glucose >200 mg/dl) in an otherwise well-controlled patient. Such patients are given human

regular insulin in small doses (5-10 units), with the dose adjusted according to glucose response.

(2) *For diabetics receiving insulin or an oral hypoglycemic drug,* it is especially important that the diet be 'diabetic' and meals given regularly along with a bedtime snack. Calories should consist of the patient's usual allotment if that has produced adequate glucose control and normal weight. If the patient has been hyperglycemic and obese, calories are reduced below that required for weight maintenance. If a procedure delays a meal, an IV should usually be started containing 5% dextrose (D) at an initial rate in adults of 80-100 cc/hour.

c. Oral hypoglycemic agents. Patients with blood glucose levels not well controlled on oral agents or who are undergoing very major surgery should be switched to insulin preoperatively. Patients in excellent control with an oral agent, who are undergoing relatively minor surgery, may have medication continued; if they are NPO, a 5%D IV should be run at 80-100 ml/hour to start, with the rate varied according to blood glucose levels. If blood glucose rises to >250 mg/dl, despite reduction of the 5%D IV rate, insulin may be given as needed.

d. Insulin. There is a large variety of insulins and insulin dosage schedules. Patients whose control is not certain should ideally be admitted 1-2 days before elective surgery. Patients receiving insulin who are well controlled as documented by daily home blood glucose monitoring may be admitted the day before elective surgery.

(1) *Subcutaneous insulin* is most reliably absorbed when given in the abdomen. Do not give insulin subcutaneously to hypotensive patients because absorption is erratic.

On the evening before surgery, patients receiving evening intermediate-acting insulin (NPH, Lente) should have the dose decreased by about one-third. The evening dose of regular is kept the same. The morning of surgery, at 6 AM, an IV line may be started with a "Y" infusion set-up so that 5%D is infused at a rate independent of normal saline used for volume replacement; 5%D should be given at about 100 ml/hour (less in children or azotemic patients). The IV rate should be closely monitored and a device used to ensure a proper infusion rate. After the IV is running, the morning insulin may be given. Ordinarily, about half the usual intermediate insulin and about one-third the usual short-acting insulin is given. Once subcutaneous insulin has been given, the 5%D IV is varied in rate to keep the blood glucose level between 150 and 250 mg/dl.

Postoperatively, a baseline insulin regimen of half the usual dosage is given while NPO. Extra supplementary insulin is used if hyperglycemia >200 mg/dl occurs after the 5%D IV has been slowed. Supplementary insulin should be used cautiously because its peak effect may coincide with that of preoperative insulin, producing hypoglycemia. Volume replacement should be done with a non–dextrose-containing solution.

Be sure diabetics continue to manage their diabetes optimally. A diabetes education course should be offered. Insulin regimens vary. A "tight control" regimen may consist of one injection of regular insulin before each meal plus an injection of intermediate-acting insulin (NPH or Lente) at bedtime. Insulin pumps providing continuous subcutaneous insulin infusion (CSII) are available.

(2) *Continuous IV insulin* is a preferred mode of treatment for insulin-dependent diabetics undergoing major surgery who are at risk for hypotension or are anticipated to require constant IV nutrition for several days postoperatively. It is also useful for patients with severe insulin resistance due to high-dose glucocorticoids or for diabetics requiring constant nasogastric or parenteral nutrition who require large constant insulin doses. The exact formulation and rate of the IV infusion vary and must be adjusted according to blood glucose. Start with: Number of units/hour = (blood glucose/150). For diabetics receiving high doses of glucocorticoids, start with: Number of units/hour = (blood glucose/100). Because a small amount of insulin does adhere to plastic tubing, run out and discard the first 20 ml. A constant infusion device is used to prevent accidental overdosage. If a patient becomes hypoglycemic or when switching to subcutaneous insulin do *not discontinue IV insulin for longer than 2 hr; decrease the insulin dose and/or give more 5%D.*

3. Ketoacidosis. The stress from an acute illness prompting surgical attention may produce ketoacidosis. All acutely ill diabetics must be quickly assessed for this with a "stat" blood glucose and serum electrolytes as well as urine for sugar and acetone. A serum bicarbonate <20 mEq/L with a urine showing "large" ketones is evidence for serious ketosis; obtain an arterial blood gas pH to assess the degree of acidosis and respiratory compensation. DKA is treated with vigorous hydration in all patients except those with serious renal insufficiency and edema. Use 0.45 NS or 0.9 NS and regular insulin, 0.1 unit/kg, IV bolus to start, then 0.1 unit/kg/hour by constant IV infusion. Monitor K^+ and glucose every 1-2 hours and supplement K^+ as required. The IV is switched to 5%D once the blood glucose drops to 250 mg/dl to avoid hypoglycemia and cerebral edema. Sodium bicarbonate is not given unless the arterial pH is <7 and then by slow infusion to avoid paradoxical CNS acidosis. After 4-8 hours of vigorous fluid and insulin infusion, parameters are usually improved enough for a patient to undergo emergency surgery.

B. ADRENAL INSUFFICIENCY. Primary adrenal insufficiency (Addison's disease) is usually autoimmune; other causes include adrenal enzyme deficiencies (congenital adrenal hyperplasia), hemorrhage, tuberculosis, and other infections. Secondary adrenal insufficiency is caused by pituitary/hypothalamic injury or suppression by prior exposure to glucocorticoids.

1. Symptoms and signs of cortisol deficiency may include weakness, nausea and vomiting, diarrhea, and even abdominal pains mimicking a "surgical abdomen." Signs may include hypotension and fever. In chronic Addison's disease, compensatory increased ACTH may cause hyperpigmentation.

2. Laboratory. *Cosyntropin test:* obtain a plasma cortisol between 6 AM and 9 AM, give ACTH 0.25 mg IM or IV and obtain another plasma cortisol 30-60 minutes later. Adrenal insufficiency is suspected if the rise in cortisol is <8 µg/dl or the maximum level is <18 µg/dl. Any serum cortisol of 20 µg/dl or greater indicates no significant adrenal insufficiency. If the test is abnormal, obtain a plasma ACTH level, which is elevated in Addison's disease and low or low-normal in secondary adrenal insufficiency.

Other laboratory abnormalities sometimes found with cortisol deficiency are hypoglycemia, hypercalcemia, and a relatively low WBC with lymphocytosis and eosinophilia. Deficiency of aldosterone in Addison's disease may produce hyperkalemia, hyponatremia, and hypotension.

Addison's disease may be associated with immune conditions, ovarian failure, diabetes mellitus, vitiligo, hypoparathyroidism, testicular failure, or pernicious anemia. Secondary adrenal insufficiency, when not due to 'suppression,' is usually associated with other pituitary hormone deficiencies: growth hormone, gonadotropins, thyrotropin, or vasopressin.

3. Radiology. CT scan of the adrenals may reveal enlarged hyperdense adrenals in cases of acute adrenal hemorrhage. Adrenal calcification may be noted in chronic adrenal insufficiency due to adrenal hemorrhage or granulomatous disease (e.g., tuberculosis).

MRI scan of the adrenals may not initially show acute hemorrhage, but T1-weighted images tend to show a hyperintense signal beginning 5-7 days after hemorrhage and lasting several days to months after the event.

4. Treatment. Chronic glucocorticoid replacement usually consists of hydrocortisone, 10-25 mg (average 15 mg) every morning and 5-15 mg (average 10 mg) every evening. Alternatively, prednisone, 4-6 mg/day, may be used. In Addison's disease, mineralocorticoid is usually replaced as fludrocortisone (Florinef), 0.05-0.1 mg, once daily.

For mild stressful illness, the usual dose of hydrocortisone is tripled for 2 days and tapered back to the usual dose over several days while the underlying condition is treated. For surgical stress, hydrocortisone is given in large doses. Usually, 100 mg is given IM "on call" to the operating room and 50 mg is given IV, IM, or orally every 6 hours thereafter for the next day. The dose may be tapered over several days. Any symptoms of adrenal insufficiency should prompt a dosage increase. If the patient has required fludrocortisone, it should be resumed once the hydrocortisone dose is reduced.

5. Addisonian crisis. Stressful illness or surgery in the presence of adrenal insufficiency may cause an exacerbation of the symptoms described above, resulting in severe intravascular volume depletion and shock. Patients have nausea, vomiting, and impaired consciousness. Such patients may be febrile as a result of an underlying infection and/or cortisol deficiency itself. This hypotension does not respond well to volume replacement alone, and thus *adrenal insufficiency should be considered in all cases of unexplained shock,* especially when poorly responsive to other treatment.

Treatment of acute adrenal crisis involves giving hydrocortisone IV in a large dose of about 200 mg to start, followed by 100 mg IV every 6 hours until symptoms abate and hypotension resolves. The dose is then tapered as outlined above for postoperative patients.

C. HYPOTHYROIDISM

1. Symptoms and signs. Symptoms frequently include fatigue, cold intolerance, weight change, constipation, myalgias, hair loss, dry skin, and brittle nails. Other symptoms may include carpal tunnel syndrome and psychiatric changes. Women may have galactorrhea and any menstrual irregularity (usually menorrhagia). Many patients have a history of prior thyroid treatment. Signs may include goiter or neck scar, puffy facies, fatigued countenance, hyperkeratotic skin, bradycardia, hypothermia, and a delayed reflex relaxation time. Children may have short stature. Hypothyroidism may progress to myxedema coma.

2. Laboratory. Because symptoms and signs of hypothyroidism are nonspecific, it is a reasonable practice to screen patients prior to surgery. The serum level of TSH is the single best screening test for primary hypothyroidism; TSH is virtually always increased in this condition, whereas serum T_4 level may be depressed by many factors including severe illness or phenytoin, and may not accurately reflect the patient's clinical thyroid status. Nevertheless, a serum **T_4RIA** and resin T_3 uptake (rT_3U, an assessment of how much T_4 is "free" and active) may be obtained; $T_4 \cdot rT_3U = FTI$. The FTI should be ordered when hypothyroidism is clinically suspected, especially when CNS pathology or any evidence of hypopituitarism is present, because the TSH is not elevated in secondary hypothyroidism.

Other laboratory abnormalities found in hypothyroidism include elevation of serum enzyme levels, anemia, hyperlipidemia, hyponatremia, hypoglycemia, hyperprolactinemia, and increased CSF protein. Antimicrosomal or antithyroglobulin antibody levels may be elevated if the patient has Hashimoto's thyroiditis.

3. Treatment of hypothyroidism should begin once the absence of concomitant hypoadrenalism is assured, because thyroid treatment might in that instance precipitate Addisonian crisis.

Patients with mild hypothyroidism actually tolerate surgery very well. Patients with more severe myxedema should receive at least partial correction prior to surgery, with the exception of patients undergoing coronary artery bypass.

In adults <50 years old without ischemic heart disease, begin treatment with L-thyroxine (Synthroid, Levothroid), 50-100 μg orally or IV daily. In adults >50 years and in patients with ischemic heart disease, begin replacement with 25 μg or 50 μg daily and increase the dose by 25 μg or 50 μg monthly until patient is euthyroid. Most adult patients require 100-200 μg daily, with younger adults usually requiring more than older individuals. Patients who are NPO may be given IV thyroxine (T_4) daily at a dose about 25% less than their usual maintenance. If coronary artery bypass or angioplasty is to be performed, delay beginning thyroid replacement until immediately following revascularization and coming off bypass; at that time, L-thyroxine 300 μg may be given IV, followed by 100 μg daily.

Myxedema coma may occur in stressed (usually infected) hypothyroid patients. Besides decreased mentation patients may exhibit hypoventilation, hypothermia, respiratory acidosis, hypotension, hypoglycemia, hyponatremia, and increased serum enzyme levels. Acute tubular necrosis and pneumonia often complicate this disorder. The diagnosis is confirmed by a low T_4 with an elevated TSH, but treatment should not be delayed while waiting for results. Myxedema coma has an extremely high mortality rate. Any surgical procedures should be avoided or done under minimal or local anesthesia when necessary.

Treatment of myxedema coma is directed at maintaining respiratory function. Patients usually need intubation and assisted mechanical ventilation.

Levothyroxine 500 μg is given IV, followed by 100 μg IV or orally daily. Hydrocortisone 100 mg is given every 8 hours and tapered as recovery occurs. Gradual external rewarming with blankets is indicated along with intensive monitoring, treatment of infection, and respiratory therapy.

VI. PREGNANCY

Edward C. Hill

Surgical procedures on the pregnant patient should be carried out promptly if the diagnosis of an acute surgical disease is made. Elective operations for conditions that do not threaten the pregnant woman's life should be postponed until the postpartum period. Special considerations in surgery on the pregnant patient are as follows:

A. ABORTION OR PREMATURE LABOR. Abortion ensues if the ovary containing the corpus luteum is removed prior to the 20th day of pregnancy, unless progesterone is administered. After the second month of pregnancy, the placental production of hormones is sufficient to maintain pregnancy.

The risks of abdominal surgery can be minimized by manipulating the uterus as little as possible during the procedure and avoiding episodes of prolonged hypotension or hypoxemia.

During the third semester, the supine position may produce hypotension from compression of the vena cava by the gravid uterus. This can be prevented by providing external lateral pressure against the uterus, displacing it to the left away from the vena cava (left lateral displacement). Operating-table attachments are available for this purpose.

B. ANESTHETICS AND DRUGS. Although systemic anesthetic agents cross the placenta and gain access to the fetal circulation, they are metabolized in the usual fashion and excreted by the mother. There are no known lasting effects on the fetus once organogenesis is complete. Before this stage, general anesthetics are best avoided if possible. Abortion rate among operating room nurses is twice as high as in the general population, and this is thought to be related to casual exposure to anesthetic gases.

Because of possible teratogenicity, certain drugs commonly used in preoperative medication should be avoided during the first 20 weeks of pregnancy. Among them are chlordiazepoxide (Librium), diazepam (Valium), and meprobamate (Equanil and Miltown).

POSTOPERATIVE COMPLICATIONS

I. NONSPECIFIC COMPLICATIONS

Theodore R. Schrock

A. FEVER
1. Causes
a. Pulmonary. Atelectasis is the most common cause of fever in the first 2 days after major abdominal or thoracic operations. Typically, the pulse and respiratory rates are elevated along with the temperature ("triple response"). Pneumonitis seldom develops before the third postoperative day unless pulmonary disease was present at the time of operation or the patient aspirated.

b. Wound infection caused by β-hemolytic streptococci or *Clostridium* can appear within hours after operation. Other bacterial wound infections require several days before they develop sufficiently to cause fever.

c. Urinary. In general, cystitis alone does not cause fever, but infection of the upper urinary tract does.

d. Infection in the operative site (deep to the incision) can cause fever (e.g., abdominal abscess, empyema, meningitis, vascular graft infection).

e. Intravenous catheters. IV plastic catheters quickly become infected unless rigid aseptic precautions are used during and after insertion.

f. Drugs. Reactions to drugs, notably antibiotics, may cause fever.

2. Diagnosis. The extent to which fever is investigated by laboratory tests and radiographs depends on the interval from operation to appearance of fever, the severity of fever, and the surgeon's certainty about the cause based on the history and physical examination.

a. Symptoms. Question the patient about symptoms (e.g., dysuria, unusual pain) that might be clues to the source of the fever.

b. Signs. Do a physical examination, including auscultation of the chest, inspection of the wound, and examination of IV sites.

c. Laboratory tests. Leukocyte count and urinalysis are ordered in most cases. Cultures of urine, sputum, blood, and drainage fluid may be indicated.

d. Radiography. Chest radiography is not necessary in patients with a clinical diagnosis of atelectasis in the first day or two after operation. Persistent fever of suspected pulmonary origin requires a chest radiograph, and radiographs of other areas (e.g., the abdomen) are obtained as indicated.

e. Special tests. The search for deep infections may require special tests such as ultrasonography, CT scan, or indium leukocyte scan.

3. Treatment. Postoperative fever is best treated by correction of the underlying cause. Because high fever (>38° C) is itself debilitating, antipyretic drugs (e.g., Tylenol 0/500) can be given by mouth or by rectal suppository while investigation of the cause is underway. Applications of ice packs or 70% alcohol to the skin surface or placement of the patient on a refrigerated blanket may be used to lower body temperature if it is very high.

If the cause of fever is not clear, IV catheters should be removed and new ones placed, and possibly causative drugs should be discontinued.

B. VOMITING immediately after operation may be an effect of the anesthesia or may be due to gastric distention (see GI Complications). The best management of gastric distention is nasogastric intubation. Drugs to suppress nausea are less effective and may have untoward side-effects.

Vomiting later in the postoperative period may be due to drugs, ileus, mechanical obstruction of the gut, or other problems that must be investigated.

C. HICCUP (SINGULTUS). Although hiccup is usually self-limited (disappearing within a few minutes to an hour), it can be sufficiently persistent and exhausting to endanger life in a debilitated patient. It may be produced by any condition that irritates the afferent or efferent phrenic nerve pathways. The causes are quite varied: CNS, cardiopulmonary, GI, renal failure, infections.

Treatment should be directed at the cause when possible but must frequently be symptomatic. Breath-holding, drinking a large glass of water, or gastric lavage with a warm 1% solution of sodium bicarbonate may be effective. Rebreathing into a paper bag or administration of 10%-15% CO_2 by face mask induces hyperventilation and may interrupt the reflex. Tranquilizing drugs such as phenothiazine preparations are worthy of trial in prolonged hiccup.

D. PSYCHOSIS. Elderly patients, and the acutely and severely ill, may become psychotic postoperatively. Causative factors include drugs, pain, sleep deprivation, isolation, and unfamiliar surroundings. Patients become disoriented, hallucinatory, agitated, combative, and fearful of personnel who are caring for them, particularly at night. The derangements are transient, and patients usually regain their former mental status as recovery from operation progresses.

Make certain that the patient is not hypoxemic; hypoxemia is a common cause of postoperative restlessness, and the administration of analgesics or sedatives to a hypoxic patient may be lethal. Discontinue possibly causative drugs (e.g., cimetidine).

Simple measures that help include keeping a light on in the room and provision of a companion. Mechanical restraints should be avoided unless the patient threatens self-injury by attempting to climb out of bed, pulling out tubes and catheters, etc. Tranquilizers (e.g., haloperidol 0.5-2 mg, orally, two or three times daily) should be used cautiously, especially in the elderly patient.

E. DECUBITUS ULCERS are caused by sustained pressure on the skin, usually over bony prominences such as the sacrum, ischium, trochanter, and heel. They occur in bedridden patients who are weak, aged, malnourished, or paralyzed and who are receiving poor nursing care. Soiling of the bed by incontinence of stools or urine frequently leads to skin irritation. Unrelieved pressure of only a few hours may be sufficient to produce a decubitus ulcer in a susceptible individual. Decubiti characteristically begin as small areas of redness and tenderness which soon break down to form indolent ulcers unless protected from further pressure. In neglected cases, large defects in skin and soft tissues may result from the combined effects of pressure, infection, and poor healing power. Osteomyelitis of underlying bone may occur.

1. Prevention. The most important elements are good nursing care, early mobilization, and good nutrition. Bedridden patients should be inspected frequently for areas of skin damage which might progress to ulceration. Prevent soiling in incontinent patients. An alternating pressure or foam rubber mattress is useful. Special washable sponge pads protect pressure points.

2. Treatment

a. General measures. Relieve pressure by frequent change of position and protection of the involved area by pillows, pads, and rubber rings. Bedclothing and skin must be kept clean and dry. Correction of malnutrition and anemia and control of infection are often essential to healing.

b. Local measures. Decubitus ulcers should be kept clean, well-drained, debrided, and either exposed or covered with dry sterile dressings. Debridement with topical hydrophilic beads (e.g., Debrisan) may help. Invasive local infection is treated by drainage, saline compression, and systemic antibiotics.

c. Surgical treatment in large, resistant lesions consists of complete debridement, including removal of any bony prominences or sequestra, and closure of the wound by a myocutaneous flap. This provides an adequate pad over the bone and avoids suture lines over the critical area of pressure. The donor area may frequently be closed by direct approximation, but a split-skin graft may be required.

II. WOUND COMPLICATIONS

Theodore R. Schrock

A. DELAYED HEALING AND DEHISCENCE

1. Causes. Many systemic factors contribute to failure of wound healing by altering collagen metabolism or impairing delivery of oxygen to the wound. Local and technical problems may impair blood supply or may provide inadequate resistance to mechanical forces.

a. Altered collagen metabolism. Malnutrition (especially protein depletion and deficiency of ascorbic acid); corticosteroids; cytotoxic drugs (by inhibiting proliferation of fibroblasts or synthesis of collagen); infection (increases collagenolysis).

b. Impaired oxygen delivery. Hypovolemia, hypoxemia, increased blood viscosity; irradiated tissues; infection; technical errors.

c. Technical errors. Wounds may dehisce because tissue is devitalized by the dissection or strangulated by placement of too many sutures or by tying sutures too tightly. This is the most common technical cause of dehiscence and is confirmed when intact sutures are found to have cut through the tissue on one side of the wound. Less commonly, too few sutures are placed, sutures are placed too far apart, sutures break or become untied, or sutures are removed too soon. Some absorbable sutures (e.g., catgut) may not remain strong long enough for secure healing, especially in debilitated patients.

d. Mechanical forces. Patients are more likely to dehisce an abdominal wound if they are obese, have a postoperative cough, vomit, become distended, or develop ascites.

2. Diagnosis. Dehiscence of skin is apparent on inspection. Abdominal fascial dehiscence is manifested by spontaneous drainage of **serosanguinous fluid** from the wound. Assume that fascia has dehisced when this type of drainage appears, especially when it persists. Fluid from a seroma or hematoma is not serosanguinous and does not continue to drain. In major abdominal dehiscences, varying amounts of intestine and omentum may be **eviscerated.**

3. Treatment. Obvious major dehiscence of fascia should be treated by resuture under anesthesia in the operating room. Often, large sutures must be placed through all layers of the abdominal wall because the fascia is friable.

Minor disruptions of fascia may be managed without resuture, but the extent of fascial disruption is often underestimated until the skin is opened and the wound explored. Do this under aseptic conditions in the operating room.

Incisional hernias result from untreated or recurrent fascial dehiscence.

B. BLEEDING from the wound usually is apparent within minutes to hours after the operation is completed. The bleeding vessel(s) may be in the skin, in the subcutaneous fat, or at the fascial level. Unless the patient has a generalized bleeding problem, the wound should be explored to control persistent bleeding. Many times this can be accomplished simply by removing a few skin sutures and ligating the bleeding point(s) with sutures or metal clips without returning the patient to the operating room.

C. HEMATOMA is a collection of clotted and/or liquid blood in or beneath the wound. A visible and palpable mass, ecchymosis, and pain are the manifestations. Large hematomas should be evacuated; usually it is necessary to open the wounds widely under aseptic conditions.

D. SEROMA. Serous fluid collects gradually over several days when a space has been left beneath a wound, particularly if large skin flaps have been created. A seroma is a fluctuant mass and is usually nontender. Small seromas may be aspirated through a needle. Large seromas, or those that recur after one or two needle aspirations, require placement of a drain through a small incision; the drain can be removed after a few days.

E. INFECTION. See Chapter 4.

F. SUTURE SINUSES. Sutures are foreign bodies that can serve as niduses for infection. Tiny abscesses form about the fascial and subcutaneous sutures in some patients. These abscesses may drain through the skin surface spontaneously or by surgical incision, thus relieving pain but resulting in persistent intermittent drainage of small amounts of pus. In time, the suture is extruded ("spit"), or the surgeon can grasp and remove the offending suture(s) by probing the wound; a crochet hook is a useful device for this. Once a suture sinus begins, it does not heal until the foreign body is removed. Sutures may be extruded for weeks, months, or even years after they were placed. Rarely, it is necessary to do a formal operation to open the wound widely and remove all of the infected sutures. Silk has a great propensity to formation of suture sinuses; less reactive materials cause fewer problems of this sort.

III. CARDIAC COMPLICATIONS

John C. Hutchinson

A. CARDIAC ARREST is the cessation of effective heart beat. The surgical patient is at risk of developing this complication during or after operation. Cardiac arrest occurs once in every 750-1000 operations, one third of which are minor procedures.

1. Causes. Special circumstances leading to cardiac arrest are electrocution, drowning, air embolism, poisoning with carbon monoxide and other gases, cardiac contusion or manipulation, and overdose of arrhythmogenic agents such as digitalis and sympathomimetics.

In the surgical patient, cardiac arrest is due to an underlying cardiac condition plus a precipitating cause. The commonest underlying condition is coronary artery disease. The commonest precipitating causes are unrecognized hypoxia due to hypoventilation; anesthetic overdose; drug effect or idiosyncrasy; vasovagal reflexes; myocardial infarction; hypovolemic shock.

Effective heart beat ceases because of arrhythmia (ventricular fibrillation or asystole) or because of marked reduction in ventricular contractility with preserved rhythm ("electromechanical dissociation").

a. Ventricular fibrillation has numerous causes including increased sympathetic stimulation, hypoxia, drug effects, electrolyte imbalances, and myocardial disease. These factors, singly or together, may cause the disordered intraventricular propagation of depolarization and/or repolarization which leads to reentry pathways. Simple reentry pathways produce premature ventricular contractions (commonly described as "irritability"); complex or multiple reentry pathways may result in ventricular fibrillation.

b. Asystole occurring as the first rhythmic abnormality ('primary asystole') generally represents the progression of prior partial atrioventricular or fascicular block.

c. Electromechanical dissociation most commonly results from profound global ventricular ischemia.

2. Prevention. ECG monitoring should be used during all surgical procedures to detect signs of impending danger and to recognize the rhythmic nature of the arrest should it occur.

- Maintain arterial oxygen tension >80 mm Hg and Pco_2 at 30-45 mm Hg.
- Maintain mean blood pressure between 60 and 100 mm Hg.
- Prevent vagal overactivity with atropine (0.4-1 mg IV).

In the presence of increasing numbers of **premature ventricular contractions,** look for light anesthesia, CO_2 retention, myocardial ischemia due to hypotension, or the combination of hypertension and tachycardia which causes increased myocardial oxygen utilization.

In the presence of **bradycardia,** look for anesthetic excess, hypoxia, A-V block, or vagal stimulation by visceral traction, carotid sinus compression, or traction on extraocular muscles.

In the presence of **falling blood pressure,** look for anesthetic excess, myocardial ischemia, or inadequate blood volume due to blood or fluid losses, obstruction of venous return, or vasodilation.

3. Diagnosis. Signs in the **surgical field** are cessation of bleeding, dark arterial blood, agonal breathing, and pulseless arteries.

Signs for the **anesthesiologist** are absent carotid pulse, absent heart tones by esophageal stethoscope, absent blood pressure, and ventricular fibrillation or asystole on the ECG monitor.

In the **postoperative patient,** the signs are absence of blood pressure, carotid pulse, or respiration.

4. Treatment. Stepwise treatment of cardiac arrest is detailed in Table 2-3. The following comments are supplementary:

a. Remove the underlying cause if recognizable.

b. Correct the fundamental abnormality as soon as possible: (1) Ventricular fibrillation requires electrical defibrillation. (2) Asystole requires cardiac massage, vagolytic or sympathomimetic drugs, or cardiac pacing. (3) Electromechanical dissociation is treated with inotropic drugs (calcium, epinephrine, or dopamine).

c. Cardiopulmonary resuscitation is used immediately and during the removal of the underlying cause and correction of the fundamental abnormality. **Act immediately!** Absence of blood flow to the brain results in a progressive ischemic injury which is fatal in about 4 minutes. Prior inadequacies in blood flow and oxygenation to the brain further shorten the time available for successful correction.

d. Open chest cardiac massage. Closed chest massage is the initial method of choice because it can be started quickly (Figure 2-1). Open chest cardiac massage is undertaken only when an operating room is available for subsequent closure (Figure 2-2). Open chest massage may be more effective and therefore is indicated when the chest is already open; there is trauma to the chest with pneumothorax, cardiac tamponade, or cardiac perforation; or the thorax is deformed.

Table 2-3. Technic of heart-lung resuscitation (modified after Safar)

PHASE I. FIRST AID (EMERGENCY OXYGENATION OF THE BRAIN). Must be instituted within 3 to 4 minutes for optimal effectiveness and to minimize the possibility of permanent brain damage.

Step 1.   Place patient in a supine position on a firm surface. A 2 × 3 foot sheet of plywood should be available at emergency care stations, or use a food tray.

Step 2.   Tilt head backward and maintain in this hyperextended position. Keep mandible displaced forward by pulling strongly at the angle of the jaw.

If victim is not breathing

Step 3.   Clear mouth and pharynx of mucus, blood, vomitus, or foreign material.

Step 4.   Separate lips and teeth to open oral airway.

Step 5.   If steps 2-4 fail to open airway, forcibly blow through mouth (keeping nose closed) or nose (keeping mouth closed) and inflate the lungs 3-5 times. Watch for chest movement. If this fails to clear the airway immediately and if pharyngeal or tracheal tubes are available, use them without delay. Tracheostomy may be necessary.

Step 6.   Feel the carotid artery for pulsations.

a. If carotid pulsations are present

Give lung inflation by mouth-to-mouth breathing (keeping patient's nostrils closed) or mouth-to-nose breathing (keeping patient's mouth closed) 12-15 times per minute—allowing about 2 seconds for inspiration and 3 seconds for expiration—until spontaneous respirations return. Continue as long as the pulses remain palpable and previously dilated pupils remain constricted. Bag-mask technics for lung inflation may be substituted. If pulsations cease, follow directions as in 6b, below.

b. If carotid pulsations are absent

Alternate cardiac compression (closed heart massage) and pulmonary ventilation as in 6a,

Table 2-3. Technic of heart-lung resuscitation (modified after Safar)—cont'd

above. Place the heel of one hand on the sternum just above the xiphoid. With the heel of the other hand on top of it, apply firm vertical pressure sufficient to force the sternum about 2 inches downward (less in children) about once every second. After 15 sternal compressions, alternate with 3-5 deep lung inflations. Repeat and continue this alternating procedure until it is possible to obtain additional assistance and more definitive care. Resuscitation must be continuous during transportation to the hospital. Open heart massage should be attempted only in a hospital. When possible, obtain an ECG, but do not interrupt resuscitation to do so. Have an assistant monitor the femoral or carotid pulse, which should be palpable with each cardiac compression as an indication of cardiac output.

PHASE II. RESTORATION OF SPONTANEOUS CIRCULATION. Until spontaneous respiration and circulation are restored, there must be no interruption of artificial ventilation and cardiac massage while steps 7-13 (below) are being carried out. Three basic questions must be considered at this point:

(1) What is the underlying cause, and is it correctable?

(2) What is the nature of the cardiac arrest?

(3) What further measures will be necessary? The physician must plan upon the assistance of trained hospital personnel,* an ECG, a defibrillator, and emergency drugs.

Step 7.   If a spontaneous effective heartbeat is not restored after 1-2 minutes of cardiac compression, have an assistant give epinephrine (Adrenalin), 1 mg (1 ml of 1:1000 or 10 ml of

---

*In the hospital, a physician able to intubate the trachea will quickly visualize the larynx, suck out all foreign material, pass a large, cuffed endotracheal tube, and attach the airway to an IPPB or anesthesia machine for adequate ventilation. Serial arterial blood gas, pH, and bicarbonate determinations are important.

Continued.

Table 2-3. Technic of heart-lung resuscitation (modified after Safar)—cont'd

	10:10,000 aqueous solution) IV or 0.5 mg (5 ml of 1:10,000 aqueous solution) by the intracardiac route. Repeat larger dose at 3-5 minute intervals if necessary. The intracardiac method is not without hazard. Inject at the cardiac apex directed toward the right scapula. Aspirate bright red blood before injecting.
Step 8.	Promote venous return and combat shock by elevating the legs or placing the patient in the Trendelenburg position, and give IV fluids as available and indicated.
Step 9.	If the victim is pulseless for more than 5 minutes, consider sodium bicarbonate solution, 1 mEq/kg IV to combat impending metabolic acidosis.
Step 10.	If pulsations still do not return, suspect ventricular fibrillation. Get ECG.
Step 11.	If ECG demonstrates ventricular fibrillation, maintain cardiac massage until just before giving an external defibrillating shock of 4 watt-seconds/kg of DC current with one electrode firmly applied to the skin over the apex of the heart and the other over the right subclavicular area. Monitor with ECG. If cardiac function is not restored, resume massage and repeat shocks at intervals of 1-3 minutes. If cardiac action is reestablished but remains weak, give calcium chloride or calcium gluconate, 5-10 ml (0.5-1 g) of 10% solution IV; it probably should not be used in patients who have been taking digitalis. Calcium must be given if hyperkalemia is suspected as cause of the arrest.
Step 12.	Thoracotomy and open heart massage may be considered (see text).
Step 13.	If cardiac, pulmonary, and CNS functions are restored, the patient should be carefully observed for shock and complications of the precipitating cause.

Table 2-3. Technic of heart-lung resuscitation (modified after Safar)—cont'd

PHASE III. FOLLOW-UP MEASURES. When cardiac and pulmonary function have been reestablished and satisfactorily maintained, evaluation of CNS function deserves careful consideration. Decision as to the nature and duration of subsequent treatment must be individualized. The physician must decide if he is "prolonging life" or simply "prolonging dying." Complete CNS recovery has been reported in a few patients unconscious up to a week after appropriate treatment.

Step 14.   If circulation and respiration are restored but there are no signs of CNS recovery within 30 minutes, hypothermia at 32° C for 2-3 days may lessen the degree of brain damage.

Step 15.   Support ventilation and circulation. Treat any other complications that might arise. Do not overlook the possibility of complications of external cardiac massage (e.g., broken ribs, ruptured viscera).

Step 16.   Meticulous postresuscitation care is required, particularly for the first 48 hours after recovery. Observe carefully for possible multiple cardiac arrhythmias, especially recurrent fibrillation or cardiac standstill.

Step 17.   Consider the use of assisted circulation in selected cases. A few patients who cannot be salvaged by conventional cardiopulmonary resuscitation may be saved by the addition of partial cardiopulmonary bypass measures.

(1) *To open the chest:* Establish positive pressure ventilation immediately. No skin preparation is necessary—speed is essential. Use gloves if available. A knife is the only necessary instrument, but a rib spreader is desirable. Make a bold submammary incision through the fourth or fifth interspace from sternum to posterior axillary line.

(2) *To massage heart:* Compress the heart rhythmically 70-80 times/minute, either against the sternum or between the thumb and fingers. Compress with a vigorous impulse, then quickly relax pressure to allow filling. Open the peri-

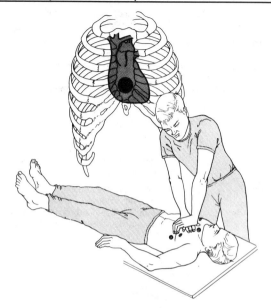

FIGURE 2-1. Technic of closed chest massage. Heavy circle in heart drawing shows area of application of force. Circles on supine figure show points of application of electrodes for defibrillation.

cardium longitudinally if response is not immediate, especially if heart trauma may have caused hemopericardium. If manual compression is effective, a distinct peripheral pulse is felt and should be monitored at the femoral or carotid artery by an assistant. The pupils should remain constricted if blood flow to the brain is adequate.

Fatigue of the hands occurs quickly, especially in the absence of a rib-spreader, and may require changes of hand position or of operator. These changes must be made as quickly as possible.

(3) *Supportive measures during open chest massage:* Be sure that the lungs are ventilating.

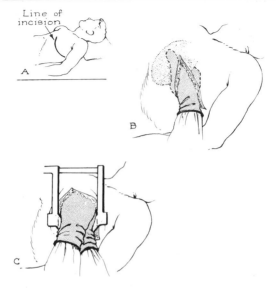

FIGURE 2-2. Open chest cardiac massage. **A,** Position of patient for cardiac massage. **B** and **C,** Insertion of one hand or two hands for rhythmic compression of heart.

Intracardiac drugs. For the soft flabby heart (with or without fibrillation), inject epinephrine into the left ventricle; inject 0.5-1.5 mg as a 1:10,000 solution, and repeat every 3-5 minutes prn. If epinephrine is ineffective in the dilated, weakly beating heart, inject calcium gluconate or chloride, 300-1000 mg of a 1:10 solution into the left ventricle.

IV drugs. As soon as possible, an IV infusion should be started by cutdown or femoral, subclavian, or internal jugular vein catheterization. Cardiac arrest and inadequate tissue perfusion during massage are accompanied by rapid development of metabolic acidosis. Correction of acidosis with sodium bicarbonate has become controversial because of potential cerebral depression due to hypercapnia and acidosis of the CSF, as well as brain dehydration due to hyperosmolarity.

(4) *Defibrillation during open chest massage.* Ventricular fibrillation may be present at the onset or may develop during manual compression. It is rarely reversible except by electric shock. Proceed as follows: Attempt defibrillation with 20-60 watt-seconds of DC discharge as soon as the defibrillator can be readied. Apply defibrillator electrodes firmly on opposite surfaces of the heart. If this attempt is unsuccessful, use cardiac compression, ventilation, and cardiotonic drugs to develop an oxygenated (pink) myocardium with good tone. Then try defibrillation again. Frequently, IV lidocaine is helpful in achieving defibrillation. The dose should be 1 mg/kg given rapidly and repeated to a maximum total dose of 3-5 mg/kg. If digitalis intoxication is possibly the cause of the arrest, avoid calcium, but guarantee that the serum potassium level is in high-normal range. Bretylium tosylate, 5-10 mg/kg IV, should be given if several attempts at defibrillation are unsuccessful.

(5) *Continuation of resuscitative efforts* is indicated as long as the heart maintains tone, color, and responsiveness and if no evidence exists of irreversible brain damage, such as widely dilated pupils, flaccid paralysis, and absence of spontaneous respiration. Resuscitation may rarely be successful after as long as 6 hours of manual compression. Recurrent ventricular fibrillation may require repeated resuscitations and may be controlled by a continuous lidocaine infusion at 1-4 mg/min (10-40 g/kg/min).

(6) *Chest closure* is routine. Begin intensive IV antibiotic therapy.

5. Care after resuscitation by closed or open method. Postresuscitative care should, if possible, be carried out in an ICU where continuous monitoring of ECG and frequent determination of central venous and arterial blood pressures are feasible. Equipment for external defibrillation should be immediately available. Recurrent cardiac arrest is common. Hypoxia and hypercapnia should be avoided by administration of oxygen and, if necessary, by ventilatory assistance with mask or endotracheal or tracheostomy tube. Determinations of arterial pH, PO_2, and PCO_2 are valuable when there is question of acidosis or inadequate ventilation. If severe acidosis is present (base deficit >10 mEq/L), sodium bicarbonate may be indicated. Hypovolemia is corrected by administration of blood and fluids as needed and urinary output is watched and maintained. Neurologic status must be closely followed, because cerebral damage is frequent. Treatment of prolonged coma is individualized.

6. Prognosis. Good results are proportional to the speed and skill of resuscitative efforts. When arrest occurs in the operating room, it is possible to save about 75% of patients. The percentage of successful resuscitations outside the operating room in cardiac arrest due to myocardial infarction and other causes is increasing with the wider application of closed chest massage. It is the responsibility of every physician to acquire the judgment, skill, and decisiveness needed to accomplish cardiac resuscitation. It is the responsibility of the hospital to provide resuscitation equipment, which should include a laryngoscope, endotracheal tubes, mask and bag for artificial ventilation, and a DC defibrillator. Along with the necessary cardiac drugs, this equipment can be conveniently stored in a special cart which can be kept available in the operating suite, or in those hospital units concerned with emergency, intensive, and coronary care.

B. ACUTE PULMONARY EDEMA (acute congestive failure) is a grave emergency. **Act immediately!** It is often precipitated by stress, transfusion of too much blood, or excess IV administration of sodium-containing fluids. Myocardial infarction or an attack of atrial fibrillation with a rapid ventricular rate may be the precipitating factor.

Treatment
a. Position. Place the patient in a sitting position in bed or in a chair in order to decrease venous return to the heart.

b. Morphine sulfate, 10-15 mg IV or IM every 2-4 hours, depresses pulmonary reflexes, relieves anxiety, and induces sleep.

c. Give oxygen in high concentrations, preferably by mask. Positive pressure breathing for short periods may be of value. Monitor CO_2 retention.

d. Vasodilation using nitroglycerin 0.4 mg sublingually, allows prompt peripheral pooling of blood volume and is immediately helpful if blood pressure does not fall <90/60. If hypertension is present, vasodilation is particularly effective and may be achieved by nitroprusside or nitroglycerin infusion.

e. Rapid digitalization is of great value. Extreme care is necessary in giving digitalis IV to a previously digitalized patient. If undigitalized, give digoxin 1 mg/m^2 body surface area in divided doses, giving 50% as the first dose, then 30% and 20% at 6-hour intervals.

f. Rapid diuresis may be accomplished with furosemide (Lasix) 40-80 mg orally or IV.

C. SUBACUTE OR CHRONIC CONGESTIVE FAILURE.

Symptoms and signs include dyspnea, orthopnea, rales at lung bases, venous and hepatic engorgement, dependent edema, increased venous pressure, and cardiac gallop.

Treatment

a. Eliminate or control precipitating factors such as stress, sepsis, anemia, excess sodium administration, arrhythmias, and thyrotoxicosis.

b. Rest in bed or chair with appropriate sedation decreases the work required of the heart.

c. The diet should be low in sodium (<0.6 g of sodium or 1.5 g of sodium chloride). With sodium restriction, fluids may be allowed ad lib.

d. Diuretics (see above).

e. Vasodilators (nitrates, hydralazine), calcium channel blockers (nifedipine, diltiazem), and angiotensin converting enzyme inhibitors (captopril, enalapril).

f. Digitalis (see above).

D. ACUTE MYOCARDIAL INFARCTION.

Prolonged, usually severe precordial or substernal pain, sometimes radiating to the neck or upper extremities, is typical, but these symptoms may be masked by anesthesia or narcotics. Infarction is often associated with shock, congestive failure, and arrhythmias. Other manifestations include fever, leukocytosis, and elevation of sedimentation rate and the serum levels of SGOT, LDH, and CPK. There are characteristic ECG changes. During the acute stage, the patient's ECG, pulse, and possibly the venous and arterial pressures should be continuously monitored in a coronary care or equivalent unit.

Treatment

a. Rest. Complete bedrest for 1 week is advocated, with gradual resumption of activity as tolerated. Use sedatives as required.

b. Relief of pain. Give morphine sulfate, 10-15 mg subcut, IM, or slowly IV, or choose an alternative narcotic.

c. Oxygen therapy is usually necessary.

d. Shock. If cardiac shock is present, treat with an inotropic drug, such as dopamine, and with cautious digitalization.

e. Digitalis and drugs to control arrhythmia are prescribed for specific indications.

E. CARDIAC ARRHYTHMIAS. Treatment of the major arrhythmias is a complex problem calling for the close collaboration of the internist and surgeon. However, the surgeon may be required to give emergency treatment or initiate treatment until the services of an internist can be obtained. The final diagnosis of the type of arrhythmia present is made from the ECG.

1. Rapid **atrial fibrillation** decreases the efficiency of the heart and may lead to congestive failure. Emergency treatment consists of slowing the rate by adequate digitalization. IV verapamil (2.5-10 mg) is a very rapid (2-minute) but short 20- to 30-minute treatment for heart rates complicated by angina, pulmonary edema, or hypotension. Conversion to normal sinus rhythm by DC countershock may be urgently required if shock or pulmonary edema ensues.

2. Rapid **atrial flutter** may also lead to congestive failure. Digitalization slows the rate, either by increasing the degree of block or by converting the flutter to sinus rhythm or atrial fibrillation. Verapamil is very useful in controlling excessive ventricular rates. DC countershock may be the treatment of choice, especially if the rhythm is poorly tolerated, because it is 99% effective.

3. Paroxysmal **supraventricular tachycardia** may occur in patients with otherwise normal hearts. In the absence of heart disease, serious effects are rare. Vagus stimulation (carotid sinus pressure, gagging, Valsalva's maneuver) should be tried initially. If mechanical measures fail, drugs should be used. Sedation alone may be sufficient. There is no unanimity regarding the most effective cardiac medication, but the following may be tried: (a) IV Verapamil, in increasing doses of 2.5, 5, 10 mg is the current drug of choice; (b) Edrophonium (Tensilon) initially 2.5 mg IV, with doubling of the dose every 5 minutes until abdominal cramps or retching occur, or until the rhythm slows or subsides. Side-effects are very brief, making this a very useful drug; (c) Vasopressor agents; (d) Digitalis orally or, if no digitalis has been given in the preceding 2 weeks, IV. Continuous ECG monitoring of heart rate and BP are essential; (e) Propranolol (Inderal), 10-30 mg three times a day before meals and at bedtime, or 1 mg IV slowly, and with continuous ECG monitoring, until therapeutic effect begins. If necessary (and there have been no untoward effects) a subsequent dose of 1 mg may be given every 2-5 minutes, to a total of 10 mg.

Rarely, cardioversion by DC countershock may be required if the patient's condition deteriorates in spite of the above measures.

4. Ventricular tachycardia is usually associated with myocardial damage, especially myocardial infarction. Digitalis toxicity may cause this arrhythmia. Lidocaine (Xylocaine) is the drug of choice for emergency treatment because of its rapid onset, short duration of action, and infrequent hypotensive effect. Give 1 mg/kg IV as a bolus and repeat the injection if the initial bolus is not effective. If the arrhythmia recurs, an IV infusion of 1-3 mg/kg/hour may be given or the IV injection repeated twice at 20-minute intervals. If lidocaine is without effect, cardioversion by DC countershock is preferred to additional pharmacologic methods of treatment. High total doses (400-600 mg) may result in seizures.

5. Ventricular fibrillation produces cardiac arrest and requires immediate electric shock defibrillation with CPR if fibrillation persists.

6. Electrical cardioversion. Conversion to normal sinus rhythm by depolarization of the entire heart with a DC shock is an important method of therapy in arrhythmias. Initial energy settings of 10-25 watt-seconds are employed for atrial flutter and supraventricular tachycardia and 100-200 watt-seconds for atrial fibrillation and ventricular tachycardia. If the initial energy is ineffective, sequential increases in energy may be required. Brief anesthesia is desirable and is induced with sodium thiopental (1.5-3 mg/kg) with preoxygenation and attention to the adequacy of ventilation.

IV. PULMONARY COMPLICATIONS

Frank R. Lewis, Jr.

A. VENTILATORY FAILURE. Some degree of ventilatory impairment is universal after abdominal and thoracic surgical procedures. In most instances, the impairment is not sufficient to prevent resumption of spontaneous breathing by the patient. However, if the operative procedures are extensive, if there has been massive trauma, if the patient is elderly, or if the patient has preexistent chronic disease or malnutrition, the ventilatory impairment may be so great that a period of mechanical ventilation is necessary.

A critical period in which acute ventilatory failure most commonly occurs is the first few hours after operation, when the effects of muscle relaxants have not worn off and muscular weakness results in reduced vital capacity. Later, during the second or third postoperative days, abdominal distention, with restriction of chest wall motion and elevation of the diaphragm, is the usual cause of ventilatory compromise. If a respiratory complication develops, decreased compliance of the lungs may contribute to inadequate ventilatory function.

1. Diagnosis. In all instances, assessment of ventilatory adequacy is best made by measurement of **forced vital capacity.** Normal values are 65-70 ml/kg of body weight. Vital capacity <12-15 ml/kg indicates borderline function. When vital capacity is less than this, the patient will not be able to breathe deeply enough to prevent atelectasis, or to cough vigorously enough to clear airway secretions.

Another test often used to evaluate mechanical lung function is **maximal inspiratory force (MIF).** This measurement is carried out in the intubated patient by asking the patient to inhale as forcefully as possible after normal expiration, with the endotracheal tube occluded. Under normal circumstances, a negative pressure of > -200 cm H_2O can be generated. In the patient with ventilatory compromise, values < -25 to -30 cm H_2O indicate inadequate mechanical function.

2. Treatment. If inadequate ventilation is indicated by the patient's clinical status and the tests described, a nasotracheal tube should be inserted and the patient placed on mechanical ventilation until the cause of the problem resolves. The nasal and pharyngeal mucosa is anesthetized with cocaine or Pontocaine, and insertion of the nasotracheal tube can be accomplished with minimal discomfort in the awake patient.

B. ASPIRATION. In patients undergoing surgery, aspiration of gastric contents is most likely to occur during the induction or termination of the general anesthetic. During the procedure itself, an endotracheal tube with a distensible cuff which seals against the tracheal wall is normally inserted, and this prevents regurgitation and aspiration.

1. Prevention. The patient undergoing elective surgery should have no oral intake for 6-8 hours prior to the procedure and may be assumed to have an empty stomach at the time of induction. Patients who require emergency operation should have a nasogastric tube inserted while awake to empty the stomach as completely as possible. Anesthesia induction technics in patients suspected of having food in the stomach are modified to minimize the hazard of aspiration. Either "awake" intubation or "crash" induction, with an assistant maintaining tracheal compression until insertion of the endotracheal tube, is commonly employed. In patients emerging from general anesthesia, the endotracheal tube is left in place until the patient has begun to react to it by coughing or straining, thus evidencing return of protective airway reflexes.

2. Treatment. If aspiration is observed, immediate endotracheal intubation, suctioning of the airways, and lavage with saline should be done. Within 10 minutes of gastric acid aspiration, the resultant bronchorrhea will neutralize the acidic pH, so lavage after an interval longer than this is probably of no benefit. Treatment otherwise is supportive, with monitoring for the development of pulmonary infiltrates, hypoxemia, and pneumonia. Steroids have been advocated, but there is no clear evidence of their benefit. Antibiotics should be reserved for treatment of specific organisms and not used prophylactically. If aspiration of solid material is suspected, bronchoscopy is indicated for inspection of the tracheobronchial tree and removal of any foreign material.

C. PNEUMOTHORAX is a relatively uncommon complication in elective surgery but should be considered in any patient who develops sudden respiratory distress or sudden deterioration intraoperatively. The **principal cause** of pneumothorax in the hospitalized patient is iatrogenic puncture of the lung during an attempt at percutaneous placement of a subclavian internal jugular venous catheter. It may also occur in the patient being anesthetized who coughs or "bucks" on the endotracheal tube, causing rupture of a pulmonary bleb.

1. Diagnosis. is classically made by a decrease in, or absence of, breath sounds on the affected side with hyperresonance to percussion and a tracheal shift away from that side. X-ray is confirmatory.

2. Treatment. Any patient who develops severe respiratory distress after insertion of a subclavian or jugular catheter should be presumed to have a pneumothorax, and a chest tube should be inserted immediately without waiting for an x-ray. If pneumothorax is suspected but the patient is comfortable, get the chest x-ray first and insert a chest tube if needed.

D. ATELECTASIS is the most common complication in the first two or three postoperative days. It is a direct result of underexpansion of portions of the lung. In the most dependent segments of the lung, and in those segments adjacent to the diaphragm (after abdominal surgery), ventilation is impaired to the greatest extent and collapse is most probable. For these reasons, the inferior and posterior portions of the lung most often become atelectatic.

1. Diagnosis. Clinical signs are fever, tachypnea, and tachycardia which develop simultaneously within the first 2 or 3 postoperative days. Chest x-ray usually shows a linear density in dependent segments or an area of lobar or sublobar collapse. There is often radiographic evidence of volume loss in the affected lung. Atelectasis may also be diffuse and miliary, in which case minimal x-ray signs will be present.

2. Treatment consists of maneuvers which cause the patient to breathe more deeply and/or cough in order to expand underventilated segments of the lung. The most conservative treatment methods consist of an aggressive "stirrup" regimen plus verbal encouragement and supervision of the patient in deep breathing and coughing. The patient should be ambulated at least every 2 hours if there are no contraindications. If the patient cannot walk, useful measures include turning every hour from supine to prone or to left and right lateral positions in bed, and if possible sitting up in a chair for short periods.

Often direct coaching of a patient, with reassurance that the abdominal incision won't be harmed by coughing, will improve the ability to ventilate. If incisional pain is severe, holding a pillow tightly against the abdomen to support it during coughing is helpful. A variety of mechanical devices, such as the incentive spirometer, blow bottles, and Triflow incentive flowmeter are available to give the patient a visual indication of the adequacy of breathing.

Intermittent positive pressure breathing has been advocated for prophylaxis and treatment of atelectasis, but in the nonintubated patient it does not achieve the objective. Simpler, and less expensive modalities are more effective. Intermittent positive pressure breathing has no role in the care of postoperative nonintubated patient.

If the above measures prove ineffective in treating atelectasis, **direct stimulation of tracheal mucosa** may be used to induce involuntary coughing and deep breathing. This is most commonly done by passing a small (size 14 Fr) suction catheter through the nose and into the trachea. In the awake patient, passage of the catheter into the trachea can be immediately recognized by the induction of coughing and the inability to phonate because the catheter separates the vocal cords. A similar effect is produced by the instillation of 5 ml of sterile water into the trachea by percutaneous tracheal puncture with a #22 needle, or by percutaneous insertion of a plastic catheter into the trachea. These methods have **risks:** the posterior tracheal wall may be lacerated when the needle is inserted, and subcutaneous emphysema may be produced from air leaking through the puncture wound in the trachea. Since these methods have no advantage over passage of a nasotracheal suction catheter, there is little justification for their use.

If all the above methods fail to reverse the atelectasis, **bronchoscopy** may be indicated to suction secretions out of the atelectatic segment. Another alternative is to insert an endotracheal tube and ventilate the patient, thus allowing expansion of the collapsed areas of lung. These modalities are rarely necessary and should be used only when the atelectasis is severe, involving an entire lobe or more, or the patient is developing respiratory distress or deteriorating blood gases.

E. PULMONARY EDEMA. Acute interstitial and alveolar edema is most likely to develop in the elderly patient with compromised cardiac function or the occasional younger patient with significant cardiac disease. It often develops on the second or third postoperative day as fluid is mobilized from third-space depots, although it can occur with excessive administration of fluid during or immediately after an operation if the patient's cardiac or renal function is compromised. The healthy patient with normal cardiac and renal function can usually tolerate fluid overload, with prompt diuresis and or pulmonary symptoms.

1. Diagnosis is made by the presence of tachypnea, tachycardia, shortness of breath, and orthopnea, coupled with an elevated central venous pressure, distended neck veins, and wet rales in the basilar lung segments. A diastolic "gallop" may be heard. The sputum is often frothy and pink. Chest x-ray shows symmetrical perihilar fluffy infiltrates, cardiac enlargement, prominent pulmonary vascular shadows, and lymphatic congestion in the costophrenic angles (Kerley's B lines).

Pulmonary edema is often difficult to diagnose in marginal cases, and confusion with bronchial asthma occurs. Pulmonary edema has been referred to as **cardiac asthma** because the findings of respiratory distress and wheezing are similar. The two conditions may be distinguished by the presence of wet rales with cardiac asthma; rales are heard bilaterally at the lung bases, and they may extend half to two-thirds of the way up the lung apex.

2. Treatment of pulmonary edema. See page 107.

F. PNEUMONIA in the postoperative patient is usually a sequela of inadequately treated atelectasis, gross airway contamination, or preexistent pulmonary disease, most commonly
from smoking. It rarely develops earlier than 4-5 days after operation unless an unusual event, such as aspiration, occurs. The
cause is nearly always bacterial, and if the patient has been
given prophylactic or therapeutic antibiotics from the time of
surgery, one may assume that the organism causing the pneumonia is resistant to the antibiotics being used.

   1. Diagnosis is made by the presence of fever, leukocytosis, increased sputum production, consolidation and/or rales
on physical examination, and a localized or diffuse infiltrate
on x-ray. Gram stain of the sputum usually reveals heavy colonization by a single organism, and a large number of polymorphonuclear leukocytes are present. If few bacteria of mixed
types are seen, and if there are minimal numbers of PMNs,
the diagnosis is open to question. *Gram stain is more valid as
an index of pulmonary infection than the culture,* as it is possible to culture some organism from the trachea in virtually
everyone.

   2. Treatment. If pneumonia is diagnosed, antibiotic therapy is begun immediately based on the Gram stain. Confirmatory culture is obtained and the antibiotic sensitivities are
checked. Therapy otherwise should be supportive and, if possible, directed at the underlying cause of the pneumonia. Blood
gases should be monitored and nasotracheal intubation and ventilation carried out if the patient's status deteriorates. If the patient is unable to eat or has had minimal caloric intake for more
than 1 week, IV hyperalimentation should be considered. Starvation causes some degree of immunologic depression within
1-2 weeks and nutritional support is mandatory if the patient is
depleted or has undergone major trauma or extensive surgery.

**G. ADULT RESPIRATORY DISTRESS SYNDROME
(ARDS).** In unusual instances, after extensive surgery or massive trauma, patients develop tachypnea, hypoxemia, diffuse
pulmonary infiltrates, and decreased compliance of the lungs.
Physical examination does not disclose rales, bronchospasm,
or evidence of alveolar edema. ARDS may differentiated from
pneumonitis by the absence of signs of infection and the absence of significant organisms or leukocytes on Gram stain of
the sputum.

   In many cases ARDS appears to be related to pulmonary
embolism, and the findings are similar to those for fat embo-

lism. Evidence of intravascular coagulation is a common accompaniment of this syndrome, but its role as a specific cause has not been proved. The most common associated condition is systemic sepsis, often from intraabdominal foci following intestinal surgery or massive trauma. Severe pancreatitis is also a common antecedent cause.

1. Diagnosis. ARDS is diagnosed by the findings described above and the exclusion of other more specific pulmonary entities. It normally does not develop until 3-4 days postoperatively, and it is usually associated with other complications, particularly sepsis.

2. Treatment. When the disease is mild to moderate, supportive care with administration of increased concentrations of oxygen by mask may be sufficient treatment. In most cases, the symptoms are relatively severe, and the degree of arterial hypoxemia necessitates endotracheal intubation and mechanical ventilation. Mechanical ventilation is indicated if the arterial PO_2 cannot be maintained at >70 mm Hg with the administration of supplemental oxygen by mask.

The patient should be closely monitored for the development of secondary pulmonary infection and should be treated with appropriate antibiotics if infection occurs. The development of intravascular coagulation should be closely monitored by standard tests, and anticoagulation with systemic heparin should be carried out if there is evidence of this disorder.

Steroids have been advocated but have not been shown to be beneficial. Potent diuretics have also been advocated; these agents are controversial, and their effects appear to be transient at best. The use of albumin in one form or another has also been advocated to "dry out" the lungs by increasing intravascular osmotic pressure, and its use for this purpose should be abandoned.

Insertion of a pulmonary catheter to monitor pulmonary wedge pressures is mandatory for careful titration of IV fluid replacement. Because of the high mortality associated with the development of renal failure in addition to respiratory failure, every effort should be made to preserve renal function by adequate hydration of the patient, but overhydration which increases the degree of pulmonary interstitial edema should be avoided. The pulmonary arterial wedge pressure should be kept as low as possible consistent with adequate peripheral perfusion and urine output of 0.5 ml/kg/hour. In no case should wedge pressure be elevated >15 mm Hg.

V. ACUTE RENAL FAILURE

Flavio Vincenti

Acute renal failure is the rapid onset of impaired renal function. The hallmark is **rapidly progressive azotemia,** usually, but not always, accompanied by oliguria (urine output <400 ml/24 hours). Causes are listed in Table 2-4. Prerenal azotemia and ATN are the most common types. Laboratory findings in these two entities are listed in Table 2-5.

A. PRERENAL AZOTEMIA is the result of renal hypoperfusion because of volume depletion (dehydration or blood loss) or decreased cardiac output from pump failure without volume depletion (congestive heart failure). The glomerular filtration rate is decreased, and there is enhanced reabsorption of sodium, water, and urea in the tubules in patients with prerenal azotemia.

It is important to diagnose prerenal azotemia because it may be easily reversible and also because persistence of renal hyperperfusion may lead to the development of ATN.

1. Diagnosis. Assess the volume status (fullness of neck veins, skin turgor, orthostatic changes in blood pressure and heart rate, peripheral perfusion). Note that central redistribution of the intravascular volume from acidosis-induced venoconstriction may result in prominent neck veins despite extra-

Table 2-4. Causes of acute renal failure

1. Prerenal azotemia
2. Renovascular disease
    Arterial occlusion
        Major emboli or thrombi
            Vasculitides and bilateral cortical necrosis
    Venous thrombosis
3. Parenchymal renal disease
    Acute tubular necrosis (ATN)
        Renal ischemia
        Nephrotoxins, radiographic contrast media
        Mixed *(a + b),* unknown
    Other causes
        Glomerulo- and interstitial nephritides
        Disorders of calcium and uric acid homeostasis
4. Postrenal azotemia (obstructive)

Table 2-5. Laboratory guidelines in the diagnosis of oliguria

	Prerenal azotemia	ATN
BUN/creatinine	>20/1	<10/1
Urine sp. gr.	≥1.020	≤1.012
U/P osm*	≥1.5	<1.5
Urine Na	<10 mEq/L	>20 mEq/L
Renal failure index†	<1	>1
Urine sediment	Unremarkable	Hematin (pigmented casts)

*U/P osm = urine to plasma osmolality.
†U_{Na} ÷ U/P creatinine.

cellular fluid depletion. (1) Examine the heart and lungs. The findings may indicate congestive heart failure. (2) Catheterize the urinary bladder to obtain a urine specimen and to monitor urine output during treatment. (3) Send blood for BUN, creatinine, electrolytes, and osmolality, and measure urine electrolytes and osmolality. (4) Examine the urine sediment (see Table 2-5).

These steps should lead to a diagnosis of prerenal azotemia on the basis of hypovolemia or congestive heart failure. In patients with borderline cardiac function, measurement of central venous or even pulmonary arterial pressures may be necessary before treatment is instituted.

2. Treatment of congestive heart failure is discussed above.

Hypovolemic patients should be given 0.9% saline solution IV at a rate of 100-500 ml/hour, depending upon the severity of volume depletion.

Do **not** give diuretics prior to correction of hypovolemia. If there is no improvement in urine output **after** blood volume has been replenished, a bolus of furosemide (80-200 mg IV) may be administered.

B. ACUTE TUBULAR NECROSIS may be a consequence of **ischemia** (usually due to hypotension), **nephrotoxins** (e.g., $HgCl_2$, CCl_4, methoxyflurane, or antibiotics—especially aminoglycosides), or **mixed** (or unknown) **mechanisms** (hemoglobinuria, myoglobinuria, radiographic contrast media).

1. The course of ATN may be divided into 3 phases:

a. Pre-ATN phase. The findings are similar to those in prerenal azotemia, and prompt treatment may prevent progression to ATN. Pre-ATN is usually a retrospective diagnosis.

b. Oliguric phase. ATN is fully established in this phase. Oliguria usually lasts 7-21 days.

c. Diuretic phase. The urine output gradually increases as the kidneys recover. In some cases, the postoliguric diuresis may be massive. The creatinine clearance returns to 80% of the baseline level in 6-12 weeks.

2. Diagnosis. ATN, despite its name, is not usually associated with necrosis of tubular cells that can be seen histologically. Renal biopsy, therefore, is not usually obtained. The clinical setting and the laboratory tests, especially urine findings (see Table 2-5), are usually sufficient to establish the diagnosis.

The severity of renal damage varies; in mild cases, there may be high urinary output rather than oliguria (nonoliguric ATN).

Anuria (urine output <50 ml/24 hours) is rare in ATN; bilateral cortical necrosis, acute glomerulonephritis, urinary obstruction, and thrombosis of the major renal vessels are more likely to cause anuria.

3. Complications. The abnormalities described in chronic renal failure (see Section III) occur in acute renal failure, frequently with greater severity because of the acuteness of the renal dysfunction. Fluid and electrolyte abnormalities are invariably present, and profound acidosis and severe hyperkalemia are common. Infection and GI bleeding are the major complications associated with ATN, and infection is the principal cause of death.

4. Treatment of ATN is supportive and is directed at preventing or treating complications until renal function returns to normal. There is no evidence that the course of established ATN is modified by the administration of furosemide or mannitol. Diuretics should not be given.

a. Fluids and electrolytes

Fluid. Measurable fluid losses (urine, GI fluids) and insensible losses (400-500 ml/day) should be replaced. Carefully record intake, output, and body weight daily.

Sodium. Replace losses of sodium from urine or other measurable sources. *Hyponatremia* developing in the course of ATN is indicative of fluid excess, rather than sodium deficit, and is best treated by fluid restriction.

Potassium. Hyperkalemia commonly occurs in these patients. A variety of factors contribute to hyperkalemia, including acidosis and potassium release from tissues secondary to excessive catabolism, trauma, or hemolysis. Be aware of the potassium content of potassium penicillin G

(1.7 mEq/million units) and salt substitutes. Monitor serum potassium concentration and the ECG.

Ion exchange resin (Kayexalate) administered orally (25 g Kayexalate and 50 g of sorbitol) or as a retention enema (50 g Kayexalate and 50 g of sorbitol with 100 ml of tap water) reduces serum potassium levels over several hours. This therapy can be repeated at 4-6 hour intervals. Potential side-effects with frequent use include excessive sodium retention and heart failure.

More urgent treatment of hyperkalemia (serum potassium >7 mEq/L) requires administration of sodium bicarbonate (44-48 mEq of sodium bicarbonate IV) or hypertonic glucose solution and regular insulin (100 ml of 50% glucose plus 10 units of regular insulin) given by IV drip over 10-20 minutes.

Life-threatening cardiac arrhythmias due to hyperkalemia are treated by IV calcium gluconate or calcium chloride (5-10 ml of 10% solution over 5 minutes with ECG monitoring).

Dialysis may be required to remove excess potassium.

Restrict *magnesium* (e.g., in antacids) and watch for low *calcium* levels in the blood.

Acidosis in ATN may result from acid produced by normal metabolic processes or in association with hypercatabolic states. Acidosis may be treated by administration of sodium bicarbonate, but this may result in sodium excess and heart failure. Acidosis associated with volume overload is best treated by dialysis and in patients with hypotension by continuous arteriovenous ultrafiltration (CAVH).

b. Diet. Adequate nutrition is fundamental in the treatment of ATN (see Nutrition section in this chapter).

c. Drugs. Dosages of drugs, including antibiotics (see Chapter 4 and Table 2-1), digoxin, and magnesium-containing antacids, must be modified in ATN. If a nephrotoxin is suspected of having caused the ATN, the nephrotoxic drug must, of course, be discontinued.

d. Dialysis. Uncontrollable hyperkalemia or acidosis, overhydration, and the development of uremic symptoms are indications for dialysis. Peritoneal and hemodialysis are equally efficacious. Early and aggressive dialysis seems to result in improved survival in ATN patients.

e. Diuretic phase. Careful observation of blood volume and electrolytes is important through the diuretic stage because the creatinine clearance may lag behind the increase in urine volume. Measurement of urine output, urine electrolyte concentrations, and serial body weights is helpful.

5. Prognosis. ATN has an overall mortality rate of 50%. Mortality is about 80% in patients with burns, trauma, or surgical procedures and only 30% in "medical ATN" (usually due to nephrotoxins) because there are more complications of the underlying condition in the surgical group.

C. POSTRENAL AZOTEMIA. Obstruction of the urinary tract should be suspected if the patient is **anuric.** Obstruction of the upper tract must be bilateral for azotemia to occur. Acute obstructions should be readily suggested by the use of the renal hippurate scan or ultrasonography. Definitive diagnosis may require antegrade or retrograde pyelography. Severe obstruction of the lower tract is easily recognized by the inability to insert a Foley catheter.

VI. URINARY RETENTION

Emil A. Tanagho

Inability to urinate after surgery is a frequent problem. It may be seen after any operation, but it is particularly common after pelvic or perianal procedures.

1. Causes
a. Reflex spasm of the voluntary sphincter because of pain or anxiety.

b. Medication—usually anticholinergics and narcotics.

c. Preexisting partial bladder outlet obstruction—e.g., enlarged prostate.

d. Detrusor atony as result of surgery and manipulation (e.g., after rectoperineal or pelvic surgery).

e. Overdistention during surgery, due to diuresis or prolonged operation.

f. Mechanical obstruction by expanding hematoma or fluid collection.

2. Prevention
a. Voiding patterns should be evaluated carefully preoperatively if one suspects bladder outlet obstruction. Obstruction can be corrected before operation, or catheter drainage may be instituted immediately after surgery.

b. Avoid excessive use of narcotics and parasympatholytic drugs.

c. Patients scheduled for lengthy operations should be catheterized preoperatively and the bladder drained throughout the procedure.

d. Avoid excessive IV fluids during and immediately after the operation. This is a common factor contributing to retention after brief, relatively minor operations (e.g., inguinal hernia repair) done under spinal anesthesia that lasts for hours after the operation is completed.

3. Diagnosis. If a patient is unable to pass urine for several hours postoperatively and there is no desire to urinate, explore the possibility of **oliguria** as a consequence of diminished fluid intake (see Section V). Sometimes a heavily sedated patient does not recognize the sensation of fullness and does not urinate for that reason.

A palpable bladder in the midline above the symphysis pubis is an almost sure sign of acute retention. Every patient who does not urinate for 6 hours after operation should be examined. In this way, overdistention of the bladder, which might induce bladder atony and perhaps myogenic damage to the bladder wall (in some cases permanent), can be avoided.

4. Treatment

a. Conservative. (1) Relieve local pain, if any, by narcotics or sedatives. (2) If the patient's condition permits, he should urinate in the standing or sitting position instead of the supine position. (3) Turning on a water faucet within the patient's hearing encourages voiding. (4) Sitting in a tub of warm water is possible after some operations, and this may make it possible to urinate. (5) Cholinergic drugs such as bethanechol chloride (Urecholine) should be given (2.5 mg subcutaneously, followed in 1 hour by another injection of 5 mg). (6) If there is no effect, the bladder should be catheterized.

b. Catheterization. When all other measures fail, the bladder is markedly distended, and the patient is experiencing severe bladder contractions without voiding, catheterization should be performed. Preferably, catheterization should be done only once and the patient then encouraged to void on his own accord. A preoperative history of any voiding difficulty is very important to help decide on the duration of catheter drainage. If there was no or only minimal preoperative obstruction, the patient should be able to resume normal voiding spontaneously. At no time should the bladder be allowed to become overdistended. If the patient cannot void spontaneously after two to three catheterizations, especially if there has been evidence of overstretching, or if there is mild mechanical obstruction, a Foley catheter might be left in for 4 to 8 days before testing spontaneous voiding again. Men older than middle aged often have an element of mechanical obstruction (prostatic enlargement). Women are more susceptible to detrusor atony after overstretching, especially if it is prolonged.

VII. BLEEDING AND THROMBOSIS

Anne E. Missavage
F. William Blaisdell

Hemostasis and thrombosis are fundamental to surgery, and all surgeons must have knowledge of the diagnosis and treatment of abnormal bleeding and abnormal clotting during and after operation.

A. FACTORS IN HEMOSTASIS. In the fresh surgical wound, three factors contribute to spontaneous cessation of bleeding: blood vessel contraction, platelet adhesion and aggregation, and coagulation. Bleeding problems are minimal if two of these three factors are functional, but if two of the three are inactive, diffuse bleeding is likely to result.

1. Blood contraction (vascular reactivity). When small blood vessels are divided, the local action of catecholamines and of the sympathetic nervous system constricts the injured vessels. Injury to larger blood vessels results in contraction, with telescoping of the layers so that the intima and media are retracted inward and the adventitia is pulled over the end of the severed vessel. Cold and ganglionic blocking agents tend to interfere with vascular reactivity; heat and sympathetic stimulation tend to increase the local vascular spasm and control or slow the rate of hemorrhage.

2. Platelet adhesion and aggregation. Exposed collagen at the site of vascular injury causes activation and adhesion of platelets to the area of injury. This triggers a secondary reaction and releases substances such as ADP and thrombin that cause aggregation of additional platelets to those already adherent. Thus, a **platelet plug** or platelet thrombus builds up rapidly. This plug is the primary factor in initial vascular hemostasis and results in the immediate cessation of bleeding. Subsequent incorporation of fibrin into the platelet plug (due to release of thrombin from aggregating platelets) consolidates the plug and prevents its dissolution. If fibrin is not incorporated, however, the platelet plug disaggregates, and platelets break loose and return to the circulation. This leads to recurrent hemorrhage from the end of the injured vessel.

Platelet adhesion and aggregation are promoted by heat, exposed collagen, catecholamines, acidosis, and stasis. Depression of platelet function interferes with formation of the platelet plug. More than 200 drugs are capable of interfering with platelet adhesion or aggregation (see Table 2-6).

3. Coagulation. The third phase of hemostasis involves the conversion of fibrinogen to fibrin. The coagulation mechanism has been described as a waterfall effect in which progressive activation of clotting factors occurs, the ultimate result being generation of fibrin (Figure 2-3). The system is activated through two alternate pathways: the extrinsic and the intrinsic systems.

a. Extrinsic system. The extrinsic system represents a short-circuiting of the usual pathway; activation occurs through a lipoprotein moiety released from damaged cells (tissue thromboplastin). Defects in the extrinsic system prolong the PT.

b. Intrinsic system. The intrinsic system, starting with factor XII (Hageman), is activated by a foreign surface (e.g., exposed collagen), by substances within the body (e.g., circu-

Table 2-6. Inhibitors of platelet aggregation

I. Antiinflammatory agents Aspirin Phenylbutazone	**IV. Antidepressants and tranquilizers** Imipramine Desipramine
II. Antihistamines Cyproheptadine Diphenhydramine Pyrilamine maleate Chlorpheniramine maleate Promethazine hydrochloride	Amitriptyline Nortriptyline Chlorpromazine Promethazine Diphenhydramine **V. Miscellaneous** Dextran
III. Local anesthetics Cocaine Lidocaine Dibucaine	Dipyridamole Clofibrate Hematoporphyrin Fibrin degradation products

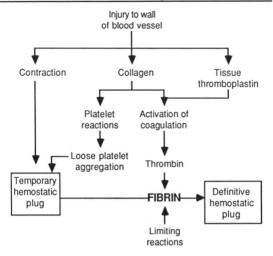

FIGURE 2-3. Summary of reaction involved in hemostasis.

lating collagen), or by exposed basement membranes. Defects in the intrinsic system result in prolongation of the PTT.

    c. Final common pathway. Defects in the final common pathway at the level of factor X or below result in prolongation of both PT and PTT.

    4. Lytic system. For every reaction in the coagulation system, there is a counterreaction designed to keep any one system in check. Intravascular clotting activates the fibrinolytic system, which is designed to clear thrombus. Plasminogen is the circulating inactive fibrinolytic agent that is incorporated into the clot. The local presence of clot stimulates the vein wall to release plasminogen activator, which invades the clot and converts plasminogen to the active enzyme plasmin, which digests the clot internally. A circulating plasminogen activator inhibitor ordinarily neutralizes any plasminogen activator that escapes into the systemic circulation.

B. OPERATIVE AND POSTOPERATIVE BLEEDING. Excessive bleeding during or immediately after an operation may be "surgical" (i.e., the surgeon failed to ligate a large blood vessel), or it may reflect some type of hemostatic defect. The differential diagnosis of hemostatic defects is listed below.

1. Platelet defects

a. Manifestations. The primary manifestation of a pre-existing platelet defect, such as might occur in association with drugs that suppress platelet function, is **oozing**; it is noted when the initial incision is made and it recurs during the operation whenever a fresh wound is made. If the coagulation mechanism is normal, this slow bleeding eventually ceases. Thus, defective platelet function rarely results in complications more serious than an increased blood loss or a greater incidence of wound hematomas.

Normally 50,000 platelets are required for effective hemostasis, assuming that 80-90% are functional. If platelets were normal in number and function preoperatively, a defect in hemostasis may develop during the operation as a result of drugs administered by the anesthesiologist that depress platelet function or because of depletion of platelets due to shock, major tissue dissection, or massive transfusion.

Platelet function is defective in uremia and may be impaired in the myeloproliferative disorders such as polycythemia, leukemia, and some cases of multiple myeloma. The congenital disorders that are associated with a history of easy bruisibility, petechiae, and bleeding after minor injury consist of thrombasthenia (Glanzmann's disease); familial platelet-ADP release dysfunction; and the most common, von Willebrand's disease. The latter problem results from a defective plasma factor that relates to Factor VIII.

b. Treatment. When bleeding due to platelet problems is recognized and the nature of the operation dictates that it be treated to prevent morbidity, the administration of **platelet transfusions** is specific therapy. One platelet pack contains the platelets from 1 unit of blood. Because the normal adult human has a blood volume equivalent to 10-12 units of blood, four to six platelet packs should normalize the defect. If use of platelets is concurrent with platelet transfusion, additional platelet packs are required as platelets are consumed.

2. Coagulation defects

a. Manifestations. Coagulation defects cause secondary bleeding from wounds. Initial hemostasis due to platelet aggregation is adequate, but massive, uncontrollable hemorrhage develops subsequently as the platelet plugs deaggregate because fibrin is not incorporated into the platelet plug. The classic example of a coagulation defect is hemophilia.

b. Differential diagnosis. Coagulation defects may be due to (1) preexisting congenital hematologic abnormalities; (2) anticoagulant drugs given deliberately or inadvertently; (3) depletion of clotting factors as a result of intravascular coagulation; (4) massive transfusion (rarely); (5) liver disease. The liver has the capability to replace labile coagulation factors V and VIII that are deficient in transfused blood. The half-life of these factors is measured in hours, and they can be turned out rapidly by the normal liver. Therefore, acquired clotting defects, when they occur, are usually generated by the consumption of clotting factors during the operation by variable degrees of intravascular coagulation.

c. Treatment. Coagulation defects are treated by the administration of fresh-frozen plasma or, if a congenital defect is present, specific factor concentrates.

3. Combined defects–consumption coagulopathy. Combined defects in platelet function and coagulation are rare. They are usually acquired secondarily to intravascular coagulation. Emergency operations, particularly those associated with shock, massive transfusion, and soft tissue injury, may be complicated by intense intravascular activation of the coagulation mechanism and result in depletion of platelets and coagulation factors. These combined depletion defects produce the hemorrhagic syndrome of DIC, the **consumption coagulopathy.**

a. Manifestations. The principal manifestation of consumption coagulopathy secondary to DIC is massive, uncontrollable, life-threatening bleeding, not only from the operative wound but also from cut-down sites or any other site of minor trauma such as the nose or mouth.

b. Treatment. (1) The initial step should be to correct or remove the factors responsible for intravascular activation of the coagulation mechanism. This may entail discontinuing a mismatched blood transfusion; debriding devitalized tissue; and, most importantly, correcting shock. When the cause is gram-negative sepsis, identification of the source of infection is imperative to permit surgical drainage and specific antibiotic treatment. (2) If the former is not successful, the patient should be anticoagulated with an IV bolus of 10,000 units of heparin to slow down consumption of clotting factors in vivo so that spontaneous regeneration of these factors can occur. In addition, platelets and clotting factors should be administered using platelet packs and fresh-frozen plasma. If fresh, warm blood is available, it may be used instead of platelets and plasma.

C. SYSTEMIC CLOTTING SYNDROMES. Surgical trauma, the stress of operation, shock, and blood loss all increase the tendency of blood to coagulate. Tissue trauma releases factors (e.g., collagen and fragments of fat) into the bloodstream, where they act as procoagulants and activate the clotting mechanism. Acidosis and release of catecholamines also increase the clotting tendency. Clotting problems may therefore arise within the vascular system; they may be categorized as mild clotting tendency (hypercoagulability), moderate intravascular coagulation, and DIC.

1. Hypercoagulability

a. Pathogenesis. The increased clotting tendency in certain types of patients (e.g., elderly, orthopedic patients in traction, and the critically ill) is well known to the clinician. A classic example of someone at increased risk for clotting complications is the older patient with a hip fracture.

Low-grade clotting occurs as a result of surgical trauma. Small amounts of fibrinogen are converted into fibrin. Then, if the fibrin does not remain localized and is diffused through the vascular system, a fibrin strand that has been formed is not able to link up with other molecules of fibrin; instead, it forms soluble complexes with molecules of fibrinogen or with fibrin degradation products. The presence of soluble fibrin monomer complexes results in a blood composition that might be considered to be a supersaturated solution, so that a little bit of additional clotting or the addition of local factors such as stasis may prime frank intravascular clotting. This is characteristically manifest by thrombosis in lower leg veins or any area of stasis within the venous system. In many instances these clots are silent and, if the lytic system is active, usually dissolve without any clinical residual. Under other circumstances, they may be responsible for overt thrombophlebitis or pulmonary embolism.

Hypercoagulability has also been defined as a "depletion of antithrombin III," a substance that circulates in the blood and neutralizes small amounts of thrombin. The clotting cascade, which can be activated as a result of mild trauma, results in consumption of antithrombin. Depletion of antithrombin III removes the check on activation of the clotting cascade and leaves the patient susceptible to clotting complications.

b. Diagnosis. Although there is little question that hypercoagulability exists, it has been difficult to identify by standard laboratory tests. Two tests, fibrin monomer assessment and antithrombin III assay, are now available to help make the diagnosis of hypercoagulability. Elevation of the former, which is positive when small amounts of thrombin produce strands of fibrin in the circulation, and depression of the latter, which results from neutralization of activated coagulation factors, are consistent with an intravascular clotting tendency.

c. Treatment. The rationale for low-dose heparin to prevent clotting complications is based on the concept of modifying this hypercoagulability. Small amounts of heparin activate and improve the efficiency of antithrombin III so that thrombin can be neutralized before it initiates the conversion of fibrinogen to fibrin. Low-dose heparin therapy has consisted of 5000 units of heparin administered subcutaneously 2-3 times daily. However, because patients at greatest risk for clotting complications are those with antithrombin III depletion, a more rational program is to administer heparin intravenously at a rate of 500-1000 units/hour or in an amount sufficient to raise the PTT 5-10 points above normal.

2. Moderate intravascular coagulation

a. Pathogenesis. Moderate intravascular coagulation is the result of major soft tissue injury or shock and is associated with the formation of moderate to large quantities of thrombin in the circulation. Fibrin generated in the microcirculation occludes locally or is swept into the systemic circulation, where it can damage other critical organs such as lung, kidney, and liver. The adult respiratory distress syndrome, renal failure, hepatic injury, and stress ulceration are complications of intravascular coagulation that develop by this mechanism. Gross evidence of clotting may be manifest also in areas of stasis such as leg veins.

b. Diagnosis. The laboratory diagnosis is associated with changes in coagulation parameters. The PTT and PT are usually slightly prolonged, and tests for fibrin degradation products and D-dimer, the breakdown products of clot lysis, are positive during the acute phase. Following the administration of radioactive-labeled fibrinogen, there is evidence of increased radioactivity in the legs in many surgical patients, which correlates well with the presence of clot as confirmed by phlebographic studies. Most patients with positive radioactive fibrinogen tests are clinically asymptomatic, but nevertheless they are at risk for subsequent pulmonary embolism (see Thrombophlebitis, below).

c. Treatment includes restoration and maintenance of circulatory blood volume and, when not contraindicated, anticoagulation. **Heparin** should be administered IV as a bolus of 150 units/kg followed by 1500-2000 units/hour, sufficient at least to raise the partial thromboplastin time to 1.5 to 2 times normal. The circulatory status should be monitored carefully and respiratory and renal support provided as necessary.

3. Disseminated intravascular coagulation

a. Manifestations. DIC in the surgical patient is inevitably associated with diffuse, uncontrollable bleeding. This is because the clotting stimulus results in the intravascular consumption of clotting factors and the activation of the fibrinolytic system. The latter results in the breakdown of any preformed clot at divided vessel ends so that previously dry wounds start to bleed uncontrollably. Transfusion reactions, septic shock, and hemorrhagic shock with massive soft tissue injury are predisposing conditions.

b. Diagnosis. The PTT and PT are markedly prolonged; fibrinogen is <100 mg/dl, platelets <100,000, D-dimer markedly elevated, and euglobulin clot lysis markedly shortened.

c. Treatment is similar to that of moderate intravascular coagulation and consists of resuscitation with careful monitoring of the circulation to control shock and removal of the predisposing factors by treatment of infection, cessation of mismatched transfusion, debridement of damaged or devitalized tissue, and resection of dead bowel. Clotting factor and platelet transfusion should be instituted. If difficulty is encountered in reversing the coagulopathy, an additional bolus injection of 10,000 units of heparin should be administered to stop clotting and prevent further fibrinogen consumption. Bleeding should not be aggravated, and build-up of clotting factors may be accomplished by preventing their utilization as they are administered.

D. THROMBOPHLEBITIS. Venous thrombosis may be categorized as **phlebothrombosis** (asymptomatic, nonobstructive clot) or **thrombophlebitis** (inflammatory, thrombotic obstruction of veins). Because one tends to blend into the other, the general term *thrombophlebitis* is often used to denote all venous clotting conditions.

Hypovolemia and recumbency during and after operation result in circulatory stasis in the lower extremities. Stasis and hypercoagulability contribute to platelet aggregation and fibrin formation, most often in the leg veins. The use of radioactive-labeled fibrinogen has documented that most thrombophlebitis starts in the valve pockets of veins in the calf and progresses proximally intraluminally into the pelvic and abdominal veins.

1. Phlebothrombosis is the formation of clot in leg veins and in other areas of stasis. Initially, the clot is not circumferentially attached to the wall of the vein and therefore does not produce venous obstruction. It usually causes no symptoms or signs. In most instances, the asymptomatic clot lyses and disappears, but in some patients the clot embolizes to the lungs (see Pulmonary Embolism).

As many as 30%-40% of patients with major medical or surgical illnesses have clots in the veins of the legs detectable by radioactive fibrinogen studies. Preventive measures include low-dose heparin therapy and avoidance of circulatory stasis by promoting active exercise of the legs or external pneumatic compression of the legs.

2. Superficial thrombophlebitis is inflammatory thrombosis in subcutaneous veins.

a. Causes. Superficial thrombophlebitis can be precipitated by trauma or by stasis in preexisting varices. It most commonly is caused by intravenous cannulation of veins or drug abuse. If there has been no break in the skin, it is safe to assume that there is no bacterial infection despite the signs of inflammation. When the vein has been invaded, however, associated infection is probable **(septic thrombophlebitis)**.

b. Diagnosis. The subcutaneous vein is a palpable, tender cord with erythema and edema of the overlying skin and subcutaneous tissue. The findings resemble those in lymphangitis. Superficial thrombophlebitis does **not** produce swelling of the limb. In fact, it is considered a benign condition and is not associated with significant risk of embolism.

c. Treatment. Warm, moist compresses and antiinflammatory agents such as aspirin or dipyridamole are usually sufficient treatment. Anticoagulants normally are **not** necessary or indicated. It is not necessary to restrict activity. Septic thrombophlebitis is treated with specific antibiotics, usually the antistaphylococcal agents. Occasionally it is necessary to ligate, excise, or drain an infected vein.

If thrombophlebitis progresses toward the junction of the involved superficial veins with the deep veins (e.g., the saphenofemoral junction), the involved superficial vein should be ligated and divided near the junction to avoid propagation of clot into the deep venous system.

3. Deep thrombophlebitis is inflammatory thrombosis of deep veins producing **obstruction** of venous return. Deep thrombophlebitis damages the veins and sets the stage for further propagation of clot and pulmonary embolism. **Postphle-**

bitic syndrome is a frequent sequela. This results from either chronic obstruction of the major deep veins or valve incompetency following recannulization (see Chapter 11).

a. Diagnosis. The primary manifestations are pain and tenderness in the involved vein and edema distal to the proximal extent of clotting. Swelling of the calf and foot is characteristic of thrombosis in the superficial femoral vein; swelling of the entire lower extremity results from thrombosis of the iliac or common femoral veins.

b. Treatment. Deep thrombophlebitis is always serious and should be treated vigorously. Systemic anticoagulation should be instituted unless there are definite contraindications. Heparin should be given in an initial bolus of 150 units/kg IV, followed by 1000-1500 units/hour by continuous IV infusion. The extremity should be elevated and immobilized until pain and swelling disappear. At this point, the patient can be mobilized progressively and converted to oral anticoagulants.

When the patient is able to remain upright for an hour or two without pain and swelling, discharge from the hospital is permissible. Elastic support from metatarsals to tibial tubercle should be used for several weeks thereafter. In most instances, oral anticoagulation should be continued for 6 weeks to 3 months, and, if episodes recur, permanent oral anticoagulation should be seriously considered. Postphlebitic syndrome is preventable by this vigorous initial treatment (see Chapter 11).

4. Phlegmasia alba dolens and phlegmasia cerulea dolens. Phlegmasia alba dolens is the term for deep thrombophlebitis with swelling; the term simply means "painful white venous inflammation." The leg edema, due to occlusion of the femoral or iliac veins, is responsible for the pale appearance of the limb.

Phlegmasia cerulea dolens is massive venous thrombosis associated with the bluish discoloration of impending gangrene. If all venous return from the extremity is obstructed, the limb becomes congested and cyanotic, arterial inflow is decreased reflexly, and gangrene follows. Thrombophlebitis associated with advanced carcinoma is likely to be of this severe type. Phlegmasia cerulea dolens is immediately life-threatening and should be treated with full doses of anticoagulants and elevation of the limb. If there is a contraindication to anticoagulation or if the condition fails to respond promptly to conservative management, surgical intervention (thrombectomy) may be indicated.

E. PULMONARY MICROEMBOLISM AND FAT EMBO-LISM. Following extensive soft tissue injury, fragments of collagen, fat, and bone marrow can be identified in the circulation. These tissue fragments activate the clotting mechanism, with aggregation of platelets and formation of fibrin microemboli. In addition, when fresh clot embolizes from leg veins, it readily fragments, ultimately lodging in the microcirculation, most commonly in the pulmonary vascular bed. In most circumstances, platelet aggregates and fibrin are rapidly disposed of by lysis and by pulmonary macrophages and result in little disability. When there is a deficit in circulating blood volume or when massive amounts of clot are generated by extensive soft tissue injury, hemolytic blood transfusion, or sepsis, the load on the pulmonary circulation may be overwhelming and the inflammatory mediators released by the propagating clot may produce endothelial damage and increased vascular permeability. Development of those secondary changes in the lungs results in the adult respiratory distress syndrome. Treatment of this syndrome is discussed under Pulmonary Complications in this chapter.

F. PULMONARY EMBOLISM. Embolism of organized clot from large systemic veins obstructs the pulmonary arteries. Manifestations depend upon the amount of pulmonary vasculature that is obstructed. Small emboli may be completely asymptomatic; multiple microemboli may cause respiratory failure described above. Moderate embolism (obstructing less than half the vasculature of previously normal lungs) is often manifest by tachycardia, transient arrhythmias, tachypnea, and a feeling of apprehension on the part of the patient.

Massive embolism (occluding two thirds of the pulmonary vasculature) causes acute pulmonary hypertension and right ventricular strain and failure. Findings are hypotension, hypoxemia, and arrhythmias; death may occur within minutes to days.

About 10% of patients with clinical evidence of pulmonary embolism develop **pulmonary infarction.** Dyspnea, pleuritic chest pain, and hemoptysis are classic symptoms. Examination may reveal decreased breath sounds, a pleural friction rub, or pleural effusion. Chest radiography typically shows a wedge-shaped density.

1. Diagnosis is based on clinical suspicion based on the above. The ECG often indicates right ventricular strain; lung scan contains areas of decreased perfusion; pulmonary angiography shows obstruction of large pulmonary arteries and is the most accurate diagnostic tool. Chest radiograph appears normal unless pulmonary infarction develops.

2. Differential diagnosis. Myocardial infarction, systemic sepsis, asthma, pneumonia, congestive heart failure, and pneumothorax are conditions that may simulate pulmonary embolism. The chest radiograph helps to differentiate these conditions by typical abnormal findings.

3. Treatment. Pulmonary embolism associated with circulatory instability requires large doses of heparin (initial bolus of 300 units/kg followed by 2000-4000 units/hour for the first 24-48 hours).

Ligation, plication, or percutaneous placement of a filter in the inferior vena cava is required if anticoagulants are contraindicated, if bleeding complications develop on anticoagulants, or if pulmonary embolism recurs in a fully anticoagulated patient.

G. ANTICOAGULATION

1. General considerations. Anticoagulation means suppression of the coagulation mechanism. The term is used loosely in clinical practice, however, and may refer to suppression of clotting or inhibition of platelet aggregation.

The **only absolute anticoagulant currently available is heparin,** a physiologic substance present in the mast cells of the body that suppresses thrombin production from prothrombin. The oral anticoagulating agents, of which warfarin is the primary example, are less effective; they indirectly block coagulation by depressing synthesis of certain coagulation factors. Antiplatelet-aggregating agents such as aspirin and dipyridamole interfere with the platelet contribution to coagulation.

Because the greater portion of clot in the venous system is composed of fibrin, anticoagulants (heparin or oral agents) are optimal for the prevention or treatment of venous thrombosis. The major portion of clot in the arterial system consists of platelets; hence, antiplatelet-aggregating drugs are often used to prevent arterial thrombosis.

2. Heparin. With the discovery and isolation of heparin in 1935, a potent therapeutic agent was made available for specific treatment of major life-threatening thrombotic conditions; heparin also has made possible the use of cardiopulmonary bypass for open heart surgery. Heparin itself is a weak antithrombin but is capable of markedly augmenting the effect of antithrombin III.

a. Routes of administration. Heparin can be administered either subcutaneously or intravenously. Intramuscular in-

jections of heparin carry an unacceptable risk of local hemorrhage. The subcutaneous route is used when only small
amounts of heparin are required, most often for prophylaxis
against clotting. Slow absorption from the subcutaneous tissues
produces, in theory, continuous low levels of activity in the
vascular system. Larger doses of heparin required to treat
thrombotic states should be administered intravenously.

   b. Dosage. Doses of heparin are measured in units; 100
units are roughly equivalent to 1 mg of heparin.

    (1) *Low-dose heparin therapy.* Sufficient amounts of hep-
       arin are administered to decrease the coagulation tendency
       without producing alterations in laboratory clotting tests.
       This (in theory) avoids the risk of systemic anticoagula-
       tion. Doses generally administered for prophylaxis in a
       low-dose heparin regimen are 5000 units subcutaneously
       2-3 times daily. However, because antithrombin III may
       be deficient in patients at highest risk for clotting, it is
       probably more effective to administer sufficient heparin
       to increase the PTT slightly (5-10 seconds) above normal.
       This can be done most easily by continuous IV infusion.

    (2) *Systemic heparin anticoagulation* requires the IV ad-
       ministration of 10,000-20,000 units as an initial bolus,
       followed by 1000-4000 units/hour, depending upon the se-
       verity of the patient's condition. Lower doses of heparin
       (1000-1500 units/hour) are administered for non–life-
       threatening conditions such as thrombophlebitis. Doses of
       2000-4000 units/hour of heparin are given for various life-
       threatening problems such as massive pulmonary embo-
       lism with cardiovascular instability.

   c. Monitoring of anticoagulation. The best means of
monitoring the anticoagulant effect of heparin is in dispute.
Clotting tests such as the Lee-White clotting time, the activated
PTT, or the activated clotting time have been used. These tests
are able to document an effect or lack of effect of a dose of
anticoagulant; the problem is that demonstrating an anticoagulant's effect on blood obtained from a peripheral vein does not
necessarily imply that a similar effect is present at the area of
vascular stasis where treatment is directed. Thus, for non–life-
threatening thrombotic conditions such as simple venous
thrombosis, conventional doses of heparin monitored by conventional tests are used, and higher doses (such as 300 units/kg
as a primary dose followed by 50 units/kg/hour by continuous
infusion) are administered for life-threatening conditions such
as acute arterial embolism and pulmonary embolism. When
high-dose heparin therapy is used, the dosage is increased un-

til the patient shows clinical improvement or the activated PTT is greater than 150 seconds (full anticoagulation).

(1) *Lee-White clotting time.* Three test tubes of blood are drawn, and all of the tubes are repeatedly tipped in sequence until clotting is observed. The presence of clotting in the third test tube is the end point. The Lee-White time is less than 10 minutes normally and should be 20-30 minutes on full anticoagulation. This test must be done at the bedside and is time-consuming, so other tests are usually used.

(2) *Activated PTT.* Blood is collected in a citrated tube, plasma isolated, calcium added, and the clotting time measured after the addition of extrinsic thrombin. The activated PTT is normally <40 seconds. Anticoagulation is assumed to be present when the activated PTT is 1.5 to 2 times normal (60-80 seconds).

(3) *Activated clotting time.* Diatomaceous earth is placed in a test tube to which blood is then added. The surface area of the tube is immeasurably increased by the presence of the foreign substance, and the clotting time is normally 2 minutes or less. Anticoagulation theoretically exists when the activated clotting time is more than 4 minutes.

d. Reversal of anticoagulation. The half-life of heparin is such that a dose of heparin is metabolized in 4-8 hours. In the presence of bleeding complications, however, it may be necessary to reverse the heparin effect immediately by giving protamine sulfate. Approximately 1.25 mg of protamine neutralizes 100 units of heparin in a test tube, but in the patient not more than 1 mg of protamine should be given for each 100 units of heparin previously administered. Too much protamine may cause hypotension or produce bleeding complications. For this reason, protamine should be administered slowly and carefully. Half of the calculated amount of protamine should be given initially, the wound should be observed for formation of clot, and half of the remaining calculated dose should be administered every 5 minutes until clot is observed or until tests of clotting become normal.

e. Complications. Anaphylactic reaction to heparin has been described but is very rare. Hemorrhage is the primary complication. Patients should have hematocrit determination at least twice daily. Usually bleeding occurs into wounds or into the retroperitoneum and is not serious if recognized promptly. Cerebral hemorrhage is the most serious complication; fortunately, it is rare.

Depression of platelet function occurs in some patients after 3-4 days of heparin therapy. Paradoxical clotting complications are the most frequent manifestation resulting from systemic platelet aggregation. The risk of hemorrhage is also greatest in these patients. These complications can be anticipated, because they are usually preceded by a fall in the platelet count below 100,000.

Heparin should be given in adequate doses. There is probably a greater risk in the administration of marginally therapeutic amounts of heparin that may not be sufficient to prevent clotting complications but may still be capable of producing hemorrhage. In systemically anticoagulated patients, no correlation exists between the amount of heparin administered and the incidence of bleeding complications.

3. Oral anticoagulants. Spontaneous hemorrhage in cattle was noted when they ate spoiled clover. From this observation has come the isolation of the oral coumarin derivatives, warfarin (Coumadin) being the principal one. This drug is less effective than heparin but is practical for prophylaxis. It is especially useful for outpatients because it is administered orally. These drugs decrease the production of vitamin K–dependent clotting factors.

a. Dosage. The dosage of warfarin required for individual patients varies considerably. The preferred regimen for initiation of oral anticoagulation in patients of average size is 10 mg of warfarin orally daily until the desired level of anticoagulation is obtained. The daily dose is then adjusted to maintain a prothrombin time of 1.5 to 2.5 times normal or an INR of 2-3. About 5 mg/day is the average maintenance dose. In some instances, an initial dose of 20 mg/day is required to achieve anticoagulation and as much as 10-12 mg daily are required subsequently.

b. Monitoring of anticoagulation. Warfarin anticoagulation is monitored by the PT, an assessment of the extrinsic clotting system. The normal PT is 10-12 seconds, and anticoagulated patients should be maintained at 1.5 to 2 times normal (INR of 2-3). PT in excess of 2½ times normal (INR of 3-4) may be necessary in high-risk cases but are associated with a higher incidence of bleeding complications. The PT should be measured daily initially; then at weekly intervals; if the PT is stable, it can eventually be measured once every 2-4 weeks.

c. Reversal of anticoagulation. The PT returns to normal within 3-4 days after warfarin is discontinued. Rapid reversal is obtained by administering 5-10 mg of vitamin K_1 intravenously.

d. Complications of oral anticoagulation are those of hemorrhage, most frequently into the retroperitoneum or into the urinary or GI tracts. The urine and stool therefore should be monitored for the presence of blood. Abdominal pain suggests the possibility of retroperitoneal hemorrhage.

4. Antiplatelet-aggregating drugs. The antiplatelet-aggregating agents are most often used to treat arterial thrombotic conditions. In special circumstances, patients who have mild venous clotting tendencies may be treated with antiplatelet-aggregating agents. These agents carry less risk of hemorrhage than do the anticoagulants, but they probably are not as effective.

Aspirin, dipyridamole, indomethacin, and related drugs depress platelet aggregation for the life of the platelet. Therefore, reversal of the drug effect depends upon generation of new platelets. The half-life of platelets is approximately 4 days, so these agents are effective for 1-2 days. The dosage of aspirin required is not more than 300 mg once daily.

The dextrans (plasma volume expanders) also depress platelet aggregation. Low–molecular weight dextran reduces viscosity, increases microcirculatory flow, and decreases the tendency toward platelet aggregation. This agent is often used postoperatively. Two units are administered IV in the first 24 hours as a priming dose in the average adult, followed by 1 unit daily for a maximum of 4 days.

VIII. GASTROINTESTINAL COMPLICATIONS*

Theodore R. Schrock

A. GASTRIC DISTENTION AND GASTRIC DILATATION

1. Gastric distention. The stomach may become distended with gas during induction of anesthesia, and further quantities of air are swallowed in the postoperative period. Gastric juice and duodenal secretions that reflux into the stomach contribute to distention also. Marked gastric distention often results in nausea and vomiting; occasionally the distended stomach impairs diaphragmatic excursion and causes tachypnea. Nasogastric intubation is sufficient treatment.

---

*See Chapter 7 for Parotitis; See Chapter 12 for Intestinal Obstruction; Pancreatitis; and Stress Ulcer.

2. Gastric dilatation. If the stomach becomes massively distended, hemorrhage from the gastric mucosa develops. This rare complication of abdominal or extraabdominal surgery is an occult cause of **shock** in the first few hours after operation. Aspiration may occur if the fluid is vomited. The distended tympanitic stomach may be visible in the epigastrium on physical examination or radiography. Nasogastric intubation returns large quantities (sometimes several liters) of dark brownish-green or black fluid containing occult blood. The losses of fluid and electrolytes must be replaced.

B. PARALYTIC ILEUS is the cessation of effective GI motility following trauma, severe illness, or operations on the abdomen or elsewhere (e.g., chest, back). The small bowel regains motility within 12-24 hours and the stomach empties well about 24 hours after operation, but the colon may remain inactive for up to 6 days. Abdominal distention is the main manifestation. Quiet bowel sounds are an unreliable observation. Abdominal radiographs show gas in the stomach, small bowel, and colon.

A nasogastric tube is inserted and left in place until the ileus resolves. Prolonged ileus should be investigated; it may be mechanical obstruction instead.

C. CONSTIPATION. Many factors contribute to postoperative constipation: Nothing by mouth eliminates gastrocolic responses and reduces fecal bulk. Dehydration encourages absorption of fluid from colonic contents, thus dessicating the stool. Ileus has a major component of impaired colonic motility.

Incisional pain makes the patient unwilling to increase intraabdominal pressure, so an important force contributing to defecation is impaired.

Physical inactivity removes important stimuli to movement of feces through the colon, i.e., positional change and the effects of gravity.

Opiates and antacids containing calcium or aluminum are constipating.

1. Manifestations. The patient may complain of abdominal distention, cramping pain, and a sensation of pressure in the rectum. **Fecal impaction** may be evidenced by frequent passage of small amounts of liquid stool around a mass of feces in the rectum; severe rectal pain or pressure may also be noted, the patient may be incontinent from the fecal mass pressing on the anal canal from above; as the patient strains to defecate, hemorrhoids may prolapse.

2. Treatment

a. A bulk agent or stool softener is added to the diet as soon as the patient can eat. Bulk agents, including methylcellulose, 1 tablespoon in water or juice 1-3 times daily, stool softeners, e.g., docusate sodium 0/05 U 3 times daily, are effective also.

b. Ambulation, regular diet, hydration, limitation of narcotics, and bathroom privileges are sufficient to reestablish bowel habits in most patients.

c. A digital rectal examination should be done if constipation appears to be a problem. If a fecal impaction is found, it must be extracted digitally; sedation may be necessary. High fecal impaction may be relieved by oil-retention enema.

d. Laxatives are contraindicated in patients with a recent colonic anastomosis and should never be given until a rectal examination has been done to exclude impaction. Milk of magnesia (30 ml) should be tried initially and more potent laxatives used thereafter if necessary. Suppositories (e.g., glycerine or a stimulant such as Dulcolax) should not be given if the rectum is empty.

e. Enemas are usually unnecessary and are contraindicated after colonic surgery. Oil-retention enemas help evacuate impacted feces. Saline or tap water (500-1500 ml) is effective in removing stool from the left colon and sometimes more proximally. Commercially available phosphosoda enemas (100-150 ml) usually reach only the rectum and sigmoid colon. Soapsuds enemas should **not** be used because they damage the colonic mucosa.

D. DIARRHEA. The first few stools after an ileus resolves may be more liquid—or more frequent—than usual, and both of these changes are interpreted as "diarrhea" by the patient. True diarrhea, the frequent passage of large quantities of liquid stool, usually has a specific cause. Loss of absorptive surface (as after right hemicolectomy), bacterial overgrowth (e.g., antibiotic-associated colitis), and drug effects (e.g., magnesium-containing antacids) are among the possibilities. Persistent diarrhea should be investigated.

E. HEPATIC COMPLICATIONS

1. Jaundice. The differential diagnosis includes all of the causes of jaundice seen in the nonsurgical patient. Especially common are hepatitis (late), hemolysis, and cholestasis from shock or drugs; anesthetic toxicity or hypersensitivity is unusual. Postoperative common duct obstruction should not be overlooked.

2. Hepatitis appears during the late postoperative period, usually 4-12 weeks after transfusion of blood.

3. Hepatic abscess (see Chapter 12).

| **FLUID AND ELECTROLYTE THERAPY** |

Donald D. Trunkey

I. WATER METABOLISM

A. BODY WATER AND ITS DISTRIBUTION. Total body water comprises 40%-65% of total body weight (mean of 55% for adult men and 45% for adult women). Body water is distributed throughout two main compartments: the **extracellular** compartment (plasma and interstitial fluid), which contains about one-fourth of the total body water, and the **intracellular** compartment, which contains about three-fourths of the total body water (Table 2-7).

The considerable variation in percentage of body weight which is made up by water is due mainly to differences in body composition. The higher the fat content of a given subject, the smaller the percentage of body weight that is water. The total body water in various subjects is relatively constant when expressed as a percentage of the so-called lean body mass, i.e., the sum of the fat-free tissue. Consideration should be given to this fact when calculating fluid requirements on the basis of body weight in order to avoid excessive administration of water to obese patients.

B. NORMAL WATER LOSSES AND WATER REQUIREMENTS. Water is lost from the body by four routes: from the **skin,** as sensible and insensible perspiration; from the **lungs,**

Table 2-7. Distribution of body water in the male

Fluid compartment	% body weight	ml of water in a 154-lb (70-kg) man
Extracellular water		
Plasma	4-5%	3200
Interstitial fluid	11-12%	7300
Intracellular water	40-45%	31,500

as water vapor in the expired gas; from the **kidneys,** as urine; and from the **intestines,** with the feces. In the absence of visible perspiration, the total losses from the skin and the lungs are generally referred to as the "insensible loss." In adults, this loss is about 0.5 ml/kg/hour (12 ml/kg/day), i.e., approximately 800 ml/day for the average adult. In children, the insensible loss is somewhat higher when estimated on the basis of body weight, varying from 1.3 ml/kg/hour in infants to 0.6 ml/kg/hour in the older child. This is due to the relatively larger increase in body surface area in children, leading to more evaporative loss. The normal daily water losses and requirements are summarized in Table 2-8.

C. ADDITIONAL WATER REQUIREMENTS IN DISEASE.

Insensible losses may rise much higher than normal postoperatively or in febrile or debilitated states. The quantity of fluid lost from the surface of the body may also be very large in the extensively burned patient.

When visible sweating occurs because of high environmental temperatures or other reasons, additional water must be provided to replace these losses. Moderate sweating results in the additional loss of about 300-500 ml/day, but with profuse sweating the losses may exceed 2000-3000 ml/day.

Water loss from the GI tract is negligible normally, but may assume great importance with prolonged diarrhea, vomiting, nasogastric suction, or drainage from fistulas or an ileostomy. If the kidney's ability to concentrate urine is impaired (e.g., chronic nephritis, nephrosclerosis, or pyelonephritis), it may be necessary to provide additional fluid.

D. ESTIMATION OF WATER LOSSES.

An accurate record of the quantity of fluid lost by all routes is of utmost importance for replacement therapy. This ordinarily includes daily measurement of urinary excretion and GI losses. It is difficult to measure fluid losses from perspiration, exudation (as in burns), diarrhea, or fluid lost into dressings. If there are major losses of these types, daily weighing of the patient is of great value. In many hospitals special bedside scales are available for patients who cannot be weighed on the usual scales.

Patients maintained on parenteral fluids (excluding TPN) do not gain weight unless they are overhydrated. Properly hydrated adults receiving only IV fluids should lose 0.25-0.5 kg/day. If rapid weight losses occur, the patient must be presumed to be dehydrated. (Patients with receding edema and those who have received diuretics are exceptions to this rule.) Table 2-9

Table 2-8. Daily water losses and water requirements for normal individuals who are not working or sweating

	Losses				Requirements	
	Urine (ml)	Stool (ml)	Insensible (ml)	Total (ml)	ml/person	ml/kg
Infant (2-10 kg)	200-500	25-40	75-300 (1.3 ml/kg/hr)	300-840	330-1000	165-100
Child (10-40 kg)	500-800	40-100	300-600	840-1500	1000-1800	100-45
Adolescent or adult (60 kg)	800-1000	100	60-1000 (0.5 ml/kg/hr)	1500-2100	1800-2500	45-30

Table 2-9. Relationship of acute weight loss to degree of dehydration

Weight loss expressed as % of normal (or preoperative) body weight	Degree of dehydration
Loss of 4% body weight	Mild
Loss of 6% body weight	Moderate
Loss of 8% body weight	Severe

shows the relationship between extent of rapid weight loss and degree of dehydration.

The amount of fluid to be replaced can be estimated from the amount of weight loss; each kilogram of weight loss is equivalent to 1 L of fluid.

E. INTERNAL LOSSES OF FLUID AND ELECTROLYTES. Extracellular fluid and electrolytes may be lost into fluid spaces newly created by a disease process. Examples are the accumulation of fluid in the edema of burns, in an area of infection, in the intestine during ileus, or intracellular shifts during severe shock. These losses are termed "third space" losses. Unless promptly replaced the effect of third space losses on the circulating plasma volume is just as serious as if the losses had been external.

Fluids lost into the third space are eventually reabsorbed unless they have been removed (as by nasogastric suction in a case of ileus), and the administration of fluid and electrolyte must be reduced to compensate. In burned patients, diuresis of fluid pooled outside the circulation usually begins after 48-72 hours; a longer interval is required in cases of infection or trauma.

II. ELECTROLYTE METABOLISM

A. ELECTROLYTE COMPOSITION OF BODY FLUIDS. Table 2-10 lists the concentrations of inorganic salts (electrolytes) in the plasma and in the cells. The electrolyte composition of intracellular fluid differs from that of the plasma in that potassium (rather than sodium) is the principal cation, and phosphate (rather than chloride) is the principal anion. There is also more protein within the cell than in the extracellular fluid.

Table 2-10. Normal electrolyte composition of body fluids

| | Atomic or radicular weight | mEq wt (mg) | Extracellular fluid (plasma) mEq/liter | | | Intracellular fluid (muscle) mEq/liter (avg) |
			(avg)	(range)	mg/dl	
Cations						
Na^+	23	23	143	135-147	310-340	13
K^+	39	39	5	4.6-5.6	18-22	140
Ca^{++}	40	20	5	4.5-5.5	9-11	Trace
Mg^{++}	24	12	2	1.5-3.0	1.8-3.6	45
Total		155				198

Continued

Table 2-10. Normal electrolyte composition of body fluids—cont'd

	Atomic or radicular weight	mEq wt (mg)	Extracellular fluid (plasma) mEq/liter			Intracellular fluid (muscle) mEq/liter (avg)
			(avg)	(range)	mg/dl	
Anions						
Cl⁻	35	35	103	100-112	350-390	3
(As NaCl)	(58)	(58)			(590-660)†	10
HCO₃⁻*	—	—	27	25-30	56-65†	
HPO₄⁼						
(as P)‡	31	17.2	2	1.8-2.3	3-4	100
SO₄ (as S)§	32	16	1			20
Org. acids§	—	—	6			Trace
Protein§	—	—	16			Trace
Total			155			198

*HCO₃⁻ is measured as CO_2 content and frequently reported in Vol.% (ml/dl plasma). To convert Vol.% to mEq/L. HCl₃⁻ divide Vol. % by 2.24.

†Vol. %.

‡The inorganic phosphorus in the serum exists as a buffer mixture in which approximately 80% is in the form of $HPO_4^=$. For this reason the mEq weight is usually calculated by dividing the atomic weight of phosphorus by 1.8. Thus, the mEq weight for phosphorus in the serum is taken as 31/1.8 = 17.2.

§The organic acids and the proteins are expressed in terms of their combining power with cations. For protein, the cation equivalence in milliequivalents is calculated by multiplying the number of grams of total protein/dl by 2.43.

The chemical reactivity of electrolytes in the body fluids cannot be evaluated when their concentrations are expressed as weight per volume (e.g., mg/dl) any more than work performance (horsepower) of an electric motor can be expressed merely in terms of its weight. For this reason, electrolyte concentrations are usually expressed in mEq per volume (mEq/liter most commonly). The mEq weight of an element is simply its atomic weight divided by its valence (number of electric changes carried by the element). In Table 2-10 the mEq weights of the electrolytes are listed. To convert a concentration of an electrolyte from mg/dl to mEq/liter, the formula shown below is used:

$$\frac{mg/dl \times 10}{mEq \text{ weight}} = mEq/L$$

For example, if the concentration of plasma sodium is reported as 322 mg/dl:

$$\frac{322 \times 10}{23} = 140 \text{ mEq/L}$$

B. COMPOSITION OF GI SECRETIONS AND SWEAT. (See Table 2-11.) Large quantities of fluid and electrolyte are secreted into the GI tract, but almost all are reabsorbed, mainly in the colon, and there are minimal losses of fluid and electrolyte in the feces. Vomiting, diarrhea, obstruction, fistulas, nasogastric suction, and an ileostomy are abnormalities that can lead to rapid depletion of fluid and electrolyte. **Note:** In surgical patients, GI losses are the principal cause of severe dehydration and electrolyte depletion.

III. VOLUME DISORDERS

A. VOLUME DEPLETION is common in surgical patients. A systematic approach to diagnosis and treatment should be developed.

1. Clinical manifestations include low blood pressure, narrow pulse pressure, tachycardia, poor skin turgor, and dry mucous membranes.

2. History may suggest the reason for volume depletion. Records of intake and output, changes in body weight, urine specific gravity, and analysis of the chemical composition of the urine are confirmatory.

3. Treatment must aim to correct the volume deficit and associated aberrations in electrolyte concentrations.

Table 2-11. Volume and composition of GI secretions and sweat

Fluid	Avg. volume (ml/24 hr)	Electrolyte concentrations			(mEq/liter)
		Na⁺	K⁺	Cl⁻	HCO₃⁻
Blood plasma*		135-150	3.6-5.5	100-105	24.6-28.8
Gastric juice	2500	31-90	4.3-12	52-124	0
Bile	700-1000	134-156	3.9-6.3	83-110	38
Pancreatic juice	>1000	113-153	2.6-7.4	54-95	110
Small bowel (Miller-Abbot suction)	3000	72-120	3.5-6.87	69-127	30
Ileostomy	100-4000	112-142	4.5-14	93-122	30
recent					
adapted	100-500	50	3	20	15-30
Cecostomy	100-3000	48-116	11.1-28.3	35-70	15
Feces	100	<10	<10	<15	<15
Sweat	500-4000	30-70	0-5	30-70	0

*Blood plasma included for purposes of comparison.

B. WATER DEFICIT. The simplest form of volume depletion is water deficit without accompanying solute deficit. In surgical patients, water and solute depletion more often occur together. Pure water deficits can develop in patients who are unable to regulate intake; examples include debilitated or comatose patients or those who have increased insensible water loss from fever. Patients given tube feedings without adequate water supplementation and those with diabetes insipidus may also develop this syndrome.

1. Pure water deficit is reflected biochemically by hypernatremia. The magnitude of the deficit can be estimated from the serum sodium. Other findings are an increase in the plasma osmolality, concentrated urine, and low urine sodium concentration (<15 mEq/L) despite the hypernatremia.

2. Clinical manifestations include depression of the CNS (lethargy or coma) and muscle rigidity, tremors, spasticity, and seizures.

3. Treatment. (1) Enough water must be given to restore the plasma sodium concentration to normal. In addition to correcting the existing water deficit, ongoing obligatory water losses (due to the diabetes insipidus, fever, and so on) must be satisfied. (2) Treat the patient with 5% dextrose and water unless hypotension has developed, in which case hypotonic saline should be used. Rarely, isotonic saline may be indicated to treat shock from dehydration even though the patient is hypernatremic.

C. VOLUME AND ELECTROLYTE DEPLETION. Combined water and electrolyte depletion may occur from GI losses due to nasogastric suction, enteric fistulas, intestinal stomas, or diarrhea. Additional causes include excessive diuretic therapy, adrenal insufficiency, profuse sweating, burns, and body fluid sequestration (third space) following trauma or surgery.

1. Clinical findings are similar to those of pure volume depletion, but hypernatremia is not so marked or the patient may be hyponatremic. The urine-sodium concentration is often <10 mEq/L, a manifestation of renal sodium conservation. The urine is usually hypertonic (specific gravity >1.020), with an osmolality >450-500 mOsm/kg. The decreased blood volume diminishes renal perfusion and produces prerenal azotemia. The BUN:creatinine ratio is increased up to 20-25:1 (see Acute Renal Failure in this chapter).

2. Treatment. Replacement therapy should be planned as follows: Calculate the sodium deficit. If serum sodium is normal, the fluid and electrolyte losses are isotonic. If serum sodium is low, subtract the sodium value from 140 and multiply by total body water (in liters) to obtain sodium deficit in mEq.

Estimate the volume deficit from clinical signs and changes in body weight. The volume deficit is replaced as isotonic saline containing added sodium chloride to correct the sodium deficit. Monitor clinical signs and serum electrolytes. Central venous or pulmonary arterial pressure should be monitored in critical cases.

D. INTRAVASCULAR VOLUME OVERLOAD. Hormonal and circulatory responses to surgery result in postoperative conservation of sodium and water by the kidneys independent of the adequacy of the ECF volume. Antidiuretic hormone released during anesthesia and surgical stress promotes water conservation by the kidneys. Renal vasoconstriction and increased aldosterone activity reduce sodium excretion. Consequently, if fluid intake is excessive in the immediate postoperative period, volume overload may occur. Distinguish intravascular volume overload from severe edema. Edematous patients may be intravascularly depleted despite such a positive fluid balance.

1. Clinical manifestations of volume overload include edema of the sacrum and extremities, jugular venous distention, tachypnea (if pulmonary edema develops), increased body weight, and elevated pulmonary arterial and central venous pressures.

2. Volume overload may precipitate prerenal azotemia and oliguria. Examination of the urine usually shows low sodium and high potassium concentrations consistent with enhanced tubular reabsorption of sodium and water.

3. Treatment depends upon the severity of the volume overload: For mild overload, sodium restriction is usually adequate. If hyponatremia is present, water restriction may also be necessary. Diuretics must be used for severe volume overload. In the presence of cardiac failure, digitalis is indicated.

4. Inappropriate secretion of antidiuretic hormone (SIADH) may occur after head injury and in some patients with cancers or burns. This syndrome is characterized by hyponatremia, concentrated urine, elevated urine sodium concentration, and a normal or mildly expanded ECF volume. Treatment with water restriction is usually successful. In some cases, diuretics and isotonic saline infusion simultaneously are necessary.

IV. SPECIFIC ELECTROLYTE DISORDERS

A. SODIUM. Regulation of the sodium concentration in plasma or urine is intimately associated with regulation of total body water. Clinically, this reflects the balance between total body solute and total body water.

1. Hypernatremia represents, chiefly, loss of water.

2. Hyponatremia may be dilutional, or it may result from isotonic dehydration. An apparent hyponatremia may be related to marked hyperlipidemia or hyperproteinemia because fat and protein contribute to plasma bulk even though they are not dissolved in plasma water. The sodium concentration in plasma water in these situations is usually normal.

3. Hyponatremia in severe hyperglycemia results from the osmotic effect of the elevated glucose concentration, which draws water from the intracellular space and dilutes the sodium in the ECF. The magnitude of this can be estimated by multiplying the blood glucose concentration in mg/dl by 0.016 and adding the result to the existing serum sodium concentration. The sum represents the serum sodium concentration if hyperglycemia were not present.

4. Hyponatremia can be treated by administering the calculated sodium needs as isotonic solutions.

5. Correction of severe sodium imbalance should be done slowly, by raising or lowering serum sodium content by no more than 1 mEq/hour. This will decrease the chances of seizures.

B. POTASSIUM. The potassium in ECF constitutes only 2% of total body potassium. The remaining 98% is within body cells. The serum potassium concentration is determined primarily by the pH of ECF and the size of the intracellular potassium pool.

With extracellular **acidosis,** a large proportion of the excess hydrogen is buffered intracellularly by an exchange of intracellular potassium for extracellular hydrogen ion. This movement of potassium may produce dangerous **hyperkalemia. Alkalosis** has an opposite effect; as the serum pH rises, potassium moves into cells, and **hypokalemia** appears.

In the absence of an acid-base disturbance, serum potassium reflects the total body pool of potassium. With excessive external losses (e.g., from the GI tract), the serum potassium falls. A loss of 10% of total body potassium drops the serum potassium from 4 to 3 mEq/L at a normal blood pH.

1. Hyperkalemia may prove fatal if not treated. Patients who may develop hyperkalemia include those with severe trauma, burns, crush injuries, renal insufficiency, or marked catabolism from other causes. It can also be found in Addison's disease.

a. Diagnosis. There are usually *no symptoms* associated with hyperkalemia, but nausea, vomiting, colicky abdominal pain, and diarrhea may occur.

ECG changes are the most helpful indicators of the severity of hyperkalemia. Early changes include peaking of the T waves, widening of the QRS complex, and depression of the ST segment. With further elevation of the blood potassium level, the QRS widens to such a degree that the tracing resembles a sine wave; this is a premonitory sign of cardiac standstill.

Etiologic factors other than those mentioned above must be considered in hyperkalemic patients, including hemolysis, leukocytosis, or thrombocytosis. Platelet counts >1 million may elevate the serum potassium. The acid-base status should be assessed.

b. Treatment. There are three general approaches to the treatment of hyperkalemia: (1) IV infusion of 100 ml of 50% dextrose solution containing 20 units of regular insulin lowers extracellular potassium by promoting its transport into cells in association with glucose. IV bicarbonate solution lowers serum potassium as acidosis is corrected. Calcium is a specific antagonist to the effects of potassium on tissues. An infusion of calcium chloride transiently reverses cardiac depression from hyperkalemia without changing the serum potassium concentration. (2) A slower method of controlling hyperkalemia is to administer the cation exchange resin sodium polystyrene sulfonate (Kayexalate) orally or by an enema at a rate of 40-80 g/day. Lasix (20-40 mg IV) can be administered if some renal function is present. (3) If hyperkalemia is a manifestation of renal failure, dialysis is often necessary.

2. Hypokalemia may be associated with alkalosis through either of two mechanisms: intracellular shifts of potassium in exchange for hydrogen, or renal wasting of potassium.

a. Clinical manifestations reflect neuromuscular dysfunction (decreased muscle contractility and muscle cell potentials). In extreme cases, death may result from paralysis of the muscles of respiration.

b. Treatment consists of correcting the cause of hypokalemia and administering potassium. Potassium is given orally if the patient is able to eat; otherwise it should be given IV. Potassium concentrations in IV solutions usually should not exceed 40 mEq/L. In *mild hypokalemia* (potassium between 3 and 3.5 mEq/L) potassium should be replaced slowly to avoid hyperkalemia. In *moderate to severe hypokalemia* (potassium <3 mEq/L), potassium may be administered at a rate of 20 mEq/hour, when monitoring is adequate.

C. CALCIUM is an important mediator of neuromuscular function and cellular enzymatic processes even though most of the body calcium is contained in the skeleton. The usual dietary intake of calcium is 1-3 g/day, most of which is excreted, unabsorbed, in the feces.

   1. The normal serum calcium concentration (8.5-10.5 mg/dl or 4.25-5.25 mEq/L) is maintained by humoral factors, mainly vitamin D, parathyroid hormone, and calcitonin.

   Approximately half of the total serum calcium is bound to plasma protein, chiefly albumin. A small amount is complexed to plasma anions such as citrate, and the remainder (approximately 40%) of the total serum calcium is free or **ionized calcium,** which is the fraction responsible for the biologic effects.

   Acidemia increases and alkalemia decreases the serum ionized calcium concentration.

   2. Hypocalcemia occurs in hypoparathyroidism, hypomagnesemia, severe pancreatitis, chronic or acute renal failure, severe trauma, crush injuries, necrotizing fasciitis, burns, and septic shock.

   a. Clinical manifestations are neuromuscular: hyperactive deep tendon reflexes, a positive Chvostek sign, muscle and abdominal cramps, carpopedal spasm, and, rarely, convulsions. Hypercalcemia is reflected in the ECG by a prolonged Q-T interval.

   b. Treatment. The initial step is to check the whole blood pH and correct alkalosis if it is present. IV calcium, as calcium gluconate or calcium chloride, may be needed for the acute problem.

   3. Hypercalcemia is caused by hyperparathyroidism, cancer with bony metastases, ectopic production of parathyroid hormone, vitamin D intoxication, hyperthyroidism, sarcoidosis, milk-alkali syndrome, or prolonged immobilization. It is also a rare complication of thiazide diuretics.

   a. Symptoms of hypercalcemia are fatiguability, muscle weakness, depression, anorexia, nausea, and constipation.

Severe hypercalcemia can cause coma and death; a serum concentration >12 mg/dl should be regarded as a medical emergency.

b. With *severe hypercalcemia* (calcium >14.5 mg/dl) IV isotonic saline should be given to expand the ECF, increase urine flow, enhance calcium excretion, and reduce the serum level of calcium.

c. Furosemide and IV sodium sulfate are other methods of *increasing renal calcium excretion.* Mithramycin is particularly useful for hypercalcemia associated with metastatic cancer. Adrenal corticosteroids are useful for hypercalcemia associated with sarcoidosis, vitamin D intoxication, and Addison's disease. Calcitonin is indicated in patients with impaired renal and cardiovascular function. If renal failure is present, hemodialysis may be required.

D. MAGNESIUM is found largely in bones and in cells where it has an important role in cellular energy metabolism. Normal plasma magnesium concentration is 1.5-2.5 mEq/L. Magnesium is excreted primarily by the kidneys. The serum magnesium concentration reflects total body magnesium.

1. Hypomagnesemia occurs with poor dietary intake, intestinal malabsorption, or excessive losses from the gut (enteric fistulas, the use of purgatives, or nasogastric suction). It may also result from excessive urinary losses, chronic alcoholism, hyperaldosteronism, and hypercalcemia. It occasionally develops in acute pancreatitis, diabetic acidosis, in burn patients, or after prolonged TPN with insufficient magnesium supplementation.

a. Clinical manifestations resemble those of hypocalcemia: hyperactive tendon reflexes, positive Chvostek sign, and tremors which may progress to delirium and convulsions.

b. Diagnosis is based on a strong index of suspicion and confirmed by measurement of the serum magnesium level.

c. Treatment consists of administering magnesium, usually as the sulfate or chloride, orally or, in serious deficiencies, IV (40-80 mEq of $MgSO_4$/L of IV fluid). When large doses are infused IV there is a risk of producing hypermagnesemia with tachycardia and hypotension. The ECG should be inspected for prolongation of the Q-T interval.

2. Hypermagnesemia usually occurs in patients with renal disease and is rare in surgical patients; it may develop in hypovolemic shock as magnesium is liberated from cells. Patients with renal insufficiency should have their serum magnesium level monitored closely.

a. Initial signs and symptoms are lethargy and weakness.

b. ECG changes resemble those in hypercalcemia (widened QRS complex, S-T segment depression, and peaked T waves). When the serum level reaches 6 mEq/L, deep tendon reflexes are lost. With levels >10 mEq/L, somnolence, coma, and death may ensue.

c. Treatment includes IV isotonic saline to increase the rate of renal magnesium excretion and may be accompanied by slow IV infusion of calcium (calcium antagonizes some of the neuromuscular actions of magnesium). Patients with hypermagnesemia and severe renal failure may need dialysis.

E. PHOSPHORUS is mainly a constituent of bone, but it is also an important intracellular ion with a role in energy metabolism. The serum phosphorus level is an approximate indicator of total body phosphorus and can be influenced by many factors including the serum calcium concentration and the pH of blood.

1. Hypophosphatemia is usually associated with poor dietary intake (especially in alcoholics), hyperparathyroidism, and antacid administration.

a. Clinical manifestations include lassitude, fatigue, weakness, convulsions, and death. Red cells may hemolyze, thus impairing oxygen delivery to tissues. White cell phagocytosis is also depressed.

b. Treatment is principally with oral phosphorus placement. In patients receiving TPN, 20-40 mEq of potassium dihydrogen phosphate should be given IV for every 1000 Cal infused.

2. Hyperphosphatemia most often develops in severe renal disease, after trauma, or with marked tissue catabolism. It is rarely caused by excessive dietary intake. Hyperphosphatemia is usually asymptomatic.

Treatment is by diuresis, to increase the rate of urinary phosphorus excretion. Aluminum-containing antacids bind phosphate and prevent absorption from the gut. In patients with renal disease, dialysis may be required.

V. ACID-BASE BALANCE

A. PHYSIOLOGY. The daily metabolism of protein and carbohydrate generates approximately 70 mEq (or 1 mEq/kg of body weight) of hydrogen ion. In addition, a large amount of carbon dioxide is formed which combines with water to make carbonic acid (H_2CO_3).

Hydrogen ions generated from metabolism are buffered through 2 major systems. The first involves intracellular protein (e.g., the hemoglobin in red blood cells). More important is the **bicarbonate/carbonic acid system,** which can be understood from the Henderson-Hasselbalch equation:

$$pH = pK + \log \frac{(HCO_3^-)}{0.03 \times PCO_2}$$

Eq(1)

where pK for the HCO_3^-/H_2CO_3 system is 6.1.

Hydrogen ion concentration is related to pH in an inverse logarithmic manner. The following transformation of Eq(1) is easier to use because it eliminates the logarithms:

$$H^+ = \frac{24 \times PCO_2}{HCO_3^-}$$

Eq(2)

There is an approximately linear inverse relationship between pH and hydrogen ion concentration over the pH range of 7.1-7.5: For each 0.01 decrease in pH, the hydrogen ion concentration increases 1 nmol. Remembering that a normal blood pH of 7.40 is equal to a hydrogen ion concentration of 40 nmol/liter, one can calculate the approximate hydrogen ion concentration of any pH between 7.1 and 7.5. For example, a pH of 7.30 is equal to a hydrogen ion concentration of 50 nmol/liter. This estimation introduces an error of approximately 10% at the extremes of this pH range.

A consideration of the right-hand side of Eq(2) demonstrates that hydrogen ion concentration is determined by the ratio of the PCO_2 to plasma bicarbonate concentration. In body fluid, CO_2 is dissolved and combines with water to form carbonic acid, the acid part of the acid-base pair. If any two of these three variables are known, the third can be calculated using this expression:

Equation (2) also illustrates how the body excretes acid produced from metabolism. Blood PCO_2 is normally controlled within narrow limits by pulmonary ventilation. The plasma bicarbonate concentration is regulated by the renal tubules by 3 major processes: (1) Filtered bicarbonate is reabsorbed, mostly in the proximal tubule, to prevent excessive bicarbonate loss in the urine. (2) Hydrogen ions are secreted as titratable acid to regenerate the bicarbonate that was buffered when these hydrogen ions were initially produced and to provide a vehicle for excretion of about one third of the daily acid production. (3) The kidneys also excrete hydrogen ion in the form of ammonium ion by a process which regenerates bicarbonate initially consumed in the production of these hydrogen ions. Volume depletion, increased P_{CO_2}, and hypokalemia all favor enhanced tubular reabsorption of HCO_3.

B. ACID-BASE ABNORMALITIES. The management of clinical acid-base disturbances is facilitated by the use of a nomogram (Figure 2-4) which relates the 3 variables in Eq(2).

Primary respiratory disturbances cause changes in the blood P_{CO_2} (the numerator in Eq(2)) and produce corresponding effects on the blood hydrogen ion concentration. Metabolic disturbances primarily affect the plasma bicarbonate concentration (the denominator in Eq(2)). Whether the disturbance is primarily respiratory or metabolic, some degree of compensatory change occurs in the reciprocal factor in Eq(2) to limit or nullify the magnitude of perturbation of acid-base balance. Thus, changes in blood P_{CO_2} from respiratory disturbances are compensated by changes in the renal handling of bicarbonate. Conversely, changes in plasma bicarbonate concentration are blunted by appropriate respiratory changes.

Because acute changes allow insufficient time for compensatory mechanisms to respond, the resulting pH disturbances are often great and the abnormalities may be present in pure form. By contrast, chronic disturbances allow the full range of compensatory mechanisms to come into play, so that blood pH may remain near normal despite wide variations in the plasma bicarbonate or blood P_{CO_2}.

C. RESPIRATORY ACIDOSIS

1. Acute respiratory acidosis occurs when respiration is suddenly inadequate. CO_2 accumulates in the blood (numerator in Eq(2) increases), and hydrogen ion concentration increases. This occurs most often in opiate overdose, acute airway obstruction, aspiration, respiratory arrest, certain pulmonary infections, and pulmonary edema with impaired gas exchange. There is acidemia and an elevated blood P_{CO_2} but little change in the plasma bicarbonate concentration. Over 80% of the carbonic acid resulting from the increased P_{CO_2} is buffered by intracellular mechanisms: about 50% by intracellular protein and another 30% by hemoglobin. Because relatively little is buffered by bicarbonate ion, the plasma bicarbonate concentration may be normal. An acute increase in P_{CO_2} from 40-80 mm Hg will increase the plasma bicarbonate by only 3 mEq/L. This is why the 95% confidence band for acute respi-

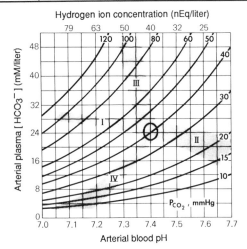

FIGURE 2-4. Acid-base nomogram for use in evaluation of clinical acid-base disorders. (Courtesy of Anthony Sebastian, MD, University of California Medical Center, San Francisco). Hydrogen ion concentration (top) or blood pH (bottom) is plotted against HCO_3^- concentration; curved lines are isopleths of CO_2 tension (Pco_2, mm Hg). Knowing any two of these variables permits estimation of the third. The circle in the center represents the range of normal values; the added bands represent the 95% confidence limits of four common acid-base disturbances: I, acute respiratory acidosis; II, acute respiratory alkalosis; III, chronic respiratory acidosis; IV, sustained metabolic acidosis. Points lying outside these shaded areas are mixed disturbances and indicate two primary acid-base disorders.

ratory acidosis (I in Figure 2-4) is nearly horizontal; i.e., increases in Pco_2 directly decrease pH with little change in plasma bicarbonate concentration.

Treatment involves restoration of adequate ventilation. If necessary, tracheal intubation and assisted ventilation or controlled ventilation with sedation should be employed.

2. Chronic respiratory acidosis arises from chronic respiratory failure in which impaired ventilation gives a sustained elevation of blood P_{CO_2}. Renal compensation raises plasma bicarbonate to the extent illustrated by the 95% confidence limits in Figure 2-4 (the area labeled III). Rather marked elevations of P_{CO_2} produce small changes in blood pH because of the increase in plasma bicarbonate concentration. This is achieved primarily by increased renal excretion of ammonium ion, which enhances acid excretion and regenerates bicarbonate, which is returned to the blood. Chronic respiratory acidosis is generally well tolerated until severe pulmonary insufficiency leads to hypoxia. At this point long-term prognosis is poor. Paradoxically, the patient with chronic respiratory acidosis appears better able to tolerate acute increases in blood P_{CO_2}.

Treatment of chronic respiratory acidosis depends largely on attention to pulmonary toilet and ventilatory status. Rapid correction of chronic respiratory acidosis, as may occur if the patient is placed on controlled ventilation, can be dangerous because the P_{CO_2} is lowered rapidly and the compensated respiratory acidosis may be converted to a severe metabolic alkalosis.

D. RESPIRATORY ALKALOSIS

1. Acute hyperventilation lowers the P_{CO_2} without concomitant changes in the plasma bicarbonate concentration and thereby lowers the hydrogen ion concentration (II in Figure 2-4). The clinical manifestations are paresthesias in the extremities, carpopedal spasm, and a positive Chvostek sign.

2. Chronic respiratory alkalosis occurs in pulmonary and liver disease. The renal response to chronic hypocapnia is to decrease the tubular reabsorption of filtered bicarbonate, increasing bicarbonate excretion with a consequent lowering of plasma bicarbonate concentration. As the bicarbonate concentration falls, the chloride concentration rises. This is the same pattern seen in hyperchloremic acidosis, and the two can be distinguished only by blood gas and pH measurements. Generally, no treatment is required.

3. Compensatory respiratory alkalosis is most commonly found in patients with acute decrease in perfusion, anaerobic metabolism, and build-up of lactate. The increased ventilatory rate eliminates more CO_2 to attempt to normalize pH. Hypovolemic shock and septic shock frequently produce compensatory respiratory alkalosis.

E. METABOLIC ACIDOSIS is caused by increased production of hydrogen ion from metabolic or other causes, or from excessive bicarbonate losses. In either case, the plasma bicarbonate concentration is decreased, producing an increase in hydrogen ion concentration (see Eq(2)).

With excessive bicarbonate loss (e.g., severe diarrhea, diuretic treatment with acetazolamide or other carbonic anhydrase inhibitors, certain forms of renal tubular disease, and in patients with ureterosigmoidostomies), the decrease in plasma bicarbonate concentration is matched by an increase in the serum chloride, so that the anion gap (the sum of chloride and bicarbonate concentrations subtracted from the serum sodium concentration) remains at the normal level, <15 mEq/L.

Metabolic acidosis from increased acid production is associated with an anion gap exceeding 15 mEq/L. Conditions in which this occurs are renal failure, diabetic ketoacidosis, lactic acidosis, methanol ingestion, salicylate intoxication, and ethylene glycol ingestion. The lungs compensate by hyperventilation, which returns the hydrogen ion concentration toward normal by lowering the blood Pco_2. In long-standing metabolic acidosis, minute ventilation may increase sufficiently to drop the Pco_2 as low as 10-15 mm Hg. The shaded area, marked IV on the nomogram (Figure 2-4) represents the confidence for sustained metabolic acidosis.

Treatment. Identifying the underlying cause and correcting it are often sufficient treatment.

In some conditions, particularly when there is an increased anion gap, **alkali administration** is required. The amount of sodium bicarbonate required to restore the plasma bicarbonate concentration to normal can be estimated by subtracting the existing plasma bicarbonate concentration from the normal value of 24 mEq/L and multiplying the resulting number by half the estimated total body water. This is a useful empirical formula. In practice, it is not usually wise to administer enough bicarbonate to return the plasma bicarbonate completely to normal. It is better to raise the plasma bicarbonate concentration by 5 mEq/L initially and then reassess the clinical situation. The administration of sodium bicarbonate may cause fluid overload from the large quantity of sodium and may overcorrect the acidosis.

The long-term management of patients with metabolic acidosis entails providing adequate alkali, either as supplemental sodium bicarbonate tablets or by dietary manipulation. In all cases, attempts should be made to minimize the magnitude of bicarbonate loss in patients with chronic metabolic acidosis.

F. METABOLIC ALKALOSIS is probably the most common acid-base disturbance in surgical patients. In this condition, the blood hydrogen ion concentration is decreased as a result of accumulation of bicarbonate in plasma. The pathogenesis is complex, but involves at least three separate factors: loss of hydrogen ion, usually as a result of loss of gastric secretions rich in hydrochloric acid; volume depletion, which is often severe; and potassium depletion, which almost always is present.

HCl secretion by the gastric mucosa returns bicarbonate ion to the blood. Gastric acid, after mixing with ingested food, is subsequently reabsorbed in the small intestine, so that there is no net gain or loss of hydrogen ion in this process. If secreted hydrogen ion is lost through vomiting or drainage, the result is a net delivery of bicarbonate into the circulation. Normally, the kidneys are easily able to excrete the excess bicarbonate load. However, if volume depletion accompanies the loss of hydrogen ion, the kidneys work to preserve volume by increasing tubular reabsorption of sodium and whatever anions are also filtered. Consequently, because of the increased sodium reabsorption, the excess bicarbonate cannot be completely excreted. This perpetuates the metabolic alkalosis. At first, some of the filtered bicarbonate escapes reabsorption in the proximal tubule and reaches the distal tubule. Here it promotes potassium secretion and enhanced potassium loss in the urine. The urine pH is either neutral or alkaline because of the presence of bicarbonate. Later, as volume depletion becomes more severe, the reabsorption of filtered bicarbonate in the proximal tubule becomes virtually complete. Now, only small amounts of sodium, with little bicarbonate, reach the distal tubule. If potassium depletion is severe, sodium is now reabsorbed in exchange for hydrogen ion. This results in the paradoxically acid urine sometime observed in patients with advanced metabolic alkalosis.

1. Assessment should involve examination of the urine electrolytes and urine pH. In the early stages, bicarbonate excretion obligates excretion of sodium as well as potassium, so the urine sodium concentration is relatively high for a volume-depleted patient, and the urine pH is alkaline. In this circumstance, the urine chloride reveals the extent of the volume depletion: A urine chloride of <10 mEq/L is diagnostic of volume depletion and chloride deficiency. Later, when bicarbonate reabsorption becomes virtually complete, the urine pH will be acid, and urine sodium, potassium, and chloride concentrations will all be low. The ventilatory compensation in metabolic alkalosis is variable, but the maximal extent of compensation can raise the blood PCO_2 only to about 55 mm Hg. A $Pco_2 > 60$ mm Hg in metabolic alkalosis suggests a mixed disturbance also involving respiratory acidosis.

2. Treatment. To treat metabolic alkalosis, fluid volume must be given, usually as sodium chloride. With adequate volume repletion, the stimulus to tubular sodium reabsorption is diminished, and the kidneys can then excrete the excess bicarbonate. Most of these patients are also substantially potassium-depleted and require potassium supplementation. This should be administered as KCl, because chloride depletion is another hallmark of this condition and potassium given as citrate or lactate does not correct the potassium deficit.

G. MIXED ACID-BASE DISORDERS.

In many situations, mixed disorders of acid-base balance develop. The most common example in surgical patients is metabolic acidosis superimposed on respiratory alkalosis. This problem can arise in patients with septic shock or hepatorenal syndrome. Because the two acid-base disorders tend to cancel each other, the disturbance in hydrogen ion concentration is usually small. The reverse situation, i.e., respiratory acidosis combined with metabolic alkalosis, is less common. Combined metabolic and respiratory acidosis occurs in cardiorespiratory arrest and obviously constitutes a medical emergency. Circumstances involving both metabolic and respiratory alkalosis are rare.

The clue to the presence of a mixed acid-base disorder comes from plotting the patient's acid-base data on the nomogram in Figure 2-4. If the set of data falls outside one of the confidence bands, then by definition the patient has a mixed disorder. On the other hand, if the acid-base data fall within one of the confidence bands, it suggests (but does not prove) that the acid-base disturbance is pure or uncomplicated.

BLOOD AND BLOOD PRODUCTS (HEMOTHERAPY)

George F. Sheldon

Modern surgery would be impossible without the capability of restoring blood volume by transfusion. Blood and blood components vary considerably from the blood that perfuses the arteries and veins of the human body. Blood products should be considered to be drugs, biological products, or transplants. This section reviews available blood products, indications for their use, and metabolic consequences of the infusion of liquid preserved blood.

A. STORAGE. All blood products undergo changes during storage. The citrate preservative of the past, ACD, has largely been replaced by CPD. A unit of whole blood contains 450-500 ml of donor blood and 63 ml of CPD anticoagulant. CPDA-1 is a newer, common component. Extra nutrients are now commonly added and labeled AS-1 or AS-2, depending on the solution.

1. Changes during storage. CPD preservative causes less of a storage lesion than ACD, but important changes still occur.

a. Potassium, lactate, and ammonia values rise.

b. Particulate matter and plasticizers increase.

c. Labile clotting factors (V, VIII) diminish.

d. Diphosphoglycerate (2,3-DPG) levels remain adequate for 14 days but are virtually absent by the end of 21 days of storage. 2,3-DPG regulates the loading and unloading of oxygen from hemoglobin; if levels of 2,3-DPG are low, oxygen does not dissociate from hemoglobin and therefore is not available to tissues perfused by such red cells.

e. Donor blood mixed with CPD or CPD-adenine preservative has an acidic pH (initially about 7), and pH falls still further to 6.5 at the end of 2 weeks in storage.

f. Platelets become functionally inadequate as soon as blood is stored at 4° C (necessary to minimize growth of bacteria); after 5 days of preservation in CPD, virtually no platelets remain.

g. Platelets that are refrigerated are not functional.

h. Freeze-thaw methods for platelet preservation are imminent.

2. Component therapy. Many of the undesirable preservation-related changes in whole blood can be avoided by precise transfusion therapy in the form of components. For that reason, most blood banks in recent years have urged conversion from frequent use of whole blood to reliance on components.

B. RED BLOOD CELLS
1. Whole blood is the transfusion product most familiar to physicians and is the standard against which components are judged.

At present, whole blood is indicated only for resuscitation of acutely bleeding patients in whom there is a need for replacement of both red cells and plasma. Because it is less viscous, whole blood can be infused more rapidly than red cell concentrates, and this is an advantage in emergency situations.

2. Red cell concentrates (packed red cells). In this product, 60%-80% of the plasma is removed immediately after collection. Red cell concentrates are metabolically similar to whole blood, except that less citrate, antigenic debris, potassium, sodium, plasma protein, and microaggregates are present. There is a lower risk of hepatitis also. Red cell concentrates are preferred for transfusion in anemic patients who are not acutely hypovolemic.

3. Washed red cells are an improved form of red cell concentrate in which most of the plasma fraction is removed by washing. Washed red cells eliminate many of the potential hazards of the plasma fraction, including transfusion of red cell antigens and transmission of bacterial and viral diseases.

4. Frozen red cells. Freezing preserves the characteristics of the red cells at the time they are frozen. Frozen cells must be washed to remove the cryopreservative before administration. Advantages include the ability to store for long periods. This method of preservation is so expensive that at present it is limited to rare red cell types.

5. Red cell rejuvenation. It is possible also to freeze red blood cells that are approaching the dating period (21 days after collection), treat the cells with inosine, glucose, and phosphate to restore the 2,3-DPG and the ATP levels, and thus "rejuvenate" a unit destined to be discarded.

C. PLATELET CONCENTRATES are obtained by centrifugation at the time of donation and can be stored up to 48 hours at room temperature, although usually they are used within 24 hours of collection. The advantage is provision of functional platelets in a small total volume of transfused fluid.

Platelets are dispensed in several different preparations. **Single-unit packs** contain the platelets from one donor and are stored in 50 ml of plasma from that donor. The 50 ml of plasma in 10 platelet packs contain equivalent or more clotting factors than fresh frozen plasma. If platelet packs are given it is usually unnecessary to give FFP also.

Platelet concentrates may contain the platelets from 8 donors in a single unit. HL-A typing reduces immunization of the recipient and probably results in longer survival of the infused platelets. When facilities for plasmapheresis are available, large quantities of platelets from a single matched donor can be given to one recipient with less destruction from isoimmunization. If platelet transfusions are anticipated over long periods, plasmapheresed platelets are preferred.

D. LEUKOCYTE CONCENTRATES are being used as an aid to control infection in patients with neutropenia.

E. CRYOPRECIPITATE is rich in factor VIII and is specific therapy for patients with hemophilia. Cryoprecipitate can be stored for long periods, and the risk of transmitting hepatitis is low.

F. PLASMA

1. Pool plasma has been removed from the market in the USA because of the high risk of hepatitis and the availability of alternatives.

2. Fresh frozen plasma contains factors V and VIII in normal concentrations, and is frequently used to reverse the coagulopathy of patients receiving massive transfusion.

3. Albumin and plasma protein fraction are used interchangeably as volume expanders and for restoration of colloid oncotic pressure. PPFs may have alpha and beta globulins as well as albumin. Both products are stored at 60° C for 10-12 hours to eliminate the risk of hepatitis.

These products are being used less frequently than previously, because of lack of advantage over crystalloid solutions and greater expense.

G. METABOLIC CONSEQUENCES OF TRANSFUSION

1. Hyperkalemia. Stored blood is acidic and hyperkalemic, but transfusion seldom causes hyperkalemia in the recipient. Transfused citrate is rapidly metabolized to yield bicarbonate, and metabolic alkalosis is the result. Metabolic alkalosis in the presence of sodium retention after injury contributes to renal excretion of potassium.

2. Loss of 2,3-DPG. Deterioration of 2,3-DPG in preserved red cells results in blood in which hemoglobin has a high affinity for oxygen. The deleterious effects of transfusion of such blood into hypoxic, hypotensive patients may be more theoretical than real, perhaps because 2,3-DPG values are restored to normal within 12-24 hours after transfusion.

3. Hypothermia is a common complication of massive transfusion of liquid blood stored at 4° C. Hypothermic patients are less able to metabolize acid and potassium; further, hypothermia increases the affinity of hemoglobin for oxygen, thus adding to the possible consequences of low 2,3-DPG values. Blood should be warmed before administration; commercial blood warmers are frequently unable to cope when large volumes of blood must be given rapidly.

4. Hypocalcemia. Citrate is a chelating agent that binds ionized calcium in the recipient and is a potential cause of hypocalcemic cardiac arrhythmia. Normothermic adults can metabolize the citrate contained in 1 unit of blood every 5 minutes without the need for exogenous calcium. However, because calcium is so essential and because ionized calcium is difficult to measure, the current recommendation is to give 13.5 mEq of calcium for every 5 units of blood if that amount of blood must be transfused in less than 30 minutes. Hypercalcemia is potentially lethal, and calcium administration should be monitored carefully with a continuous ECG.

5. Defective hemostasis is a complication of massive transfusion, although the exact mechanism is incompletely defined. The labile factors (V and VIII) are the only coagulation factors that decay to any great extent during preservation of liquid blood. Moreover, in the patient who has been resuscitated adequately, factor VIII levels actually rise to higher than normal because of accelerated manufacture of factor VIII by the liver. Therefore, factor V is the only clotting factor that is significantly lowered by massive transfusion. FFP provides clotting components, but its effectiveness in correcting the hemostatic defect caused by massive transfusion has not been established.

It should be assumed that all blood routinely dispensed from the blood bank lacks functioning platelets. Platelets lose their aggregability in cold storage, and preservatives do not maintain platelet viability beyond 72 hours. In addition, most blood banks with component programs remove the platelets from the donated unit as a routine procedure. Absent or nonfunctioning platelets contribute to posttransfusion bleeding, and the magnitude of the problem is roughly proportional to the number of units of blood administered. It is a good policy to give platelet concentrates (or platelet packs) to patients who receive 10 units of blood or more in less than 1 hour.

H. COMPLICATIONS OF TRANSFUSION. Blood is the most dangerous drug used by most physicians. Complications are common and potentially fatal.

1. Infections. Transmissions of syphilis, malaria, bacteria, viruses, and acquired immune deficiency syndrome (AIDS) are infrequent with current banking practices. **Hepatitis,** however, remains a problem. Blood products carry a hepatitis risk proportional to the number of donors contributing blood to the pool. Recently available assays for hepatitis have greatly reduced the potential of dispensing blood from hepatitis carriers, but most cases of hepatitis which follow transfusion in the United States are not due to hepatitis B or other known viruses and may represent infection by an unidentified hepatocellular virus. The statistical risk of hepatitis is unknown because many cases are subclinical. Blood acquired from volunteer donors has a lower risk than blood from paid donors. AIDS can be transmitted, but current screening methods make AIDS transmission of HIV extremely rare. Hepatitis is a more serious problem (Table 2-12).

2. Isoimmunization. Blood is an allograft, and the recipient may become immunized against HLA antigen, platelet antigens, and red cell antigens.

Reactions to leukocyte antigens are the probable cause of many febrile responses to transfusions. Reactions to transfusions of proteins, especially IgA, are frequently severe and may be hemolytic in nature.

3. Mismatched blood. Administration of blood to the wrong recipient is the most common immunologic complication; usually it is due to incorrect labeling of blood specimens. Massive hemolysis may occur, leading to renal failure and death. Symptoms of early hemolysis are chills, fever, back pains, circulatory collapse, and hemorrhage. Delayed hemolysis occurs from several days to 1 month after transfusion and is manifested by anemia or mild jaundice.

Table 2-12. Risk of transfusion-transmitted infection in general blood supply (i.e., community volunteer donors)

Infection	Risk per unit
HIV	1 in 225,000
Hepatitis B	1 in 200,000
Hepatitis C	1 in 3,300
HTLV-I/II	1 in 50,000
Yersinia enterocolitica, malaria, *Babesia microti, Trypanosoma cruzi*	<1 in 1,000,000

From: Dodd R: The risk of transfusion-transmitted infection, *N Engl J Med* 327:419, 1992.

4. Management of transfusion reactions

a. Stop the transfusion and send the remaining blood to the blood bank for investigation of the appropriateness of the cross match, Rh compatibility, and Coombs test.

b. Maintain hydration.

c. Send samples of plasma and urine for hemoglobin determination; hemoglobin in these fluids implies that hemolysis has occurred.

d. Obtain cultures of the recipient's blood and the donor blood.

e. If a severe reaction has occurred, renal function should be evaluated and protected by giving mannitol and bicarbonate.

f. Febrile reactions, without hemolysis, are treated with antihistamines.

g. Isoimmunized patients who require subsequent transfusions should receive washed red cells.

I. HEMOTHERAPY IN SURGICAL PRACTICE. Surgical patients usually receive blood transfusions for the restoration of red cell mass or blood volume.

1. Preoperative anemia. Anemic patients who are asymptomatic are able to tolerate operations of almost any magnitude if operative blood loss is minimal. If a surgical procedure commonly associated with large losses of blood is planned, anemia should be corrected 1-2 days prior to operation so that the storage-related defects of transfused blood can be restored to normal. Moreover, preoperative transfusion permits transfusion reactions to be detected, a difficult task in an anesthetized patient. Red cell concentrates are preferred for correction of preoperative anemia in stable patients.

2. Postoperative anemia. The need for transfusion to correct postoperative anemia is assessed by measurement of the reticulocyte count; if it is elevated, and if the patient does not have postural hypotension or dyspnea, transfusion is unnecessary. If the reticulocyte count is low, the response to total or parenteral iron should be determined before concluding that transfusions must be given. Chronically ill patients (e.g., those with persistent sepsis) frequently have aregenerative anemia and may require periodic transfusion of blood. Red cell concentrates are recommended for this purpose.

3. Exsanguinating hemorrhage. Whole blood is the transfusion product of choice; red cell concentrates are too viscous to be administered rapidly.

4. Autotransfusion. There are two forms of autotransfusion. In one type, a patient donates blood 2 weeks in advance of elective operation, and this blood is stored for transfusion back into the donor should it be required. This practice permits stimulation of erythropoiesis and results in restoration of red cell mass nearly to normal by the time of operation. A further advantage is the availability of the safest possible blood when the patient needs it (the patient's own blood).

The other kind of autotransfusion is useful in emergencies. Blood lost by the patient is collected into apparatus designed for this purpose, anticoagulated, and returned immediately to the circulation. The method is more complicated than it appears at first glance, and this fact makes autotransfusion impractical for wide use. It is most applicable in cases of bleeding into the pleural space, and it may be life-saving when compatible blood is unavailable. Coagulopathies may develop with reinfusion of large amounts of blood.

METABOLISM AND NUTRITION

George F. Sheldon

Increased attention to nutrition and the development of methods of nutritional support are among the most important surgical advances in recent years. The fundamentals of surgical metabolism and nutrition are discussed briefly in this section. Table 2-13 lists some useful numerical constants. Daily nutritional requirements for normal children and adults are listed in Table 2-14.

A. METABOLIC EFFECTS OF STARVATION AND INJURY

1. Starvation. During a brief period of starvation (<3 days), muscle protein is catabolized to fulfill energy requirements by gluconeogenesis. About 10-15 g of nitrogen are excreted in the urine daily during this phase.

By the end of 2 weeks of starvation, lipolysis has increased seven-fold, and fat is the primary source of energy. Ketosis is present, and the brain and heart adapt to utilize ketones as the energy substrate. Minimal amounts of nitrogen (<2 g daily) are excreted in the urine. The basal metabolic rate is lowered. Death occurs after 2-3 months of total starvation.

During starvation, the provision of small amounts of carbohydrate orally or IV has a remarkable sparing effect on pro-

Table 2-13. Some numerical constants useful in estimates of metabolic changes

Protein catabolized = Urinary nitrogen × 6.25

Wet lean tissue broken down = Urinary nitrogen × 30 or protein × 4.75

Wet lean tissue is assumed to be 73% water and 27% protein

In muscle tissue:
Extracellular potassium = 3.8-4.3 mEq/L

Intracellular potassium = 148-155 mEq/L

Potassium content = 100 mEq/kg wet weight

Zinc content = 58.5 $\mu g/g_N$

Energy considerations:
Caloric equivalents of nutrients:

Carbohydrate = 4 Cal/g	Protein = 4 Cal/g
Fat (triglycerides) = 9 Cal/g	Ethyl alcohol = 7 Cal/g

Respiratory quotient (RQ) = CO_2/O_2 ratio

RQ for oxidation of carbohydrates = 1.00

RQ for oxidation of fat = 0.70

When carbohydrate is being converted to fat, RQ >1.00

On the usual mixed diet, RQ = 0.75-0.85

Basal Metabolic Rate (adults) = 36-41 Cal/m² hour (approx. 1600-1800 Cal/day)

For 1800 Cal energy expenditure, oxygen consumption = 250 ml/minute

Carbohydrate consumption	= 400 Cal (100 g)
Fat consumption	= 1160 Cal (130 g)
Protein consumption	= 240 Cal (60 g)
Total	= 1800 Cal/day

From Way LW, editor: *Current Diagnosis and Treatment,* Jefferson City, MO, Lange E. N. T. Publishing.

tein in the body, and the feeding of a balanced diet results in rapid resynthesis of tissue. These effects are in sharp contrast to those seen in injured patients.

2. Injury. Accidental or planned surgical injury causes profound metabolic alterations that are different from the changes in simple starvation.

The metabolic rate is normal or high, protein catabolism is immediate and rapid, and although oxidation of fat occurs promptly, the body does not adapt to the use of lipid for energy. Infusion of small amounts of glucose has little sparing

Table 2-14. Recommended daily dietary allowances of the Food and Nutrition Board, National Academy of Sciences–National Research Council.* Designed for the maintenance of good nutrition of practically all healthy people in the United States

Age (years)	Energy (kcal)†	Protein (g)	Fat-soluble vitamins A activity (RE)‡	A activity (IU)	D activity (IU)	E activity‖ (IU)	Water-soluble vitamins C (mg)	Fola-cin¶ (µg)	Nia-cin# (mg)	Ribo-flavin (mg)	Thia-mine (mg)	B₆ (mg)	B₁₂ (µg)	Biotin (µg)	Panto-thenic acid (mg)	Minerals** Ca (mg)	P (mg)	I (µg)	Fe (mg)	Mg (mg)	Zn (mg)	Cu (mg)	Mn (mg)
Infants																							
0-0.5	kg × 115	kg × 2.2	420§	1400	400	4	35	30	6	0.4	0.3	0.3	0.5	35	3	360	240	40	10	50	3	0.6	0.6
0.5-1	kg × 105	kg × 2	400	2000	400	5	35	45	8	0.6	0.5	0.6	1.5	50	3	540	360	50	15	70	5	0.6	0.6
Children																							
1-3	1300	23	400	2000	400	5	45	100	9	0.8	0.7	0.9	2	65	3	800	800	70	15	150	10	1	1
4-6	1700	30	500	2500	400	6	45	200	11	1	0.9	1.3	2.5	85	3	800	800	90	10	200	10	1.5	1.5
7-10	2400	34	700	3300	400	7	45	300	16	1.2	1.2	1.6	3	120	5	800	800	120	10	250	10	2	2
Males																							
11-14	2700	45	1000	5000	400	8	50	400	18	1.6	1.4	1.8	3	200	10	1200	1200	150	18	350	15	2	4
15-18	2800	56	1000	5000	400	10	60	400	18	1.7	1.4	2	3	200	10	1200	1200	150	18	400	15	2	4
19-22	2900	56	1000	5000	300	10	60	400	19	1.7	1.5	2.2	3	200	10	800	800	150	10	350	15	2	4
23-50	2700	56	1000	5000		10	60	400	18	1.6	1.4	2.2	3	200	10	800	800	150	10	350	15	2	4
51+	2400	56	1000	5000		10	60	400	16	1.4	1.2	2.2	3	200	10	800	800	150	10	350	15	2	4
Females																							
11-14	2200	46	800	4000	400	8	50	400	15	1.3	1.1	1.8	3	200	10	1200	1200	150	18	300	15	2	4
15-18	2100	46	800	4000	400	8	60	400	14	1.3	1.1	2	3	200	10	1200	1200	150	18	300	15	2	4
19-22	2100	44	800	4000	300	8	60	400	14	1.3	1.1	2	3	200	10	800	800	150	18	300	15	2	4
23-50	2000	44	800	4000		8	60	400	13	1.2	1	2	3	200	10	800	800	150	18	300	15	2	4
51+	1800	44	800	4000		8	60	400	13	1.2	1	2	3	200	10	800	800	150	10	300	15	2	4
Pregnant	+300	+30	1000	5000	600	10	80	800	+2	+0.3	+0.4	2.6	4	200	10	1200	1200	175	18+††	450	20	2	4
Lactating	+500	+20	1200	7000	600	10	100	500	+5	+0.5	+0.5	2.5	4	200	10	1200	1200	200	18	450	25	2	4

*The allowances are intended to provide for individual variations among most normal persons as they live in the United States under usual environmental stresses. Diets should be based on a variety of common foods in order to provide other nutrients for which human requirements have been less well defined.

†Kilojoules (kJ) = 4.2 × kcal.

‡Retinol equivalents.

§Assumed to be all as retinol in milk during the first 6 months of life. All subsequent intakes are assumed to be one-half as retinol and one-half as β-carotene when calculated from international units. As retinol equivalents, three-fourths are as retinol and one-fourth as β-carotene.

‖Total vitamin E activity, estimated to be 80% as α-tocopherol and 20% other tocopherols.

¶The folacin allowances refer to dietary sources as determined by *Lactobacillus casei* assay. Pure forms of folacin may be effective in doses less than one-fourth of the recommended dietary allowance.

#Although allowances are expressed as niacin, it is recognized that on the average 1 mg of niacin is derived from each 60 mg of dietary tryptophan.

**Recommended daily allowances are now available for fluoride, selenium, molybdenum, and chromium.

††This increased requirement cannot be met by ordinary diets; therefore, the use of supplemental iron is recommended.

effect on protein, and oral or IV feedings of protein alone are ineffective because carbohydrate is the preferred source of energy.

Accelerated protein catabolism from trauma, particularly if the injury was a thermal burn or if there is associated sepsis, can result in the loss of 30% of lean body mass within a month if nutritional support is not provided. Lean body mass is protein that is essential for structure and function. If 30%-50% of lean body mass is catabolized to supply energy, death usually ensues.

The consequences of these metabolic changes depend upon the severity and duration of the illness. Routine major operations are followed by a transient phase of protein catabolism, but if food can be taken orally within a few days, metabolism returns toward normal, and the patient recovers. Multiple injuries, sepsis, malignancy, inability to resume eating, malabsorption, and other complications allow the metabolic derangements to persist and worsen.

B. ASSESSMENT OF NUTRITION. Pronounced malnutrition is clinically obvious, but evidence of less severe nutritional deprivation may be subtle.

1. History. Duration of illness, weight loss, eating habits, age, habitus, and economic status are important data in assessing adequacy of nutrition.

2. Hospital course. Hospitalized patients may become nutritionally depleted while undergoing diagnostic or therapeutic procedures. Patients of different nationalities and backgrounds may not eat institutional diets, and they may become malnourished in the hospital.

3. Weight loss reflects changes in body water and/or tissue mass. Weight should be obtained daily during acute illness and at least weekly in more stable disease states.

a. Starvation alone results in the loss of about 0.5 kg/day; in the early stages of starvation, 0.2-0.3 kg of this loss is protein.

b. Stress (infection, injury) increases losses of protein by four- to tenfold.

4. Laboratory tests. Hemoglobin, serum albumin, serum iron, and serum transferrin levels reflect the nutritional state.

Nitrogen balance is a useful test for protein catabolism.

a. Measure urea nitrogen in a 24-hour collection of urine. Add an arbitrary 2 g nitrogen to total urinary loss to allow for unmeasured protein byproducts.

b. Measure the amount of protein taken orally or IV during the same period. Divide the protein by 6.25 to determine nitrogen intake.

c. The nitrogen balance is positive if more nitrogen is taken in than is excreted during the 24-hour period.

C. NUTRITIONAL SUPPORT

1. Indications. Nutritional support should be provided by enteric and/or parenteral feeding if the postoperative or postinjury patient is not expected to resume a normal diet within 5 days. A patient who has lost 10% of body weight or has a serum albumin level <3 g/dl should receive total parenteral nutrition for 2-3 weeks before major elective surgery. Other indications for nutritional therapy are loosely defined; in general, if a question arises about the adequacy of nutrition in an acutely ill patient it is advisable to provide nutritional support.

2. Caloric requirements. Patients' caloric needs should be estimated.

a. About 1800 Cal/day is required to support biochemical functions; <100 Cal/day results in gradual starvation.

b. Add 12% for each degree of fever above 37° C.

c. Allow for caloric expenditure from muscular activity; in general, this raises total requirements to about 2500-3000 Cal/day.

d. Septic or burned patients may need as much as 6000 Cal/day.

e. Malnourished patients, e.g., those about to undergo elective surgery, require 45 Cal/kg/day to establish positive nitrogen balance.

3. Selection of method. If the absorptive surface of the small intestine is intact and functional, enteric feeding is preferred. If caloric requirements exceed what can be delivered into the gut, total parenteral nutrition is necessary.

D. ENTERIC FEEDING (TUBE FEEDING)

1. Diets. Commercially available special liquid diets for tube feeding fall into 3 categories: Complete meal, supplements, and defined formula diets.

a. Meal replacement formulas are products low in residue with approximately 30% of calories as fat and 12%-16% of calories as protein with varying quantities of lactose. In calorically adequate volume, the RDAs for vitamins and minerals are met or exceeded. Added flavoring enhances acceptance for oral use. If unflavored, the osmolalities vary from 300-450 mOsm.

b. Supplements are nutritionally incomplete products administered to increase the intake of one or more nutrients. They may be concentrated sources of a single nutrient, e.g., fat (McToil), or "feeding module" products to increase various components to meet specific requirements (Amin-AID).

c. Defined formula diets usually are clear liquid, contain minimal residue, and are lactose free. Protein content varies from 8%-16% of total calories, and carbohydrate varies from 50%-90% of calories. If provided in sufficient volume, the RDAs for vitamins and minerals are met.

2. Insertion of tube. A polyethylene feeding tube (2-3 mm in diameter) and a 16 Fr nasogastric tube are introduced together, with the tips of both tubes inserted into one gelatin capsule. Recently, weighted Silastic tubes have become available and have the advantage of increased comfort as well as the ease with which they enter the jejunum. After tubes have been passed through the nose into the stomach, wait 30 minutes for the capsule to dissolve, then remove the nasogastric tube. Tape the feeding tube to the side of the face.

3. Technic of administration

a. Begin tube feeding with a balanced or low-residue diet. Dilute the formula to one third Cal/ml and infuse at the rate of 50 ml/hour. After 500 ml have been given, aspirate the contents of the stomach; if most of the administered volume is still in the stomach, reduce the rate of infusion.

b. Tube feedings should be delivered with an infusion pump at a constant rate over 24 hours. Boluses of fluid often cause vomiting and aspiration.

c. Observe the patient for glycosuria, gastric distention, and diarrhea. If the patient tolerates the dilute formula, increase the concentration to two thirds Cal/ml and then to 1 Cal/ml—the maximal concentration tolerated by most patients.

d. Maintain a balance sheet to record the amounts of fluid and calories administered. It is seldom possible to deliver >300 Cal daily by tube feeding. Larger requirements must be met by supplementary parenteral nutrition.

4. Other enteric routes

a. Tube gastrostomy is useful for prolonged feeding in patients with neurologic disease or other causes of inability to swallow.

b. Tube jejunostomy is constructed by inserting a 14 Fr catheter into proximal jejunum. "Needle" jejunostomy catheters have the disadvantage of small lumens that plug easily. If operation is performed for another purpose, a jejunostomy can be established at the same time; this is recommended if the need for nutritional support is anticipated. In general, the availability of TPN makes it unnecessary to operate solely to construct a feeding jejunostomy.

5. Dietary supplements. Commercially available preparations can be used to supplement the diets of patients who are eating food but need to take in more nutrition than is provided by standard hospital diets. Examples are Citrotein, Lanolac, Meritene, and Sustecal.

E. TOTAL PARENTERAL NUTRITION (TPN) (also termed IV hyperalimentation) is the IV administration of solutions containing amino acids and large amounts of calories in the form of fat and carbohydrate.

1. Clinical application of TPN is empirical and is used in the treatment of many illnesses that are complicated by nutritional deprivation, enhanced catabolism, or loss of GI function. Prevention of muscle breakdown, rather than treatment of fully developed malnutrition, is the goal in patients who are well-nourished when the illness or injury strikes.

2. Solutions. Table 2-15 lists the composition of typical TPN solutions; these should be prepared by a trained pharmacist under a laminar flow hood.

Table 2-15. Average daily composition of adult TPN solution*

Water	2500-3000 ml	Protein (amino acids)	100-130 g
Nitrogen	18-20 g	Carbohydrate (dextrose)	525-625 g
Kilocalories	2500-3000	Sodium	125-150 mEq
Potassium	75-120 mEq	Phosphorus	20-25 mEq/1000 kcal
Magnesium	4-8 mEq	Calcium	13.5 mEq
Zinc	5 mg/L	Copper	2 mg/L
Manganese	1 mg	Chromium	20 μg

*Trace metal additives are a routine part of TPN. Zinc and copper should be administered as routine and adjusted on the basis of abnormal needs, losses, and serum values. Chromium and manganese are added when the duration of TPN exceeds 40 days or for patients on home hyperalimentation.

a. Protein. Commercially available protein sources are either hydrolysates of casein or fibrin (supplied as 5% or 10% solutions) or synthetic L-amino acids (prepared as 3.5%-8.5% solutions). The hydrolysates contain large amounts of oligo-peptides and various amounts of nonessential amino acids. Except for the conditions described below, any of the preparations may be used with no particular advantage of one over another.

b. Dextrose is added to the protein base in concentrations of 20%-50%. Nitrogen balance is a function of the calorie:nitrogen ratio in the solution. This ratio should be 100-150:1 nonprotein Cal/g of nitrogen in most patients who receive TPN.

c. Electrolytes and vitamins are added to the desired concentrations. Usually "maintenance" electrolyte concentrations are insufficient for a malnourished patient.

d. Special considerations. Patients in acute renal failure are both catabolic and unable to excrete urea. TPN decreases urea production by providing amino acids and dextrose. Because hydrolysates contain excess nitrogen, a solution of amino acids (preferably essential amino acids, e.g., Nephramine) should be used instead. Limitations on the amount of fluid that can be safely infused in renal failure are met by increasing the dextrose concentration to 50%. A calorie:nitrogen ratio of 800-900:1 is required to suppress urea formation.

Patients with hepatic disease should receive amino acid solutions, because the protein hydrolysates provide excessive nitrogen.

3. Technic of administration

a. TPN should be administered into a large central vein because the solutions are hypertonic. **Subclavian vein** is the preferred site. Sterile precautions should be observed during percutaneous insertion of the catheter. Povidone-iodine ointment is applied after insertion, and the area is dressed sterilely. The catheter site should be inspected under aseptic conditions and cleansed with povidone-iodine solution every other day.

b. The IV tubing should contain a bacterial filter, and the tubing connecting the bottle to the subclavian catheter should be changed daily. The tubing used for delivery of TPN must **not** be used for any other purpose (e.g., drawing blood samples, administration of drugs). A constant infusion pump is recommended for administration.

c. Studies to be obtained before starting TPN and parameters to monitor are listed in Table 2-16.

d. The amount of glucose infused should be increased gradually. One method is to keep the dextrose concentration constant in the TPN solution and slowly increase the volume of solution. A recommended program of this type is to give 2 liters of solution containing 25% dextrose each day for 3 days initially, then increase the volume as the patient's condition warrants. Additional fluid should be given through a periph-

---

Table 2-16. Monitoring protocol for total parenteral nutrition

1. Baseline studies before starting TPN:

Hemoglobin	Fasting blood sugar	SGOT
Hematocrit	BUN	Alkaline phosphatase
Red blood cell indices	Creatinine	Platelet count
	Cholesterol	Na^+ Ca^{2+}
Uric acid	Triglycerides	K^+ PO_4^{3-}
Total protein	Serum osmolality	Cl^- Mg^{2+}
Albumin	CO_2	Bilirubin
Prothrombin time	Serum iron and iron-	Chest radiograph
Urinalysis	binding capacity	
ECG		

2. Daily studies until the patient is stabilized (5-7 days):
Fractional urine for glucose every 6 hours (with simultaneous blood glucose determinations for the first 24-48 hours)
Blood glucose in the afternoon to correlate with urine sugar
Serum electrolytes
Accurate records of intake and output
Body weight
Nitrogen balance

3. Routine studies after the patient is stabilized:
Daily: Intake and output, body weight, fractional urines for glucose 2-3 times weekly; electrolytes (Na^+, K^+, Cl^-, CO_2).
Once weekly: Complete platelet count, prothrombin time, BUN, serum creatinine, calcium, phosphorus, red blood cell indices.
Once monthly: Repeat baseline studies and also measure serum vitamin B_{12} and folate.

4. Measurement of nitrogen balance indicates whether anabolism has been achieved. If the patient is not gaining weight, oxygen consumption may be measured to calculate caloric needs.

eral vein to meet basal fluid requirements until the volume of TPN solution reaches about 3000 ml/day.

e. Do not discontinue TPN suddenly; taper the infusion gradually over 12 hours to avoid hypoglycemia

4. Mechanical complications. Complications of inserting subclavian catheters include air embolism, hemothorax, pneumothorax, hydrothorax, and injury to any of the other structures in the vicinity of the subclavian vein.

5. Septic complications. With strict aseptic precautions, incidence of infection in the IV catheter is about 3%. If fever develops, IV catheter should be removed and cultures should be obtained of catheter tip, TPN solution, and blood. Another catheter should be inserted in a new site 48 hours later, and new solution and tubing should be used. Indiscriminate use of antibiotics contributes to fungemia (e.g., candidiasis). See Table 2-17.

6. Metabolic complications

a. Hyperosmolar nonketotic dehydration and coma is the result of infusion of dextrose at a rate which exceeds the ability of endogenous insulin to cope with it. Careful monitoring of glucose in blood and urine avoids this complication; if glycosuria appears, measure blood osmolarity. About 15% of patients receiving TPN require exogenous insulin; it is added directly to the solution. Diabetics can receive TPN safely. Sudden hypoglycemia in a previously stable patient suggests resistance to insulin caused by infection; chromium deficiency may also be responsible.

Table 2-17. Indications for removal of TPN catheter

Relative indications

Fever

Glycosuria

Persistent sepsis after apparently adequate treatment for an infection unrelated to the TPN

Appearance of *Candida* infections at sites unrelated to the TPN catheter

Contamination of the TPN line

Absolute

Septicemia or septic shock

Proved or suspected infection at the catheter insertion site *b. Azotemia* results from administering hypertonic solutions to dehydrated patients or infusing a solution with a low (<50:1) calorie:nitrogen ratio. Azotemia from osmotic dehydration may occur if the infusion is too rapid.

c. Electrolyte abnormalities can develop from the intracellular shift of potassium, magnesium, phosphate, and calcium as anabolism begins. Hyperkalemia results from acidosis or sudden cessation of the infusion. Hypocalcemia is unusual if calcium is given routinely. Hypercalcemia occurs if excessive amounts of vitamin D are administered.

d. Hypophosphatemia. Deficiency of inorganic phosphate develops within 10 days after starting TPN if supplemental phosphate is not provided. Hypophosphatemia decreases levels of ATP and 2,3-DPG in red cells and causes impaired delivery of oxygen to tissues. The problem is prevented by including 20-25 mEq of phosphate/1000 Cal in the TPN solution.

7. Home parenteral nutrition. Chronic TPN in ambulatory patients is available at several centers. Patients with short bowel syndrome are prime candidates; they can receive TPN at home through a special type of subclavian catheter (Hickman or Broviac shunt). Solution is infused at night or around the clock, depending upon the patient's requirements. Special training and surveillance of these patients are essential.

F. INTRAVENOUS FAT EMULSION (Intralipid 10%) is prepared from soybean oil. Recently, a 10% safflower emulsion has become available. IV fat as safflower or soybean can be considered generic. A 20% soybean emulsion is now available and provides a higher calorie density than the 10% emulsion. Fat should provide 2-4% of daily calories to prevent EFAD. EFAD may be avoided by giving 10% fat 3 times a week. Fat as the primary energy source is used for neonates and for patients with respiratory insufficiency. Patients with respiratory insufficiency may develop hypercapnia from hypertonic glucose infusion and are better treated with fat while being withdrawn from mechanical ventilators.

IV fat emulsion contains 11 Cal/g and can be infused through a peripheral vein. Intralipid should not comprise >60% of the daily caloric input. The principal use of this preparation is to prevent deficiency of essential fatty acid which begins 3 days after initiation of TPN and is clinically evident within 10 days. Patients who receive TPN should be given 500 ml of Intralipid 10% every other day for this reason.

3

Anesthesia

Martin S. Bogetz
Barbara S. Gold

The anesthesia care team consists of physician anesthesiologists, anesthesia residents, nurse-anesthetists, and anesthesia assistants. Traditionally, the team's responsibility begins with the preoperative visit and ends after the patient has completely recovered from the anesthetic and any postanesthetic complications. The field of anesthesia has expanded its focus to include acute pain management after surgery.

Increasingly, members of the anesthesia team are caring for patients, especially children, outside the operating room. The quality of sophisticated diagnostic tests such as CT and MRI scans demands that the patient remain motionless. Children (and some adults) benefit from monitored anesthesia care (conscious sedation) or general anesthesia in this setting. Similarly, more invasive radiologic procedures, radiation therapy, and painful procedures such as bone marrow biopsy and lumbar puncture provide unique opportunities for the anesthesiologist to use his or her expertise to help facilitate needed procedures with minimal psychological harm and pain.

Anesthetic management includes (1) evaluation and preparation of the patient before surgery; (2) familiarity with the action and side effects of anesthetic drugs; (3) ability to competently apply recommended techniques; (4) ability to administer supportive measures as necessary (e.g., maintenance of adequate pulmonary ventilation); and (5) care of the patient in the postanesthetic period.

I. PATIENT EVALUATION

The preoperative visit is an essential component of anesthetic care which enables the anesthesiologist to address the patient's concerns as well as become familiar with the patient's history, physical examination, and laboratory data. Information gathered from this visit is used to formulate the anesthetic plan and anticipate complications. Usually the preoperative visit takes place before the day of surgery. When emergencies arise, a complete and efficient assessment must be made just before surgery.

The American Society of Anesthesiologists (ASA) has developed a scale (range 1-5) for categorizing the relative physical condition of surgical patients. Physical status (PS) 1 patients have no systemic disease; PS 2 patients have mild systemic disturbances; PS 3 patients have severe underlying illness; PS 4 patients have life-threatening disorders; PS 5 patients are moribund.

A. HISTORY. The history should focus on the presence of underlying illness, previous anesthetic experiences, drug use, and allergies. In particular, the cardiovascular and pulmonary systems should be reviewed in detail.

1. Cardiac system
a. Exercise tolerance

b. Anginal pattern; presence of unstable angina; history of myocardial infarction

c. Symptoms of congestive heart failure

d. Arrhythmias (palpitations, syncope)

e. Valvular disease; mitral valve prolapse; need for prophylactic antibiotics

f. Hypertension; degree of control

g. Transient ischemic episodes; history of cerebrovascular accident

2. Pulmonary system
a. Exercise tolerance

b. Obstructive versus restrictive disease; results of pulmonary function tests and arterial blood gases

c. Presence of wheezing; baseline pulmonary examination

d. History of bronchospasm; use of bronchodilators and/or corticosteroids

e. Recent pulmonary infections; change in sputum character or production

3. History of previous anesthetics and complications

4. Family history of anesthetic-related problems (e.g., malignant hyperthermia, nausea)

5. Drugs. In general, most drugs should be continued up

to the time of surgery. Drugs that can have an effect on anesthetic management include:

a. CNS depressants. Sedatives, amphetamines, narcotics, and ethanol may alter anesthetic requirement.

b. Psychotropic drugs. Phenothiazines, MAO inhibitors, and tricyclic antidepressants may predispose to intraoperative hypotension, arrhythmias, and reactions with narcotics (see below).

c. Diuretics. Patients taking diuretics can be hypokalemic. They also may become hypotensive during induction of anesthesia owing to relative intravascular volume depletion. Diuretics are often omitted the day of surgery.

d. Corticosteroids. Chronic steroid use impairs the physiologic response of the adrenal cortex to perioperative "stress." Such patients often receive additional "stress doses" of hydrocortisone perioperatively.

e. Insulin. Management of the insulin-dependent diabetic patient depends on many factors. These include the individual's normal degree of control, the nature of the surgical procedure, the type of anesthetic, the time of day, and the expectation for renewed food intake after surgery. All options involve monitoring the blood glucose level at appropriate intervals. Depending on these factors, insulin can be continued, given in a smaller dose, given as needed, or given as a continuous infusion.

6. Drug allergies and side effects and untoward responses to drugs (e.g., nausea from narcotics)

7. Smoking history. Presence of bronchospasm, chronic obstructive pulmonary disease, change in sputum characteristics

8. Last oral intake. Presence of food in the stomach places patients at additional risk for regurgitation and aspiration, which can be fatal. Usually, patients fast for >8 hours ("NPO after midnight") to minimize this risk. However, pain, anxiety, and narcotics may delay gastric emptying. In emergency cases, special techniques such as a rapid intravenous induction of anesthesia coincident with the application of cricoid pressure and immediate endotracheal intubation, or awake intubation, are used to decrease the possibility of aspiration. Given the evidence that clear liquids leave the stomach very quickly, children have recently been allowed to drink clear liquids (e.g., water, tea, filtered juice) until 2-3 hours before surgery. Liberalization of clear liquid intake may become acceptable for teenagers and adults in the near future.

B. PHYSICAL EXAMINATION. Although the physical examination should be comprehensive, special attention should be placed on:

1. Airway. Conditions such as superior larynx, short neck, limited neck flexion/extension, abnormal dentition, or small mouth opening may make mask ventilation and tracheal intubation difficult. If the faucial pillars and uvula cannot be seen with the patient in the sitting position with the tongue protruding, direct laryngoscopy is likely to be difficult.

2. Cardiac system. Congestive heart failure, arrhythmias, and diminished cardiac reserve may affect choice of anesthetic technique, intensity of monitoring, and intensity of postoperative care.

3. Pulmonary system. Wheezes, rales, and labored breathing should be treated preoperatively to reduce the likelihood of intraoperative and postoperative respiratory complications.

4. Body habitus, presence of physical deformities, and obesity influence anesthetic management. This is especially important for safe positioning of the patient during anesthesia and surgery. For example, obese patients may require a rapid intravenous induction and intubation owing to their increased risk of aspiration. Patients with kyphoscoliosis may require postoperative ventilatory support. If spinal or epidural anesthesia is contemplated, patients should be examined for spinal deformities and skin lesions at the site of needle insertion.

5. Neurologic. A baseline neurologic examination should be established on all patients before receiving anesthesia. This is especially important in patients who are to receive regional anesthesia.

C. LABORATORY TESTS. The patient's history and physical examination are the most important determinants for laboratory tests before surgery. Screening batteries of laboratory tests provide little benefit given their great cost. Nevertheless, hospital and state requirements for laboratory tests need to be checked as the trend away from screening tests proceeds.

D. AMBULATORY SURGERY. More than 50% of all surgical procedures are now performed on an outpatient basis. In the past, only patients in good health undergoing simple surgical procedures were considered candidates for outpatient surgery. Now, patients at the extremes of age and those with substantial medical illness are successfully having relatively straightforward surgery on an outpatient basis. To qualify for ambulatory surgery, the patient must be able to follow perioperative instructions, have a responsible escort and caretaker after surgery, and have access to emergency care.

II. PATIENT PREPARATION

A. PSYCHOLOGICAL PREPARATION. The preoperative visit, when conducted in an unhurried, informative, and reassuring manner, is important for the patient's psychological preparation. Questions should be answered in appropriate depth and the anesthetic plan should be agreeable to both anesthesiologist and patient. Many believe that the personal interview is invaluable for reducing preoperative anxiety.

B. MEDICAL PREPARATION. In order to minimize risk, patients should be in their best possible medical condition before proceeding with anesthesia and surgery. However, consideration must be given to issues such as the urgency of the proposed procedure and the limitations of access to the health care system. Except in the case of extreme emergency, conditions that should be treated prior to induction of anesthesia include shock, hypovolemia, electrolyte imbalance, heart failure, unstable angina, diabetic ketoacidosis, and acute respiratory infections. Patients who have had a complicated myocardial infarction within 6 months before surgery may be at an increased risk for reinfarction. Consequently, elective surgery should be deferred for 6 months following a complicated myocardial infarction. Elective surgery should also be postponed during pregnancy, especially during the first trimester, because of the possible teratogenicity of anesthetics and risk of spontaneous abortion.

C. PREMEDICATION. Although a thorough and reassuring preoperative visit often allays a patient's concerns, premedication is a useful adjunct for minimizing preoperative anxiety, producing amnesia, and decreasing autonomic reflexes. Such drugs are often administered intravenously just before the patient is moved to the operating room. After premedication, the patient should be drowsy but cooperative with minimal respiratory depression. Some undesirable side effects of premedication are respiratory depression and delirium. Commonly used premedicants include:

    1. Benzodiazepines (midazolam IV, diazepam PO, triazolam PO) produce sedation and amnesia and allay anxiety but are not analgesic.

2. Barbiturates (pentobarbital, secobarbital) produce sedation but no analgesia.

3. Narcotics (morphine, meperidine, fentanyl, methadone) produce analgesia and some sedation.

4. Anticholinergics (atropine, glycopyrrolate, scopolamine) are given to dry secretions and blunt vagal responses.

III. SELECTION OF ANESTHETIC TECHNIQUES

A. COMMONLY USED TECHNIQUES

1. General anesthesia with or without tracheal intubation

2. Regional anesthesia (e.g., spinal, epidural, axillary block, IV regional)

3. Local anesthesia with or without sedation/analgesia (monitored anesthesia care)

B. FACTORS AFFECTING THE CHOICE OF TECHNIQUE

1. Patient preference. Some patients, for example, are adamantly opposed to regional anesthesia and prefer to be unconscious, or vice versa.

2. Surgical requirements. Site of procedure, patient position, duration of procedure, expected blood loss, fluid shifts, open body cavities.

3. Coexisting medical conditions. Sepsis, neurologic deficit, or impaired coagulation status may preclude regional anesthesia.

4. Expertise of the individual anesthesiologist or surgeon.

5. Discharge plan. Ambulatory surgery requires technics that produce relatively rapid recovery with minimal side effects. In contrast, a critically ill patient undergoing major surgery followed by ventilatory support in the ICU may be heavily sedated on purpose.

IV. GENERAL ANESTHESIA

General anesthesia is a state of drug-induced CNS depression characterized by amnesia, loss of consciousness, analgesia, depression of physiologic reflexes, and depression of muscle tone.

A. MANAGEMENT OF GENERAL ANESTHESIA. The anesthetist balances the depressive effects of anesthetic agents against the physiologic stimulation of surgery. General anesthetics also depress the physiologic responses to hypoxemia, hypercarbia, and hypotension. In general, the higher the dose of anesthetic, the greater the depression. As a result, vital functions of respiration and circulation must be monitored intensively and supported. Unfortunately, no one vital or physical sign reliably reflects the "depth" of anesthesia for all drugs, in all patients, all the time.

B. MONITORING DURING ANESTHESIA

   1. Basic monitoring. The ASA has established standards for basic monitoring during surgery. Except in the event of a direct known hazard (e.g., radiation during radiation therapy), qualified anesthesia personnel are to be continuously present to monitor the patient and provide anesthesia care. Continual evaluation of oxygenation, ventilation, circulation, and temperature is required. The monitors commonly used include a pulse oximeter, oxygen analyzer, spirometer, capnometer, ECG, noninvasive blood pressure device, temperature sensor, and precordial or esophageal stethoscope. When an endotracheal tube is inserted, its correct positioning in the trachea must be verified by clinical assessment and by identification of carbon dioxide in the expired gas.

   2. Invasive (advanced) monitoring. Invasive intravascular monitors include the measurement of cardiac output and central venous, intra-arterial, pulmonary artery, and pulmonary capillary wedge pressures. Two-dimensional transesophageal echocardiography is particularly useful for monitoring cardiac wall motion for ischemic changes, cardiac contractility, ventricular volume, valve function, and air embolism. A Doppler device can also be used to detect venous air embolism when the site of surgery is above heart level (e.g., neurosurgery). Computer-processed EEG devices monitor cerebral function, and evoked potential devices monitor the integrity of somatosensory, auditory, and visual neuropathways. Mass spectrometry or infrared technology permits on-line analysis of carbon dioxide, nitrogen, nitrous oxide, and the volatile anesthetic agents.

C. AIRWAY MANAGEMENT. Anesthetics cause loss of airway tone which can lead to airway obstruction. Signs of airway obstruction are paradoxical chest movement and stertorous breathing. If obstruction is not relieved, hypoxemia, hypercarbia, bradycardia, hypotension, and cardiac arrest occur. Technics of airway management include:

1. Manual. Hyperextension of the neck and anterior displacement of the mandible pull the tongue off the posterior pharynx.

2. Airway devices. Oral or nasal airways can be inserted to force the tongue off the posterior pharynx.

3. "Bag and mask." A tight-fitting face mask connected to an oxygen/anesthetic gas source allows positive pressure to be generated in the airway. This "expands" airway soft tissue and counteracts the collapse of soft tissue that occurs with inspiration.

4. Laryngeal mask. The LM consists of a conventional silicone tracheal tube that has been cut diagonally across to remove the cuff. An elliptical cuff in the shape of a pediatric face mask is attached to the distal end, which can be inflated through a pilot tube. After the patient is anesthetized, the laryngeal mask is inserted into the hypopharynx. Its primary contraindication remains the patient at risk for passive or active regurgitation and aspiration because the LM cannot guarantee a seal against the inhalation of gastric contents or other fluids. An additional advantage of the LM is its use in the failed intubation drill because the LM can often be easily placed in patients who have difficult airways or who cannot have their tracheas intubated by conventional means.

5. Tracheal intubation (Figure 3-1). Cuffed or uncuffed (for children) endotracheal tubes can be inserted through the mouth or nose into the trachea. This provides a direct and reliable connection between the anesthesia machine and the lungs. Tracheal intubation is indicated when (1) ventilation must be manually or mechanically controlled; (2) the nature of surgery does not permit the use of an anesthesia mask (e.g., intraoral); (3) the patient is in the lateral, prone, or head-down position during surgery and the airway is not accessible; (4) muscle relaxants are administered; (5) the patient is at risk for aspiration of gastric contents; or (6) airway obstruction must be overcome.

D. DRUGS FOR GENERAL ANESTHESIA. Modern anesthetic agents produce general anesthesia, usually without causing tissue damage. Many different drugs, classified by their route of administration, are used to produce general anesthe-

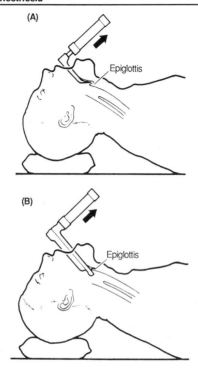

FIGURE 3-1. Schematic diagram depicting proper position of the laryngoscope during direct laryngoscopy for exposure of the glottic opening. **A,** The distal end of the curved blade is advanced into the space between the base of the tongue and pharyngeal surface of the epiglottis (vallecula). **B,** The distal end of the straight blade (Jackson-Wisconsin or Miller) is advanced beneath the laryngeal surface of the epiglottis. Regardless of blade design, forward and upward movement exerted along the axis of the laryngoscope blade, as denoted by the arrows, serves to elevate the epiglottis and expose the glottic opening. (From Stoelting RK: Endotracheal intubation. In Miller RD, editor: *Anesthesia,* Vol 1, 2nd ed., New York, 1986, Churchill Livingston.)

sia. To take advantage of the pharmacodynamics and pharmacokinetics of the various classes of drugs, a general anesthetic is usually made up of a combination of drugs, rather than only one class.

1. Inhalation anesthesia. Anesthetic gases are delivered to the patient's lungs, where they are taken up by blood and carried to the brain, their primary site of action. These agents also can be administered in subanesthetic concentrations to produce analgesia and amnesia without loss of consciousness. Modern anesthesia machines facilitate the administration of known amounts of the anesthetic agents and have safety systems to prevent the administration of a gas mixture with insufficient O_2.

a. Nitrous oxide. N_2O is the most commonly used inhalation agent. It has no odor and a rapid onset and offset. Consequently, it is commonly used when anesthesia is induced with an inhalation agent rather than IV (e.g., in children). Although it is an excellent analgesic, it does not reliably produce "sleep" or amnesia at its limit of useful concentrations, i.e., 70%. Consequently, more potent volatile anesthetics, such as halothane, enflurane, and isoflurane, or IV drugs, are usually combined with N_2O to reliably produce anesthesia. N_2O is particularly contraindicated when a high concentration of inspired O_2 is necessary and when air is present in an enclosed space, such as in cases of pneumothorax and intestinal obstruction.

b. Volatile inhalational anesthetics. At present, 3 common inhalation anesthetics are 50-100 times more potent than N_2O in producing general anesthesia. Halothane, enflurane, and isoflurane are volatile liquids that are vaporized in the anesthesia machine and delivered to the lungs by the carrier gas, usually a combination of O_2 and N_2O. In contrast to N_2O, they are excellent amnesiacs but relatively poor analgesics. Each has a pungent odor, which can be objectionable to the patient and irritating to the airway. Although each agent has different pharmacokinetics and pharmacodynamics, given in a large enough dose, all eventually cause respiratory and cardiovascular depression. Halothane is commonly given to children because it causes less airway irritation and children are very rarely affected by its metabolites. Isoflurane is commonly given to adults because it is minimally metabolized. Two new volatile anesthetics, desflurane and sevoflurane, are undergoing clinical trials at present.

2. Intravenous anesthetics. Intravenous agents are commonly used to induce anesthesia because of their rapid onset. Intravenous access is an obvious prerequisite. Agents can be administered as a bolus, intermittently, or by continuous infusion.

a. Sedative-hypnotics

(1) *Barbiturates.* Thiopental (Pentothal), thiamylal (Surital), and methohexital (Brevital) are administered to induce, and sometimes to maintain, general anesthesia. Side effects include pain at the IV site, involuntary muscle movement, respiratory depression, tachycardia, and cardiac depression.

(2) *Propofol.* This relatively new drug is an alkylphenol that is virtually insoluble in water. Its solubilization in an intralipid emulsion gives it its characteristic milklike appearance. The drug is rapidly redistributed and eliminated, making it very short acting and especially useful in the outpatient setting. Side effects include pain at the IV site, involuntary muscle movement, respiratory depression, and cardiac depression.

(3) *Benzodiazepines.* Midazolam, triazolam, and diazepam are administered before surgery to reduce anxiety and produce amnesia. They can also be used to accomplish the same goal during surgery under local or regional anesthesia. Midazolam is water-soluble and causes less irritation than diazepam during injection. Both are respiratory depressants, especially when given with narcotics. Flumazenil can be administered to antagonize unwanted side effects or an overdose.

b. Narcotics.

Morphine, meperidine, and fentanyl are administered to provide analgesia during and after surgery. The shorter-acting narcotics, sufentanil and alfentanil, are commonly administered as continuous infusions during surgery. Even in high doses, narcotics must be combined with a sedative-hypnotic agent or volatile anesthetic to reliably produce amnesia. Respiratory depression and nausea are the common side effects. Naloxone can be used to antagonize unwanted side effects or an overdose.

c. Ketamine.

Ketamine is a "dissociative" anesthetic that produces a unique and characteristic state of analgesia and amnesia. This state has the appearance of mild sedation because of intact body tone, movement, and the tendency to vocalize to pain. Ketamine is most often administered when the patient is uncooperative, e.g., a mentally handicapped adult or an extremely uncooperative child. It causes little respiratory and cardiovascular depression, but it may produce copious oral secretions that can be reduced by pretreatment with an anti-cholinergic.

3. Muscle relaxants. Muscle relaxants are administered during anesthesia to facilitate endotracheal intubation, provide optimal operating conditions, and prevent patient movement in critical situations.

a. Depolarizing drugs. Succinylcholine is used to facilitate tracheal intubation, but it can be given as a continuous infusion to maintain muscle relaxation. Its major attribute is its rapid onset. Side effects include bradycardia with repeated administration, myalgias, myoglobinuria, excessive intracellular potassium release when the myoneural junction is abnormal (after burn injury), and the potential to trigger malignant hyperthermia.

b. Nondepolarizing drugs. These drugs are also used to facilitate tracheal intubation and maintain muscle relaxation. Pancuronium, doxacurium, *d*-tubocurarine, metocurine, atracurium, vecuronium, and mivacurium are the drugs in use currently. Volatile anesthetics potentiate the action of these drugs, and their dosage must be guided by clinical signs and a neuromuscular stimulator.

c. Antagonism of nondepolarizing drugs. Nondepolarizing muscle relaxant drugs are antagonized by the cholinesterase inhibitors edrophonium and neostigmine. To minimize the muscarinic effects of these drugs, atropine or glycopyrrolate is given. Before the trachea is extubated, adequate antagonism must be assessed by the use of a neuromuscular stimulator and clinical signs of sustained muscle strength, e.g., head lift and hand grip.

E. COMPLICATIONS OF GENERAL ANESTHESIA

1. Hypoxemia. Hypoxemia is the commonest cause of serious anesthesia-related morbidity and mortality.

a. Signs. The early signs of hypoxemia, e.g., tachycardia and hypertension, may be suppressed by anesthetics or misinterpreted as "light" anesthesia. Skin and blood color are insensitive indicators of hypoxemia. Late signs include bradycardia, hypotension, and cardiac arrest. The pulse oximeter is an excellent noninvasive monitor to detect oxyhemoglobin desaturation.

b. Etiology

(1) *Inadequate oxygen delivered to lungs.* Esophageal intubation, oxygen supply failure, blocked endotracheal tube, breathing circuit disconnection

(2) *Hypoventilation*
(a) *Upper airway obstruction.* Relaxation of the tongue muscles, foreign material, laryngospasm, obstructed endotracheal tube
(b) *Lower airway obstruction.* Foreign material within tracheobronchial tree (e.g., blood, secretions), bronchospasm, mucosal edema, tension pneumothorax, mediastinal tumor
(c) *Drug depression.* Anesthetics and muscle relaxants
(3) *Intubation of a mainstem bronchus*
(4) *Pulmonary disorders.* Atelectasis, aspiration, bronchospasm, pulmonary edema, pulmonary embolism
(5) *Decreased cardiac output.* Low mixed-venous oxygen content
(6) *Extrapulmonary mechanical disorders.* Pneumothorax and abdominal distention

2. Physical injury during surgery. The unconscious patient cannot protect himself or herself from physical harm. Meticulous attention must therefore be paid to positioning during surgery to prevent nerve injury caused by stretching or compression. Patients must be electrically grounded properly and electrical equipment maintained to prevent electrical burns and shock. More common, but less serious, injuries include damage to teeth and lips during tracheal intubation.

V. REGIONAL ANESTHESIA

Regional anesthesia involves reversibly blocking nerve conduction, either centrally (e.g., spinal, epidural) or peripherally (e.g., plexus block, single nerve block, intravenous regional block, local infiltration). Regional anesthesia is versatile because it can be used as the sole anesthetic, as an adjunct to general anesthesia, or as a method of providing pain relief after surgery.

A. AGENTS. Local anesthetics used for regional anesthesia produce reversible blockade of nerve conduction without causing permanent damage. The most useful drugs have a high therapeutic index; i.e., the therapeutic dose is much less than the toxic dose. There are two chemical types of local anesthetics: esters (metabolized in the plasma) and amides (metabolized in the liver). The choice of which local agent to use depends on the type of regional block, the length of time anesthesia is needed (duration of surgery) or desired (pain relief after surgery), and the anticipated amount of drug necessary for the anesthetic (Table 3-1).

B. TOXICITY. The central nervous system (CNS) is most affected by a toxic level of local anesthetic.

1. Signs of toxicity

a. Early. Lightheadedness, numbness of the tongue, slurred speech

b. Late. Visual and auditory disturbances, muscle twitching, convulsions, coma

2. Types of toxic reactions

a. Immediate reactions are due to direct or near-direct intravascular injection. This can be minimized by aspirating for blood before and during any injection of local anesthetic. If the anesthetic solution contains epinephrine (1:200,000 or 5 μg/ml), an increase in heart rate within 20 seconds of injection indicates intravascular injection.

b. Delayed reactions (5-15 minutes) are due to absorption of the anesthetic. This can be minimized by the use of a vasoconstrictor (epinephrine) and administering less than the toxic dose.

c. Reaction to the vasoconstrictor is manifested by hypertension, tachycardia, headache, and apprehension. It is caused by intravascular injection or absorption of the vasoconstrictor (epinephrine). Treatment is sedation and time.

d. Vasovagal reactions are characterized by bradycardia, hypotension, pallor, and faintness. Ephedrine is given for treatment.

e. Allergic reactions can be immediate and are almost always associated with an ester type of anesthetic. The allergen PABA is a common metabolite of the ester-type drugs. Furthermore, methylparaben (chemically similar to PABA) is the preservative used in multidose preparations of all types of local anesthetics. Preservative-free solutions of amide anesthetics should be used when the patient is allergic to ester anesthetics. Anaphylaxis is the most serious allergic reaction and is treated with epinephrine and IV fluids.

3. Factors associated with toxicity. Because the anesthetic concentration in the CNS is directly related to the concentration in blood, factors that lead to a high blood concentration are more likely to cause CNS toxicity. These factors include type of anesthetic, site of injection (proximity to blood vessels), speed of injection, amount of drug administered, con-

Table 3-1. Local anesthetic agents in common clinical use

Generic name (proprietary)	Main anesthetic utility	Representative commercial preparation	Max dose (mg/70-kg)
Cocaine*	Topical	Bulk powder	200
Benzocaine* (Americaine)	Topical	20% ointment	—
	Topical	20% aerosol	
Procaine* (Novocain)	Infiltration	10 and 20 mg/ml solutions	1000
	Spinal	100 mg/ml solution	
Dibucaine† (Nupercaine)	Spinal	0.667, 2.5, and 5 mg/ml solutions	100
Tetracaine* (Pontocaine)	Spinal	Niphanoid crystals—20 mg/ml	200
	Spinal		
Lidocaine† (Xylocaine)	Infiltration	10 mg/ml solutions	500
	Peripheral nerve blocks	5 and 10 mg/ml solutions	
		10, 15, and 20 mg/ml solutions	
	Epidural	10, 15, and 20 mg/ml solutions	

			Maximum dose (mg)
	Spinal	50 mg/ml solution	
	Topical 2% jelly, viscous		
	Topical	2.5%, 5% ointment	
Chloroprocaine* (Ne-sacaine)	Infiltration	10 mg/ml solution	1000
	Peripheral nerve blockade	10 and 20 mg/ml solutions	
	Epidural	20 and 30 mg/ml solutions	
Mepivacaine† (Carbocaine)	Infiltration	10 mg/ml solution	500
	Peripheral nerve blockade	10 and 20 mg/ml solutions	
	Epidural	10, 15, and 20 mg/ml solutions	
Prilocaine† (Citanest)	Infiltration	10 and 20 mg/ml solutions	900
	Peripheral nerve blockade	10, 20 and 30 mg/ml solutions	
	Epidural	10, 20 and 30 mg/ml solutions	
Bupivacaine† (Marcaine)	Infiltration	2.5 mg/ml solutions	200
	Peripheral nerve blockade	2.5 and 5 mg/ml solutions	
	Epidural	2.5 and 5 mg/ml solutions	
Etidocaine† (Duranest)	Infiltration	2.5 and 5 mg/ml solutions	300
	Peripheral nerve blockade	5 and 10 mg/ml solutions	
	Epidural	5 and 10 mg/ml solutions	

*Ester.
† Amide.

comitant use of a vasoconstrictor (epinephrine, 1:200,000 or 5 μg/ml), and rate of drug clearance and metabolism. The toxic ceiling is slightly raised in sedated patients.

4. General precautions. Administer less than the toxic dose, aspirate before and frequently during injection, communicate with the patient in order to detect early signs of toxicity, and ensure that trained personnel, resuscitative equipment, drugs, oxygen, and suction are immediately available.

5. Monitoring. Verbal conversation with patient, heart rate, ECG, pulse oximetry, blood pressure

6. Treatment. CNS depressant (thiopental, diazepam, or midazolam), oxygen, and airway support (including paralysis and tracheal intubation, if necessary), IV fluids, and vasoactive drugs (atropine, ephedrine).

C. REGIONAL ANESTHETIC TECHNIQUES

1. General precautions. Use aseptic technic, do not inject into infected areas, and aspirate before and during injection. Anticoagulation, generalized sepsis, and skin lesions at the site of injection are contraindications to the use of a regional anesthetic technic. Many patients are given sedatives and/or narcotics during a regional anesthetic. As a result, communication with the patient and physiologic monitoring are essential. The pulse oximeter is a particularly useful monitor in this setting. Supplemental oxygen should be administered if indicated.

2. Topical anesthesia. Readily absorbed local anesthetics (cocaine, lidocaine, tetracaine) are applied to mucosal surfaces such as the nose, mouth, and trachea. Cocaine is unique in that it causes vasoconstriction.

3. Infiltration anesthesia. Local anesthetic (e.g., lidocaine, bupivacaine) is injected *directly into* a wound or surgical site.

4. Field block. Local anesthetic is injected *around* the perimeter of the surgical site.

5. Nerve blocks. Local anesthetic is injected around the peripheral nerve(s) associated with the site of surgery. Correct placement of the needle can be achieved by eliciting paresthesias or using a nerve stimulator.

6. Plexus blocks. A relatively large volume of local anesthetic (e.g., lidocaine, bupivacaine, mepivacaine) is placed in the neurovascular sheath that envelopes proximal nerves.

Examples include axillary, interscalene, and lumbar plexus blocks.

7. Intravenous block (Bier). The affected limb is first exsanguinated by gravity and then by wrapping it with an elastic bandage. Blood is kept out of the limb by a pneumatic double tourniquet. Local anesthetic (e.g., lidocaine 0.5%) is then injected into a peripheral vein in the affected limb. Anesthesia persists until the cuff is deflated (up to 90 minutes).

8. Spinal anesthesia. Local anesthetic (e.g., lidocaine, bupivacaine, tetracaine, procaine) is placed into the CSF using a spinal needle. Because the spinal cord terminates at L2, the needle is usually inserted in the lumbar area at or below the L3,4 vertebral interspace. The site of surgery determines the dermatomal level of anesthesia needed. The level of anesthesia is affected by the baricity of the anesthetic solution (hyperbaric, isobaric, hypobaric) compared with CSF, the position the patient is placed in, and the mass (concentration × volume) of anesthetic administered. The duration of anesthesia is affected by the choice and dose of anesthetic agent, and the use of vasoconstrictor (epinephrine, phenylephrine). **Continuous spinal anesthesia** involves the insertion of a catheter into the CSF, thus permitting the intermittent administration of small doses of anesthetic as demanded by the duration and site of surgery.

9. Epidural. Local anesthetic (e.g., lidocaine, chloroprocaine) is placed into the epidural space in either the lumbar or the thoracic area or through the sacral hiatus (caudal). The dermatomal level of anesthesia is determined by the volume of anesthetic. By carefully choosing the anesthetic concentration and volume, a segmental "band" of analgesia, with minimal muscle relaxation, can be achieved. The anesthetic can be administered as a single dose through the epidural needle, or a catheter can be inserted into the epidural space, thus permitting intermittent or continuous administration of local anesthetic. The latter is most commonly used to provide analgesia during labor and to deliver narcotics for analgesia after surgery. Because a much greater amount of anesthetic is needed for this block vis-à-vis a spinal anesthetic, caution must be exercised so that the drug is not injected into the CSF or into an epidural blood vessel.

10. Physiologic effects of spinal and epidural anesthesia

a. Hypotension is the most common side effect. It is caused by loss of sympathetic "tone" over an area a few segments higher than that of the sensory block. Venous capacitance increases, venous return decreases, and cardiac output decreases. Hypotension is likely if the anesthetic is "high" (e.g., above T3) or the patient is dehydrated or hypovolemic. Similarly, *bradycardia* occurs with the sympathetic block. Hydration before the block and the use of sympathomimetics (ephedrine) before or during the block keep blood pressure and heart rate at an acceptable level.

b. Respiratory. Some patients "sense" their breathing through chest wall movement. When this area becomes anesthetized, such patients may have the sensation of dyspnea. Patients who use their abdominal muscles to facilitate expiration (e.g., asthmatics) may have difficulty breathing during spinal or epidural anesthesia. If sufficient anesthetic enters the CSF surrounding the medulla, respiratory support is necessary. Similarly, if the reticular activating system or the cerebral cortex is exposed to anesthetic, the patient becomes unconscious and respiratory support is necessary.

11. Complications of spinal and epidural anesthesia

a. Post—dural puncture headache is the most common complication of spinal anesthesia, being most common in young women. The headache is due to leakage of CSF through the puncture site, causing traction on pain-sensitive structures when the patient sits or stands. Onset of the headache usually occurs within 24 to 48 hours after dural puncture. With bedrest, most headaches resolve in a few days. When the headache is prolonged or incapacitating, autologous blood can be placed into the epidural space adjacent to the dural puncture site. This "epidural blood patch" is very efficacious. Factors that help to reduce the incidence of post—dural puncture headache include use of the smallest needle practical, piercing the dura with the bevel of the spinal needle parallel to the longitudinal orientation of the dural fibers, and use of a "pencil point" needle. Bed rest does not prevent headache but simply delays its onset. Because the epidural block is performed using a larger needle than a spinal block, inadvertent dural puncture during an epidural block results in a higher incidence (20%-80%) of headache.

b. Nerve injury, transverse myelitis, and arachnoiditis may cause temporary or permanent disability ranging from minor paresthesias to paraplegia. Fortunately rare, injury can be due to direct surgical trauma, contaminants, and drug sensitivity.

VI. CONSCIOUS SEDATION/MONITORED ANESTHESIA CARE

Benzodiazepines, propofol, and narcotics are often used to supplement local anesthesia for surgical procedures. When used appropriately, these agents can reduce patient anxiety and produce mild analgesia, which results in a cooperative and comfortable patient with minimal respiratory depression. These drugs can be administered in small bolus doses and/or given as continuous infusions.

A. BENZODIAZEPINES

1. CNS effects include anterograde amnesia and sedation, which progress to hypnosis and stupor at higher doses. Benzodiazepines inhibit seizure activity. They do not produce analgesia.

2. Respiratory effects. With sedative doses ventilation is slightly depressed, but CO_2 narcosis may occur in patients who have baseline CO_2 retention. Use of benzodiazepines with narcotics can result in apnea.

3. Cardiovascular effects are relatively minor and include a slight decrease in blood pressure and increase in heart rate.

4. Other side effects include lightheadedness, incoordination, ataxia, confusion, slurred speech, headache, blurred vision, nausea, and vomiting. Because the elderly are especially sensitive to benzodiazepines and prone to these side effects, their dose should be reduced by 30%-50%.

5. Antagonism. Flumazenil can be given to antagonize an overdose of benzodiazepine.

B. PROPOFOL.
This relatively new drug is an alkylphenol that is virtually insoluble in aqueous solution. Its solubilization in an intralipid emulsion gives it its characteristic milklike appearance. The drug is rapidly redistributed and eliminated, making it very short acting and especially useful in the outpatient setting. These same properties make it very useful in providing IV sedation. Most commonly, it is administered as a continuous IV infusion.

C. OPIATES

1. Cardiovascular effects

a. Morphine. Cardiovascular effects occur with relatively small doses (e.g., 5-10 mg IV) and include histamine-mediated vasodilatation and consequently hypotension. Hypotensive effects are minimized if patients are in the supine position.

b. Meperidine (Demerol). Hypotension can occur, especially in volume-depleted patients. Meperidine is contraindicated in patients taking MAO inhibitors owing to adverse reactions which include hypotension, coma, cyanosis, and hyperpyrexia.

c. Fentanyl. Although blood pressure usually remains stable, bradycardia may occur.

2. Respiratory effects

a. Respiratory depression is common to all opioids.

b. Peak onset of respiratory depression: morphine, 10-45 minutes; fentanyl, 5-10 minutes

c. Respiratory depression lasts for hours.

d. Factors that promote respiratory depression: old age, use of other sedatives (e.g., diazepam, midazolam)

e. Muscular (especially respiratory) rigidity with fentanyl can be minimized by *slow* intravenous injection.

3. Signs of overdose. Constricted pupils, respiratory depression, hypotension, seizures (especially with meperidine)

4. Antagonism: Naloxone (Narcan)

a. Primary indication: Reverse respiratory depression

b. Dose: 1-2 μg/kg or 0.04-0.08 mg IV; doses may need to be repeated after 5-10 minutes.

c. Side effects: Hypertension, pulmonary edema, arrhythmias, cardiac arrest

d. Half-life of naloxone (1-2 hours) is less than that of fentanyl, morphine, or meperidine (2-4 hours), therefore patients should be observed for renarcotization.

D. MIXED OPIATE AGONISTS/ANTAGONISTS. These agents, such as nalbuphine, butorphanol, and dezocine, are promoted as having limited respiratory depressant effects, but their analgesic effects are also limited.

VII. RECOVERY FROM ANESTHESIA

After surgery, patients are taken to a recovery room, where they are observed and monitored with an intensity proportional to their preexisting health status and surgical procedure. The degree of recovery necessary before discharge from the recovery room depends on whether the patient is returning home (outpatient surgery), to a hospital room, or to an ICU.

A. PROBLEMS DURING RECOVERY

1. Hypoxemia. The availability of the pulse oximeter makes hypoxemia easier to detect in the recovery room. The site of surgery (e.g., thoracic, abdominal) and the residual effects of anesthetic agents (e.g., narcotics, volatile anesthetics, muscle relaxants) combine to adversely affect oxygenation and the physiologic response to hypoxemia. As a result, supplemental oxygen is commonly administered after surgery. Airway obstruction, the most common cause of hypoxemia, can be caused by residual sedation, incomplete reversal of muscle relaxants, and secretions.

2. Hypotension after surgery can be caused by continued hemorrhage, residual effect of anesthetic drugs, residual autonomic block following a spinal or epidural block, cardiac failure, or hypoxemia.

3. Pain after surgery should be anticipated. Narcotic administration or local infiltration with long-acting local anesthetics (e.g., bupivacaine) provides relief.

a. Spinal opiates. With the development of the "postoperative pain management team," narcotics (morphine, fentanyl) can be continuously infused into the epidural or subarachnoid space via an indwelling catheter. This provides excellent pain relief and substantially reduces the dose of narcotic needed. Side effects include pruritus, urinary retention, and most importantly, respiratory depression. As a result, patients must be monitored closely. Small doses of naloxone (1 μg/kg IV) can be given to treat these side effects.

b. Patient-controlled analgesia. After proper instruction, patients can self-administer potent narcotics within dose and time limits controlled by the physician. Although actual drug use is similar to intermittent IM or IV regimens, patients feel that the psychological benefit of being more "in control" is a distinct advantage.

B. DISCHARGE CRITERIA

1. Critically ill patients may be taken directly to an ICU or special care unit such as a neurosurgical or cardiac ICU. Such patients may be heavily sedated so that wakening can occur gradually. Tracheal extubation is delayed until pulmonary function and mental status are sufficient.

2. Surgical inpatients are discharged from the recovery room when vital signs are stable, the wound is intact, the patient is comfortable, and perioperative problems are addressed.

3. Surgical outpatients are discharged from the facility when psychomotor and physiologic status have returned to a level close to that before surgery. Vital signs should be stable and approximate preoperative values. Nausea and pain should be minimal, the surgical site intact and dry, and the patient able to urinate if a spinal or epidural anesthetic was given. A responsible adult must accompany the patient after discharge if anything more than a simple local anesthetic is administered. Postoperative instructions must be communicated and understood.

4

Surgical Infections

I. STERILIZATION AND ANTISEPSIS

Ernest Jawetz
Dennis J. Flora

Protection of the surgical patient from infection is a primary consideration throughout preoperative, intraoperative, and postoperative phases of care. Host resistance, which determines the individual patient's susceptibility to infection, is discussed in Chapter 2. Incidence and severity of infection, particularly wound sepsis, are related also to the hospital environment and to the care with which basic principles of asepsis, antisepsis, and surgical technic are implemented.

A. STERILIZATION. The only completely reliable methods in wide use are steam under pressure (autoclaving), dry heat, and ethylene oxide gas.

1. Autoclaving. Saturated steam at a pressure of 750 mm Hg (15 lb/in^2) at 120° C destroys all vegetative bacteria and most resistant dry spores in 13 minutes. Additional time (usually a total of 30 minutes) must be allowed for penetration of heat and moisture into the centers of packages. Modern high-vacuum or high-pressure autoclaves markedly shorten sterilization time.

2. Dry heat. Exposure to continuous dry heat at 170° C for 1 hour sterilizes articles that would be spoiled by moist heat or are more conveniently kept dry. If grease or oil is present on instruments, safe sterilization calls for 4 hours of exposure at 160° C.

3. Gas sterilization. Liquid and gaseous ethylene oxide destroys all infectious agents and spores. It is also flammable and toxic and causes severe burns if it comes in contact with the skin. This is the method of choice for most materials that cannot withstand autoclaving (e.g., telescopic instruments, plastic and rubber goods, sharp and delicate instruments, electric cords, sealed ampuls). Some materials (acrylics, polystyrene, pharmaceuticals) interact chemically with the ethylene oxide mixture and may be damaged, so alternative methods of sterilization must be used.

Gas sterilization requires 1 hour and 45 minutes in a gas autoclave using a mixture of 12% ethylene oxide and 88% dichlorodifluoromethane (Freon 12) at 55° C and a pressure of 410 mm Hg. Following sterilization, a variable period of time is required for dissipation of the gas from the materials.

4. Boiling. Instruments should be boiled only if autoclaving, dry heat, or gas sterilization are not available. Minimum period for sterilization in boiling water is 3 minutes at altitudes <300 meters. At higher altitudes, the period of boiling must be prolonged.

5. Soaking in antiseptics. Sterilization by soaking is rarely indicated and should never be relied upon if steam autoclaving, dry heat, or gas sterilization is suitable and available. Under some circumstances, it may be necessary to sterilize lenses or delicate cutting instruments by soaking in a liquid germicide such as glutaraldehyde in 2% aqueous alkaline concentration. This solution is bactericidal and virucidal in 10 minutes and sporicidal in 3 hours.

B. ANTISEPSIS. Antiseptics are chemical agents that kill bacteria or arrest their growth; they may or may not be sporicidal. Antiseptics (with the possible exception of the iodophors) must not be placed in wounds because their toxicity to host cells far outweighs the possible advantages of their antibacterial effects.

1. Antiseptics for general purposes are used for cleaning floors, furniture, and operating room equipment and for soaking contaminated articles.

a. Soap solution is an excellent cleansing agent but a weak antiseptic.

b. Phenol compounds. Phenol and creosol are potent bactericidal chemicals but are too caustic for safe use. They have been superseded by synthetic phenolic germicides such as Lamar SP-63, Vestal Vasphene, and Western Polyphene. They kill gram-positive and gram-negative bacteria (including tubercle bacilli) and fungi. Surfaces treated with these compounds may retain antibacterial properties for 10-14 days, but this must not be relied on as a substitute for routine frequent disinfection. Synthetic phenolic compounds, like PBS (below), are compatible with many other anionic and alkaline agents used in hospitals, and they resist deactivation by organic matter.

c. Polybrominated salicylanilide. This class of chemicals is similar to synthetic phenols with respect to antimicrobial spectrum, residual surface action, compatibility with other anionic and alkaline agents, and resistance to deactivation by organic matter. When PBS preparations are used in laundries, textiles take on a self-sanitizing antibacterial finish. A disadvantage of PBS is the white powdery film that remains on metal and other surfaces. PBS is the essential ingredient in Lamar L-300.

d. Iodophors. In these chemicals, iodine is combined with a detergent (Wescodyne, Surgidine) or with polyvinylpyrrolidone (Betadine, Prepodine, Isodine). The toxicity of the iodine is practically eliminated, but surface and skin disinfection is efficient. Iodophors are rapidly diminished in activity by anionic or alkaline materials and are subject to a certain degree of volatilization.

e. Alcohols. 70% ethyl alcohol is a powerful germicide. Isopropyl alcohol should be used as 70%-90% solution. Neither is effective against spores.

f. Quaternary ammonium compounds are less effective and are inactivated by soap and absorbed by fibers. Benzalkonium chloride is the prototype. It has given rise to outbreaks of gram-negative sepsis.

g. Formaldehyde and glutaraldehyde. Aqueous solutions of 40% formaldehyde (20% formalin) are effective but irritating. A combination of 8% formaldehyde (20% formalin) in 70% alcohol is even more rapidly bactericidal and is sporicidal within 3 hours. Glutaraldehyde has the germicidal properties of formaldehyde but has a low tissue toxicity and no irritating odor. Glutaraldehyde in 2% aqueous alkaline concentration (Cidex) is equivalent to 8% formaldehyde in alcohol and is a good agent for soaking instruments.

2. Skin antisepsis. The most important applications are the hand scrub of the operating team and the preparation of the operative field.

a. Skin antiseptics

Tincture of iodine is 1%-2% iodine in 70% ethyl alcohol. It is the most efficient and economical skin antiseptic, but it occasionally causes skin reactions and should not be used on irritated or delicate skin.

Iodophors (see above) are useful for the hand-scrub and for preparation of the operative site in situations in which tincture of iodine is inadvisable.

Hexachlorophene in combination with a detergent (e.g., pHiso-Hex) or soap (Septisol, Gamophen, Dial) is also used for the hand-scrub and sometimes for the operative site. Daily use produces a sustained lowering of the bacterial count on the skin. Four percent chlorhexidine in soap is equally effective and is less toxic than hexachlorophene if absorbed. Alcohol dissolves hexachlorophene and should not be applied to skin if a prolonged surface effect is desired.

b. Hand-scrub. Put on a cap and mask. Wash hands and forearms thoroughly with an iodophor or hexachlorophene preparation. Clean fingernails. Scrub for 8 minutes (5 minutes between clean cases) with a sterile brush, covering the hands and forearms repeatedly. Most institutions use brushes impregnated with antiseptic and packaged individually; it is not possible to change brushes without contaminating the hands, so it is best to use just one brush and add more antiseptic from a dispenser.

Dry with a sterile towel and immediately don gown and gloves aseptically.

c. Preparation of the operative field. Patient should bathe the evening before operation using soap and water. Umbilicus should be cleansed with particular care in abdominal cases, for it can be the repository of dirt.

Shaving is required if hair is present at the operative site. It should be done immediately before operation; if skin is shaved the evening before, folliculitis or infection in nicks and scratches may develop.

After the patient is anesthetized and positioned, the operative site is painted with antiseptic. Tincture of iodine is used in most cases; it is not necessary to remove the iodine with alcohol until the operation is completed. Iodophors are preferable on the face, perineum, or delicate skin (e.g., in small children). Hexachlorophene compounds are used if the patient is sensitive to iodine. 70% alcohol is another alternative in iodine-sensitive patients.

II. ANTIMICROBIAL THERAPY OF SURGICAL INFECTIONS

Ernest Jawetz
Dennis J. Flora

Microbial infection has always been an accompaniment of surgical procedures and has often delayed or prevented successful results. Conversely, localized infections of many types have required surgery for cure. The first major development in the control of infectious complications of surgery was the concept of antisepsis, sterilization of instruments, and asepsis. The second was the development of effective antimicrobial drugs that could be used for the control of infections.

A. PRINCIPLES OF ANTIMICROBIAL CHEMOTHERAPY.
Antimicrobial drugs are never a substitute for sound surgical technic but they can be of help in the management of local infections, and they may be lifesaving in systemic disseminated infections. Improper application of antimicrobials may contribute to patient morbidity and mortality.

1. Selection of an antimicrobial drug on clinical grounds. For optimal treatment of an infectious process, a suitable antimicrobial must be administered as early as possible. This involves a series of decisions:

a. The surgeon decides, on the basis of a clinical impression, that a microbial infection probably exists.

b. Analyzing the symptoms and signs, the surgeon makes a guess at the most likely microorganism causing the suspected infection; i.e., he attempts an etiologic diagnosis on clinical grounds.

c. The surgeon selects the drug most likely to be effective against the suspected organism; i.e., he aims a specific drug at a specific organism.

d. Before starting the drug, the surgeon must secure specimens that are likely to reveal the causative agent by laboratory examination.

e. He observes the clinical response to the prescribed antimicrobial. Upon receipt of laboratory identification of a possibly important microorganism, he weighs this new information against his original empiric choice.

f. The surgeon may choose to change his drug regimen then or upon receipt of further laboratory information on drug susceptibility of the isolated organism. However, laboratory data need not always overrule a decision based on clinical and empiric grounds, especially when the clinical response supports the initial diagnosis and drug selection.

2. Selection of an antimicrobial by laboratory tests. When a pathogen has been isolated from a representative specimen, it is often possible to select the drug of choice on the basis of current clinical experience. A listing of drug choices is given in Table 4-1. At other times, laboratory tests for an-

Text continued on p. 213.

Table 4-1. Drugs of choice for suspected or proved microbial pathogens, 1990–1991
(± = alone or combined with)

Suspected or proved etiologic agent	Drug(s) of first choice	Alternative drug(s)
Gram-negative cocci		
Moraxella (Branhamella) catarrhalis	Amoxicillin-clavulanic acid or TMP-SMZ*	Newer cephalosporins,† erythromycin,‡ tetracycline§
Gonococcus	Ceftriaxone	Penicillin,‖ ampicillin, or amoxicillin + probenecid
Meningococcus	Penicillin‖	Newer cephalosporins,† ampicillin, chloramphenicol
Gram-positive cocci		
Pneumococcus (*Streptococcus pneumoniae*)	Penicillin‖	Erythromycin,‡ cephalosporin,¶ vancomycin
Streptococcus, hemolytic, groups A, B, C, G	Penicillin‖	Erythromycin,‡ cephalosporin,¶ vancomycin
Streptococcus viridans	Penicillin‖ ± aminoglycosides#	Cephalosporin,¶ vancomycin
Staphylococcus, methicillin-resistant	Vancomycin ± gentamicin or rifampin (or both)	TMP-SMZ, ciprofloxacin
Staphylococcus, non–penicillinase producing	Penicillin	Cephalosporin, vancomycin
Staphylococcus, penicillinase-producing	Penicillin-resistant penicillin**	Vancomycin, cephalosporin¶
Streptococcus faecalis (enterococcus)	Ampicillin + gentamicin	Vancomycin + gentamicin

Gram-negative rods

Acinetobacter	Aminoglycoside# ± imipenem	Minocycline, TMP-SMZ*
Bacteroides, oropharyngeal strains	Penicillin,‖ clindamycin	Metronidazole, cephalosporin†¶
Bacteroides, gastrointestinal strains	Metronidazole	Cefoxitin, chloramphenicol, clinda-mycin
Brucella	Tetracycline§ ± streptomycin	TMP-SMZ*
Campylobacter	Erythromycin‡	Tetracycline,§ ciprofloxacin
Enterobacter	TMP-SMZ,* aminoglycoside#	Imipenem, newer cephalosporin†

From Jacobs RA and Jawetz E: In Schroeder S, et al (eds): Current Medical Diagnosis and Treatment, 30th ed. Norwalk, CT, Appleton & Lange, 1991.

*TMP-SMZ is a mixture of one part trimethoprim and five parts sulfamethoxazole.

†Newer cephalosporins (1990) include cefotaxime, cefuroxime, ceftriaxone, ceftazidime, ceftizoxime, and others.

‡Erythromycin estolate is best absorbed orally but carries the highest risk of hepatitis; erythromycin stearate and erythromycin ethylsuccinate are also available.

§All tetracyclines have similar activity against microorganisms. Dosage is determined by rates of absorption and excretion of various preparations.

‖Penicillin G is preferred for parenteral injection; penicillin V for oral administration—to be used only in treating infections due to highly sensitive organisms.

¶Older cephalosporins are cephalothin, cefazolin, cephapirin, and cefoxitin for parenteral injection; cephalexin and cephradine can be given orally.

#Aminoglycosides—gentamicin, tobramycin, amikacin, netilmicin—should be chosen on the basis of local patterns of susceptibility.

**Parenteral nafcillin or oxacillin; oral dicloxacillin, cloxacillin, or oxacillin.

††Oral sulfisoxazole and trisulfapyrimidines are highly soluble in urine; parenteral sodium sulfadiazine can be injected intravenously in treating severely ill patients.

‡‡Antipseudomonal penicillins: ticarcillin, carbenicillin, mezlocillin, azlocillin, piperacillin.

§§First choice for previously untreated urinary tract infection is a highly soluble sulfonamide (see Note *). TMP-SMZ (see Note *) is acceptable.

Continued.

Table 4-1. Drugs of choice for suspected or proved microbial pathogens, 1990-1991
(± = alone or combined with)—cont'd

Suspected or proved etiologic agent	Drug(s) of first choice	Alternative drug(s)
Gram-negative rods—cont'd		
Escherichia coli (sepsis)	Aminoglycoside,# newer cephalosporin†	Ampicillin, TMP-SMZ*
Escherichia coli (first urinary infection)	Sulfonamide,†† TMP-SMZ*	Ampicillin, cephalosporin¶
Haemophilus (meningitis, respiratory infections)	Newer cephalosporin†	Ampicillin and chloramphenicol
Klebsiella	Newer cephalosporins†	TMP-SMZ,* aminoglycoside#
Legionella sp (pneumonia)	Erythromycin‡ ± rifampin	TMP-SMZ*
Pasteurella (*Yersinia*) (plague, tularemia	Streptomycin, tetracycline§	Chloramphenicol
Proteus mirabilis	Ampicillin	Newer cephalosporins,† aminoglycoside#
Proteus vulgaris and other species	Newer cephalosporins†	Aminoglycoside#
Pseudomonas aeruginosa	Aminoglycoside# + antipseudomonal penicillin§§	Ceftazidime or cefoperazone ± aminoglycoside; imipenem ± aminoglycoside; aztreonam
Pseudomonas pseudomallei (melioidosis)	Ceftazidime	Chloramphenicol, tetracycline,§ TMP-SMZ*
Pseudomonas mallei (glanders)	Streptomycin + tetracycline§	Chloramphenicol + streptomycin

Organism	First choice	Alternative(s)
Salmonella	Ceftriaxone	TMP-SMZ,* ciprofloxacin, ampicillin, chloramphenicol
Serratia, Providencia	Newer cephalosporins,† aminoglycoside#	TMP-SMZ*
Shigella	TMP-SMZ*	Ampicillin, tetracycline,§ ciprofloxacin, chloramphenicol
Vibrio (cholera, sepsis)	Tetracycline§	TMP-SMZ*
Gram-positive rods		
Actinomyces	Penicillin||	Tetracycline§
Bacillus (e.g., anthrax)	Penicillin||	Erythromycin‡
Clostridium (e.g., gas gangrene, tetanus)	Penicillin||	Metronidazole, chloramphenicol, clindamycin
Corynebacterium diphtheriae	Erythromycin‡	Penicillin||
Corynebacterium, JK strain	Vancomycin	Ciprofloxacin
Listeria	Ampicillin ± aminoglycoside#	TMP-SMZ*
Acid-fast rods		
Mycobacterium tuberculosis	INH + rifampin + pyrazinamide	Other antituberculous drugs
Mycobacterium leprae	Dapsone + rifampin, clofazimine	Ethionamide
Mycobacterium kansasii	INH + rifampin + ethambutol	Other antituberculous drugs
Mycobacterium avium-intracellulare	Ethambutol + rifampin + clofazimine + ciprofloxacin + amikacin	Other antituberculous drugs

Continued.

Table 4-1. Drugs of choice for suspected or proved microbial pathogens, 1990-1991 (± = alone or combined with)—cont'd

Suspected or proved etiologic agent	Drug(s) of first choice	Alternative drug(s)
Acid-fast rods—cont'd		
Mycobacterium fortuitum-chelonei	Amikacin + doxycycline	Cefoxitin, erythromycin, sulfonamide
Nocardia	Sulfonamide,†† TMP-SMZ*	Minocycline
Spirochetes		
Borrelia (Lyme disease, relapsing fever)	Tetracycline,§ ceftriaxone	Penicillin,‖ erythromycin‡
Leptospira	Penicillin‖	Tetracycline§
Treponema (e.g., syphilis, yaws)	Penicillin‖	Erythromycin,† tetracycline§
Mycoplasmas	Erythromycin‡ or tetracycline§	
Chlamydiae (*C. trachomatis, C. psittaci, C. pneumoniae*)	Tetracycline§	Erythromycin‡
Rickettsiae	Tetracycline§	Chloramphenicol

timicrobial drug susceptibility are necessary, particularly if the isolated organism is of a type that varies greatly in response to different drugs.

Antimicrobial drug susceptibility tests may be done on solid media as 'disk tests,' in broth in tubes, or in wells of microdilution plates. The latter methods yield results expressed as MIC (minimal inhibitory concentration) and the technic can be modified to provide MBC (minimal bactericidal concentration). Values for MIC or MBC may permit a better estimate of the amount of drug required for therapeutic effects.

In general, controlled disk or microdilution tests give valuable results. At times, however, there is a marked discrepancy between the results of the test and the clinical response of the patient treated with the chosen drug. Some possible explanations for such discrepancies are listed below:

a. The organism isolated from the specimen may not be the one responsible for the infectious process.

b. Failure to drain a collection of pus, debride necrotic tissue, or remove a foreign body. Antimicrobials can never replace essential surgical procedures.

c. Sometimes two or more microorganisms participate in an infectious process but only one may have been isolated from the specimen. The antimicrobial drug in use may be effective only against the less virulent organism.

d. Superinfection occurs fairly often in the course of prolonged chemotherapy. New microorganisms may have replaced the original infectious agent. This is particularly common with open wounds or sinus tracts.

e. The drug may not reach the site of active infection in adequate concentration. Certain drugs penetrate poorly into abscesses, the eye, or pleural space unless injected locally. Other drugs penetrate cells poorly and do not affect intracellular organisms.

3. Assessment of drug and dosage. Clinical response is an important but not always sufficient indication that the right drug is being given in the right dosage. Proof of drug activity in serum or urine against the original infecting organisms may provide important support for a selected drug regimen even if fever or other signs of infection are continuing. If drug therapy is adequate, the patient's serum is markedly bactericidal in vitro against the organism isolated from that patient prior to therapy. In infections limited to the urinary tract, the patient's urine must exhibit marked activity against the original organism.

4. Duration of therapy is determined in part by clinical response and past experience, and in part by laboratory indications of suppression or elimination of infection. Ultimate recovery must be verified by careful follow-up. In evaluating the patient's clinical response, the possibility of adverse reactions to antimicrobial drugs must be kept in mind. Such reactions may mimic continuing activity of the infectious process by causing fever, skin rashes, CNS disturbances, and changes in blood and urine. In the case of many drugs, it is desirable to examine blood and urine and to assess liver and kidney function at intervals. Abnormal findings may force the surgeon to reduce the dose or even discontinue a given drug.

5. Impaired renal function has an important influence on antimicrobial drug dosage, because many of these drugs are excreted by the kidneys. Only minor adjustment in dosage or frequency of administration is necessary with relatively non-toxic drugs. (e.g., penicillins) or with drugs that are detoxified or excreted mainly by the liver (e.g., erythromycins or chloramphenicol). On the other hand, aminoglycosides, tetracyclines, and some other drugs must be reduced in dosage or frequency of administration to avoid toxicity in renal failure. Some general guidelines are given in Table 4-2. Administration of particularly nephrotoxic antimicrobials may have to be guided by frequent direct assay of drug concentration in serum.

In the newborn or premature infant, excretory mechanisms for some antimicrobials are poorly developed, and special dosage schedules must be used in order to avoid toxic accumulation of drugs.

B. PROPHYLAXIS IN SURGERY. The incidence of infection following certain procedures can be significantly reduced if an effective drug is present at the site at time of incision, during the procedure, and for a few hours thereafter. Drugs started only after the procedure are without value in prevention. Drugs continued for more than 48 hours cause side effects and superinfection with resistant organisms to outweigh the benefit provided. Such prophylaxis is recommended for many clean-contaminated procedures and clean procedures that involve implantation of a prosthesis or transplant of an organ. Drugs such as cefazolin (0.5-1 g), cefonicid (0.5 g) or cefoxitin should be injected IV within the 2 hours preceding the incision and repeated once or twice in the next 12-24 hours to provide high drug levels for 24-48 hours. This can be effective in orthopedic, cardiothoracic, vascular, abdominal, and gynecologic surgery.

Table 4-2. Use of antibiotics in patients with renal failure* and hepatic failure

	Principal mode of excretion or detoxification	Approximate half-life in serum	
		Normal	Renal failure†
Penicillin G	Tubular secretion	0.5 hour	7-10 hours
Ampicillin	Tubular secretion	0.5-1 hour	8-12 hours
Carbenicillin	Tubular secretion	1 hour	16 hours
Ticarcillin	Tubular secretion	1.1 hour	15-20 hours
Azlocillin, mezlocillin, piperacillin	Renal, 50%-70%; biliary, 20%-30%	1 hour	3-6 hours
Nafcillin	Liver, 80%; kidney, 20%	0.75 hour	1.5 hours
Vancomycin	Glomerular filtration	6 hours	6-10 days
Chloramphenicol	Mainly liver	3 hours	4 hours
Erythromycin	Mainly liver	1.5 hours	1.5 hours
Clindamycin	Liver	2-4 hours	2-4 hours
Trimethoprim-sulfamethoxazole	Some liver	TMP 10-12 hours; SMZ, 8-10 hours	TMP 24-48 hours; SMZ 18-24 hours
Metronidazole	Liver	6-10 hours	6-10 hours

Modified from Jacobs RA and Jawetz E: In Schroeder S, et al, editors: *Current Medical Diagnosis and Treatment.* ed 30, Norwalk, CT, Appleton & Lange, 1991.

*For cephalosporins, see Table 4-3.

†Considered here to be marked by creatinine clearance of 10 mL/min or less.

‡For a 70-kg adult with a serious systemic infection.

§When serum levels reach 5-10 μg/ml, another dose should be given.

Table 4-2. Use of antibiotics in patients with renal failure and hepatic failure—cont'd

	Proposed dosage regimen in renal failure†	
	Initial dose‡	**Maintenance dose**
Penicillin G	1-2 million units	1 million units every 8 hours
Ampicillin	1 g	1 g q8-12h
Carbenicillin	4 g	2 g q12h
Ticarcillin	3 g	2 g q6-8h
Azlocillin, mezlocillin, piperacillin	3 g	2 g q6-8h
Nafcillin	1.5 g	1.5 g q5h
Vancomycin	1 g	1 g q6-10 days based on serum levels§
Chloramphenicol	0.5 g	0.5 g q6h
Erythromycin	0.5-1 g	0.5-1 g q6h
Clindamycin	0.6 g IV	0.6 g q8h
Trimethoprim-sulfamethoxazole	320 mg TMP + 1600 mg SMZ	80 mg TMP + 400 mg SMZ q12h
Metronidazole	0.5 g IV	0.5 g q8h

In elective procedures on the lower intestinal tract, it is customary to lower the microbial flora by administering insoluble drugs by mouth (bowel prep) in addition to mechanical cleansing. This effect is transient and the drugs must be properly timed, e.g., neomycin 1 g plus erythromycin base 0.5 g orally every 4-6 hours for 1-2 days before operation.

Grossly contaminated wounds, compound fractures, spillage of pus or gut contents into the peritoneal cavity, etc. require immediate treatment, sometimes called "prophylaxis." Drugs are chosen to suppress likely contaminating organisms such as anaerobes (metronidazole, clindamycin, penicillin), gram-negative enteric aerobes (aminoglycoside, cephalosporin), or staphylococci (nafcillin). This early therapy is often continued for several days while patient observation and laboratory results may give a clue as to the predominant organism maintaining the infection.

Table 4-2. Use of antibiotics in patients with renal failure and hepatic failure—cont'd

	Removal of drug by hemodialysis	Dose after hemodialysis	Dosage in hepatic failure
Penicillin G	Yes	500,000 units	No change
Ampicillin	Yes	1 g	No change
Carbenicillin	Yes	2 g	No change
Ticarcillin	Yes	1 g	No change
Azlocillin, mezlocillin, piperacillin	Yes	1 g	1-2 g q8h
Nafcillin	No	None	1-1.5 g q12h
Vancomycin	No	None	No change
Chloramphenicol	Yes	0.5 g	0.25-0.5 g q12h
Erythromycin	No	None	0.25-0.5 g q6h
Clindamycin	No	None	0.3-0.6 g q8h
Trimethoprimsulfamethoxazole	Yes	80 mg TMP + 400 mg SMZ	No change
Metronidazole	Yes	0.25 g	0.25 g q12h

III. ANTIMICROBIAL DRUGS

Ernest Jawetz
Dennis J. Flora

A. PENICILLINS. All penicillins share a chemical nucleus that contains a beta-lactam ring that is essential to antibacterial action. The penicillins can be arranged according to several major criteria: (1) Susceptibility to destruction by penicillinase, (2) Stability to gastric acid and suitability for oral administration; (3) Relative efficacy against gram-positive versus gram-negative bacteria.

1. Antimicrobial activity. All penicillins specifically inhibit the synthesis of rigid bacterial cell walls which contain peptidoglycan. Penicillins are inactive against bacteria that are not actively multiplying and not forming cell walls.

One million units of penicillin G equal 0.6 g. Other penicillins are prescribed in grams. A serum level of 0.01-1 µg/ml penicillin G or ampicillin is lethal for a majority of susceptible microorganisms; nafcillin and other β-lactamase–resistant penicillins are 5-50 times less active. Blood levels of penicillins can be raised by giving probenecid 0.5 g orally every 6 hours.

2. Resistance to penicillins falls into several categories:

a. Production of β-lactamase, e.g., by staphylococci, gonococci, *Hemophilus* sp., coliform and other gram-negative organisms.

b. Lack of penicillin receptors (e.g., pneumococci) or impermeability of cell envelope so that penicillins cannot reach receptors.

c. Failure of activation of autolytic enzymes in the cell wall; e.g., staphylococci may be inhibited but "tolerant" and thus not killed by penicillins.

d. Cell-wall deficient (L) forms or mycoplasmas that do not synthesize a cell wall; they may perpetuate infection.

3. Indications, dosages, and routes of administration. The penicillins are by far the most effective and the most widely used antimicrobial drugs. All oral penicillins must be given away from meal times.

a. Penicillin G is drug of choice for infections caused by pneumococci, streptococci, meningococci, non–β-lactamase-producing staphylococci, and gonococci, *Treponema pallidum* and other spirochetes, anthrax bacilli and other gram-positive rods, *Clostridia, Listeria,* and *Bacteroides* (except *Bacteroides fragilis*).

Intramuscular or intravenous. Most of the above-mentioned infections respond to aqueous penicillin G in daily doses of 0.6-20 million units (0.36-12 g) given by intermittent IV injection. Sites for such IV administration are subject to thrombophlebitis and superinfection and must be rotated every 2-3 days and kept scrupulously aseptic. In enterococcus and some gram-negative infections, aminoglycosides are given simultaneously.

Oral. Penicillin V is indicated only in minor infections (e.g., respiratory tract or associated structures) in daily doses of 1-4 g (1.6-6.4 million units). Oral administration is subject to so many variables that it should not be relied upon in seriously ill patients.

Intrathecal. With high serum levels of penicillin, adequate concentrations reach the CNS and CSF for the treatment of meningitis. Therefore, intrathecal injection has been virtually abandoned.

Topical. Penicillins have been applied to skin, wounds, and mucous membranes by compress, ointment, and aerosol. These applications are highly sensitizing and rarely warranted. Rarely, solutions of penicillin (e.g., 100,000 units/ml) are instilled into infected joint or pleural spaces.

b. Benzathine penicillin G is a salt of very low water solubility. It is injected IM to establish a depot which yields low but prolonged drug levels. A single injection of 1.2 million units IM is satisfactory for treatment of beta-hemolytic streptococcal pharyngitis. An injection of 1.2-2.4 million units IM every 3-4 weeks provides satisfactory prophylaxis for rheumatics against reinfection with group A streptococci. Early syphilis can be treated with benzathine penicillin, 2.4 million units IM once weekly for 1-3 weeks. Procaine penicillin 600,000 unit IM once daily is another repository form for maintaining drug levels for up to 24 hours.

c. Ampicillin, amoxicillin, carbenicillin, ticarcillin, piperacillin, mezlocillin, azlocillin have greater activity against gram-negative aerobes than penicillin G but are also destroyed by penicillinases. Ampicillin, 0.5 g orally every 6 hours, or amoxicillin, 0.5 g every 8 hours, is used to treat common urinary tract infections with gram-negative coliform bacteria or secondary bacterial infections of the respiratory tract (sinusitis, otitis, bronchitis). In typhoid or bacteremic salmonella infections ampicillin, 4-12 g IV daily, is given, but it usually has no effect in salmonella gastroenteritis. The other drugs are all somewhat more active against gram-negative enteric aerobic bacteria, including pseudomonas, and are used in sepsis (e.g., burns, leukemia) often in combination with an aminoglycoside. Ticarcillin, 18 g daily IV, is representative.

d. Penicillinase-resistant penicillins are relatively resistant to destruction by β-lactamase. The only indication for their use is in infection by β-lactamase–producing staphylococci.

Oral. Cloxacillin, nafcillin, and others may be given in doses of 0.25-0.5 g every 4-6 hours in mild or localized staphylococcal infections (50-100 mg/kg/day for children). Food must not be given in proximity to these doses.

Intravenous. For serious systemic staphylococcal infections, nafcillin, 6-12 g, is administered IV, usually by injecting 1-2 g during 20-30 minutes every 2 hours into a continuous infusion of 5% dextrose in water. The dose for children is nafcillin 50-100 mg/kg/day.

4. Adverse effects. The penicillins undoubtedly possess less direct toxicity than any other antibiotics. Most side effects are due to hypersensitivity.

a. Allergy. All penicillins are cross-sensitizing and cross-reacting. Any preparation containing penicillin may induce sensitization, including foods or cosmetics. Skin tests with penicilloylpolylysine, with alkaline hydrolysis products, and with undegraded penicillin will identify many hypersensitive individuals. Among positive reactors to skin tests, the chance of subsequent severe immediate penicillin reactions is high. Although many persons develop IgG antibodies to penicillin, such antibodies are not correlated with allergic reactivity except rare hemolytic anemia. The presence of cell-bound IgE antibodies is far more significant but is not detected by available serologic tests. A history of a penicillin reaction in the past is not reliable; however, in such cases the drug should be administered with caution or a substitute drug used.

Allergic reactions may occur as anaphylactic shock (rare—0.05%), serum sickness (urticaria, fever, joint swelling, angioneurotic edema, intense pruritus, and respiratory embarrassment occurring 7-12 days after exposure), skin rashes, fever, nephritis, eosinophilia, hemolytic anemia, other hematologic disturbances, and vasculitis. Incidence of hypersensitivity to penicillin is about 2%-8% among adults in the United States, but is negligible in small children.

b. Toxicity. The toxic effects of penicillin G are due to the direct irritation caused by IM or IV injections of exceedingly high concentrations (e.g., 1 g/ml). Such concentrations may cause local pain, induration, thrombophlebitis, or degeneration of an accidentally injected nerve. All penicillins are irritating to the CNS. There is no indication for intrathecal administration at present. In rare cases, a patient receiving >5 g of penicillin G daily parenterally has exhibited signs of of cerebrocortical irritation. Direct cation toxicity (Na^+, K^+) can also occur with very large doses. Potassium penicillin G contains 1.7 mEq of K^+ per million units (2.8 mEq/g), and potassium may accumulate in the presence of renal failure. Carbenicillin contains 4.7 mEq/g Na^+.

Large doses of penicillins given orally may lead to nausea and diarrhea. Oral therapy may also be accompanied by luxuriant overgrowth of staphylococci, pseudomonas, proteus, clostridia, or yeasts which may occasionally cause enterocolitis. Superinfections in other organ systems may occur with penicillins as with any antibiotic therapy.

Methicillin causes interstitial nephritis more often than nafcillin. Carbenicillin can cause hypokalemic alkalosis and hemostatic defects leading to bleeding tendency. It and others may induce granulocytopenia.

B. CEPHALOSPORINS are a group of β-lactam drugs related to penicillins, with similar mechanisms of antibacterial action and varying resistance to beta-lactamases (Table 4-3). New cephalosporins with increased activity especially against resistant gram-negative bacteria appear frequently. Enterococci and some other gram-positive bacteria are often resistant and may produce superinfections.

Many cephalosporins are excreted mainly by the kidney and may cumulate and induce toxicity in renal insufficiency.

1. First-generation cephalosporins are very active against gram-positive cocci (except enterococci and methicillin-resistant staphylococci) and moderately active against some gram-negative rods (except pseudomonas, proteus, enterobacter, serratia, and acinetobacter). Anaerobic cocci are often sensitive but *B. fragilis* is not.

Cephalexin, cephradine, and cefadroxil are absorbed from the gut to a variable extent and can be used in doses of 0.25-0.5 g orally four times daily to treat urinary and respiratory tract infections. Other members must be injected to give levels in blood and tissues. Cefazolin, 1-2 g IV every 8 hours, is a choice for surgical prophylaxis because it gives high (90-120 μg/ml) levels. None of the first-generation drugs penetrate into the CNS, and they are not drugs of first choice for any infection.

2. Second-generation cephalosporins are a heterogeneous group. All are active against organisms covered by first-generation drugs, but have an extended coverage against gram-negative rods, including klebsiella, enterobacter, and proteus, but not *Pseudomonas aeruginosa.*

Only cefaclor can be given orally (0.25-0.5 g, 3-4 times daily) to treat sinusitis and otitis caused by *Haemophilus influenzae,* including β-lactamase–producing strains. The other members of the group are injected IV.

Cefoxitin (2 g every 6 hours) and cefotetan (1-2 g every 8 hours) are particularly active against *B. fragilis* and thus are used in mixed anaerobic infections, including peritonitis or pelvic inflammatory disease. Cefamandole (2 g), cefuroxime (1.5 g), cefonicid (1 g), ceforanide (2 g), are injected IV at 6-12 hour intervals in the treatment of gram-negative bacterial pneumonias or other community-acquired infections. Dosage must be reduced in renal failure.

3. Third-generation cephalosporins have little activity against gram-positive cocci; enterococci and staphylococci often produce superinfections during their use. The major advan-

Table 4-3. Pharmacology of the cephalosporins

Drug	Peak serum level (μg/ml) after 1 g IV	Serum half-life (min)	Total daily dose (mg/kg)	Dosage interval (hours)	Dosage adjustments in renal failure		
					Moderate (Cl_{cr} 10-50 ml/min)	Severe ($Cl_{cr} < 10$ ml/min)	Post-hemodialysis dose
Cephalothin, cephapirin	40-60	40	50-200	4-6	1-2 g q6-12h	1 g q12h	1 g
Cefazolin	90-120	90	25-100	8	0.5-1 g q12h	0.5 g daily	0.5 g
Cephalexin, cephradine*	15-20	50-60	15-30	6	0.25-0.5 g q8-12h	0.25-0.5 g daily	0.5 g
Cefadroxil*	15	75	15-30	12-24	1 g daily	0.5 g daily	0.5 g
Cefamandole	60-80	45	75-200	6-8	1 g q12h	1-2 g daily	0.5 g
Cefuroxime	80-100	80	50	6-12	1 g q12h	1-2 g daily	0.5 g
Cefuroxime axetil*	6-8	75	5-15	12	0.5 g q24h	0.25 g daily	0.25 g
Cefonicid	200-250	240	15-30	24	0.5 g daily	1 g q72h	0.25 g
Ceforanide	125	180	15-30	12	1 g daily	1 g q48h	0.25 g
Cefaclor*	15-20	50	20-40 children, 10-15 adults	6-8	0.5 g q8-12h	0.25-0.5 g q12-24h	0.25-0.5 g

Cefixime*	3-5	180-240	8 (with maximum of 0.4 g/d total)	12-24	0.4 g daily	0.1 g daily	None
Cefotetan	60-80	150	50-100	8-12	1 g q8-12h	0.5-1 g daily	0.5 g
Cefotaxime	40-60	60	50-75	6-8	1-2 g q6-8h	1-2 g q12h	1-2 g
Cefoxitin	60-80	60	50-100	6-8	1 g q12h	1-2 g daily	0.5 g
Cefmetazole	70-100	60-80	50-100	6-8	1-2 g q12-24h	1-2 g q24-48h	1 g
Ceftizoxime	80-100	100	5-75	8-12	0.5-1 g q8-12h	0.25-0.5 g q12-24h	0.5 g
Ceftriaxone	150	480	30-50	12-24	1-2 g daily	1-2 g daily	None
Ceftazidime	100-120	120	50-75	8-12	1 g q8-12h	0.5-1 g daily	0.5 g
Cefoperazone	150	120	30-200	8-12	1-2 g q12h	1-2 g q12h	None
Moxalactam	60-100	120	50-200	6-12	0.5-1 g q12h	0.25-0.5 g q12h	0.5 g

From Jacobs RA, Jawetz E: In Schroeder S, et al editors: *Current Medical Diagnosis and Treatment*, ed 30, Norwalk, CT, 1991, Appleton & Lange.
*Oral agents. Serum levels based on 0.5 g oral dose.

tage of third-generation drugs is their expanded coverage of gram-negative rods. Ceftazidime and cefoperazone are often effective against *P. aeruginosa,* the other members only occasionally. Thus, a major use of third-generation drugs is the management of hospital-acquired gram-negative bacteremia. In immunocompromised patients these drugs are often combined with an aminoglycoside.

A distinguishing feature is the ability of several third-generation drugs (except cefoperazone) to reach the CNS, and appear in CSF in sufficient concentrations to treat meningitis caused by gram-negative rods. Cefotaxime (2 g), ceftriaxone (2 g), ceftizoxime (2 g) given IV every 8 hours are choices for the management of gram-negative bacterial sepsis and meningitis. Cefoperazone and ceftriaxone are excreted primarily by the liver; the others are excreted by the kidney and require dosage adjustment in renal insufficiency.

4. Adverse effects of cephalosporins

a. Allergy. Cephalosporins are sensitizing and can elicit a variety of hypersensitivity reactions, including anaphylaxis, fever, skin rashes, nephritis, granulocytopenia, and hemolytic anemia. The frequency of cross-allergy between cephalosporins and penicillins remains uncertain (6%-12%). Patients with minor penicillin allergy can often tolerate cephalosporins, but those with a history of anaphylaxis must not receive cephalosporins.

b. Toxicity. Thrombophlebitis can occur after IV injection. Hypoprothrombinemia is frequent with cephalosporins that have a methylthiotetrazole group, e.g., cefamandole, moxalactam, cefoperazone; administration of vitamin K, 10 mg twice weekly, can prevent this complication. These same drugs can also cause severe disulfiram-like reactions, and use of alcohol must be avoided. Moxalactam interferes with platelet function, has been associated with severe bleeding, and has therefore fallen into disuse.

c. Superinfection. Many second- and third-generation cephalosporins have little activity against gram-positive organisms, particularly staphylococci and enterococci, so superinfection with these organisms and fungi may occur (Table 4-4).

C. OTHER β-LACTAM DRUGS. *Aztreonam* (1-2 g IV every 6-8 hours), a monocyclic drug, is resistant to β-lactamases and has activity similar to aminoglycosides. *Imipenem* has a broad antibacterial spectrum and is resistant to β-lactamases. It is given IV (0.5-1 g every 6 hours) together with cilastatin, an

Table 4-4. Major groups of cephalosporins

First generation	Second generation	Third generation
Cephalothin	Cefamandole	Cefotaxime
Cephapirin	Cefuroxime	Ceftizoxime
Cefazolin	Cefonicid	Ceftriaxone
Cefalexin*	Ceforanide	Ceftazidime
Cephradine*	Cefaclor*	Cefoperazone
Cefadroxil*	Cefoxitin	Moxalactam
	Cefotetan	

*Oral agents

inhibitor of renal dipeptidase. Bacterial resistance may emerge rapidly, and its place in therapy is not well defined.

D. ERYTHROMYCIN GROUP (MACROLIDES). The erythromycins are compounds that are active against gram-positive organisms (especially pneumococci, streptococci, staphylococci, and corynebacteria). Chlamydiae and mycoplasmas are also susceptible. Resistant mutants occur in most microbial populations and tend to emerge during prolonged treatment. Absorption varies greatly. There is wide distribution of the drug in all tissues except the CNS. Erythromycins are excreted largely in bile; only 5% of the dose is excreted into the urine.

Erythromycins are the drugs of choice in corynebacterial infections (diphtheroid sepsis, erythrasma). They are also effective in mycoplasmal pneumonia, *Legionella,* and *C. trachomatis* infections. They are useful for streptococcal and pneumococcal infections in persons allergic to penicillin.

For oral administration, give erythromycin stearate, succinate, or estolate, 0.5 g every 6 hours (for children, 40 mg/kg/day). For IV administration, give erythromycin lactobionate or glucepate, 0.5 g every 12 hours.

Such **adverse effects** as nausea, vomiting, and diarrhea may occur after oral intake. Erythromycins, particularly the estolate, can produce cholestatic hepatitis as a hypersensitivity reaction. Although most patients recover completely, it may recur upon readministration of the drug.

E. TETRACYCLINE GROUP. The tetracyclines constitute a large group of drugs with common basic chemical structures, antimicrobial activity, and pharmacologic properties. Microorganisms resistant to this group show complete cross-resistance to all tetracyclines.

1. Antimicrobial activity. Tetracyclines are inhibitors of protein synthesis and are bacteriostatic for many gram-positive and gram-negative bacteria, including anaerobes, mycoplasmas, rickettsiae, chlamydiae, and some protozoa (e.g., amebas). Equal concentrations of all tetracyclines in blood or tissue have approximately equal antimicrobial activity. Because of the emergence of resistant strains, tetracyclines have lost some of their former usefulness. Proteus and pseudomonas are regularly resistant; among coliform bacteria, pneumococci, and streptococci, resistant strains are increasingly common.

2. Indications, dosages, and routes of administration. At present, tetracyclines are the drugs of choice in mycoplasmal, chlamydial, rickettsial, and vibrio infections. They may be used in various bacterial infections (provided the organism is susceptible) and in amebiasis.

a. Oral. Tetracycline hydrochloride, oxytetracycline, and chlortetracycline are dispensed in 250-mg capsules. Give 0.25-0.5 g orally every 6 hours (for children, 20-40 mg/kg/day). In acne vulgaris, 0.25 g once or twice daily for many months is prescribed by dermatologists.

Demeclocycline and methacycline are slowly excreted. Give 0.15-0.3 g orally every 6 hours (12-20 mg/kg/day for children). Doxycycline is available in capsules of 50 or 100 mg. Give 100 mg every 12 hours on the first day, then 100 mg/day.

b. Intramuscular or intravenous. Several tetracyclines are formulated for IM or IV injection. Give 0.1-0.5 g every 6-12 hours in individuals unable to take oral medication (for children, 10-15 mg/kg/day).

c. Topical tetracycline, 1% in ointments, can be applied to conjunctival infections.

3. Adverse effects

a. Allergy. Hypersensitivity reactions with fever or skin rashes occur.

b. Gastrointestinal side-effects. Diarrhea, nausea, and anorexia are common. These can be diminished by reducing the dose or by administering tetracyclines with food or carboxymethylcellulose, but sometimes they force discontinuance of the drug. After a few days of oral use, the gut flora is modified so that drug-resistant bacteria and yeasts become prominent. This may cause anal pruritus, vaginitis, or even enterocolitis.

c. Bones and teeth. Tetracyclines are bound to calcium deposited in growing bones and teeth, causing fluorescence, discoloration, enamel dysplasia, deformity, or growth inhibition. Therefore, tetracyclines should not be given to pregnant women or children under age 6 years.

d. Liver damage. Tetracyclines can impair hepatic function or even cause liver necrosis, particularly during pregnancy, in the presence of preexisting liver damage or with doses of more than 3 g IV.

e. Other. Tetracyclines, principally demeclocycline, may induce photosensitization, especially in blonds. IV injection may cause thrombophlebitis, and IM injection may induce local inflammation with pain. Minocycline can produce severe vestibular reactions.

F. CHLORAMPHENICOL inhibits bacterial protein synthesis and blocks growth. There is no cross-resistance with other drugs. It penetrates well into the CNS. Because of its potential toxicity, it is at present a possible drug of choice only in (1) Symptomatic salmonella infection, e.g., typhoid fever; (2) *H. influenzae* meningitis, laryngotracheitis, or pneumonia that does not respond to ampicillin; (3) Severe rickettsial infections; (4) Meningococcal infection in patients hypersensitive to penicillin; (5) Anaerobic or mixed infections, especially in the CNS. It is occasionally used topically in ophthalmology.

In serious systemic infection, the dose is 0.5 g orally every 4-6 hours (children, 30-50 mg/kg/day) for 7-21 days. Similar amounts can be given IV.

Nausea, vomiting, and diarrhea occur infrequently. The most serious **adverse effects** pertain to the hematopoietic system. Adults taking chloramphenicol in excess of 50 mg/kg/day regularly exhibit disturbances in red cell maturation after 1-2 weeks of blood levels above 25 μg/ml. There is anemia, rise in serum iron concentration, reticulocytopenia, and the appearance of vacuolated nucleated red cells in the bone marrow. These changes regress when the drug is stopped and are not related to aplastic anemia.

Serious aplastic anemia is a rare consequence of chloramphenicol administration and represents a specific, probably genetically determined individual defect. It tends to be irreversible. Fatal aplastic anemia occurs in one of 25,000-40,000 courses of chloramphenicol therapy. Hypoplastic anemia may be followed by the development of leukemia.

Chloramphenicol is specifically toxic for newborns, producing the highly fatal "gray syndrome" with vomiting, flaccidity, hypothermia, and collapse. Chloramphenicol should only rarely be used in infants, and the dose must be limited to

<50 mg/kg/day in full-term infants and <30 mg/kg/day in prematurely born infants.

G. AMINOGLYCOSIDES are a group of drugs which share chemical antimicrobial, pharmacologic, and toxic characteristics. In 1992, the group includes streptomycin, neomycin, kanamycin, amikacin, gentamicin, tobramycin, Netilmicin, and others. These drugs are bactericidal by inhibiting protein synthesis in bacteria. Resistance develops through transmissible plasmids which spread among bacteria and control enzymes that destroy the drugs or make the organisms impermeable to them. Anaerobic bacteria and streptococci are usually resistant.

Aminoglycosides are employed most often against gram-negative bacteria, especially in combination with a penicillin or cephalosporin which facilitates the entry of the aminoglycoside into cells. Combinations of an aminoglycoside and a penicillin can be bactericidal for enterococci in sepsis or endocarditis. All aminoglycosides are ototoxic and nephrotoxic in varying degrees. Individual drugs are selected according to recent susceptibility patterns in a given area or hospital until laboratory tests become available on a specific isolate. In renal insufficiency, the dose or drug interval has to be adjusted (see Table 4-3).

1. Streptomycin. Resistance to streptomycin emerges so rapidly and has become so widespread that only the following indications remain:

a. Plague, tularemia, brucellosis where it is used singly or in combination with tetracycline.

b. Severe, active tuberculosis, used with other antituberculosis drugs, usually INH or rifampin.

Streptomycin should not be used concurrently with other drugs of similar toxicity; the usual dose is 0.5 mg IM every 6 hours.

2. Neomycin and kanamycin are closely related, with similar activity and complete cross-resistance. Because of ototoxicity and nephrotoxicity they are now used only topically or orally. They are not absorbed from the gut.

Ointments containing 1-5 mg/g of neomycin, often combined with bacitracin and polymyxin, can be applied to infected superficial skin lesions, although their efficacy is limited. Solutions of neomycin or kanamycin, 1-5 mg/ml, have been used for irrigation of infected wounds or cavities. The total amount of drug must be kept <15 mg/kg/day to avoid systemic toxicity. Neostigmine or calcium gluconate acts as an antidote.

Oral kanamycin or neomycin, 1 g every 4-6 hours (often combined with erythromycin 1 g), serves to reduce the aerobic bowel flora in preparation for colon surgery 1-2 days later.

3. Amikacin is a derivative of kanamycin and is relatively resistant to some microbial enzymes that destroy other aminoglycosides. However, impermeability to amikacin is spreading among gram-negative bacteria. Many infections caused by gram-negative bacteria resistant to other aminoglycosides can be treated with amikacin, 0.5 mg IM every 8-12 hours (15 mg/kg/day). Like all aminoglycosides, amikacin is ototoxic (especially producing deafness) and nephrotoxic. Levels should be monitored in patients with renal insufficiency.

4. Gentamicin and tobramycin are very similar aminoglycosides, with the latter perhaps somewhat less toxic. The dose is 5-7 mg/kg/day in divided doses, given IV or IM for burns, sepsis, pneumonia, and other serious gram-negative rod infections. They are often combined with a penicillin or a cephalosporin in infections with pseudomonas, serratia, klebsiella, proteus, enterobacter, or fecal streptococci. Resistance to these drugs has emerged widely and in proportion to the level of use. Gentamicin 0.1% cream has been applied to infected surface lesions but rapidly selects resistant bacteria. To minimize the ototoxic and nephrotoxic effects of either drug, it is desirable to monitor serum levels, particularly in patients with renal insufficiency.

5. Spectinomycin. This aminocyclitol drug is used in gonorrhea if the gonococci produce β-lactamase. Inject 2 g of spectinomycin IM in a single dose. Local pain, fever, and nausea may be side effects.

H. POLYMYXINS. These basic polypeptides are bactericidal for many gram-negative bacteria, especially pseudomonas. Systemic administration has been largely abandoned because of significant toxicity.

Topical. Solutions of polymyxin B sulfate, 1 mg/ml, can be applied to infected surfaces, or injected into joint or pleural spaces or beneath the conjunctivae. Ointments containing 0.5 mg/g polymyxin B sulfate in a mixture with neomycin or bacitracin are often applied to infected skin lesions. Solutions containing polymyxin B, 20 mg/L, and neomycin, 40 mg/L, can be used for continuous irrigation of the bladder with an indwelling catheter and a closed drainage system.

Adverse effects. Systemic administration resulted in neurotoxicity and nephrotoxicity. This rarely occurs with topical administration.

I. ANTIMYCOBACTERIAL DRUGS. Tuberculosis and other mycobacterial infections tend to be exceedingly chronic but may give rise to hyperacute lethal complications. The organisms are frequently intracellular, have long periods of metabolic inactivity, and tend to develop resistance to any one drug. Combined drug therapy is often employed to delay the emergence of this resistance.

1. Isoniazid (INH) is the most active and the most widely used drug. INH inhibits most tubercle bacilli. Most "atypical" mycobacteria are resistant, and in large populations of *Mycobacterium tuberculosis*. INH-resistant mutants also occur; their emergence is delayed in the presence of a second drug. There is no cross-resistance between INH, and other antimycobacterial drugs.

In active, clinically manifest disease, INH is given in conjunction with rifampin or ethambutol. The initial dose is 8-10 mg/kg/day orally; later, the dosage is reduced to 5-7 mg/kg/day.

Children (or young adults) converting from a tuberculin-negative to a tuberculin-positive skin test may be given 10 mg/kg/day (maximum: 300 mg/day) for 1 year as prophylaxis against the 5%-15% risk of meningitis or miliary dissemination. For this "prophylaxis" INH is given as the sole drug.

Toxic reactions to INH include insomnia, restlessness, dysuria, hyperreflexia, and even convulsions and psychotic episodes. Many of these effects are attributable to peripheral neuritis from relative pyridoxine deficiency and can be prevented by the administration of pyridoxine, 100 μg/day. INH can produce liver damage, especially in persons >50 years or alcoholics.

2. Rifampin, a first-line antituberculosis drug, also inhibits other bacteria. In combination with INH or ethambutol, rifampin 600 mg is given as a single oral dose daily or twice weekly. It should not be given singly in respiratory or urinary tract infections, because resistance emerges rapidly. Rifampin imparts a harmless orange color to urine and sweat. It has an important use for short-term prophylaxis of infections due to *N. meningitides* and *H. influenzae.*

3. Ethambutol is well-absorbed from the gut and widely distributed (including CNS and CSF). It is given as a single daily dose (15 mg/kg) for months, combined with rifampin or INH, in the treatment of tuberculosis or infections with atypical mycobacteria. The commonest side effects are visual disturbances (optic neuritis) that regress when the drug is stopped.

4. Streptomycin (1-10 µg/ml) is inhibitory and bactericidal for most tubercle bacilli. Most "atypical" mycobacteria are resistant, and resistant strains of tubercle bacilli emerge within 2-4 months if streptomycin is used alone. So, it is used in combination with the other antituberculosis drugs. Doses and adverse effects of streptomycin are listed above. Streptomycin penetrates poorly into cells and exerts its action mainly on extracellular tubercle bacilli.

5. Pyrazinamide is bactericidal for most *M. tuberculosis* and many atypical mycobacteria. Oral doses of 1.5-2 g are given once daily. It is beneficial especially in the early months of short-course antituberculosis therapy.

6. Alternative drugs (e.g., cycloserine, ethionamide, viomycin) are chosen in cases of resistance to "first-line" drugs, but expert guidance is needed.

J. SULFONAMIDES AND TRIMETHOPRIM

1. Activity. Sulfonamides inhibit bacterial growth by competing with para-amino-benzoic acid for the enzyme that synthesizes folate. This is a reversible reaction and mammalian cells are independent of it. Trimethoprim binds dihydrofolate reductase of bacteria 10,000 times more effectively than the same enzyme of mammalian cells. These two drugs thus can inhibit sequential steps in the metabolic pathway which leads to nucleic acid synthesis in bacteria and some parasites.

2. Indications. The widespread emergence of resistance to sulfonamides has curtailed their usefulness. Only the following are valid indications in 1992.

a. First (previously untreated) *infection of the urinary tract* due to coliform or other susceptible bacteria. Trimethoprim alone may be similarly useful.

b. Parasitic infections, most prominently *Pneumocystis carinii* pneumonia.

c. Bacterial infections, e.g., due to *Nocardia* and susceptible strains of pneumococcus, meningococcus, shigella, and salmonella strains and others.

d. Certain sulfones (e.g., dapsone) are widely used in leprosy.

3. Dosages and routes of administration

a. Topical application of sulfonamides is highly sensitizing. Current uses include sodium sulfacetamide solution (30%) or ointment (10%) to the conjunctivae, and mafenide acetate (Sulfamylon) or silver sulfadiazine to burns.

b. Oral. For systemic diseases, the soluble, rapidly excreted sulfonamides (e.g., sulfadiazine, sulfisoxazole, trisulfapyrimidines) are given in an initial dose of 2-4 g (40 mg/kg) followed by a maintenance dose of 0.5-1 g (20 mg/kg) every 4-6 hours. Keep urine alkaline to avoid precipitation of crystals.

For uncomplicated, previously untreated symptomatic UTIs (e.g., cystitis) in nonpregnant women, a single dose of sulfisoxazole 1 g, or of trimethoprim 320 mg plus sulfamethoxazole 1600 mg (i.e., two tablets twice in one day), is effective in 80%-90% of cases. Half a tablet of the TMP-SMX combination 3 times weekly serves as prophylaxis for recurrent UTIs in some women. The combination may also be effective in respiratory or enteric infections. Trimethoprim alone, 100 mg orally every 12 hours, may be effective in some first UTIs.

Sulfasalazine (6 g/day) is commonly used in inflammatory bowel disease.

"Long-acting" sulfonamides (e.g., sulfamethoxypyridazine) have a significantly higher rate of toxic effects than the "short-acting" sulfonamides.

c. Intravenous. Sodium sulfadiazine can be injected IV in 0.5% concentration in D_5W for a total dose of 6-8 g/day (120 mg/kg/day). This route is reserved for individuals unable to take oral medication.

IV TMP-SMX contains 80 mg of trimethoprim and 400 mg of sulfamethoxazole per 5-ml ampule in 40% propylene glycol to be diluted with 125 ml of D_5W. Up to 6-12 ampules are given in three to four divided doses in *P. carinii* pneumonia or gram-negative bacterial sepsis.

4. Adverse effects. Sulfonamides produce a wide variety of side effects, due partly to hypersensitivity and partly to direct toxicity.

a. Systemic side effects. Fever, skin rashes, urticaria, vomiting, or diarrhea; conjunctivitis, arthritis, exfoliative dermatitis; hematopoietic disturbances, including thrombocytopenia, hemolytic (in G6PD deficiency) or aplastic anemia, granulocytopenia, leukemoid reactions; hepatitis, polyarteritis nodosa, vasculitis, Stevens-Johnson syndrome; psychosis; and many others.

b. Urinary tract disturbances. Sulfonamides may precipitate in urine, especially at neutral or acid pH, producing hematuria, crystalluria, or obstruction. They have been implicated in various types of nephritis and nephrosis.

5. Precautions in the use of sulfonamides

a. There is cross-allergenicity among all sulfonamides. Obtain a history of past administration or reaction. Observe for possible allergic responses.

b. Keep the urine volume >1500 ml/day. Check urine pH; it should be 7.5 or higher. Give alkali by mouth (sodium bicarbonate or equivalent 5-15 g/day). Examine fresh urine for crystals and red cells once weekly.

c. Check hemoglobin, WBC, and differential count every 5-10 days to detect possible disturbances early.

d. If adverse effects appear, discontinue the sulfonamide drugs.

K. SPECIALIZED DRUGS AGAINST GRAM-POSITIVE BACTERIA

1. Bacitracin. This polypeptide antibiotic is selectively active against gram-positive bacteria. Because of severe nephrotoxicity upon systemic administration, its use is limited to topical application on surface lesions. Occasionally, it is given orally for pseudomembranous antibiotic-associated colitis, in lieu of oral vancomycin.

2. Clindamycin and lincomycin are active against staphylococci and streptococci, but not enterococci. They are alternatives to erythromycin as substitutes for penicillin. However, the principal indication for clindamycin is anaerobic infection (e.g., abdominal or pelvic sepsis) involving *B. fragilis*. The dose in serious illness is clindamycin 600 mg IV every 8 hours (20-30 mg/kg/day). Common side effects are diarrhea, nausea, and skin rashes. Most seriously, clindamycin has been associated with the development of pseudo-membranous colitis often caused by the necrotizing toxin of *C. difficile*. That may require oral vancomycin, bacitracin, or metronidazole.

3. Vancomycin is bactericidal for many gram-positive bacteria, such as staphylococci (including methicillin-resistant staph) and enterococci. The major indications for vancomycin are serious staphylococcal sepsis or endocarditis. Vancomycin, 0.5 g, is given IV during a 20-minute period, every 8 hours (20-40 mg/kg/day for children). In renal failure, the half-life of vancomycin is very greatly prolonged (Table 4-3). Oral vancomycin is not absorbed from the gut. It is given orally, 0.2-0.5 g 2-4 times daily for pseudo-membranous colitis. IV vancomycin may produce fever and thrombophlebitis and occasionally some oto- or nephrotoxicity.

L. METRONIDAZOLE is a drug of choice in treating trichomonas and amoeba infection. It is also very effective in anaerobic bacterial infections (500-750 mg orally, 3-4 times daily) and in Gardnerella (nonspecific) vaginitis. Metronidazole may be effective in preparation of the colon for surgery. Adverse effects include nausea, diarrhea, and stomatitis with prolonged use.

M. QUINOLONES are synthetic analogues of nalidixic acid (below), which are active against many gram-positive and gram-negative bacteria. All quinolones inhibit DNA synthesis in bacteria by blocking DNA gyrase. Newer fluorinated quinolones (e.g., norfloxacin, ciprofloxacin, ofloxacin) have much enhanced antibacterial potency and achieve clinically useful blood and tissue levels. Norfloxacin 400 mg or ciprofloxacin 500 mg orally twice daily can be effective not only in UTIs, but in enteritis caused by *Salmonella sp* or *Campylobacter* sp., in traveler's diarrhea caused by toxigenic *E. coli*, in gonococcal urethritis and pharyngitis, and perhaps in a variety of respiratory, gynecologic, and soft tissue infections. They may be useful for the prophylaxis of infection in neutropenic patients.

Adverse effects include vomiting, diarrhea, headache, dizziness, insomnia and seizures. Superinfections with streptococci or *Candida* have been observed.

N. URINARY ANTISEPTICS. The following are often used:

1. Nitrofurantoin (Furadantin) is active against many types of bacteria, particularly at acid pH in urine. The usual dose is 100 mg orally 4 times daily (children 5-10 mg/kg/day) taken with food. GI side effects are common; hypersensitivity causes rashes and pneumonic infiltrates; hemolytic anemia occurs in G6PD deficiency.

2. Nalidixic acid is a quinolone effective only in urine. It is readily absorbed with oral doses of 1 g 4 times daily, but bacterial resistance tends to emerge rapidly.

3. Methenamine mandelate or hippurate acidifies urine and liberates formaldehyde there. Oral dose is 2-6 g daily. Other drugs that acidify urine, e.g., methionine, ascorbic acid, can provide bacteriostasis in chronic UTIs.

O. ANTIFUNGAL DRUGS

1. Amphotericin B (Fungizone) inhibits several organisms producing systemic mycotic disease in man, including *Histoplasma*, *Cryptococcus*, *Coccidioides*, *Candida*, *Blastomyces*, *Sporothrix*, and others.

Amphotericin B solutions, 0.1 mg/ml in D_5W, are given IV by slow infusion. The initial dose is 1-5 mg/day, increasing daily by 5-mg increments until a final dosage of 0.4-0.8 mg/kg/day is reached. Treatment is usually continued for many weeks. In fungal meningitis, amphotericin B (0.5 mg) is injected intrathecally three times weekly; continuous treatment for many weeks with an Ommaya reservoir is sometimes employed.

The IV administration of amphotericin B usually produces chills, fever, vomiting, and headache. Tolerance may be enhanced by temporary lowering of the dose or administration of corticosteroids, aspirin, phenothiazines, or antihistaminics. Therapeutically active amounts of amphotericin B commonly impair kidney and liver function and can produce anemia, hypokalemia, shock, and a variety of neurologic symptoms.

2. Griseofulvin (Fulvin, Grifulvin) can inhibit growth of some dermatophytes but has no effect on bacteria or on the fungi that cause deep mycoses. The absorbed drug has an affinity for skin and is deposited there, bound to keratin. Thus, it makes keratin resistant to fungal growth and the new growth of hair or nails is first freed of infection. As keratinized structures are shed, they are replaced by uninfected ones. Topical application has little effect.

The best absorbed preparation consists of ultramicrosize particles (Gris-PEG). Oral doses of 0.3-0.5 g daily must be given for 6 weeks if only the skin is involved and for 3-6 months or longer if the hair and nails are involved. Griseofulvin is most successful in severe dermatophytosis, particularly if caused by trichophyton or microsporon.

Side effects include headache, nausea, diarrhea, photosensitivity, fever, skin rashes, and disturbances of nervous and hematopoietic systems. Griseofulvin increases the breakdown of coumarin anticoagulants.

3. Nystatin (Mycostatin) inhibits *Candida* sp. upon direct contact. It is not absorbed from mucous membranes or the gut. Nystatin in ointments, suspensions, and so on, can be applied to buccal or vaginal mucous membranes to suppress a local candida infection.

4. Flucytosine has been used (150 mg/kg/day) orally in various fungus infections, including *Cryptococcus, Candida,* and *Torulopsis*. The efficacy of the drug is limited by the emergence of resistance, which can be delayed by simultaneous administration of amphotericin B. Treatment with this drug combination is beneficial in cryptococcal meningitis and disseminated candidiasis. Flucytosine can produce depression of bone marrow and loss of hair.

5. Antifungal imidazoles inhibit lipid synthesis in fungal cell membranes and inhibit growth. **Clotrimazole,** 10-mg troches taken by mouth five times daily, can suppress oral candidiasis. **Miconazole** is effective as 2% cream in suppressing dermatophytosis and vaginal candidiasis. Systemic miconazole is difficult to administer and has marginal effects in mycoses. **Ketoconazole** is given orally in a single daily dose of 200-600 mg and is well absorbed. It can dramatically improve mucocutaneous candidiasis and paracoccidioidomycosis and is the drug of choice in blastomycosis. The benefits in pulmonary coccidioidomycosis and histoplasmosis are more limited, and in meningitis due to these fungi there appears to be no effect. **Fluconazole** can be given orally (200 mg/day) and reaches the CNS to suppress cryptococcal meningitis.

Adverse effects of imidazoles include nausea, vomiting, skin rashes, and elevations of transaminase levels. There may be a block of synthesis of adrenal steroids, leading to gynecomastia.

IV. SPECIFIC TYPES OF SURGICAL INFECTIONS

William P. Schecter
Dennis J. Flora

A. CELLULITIS, LYMPHANGITIS, AND LYMPHADENITIS.

Cellulitis is a common infection of the skin and subcutaneous tissues, with prominent infiltration of polymorphonuclear leukocytes but no gross suppuration except, perhaps, at the portal of entry. **Lymphangitis** is an infection ascending the lymphatic channels in the arms and legs. **Lymphadenitis** is infection of the regional lymph nodes as a result of cellulitis and lymphangitis; rarely these nodes suppurate and form abscesses.

Most cases are caused by aerobic hemolytic streptococci. *Staphylococcus aureus* and *Staphylococcus epidermidis* as well as anaerobic streptococci also can be responsible. Diabetes, alcoholism, and the postphlebitic syndrome are often associated with these infections.

1. Diagnosis
a. Symptoms and signs
(1) There may be a surgical wound, puncture, skin ulcer, or patch of dermatitis, but often a portal of entry is not seen.

(2) Moderately high fever.

(3) Cellulitis on an extremity is a rapidly advancing warm, tender, red or reddish-brown area of edematous skin.

(4) Lymphangitis produces red, tender, warm streaks 1-2 cm wide leading from the cellulitis toward the regional lymph nodes.

(5) Lymphadenitis is diagnosed by the presence of enlarged, tender regional lymph nodes.

(6) *Erysipelas* is a severe form of cellulitis, actually an acute lymphangitis of the skin, with a well-demarcated raised advancing edge. It is caused by group A β-hemolytic streptococci and is most common in children and the elderly.

(7) *Acute hemolytic streptococcal gangrene* is a rare, intense form of streptococcal cellulitis that progresses to necrosis of the skin and subcutaneous tissue. It is most likely to occur if the blood supply to the part is diminished.

b. Laboratory tests

(1) Leukocytosis is usually present.

(2) Material for culture is difficult to obtain from the infected area; blood cultures may be positive.

2. Differential diagnosis

a. Thrombophlebitis can resemble cellulitis; swelling is usually greater in phlebitis, and tenderness may be localized over a vein. Fever is higher in cellulitis. Suppurative thrombophlebitis occurs most often in association with intravenous drug use. Pus is present within the lumen of the vein. Surgical excision of the vein is required.

b. Contact allergy such as poison oak or poison ivy may be indistinguishable from cellulitis in its early phase; nonhemorrhagic vesiculation is characteristic of the allergic process later.

c. Chemical inflammation can mimic cellulitis.

d. Cat scratch fever can cause local inflammation, lymphangitis, and suppuration of regional lymph nodes.

e. Intense pain with marked edema, with or without hemorrhagic bullae and skin necrosis, suggests *necrotizing fasciitis* as the correct diagnosis.

3. Treatment.
The affected part is immobilized and elevated, and hot packs are applied. Antibiotic therapy is based on Gram stain and culture if available; usually the surgeon must select an antibiotic without this information.

a. Clear-cut streptococcal cellulitis

(1) *Mild disease:* 2.4 million units of procaine penicillin G IM daily or penicillin V, 1-4 g/day orally.

(2) *Moderate or severe disease* (including all patients with lymphangitis or lymphadenitis): 1.5-20 million units of aqueous penicillin G IV daily in divided doses every 4 hours.

b. Staphylococcal cellulitis (localized, spreads slowly, tends to suppurate) alone or mixed with streptococcal infection: Penicillinase-resistant penicillin orally or IV, depending upon the severity of the infection.

Examine the patient one or more times daily to look for hidden abscess and to determine response to treatment.

B. BURSITIS. Bursitis is an inflammation of one or more synovial bursae. Bacterial infection of the prepatellar and epithrochlear bursae is a common problem in patients with a history of alcoholism or intravenous drug use. Streptococci and staphylococci are the most common offending bacteria.

1. Diagnosis. A painful red swollen area over the prepatellar and epitrochlear bursae is often associated with a skin abrasion. Sometimes the bursa spontaneously drains pus through a small opening in the skin.

2. Differential diagnosis. Gout, pyarthrosis, and sterile "traumatic" bursitis.

3. Complications. Skin loss, chronic open draining bursae, necrotizing soft tissue infection, and knee or elbow stiffness.

4. Treatment. Swollen bursae should be aspirated and the fluid Gram stained, cultured, and examined for crystals. Antibiotic therapy should be guided by the results of the Gram stain and culture. Empiric coverage against streptococci is the general rule. Drainage of partial abscesses should usually be accomplished through a small incision, to avoid the complication of a chronically draining bursa. Alternatively, the bursa can be drained and closed over tubes. Ultimately, infected bursae may require excision with or without flap coverage to achieve healing.

C. FURUNCLE. A furuncle or boil is an abscess of a sweat gland or hair follicle. Furuncles can be serious when multiple and recurrent (furunculosis). This condition usually occurs in adolescents or in uncontrolled diabetics and is due to dermatologic disease, altered glandular secretions, or impaired resistance to common skin organisms. *S. aureus* and diphtheroids are the organisms recovered from the furuncle most commonly.

1. Diagnosis. Furuncles produce pain and itching. The skin is red and indurated initially and then turns white over the center of the abscess. Systemic symptoms are rare except in furunculosis in poorly controlled diabetics.

2. Differential diagnosis: Gout, bursitis, inflamed Baker's cyst, fungal infections, malignant skin tumors, and inflamed sebaceous or inclusion cysts.

3. Complications. Suppurative thrombophlebitis may develop when furuncles are located near major veins. A furuncle on the face may lead to intracranial venous thrombosis.

4. Treatment: Hot packs and then incision and drainage after the process had localized. Squeezing or incision before localization must be avoided. Antibiotics are rarely indicated except in patients with furuncles on the nose or face or in the immunosuppressed host. An appropriate antibiotic is dicloxacillin, 500 mg orally every 6 hours. The antibiotic regimen should be altered depending on sensitivities of the organism(s).

Patients with furunculosis should be checked for diabetes or immune deficiencies. Have the patient bathe all over once or twice daily with soap containing hexachlorophene or other antiseptics.

D. CARBUNCLE. A carbuncle is an infection that dissects through the dermis and subcutaneous tissue to form myriad connecting tunnels. Some of the small extensions open to the surface, giving the appearance of partially confluent furuncles with many pustular openings. There is considerable surrounding induration. The common cause is *S. aureus*. The patient usually has fever and malaise. The back of the neck is a typical site. In debilitated or diabetic patients, carbuncles may extend locally, may disseminate, may result in an epidural abscess or meningitis, and may become life-threatening.

1. Treatment

a. Carbuncles are best treated by excision of the entire process, including all of the sinus tracts; these tracts usually extend far beyond the cutaneous evidence of suppuration. A large open wound results, but failure to excise all of the sinuses allows infection to persist.

b. Specific antibiotic therapy directed against penicillinase-producing staphylococci frequently helps localize the process and reduces the extent of surgical excision. Antibiotic therapy is indicated in the compromised host (diabetics and immunosuppressed patients) with or without systemic manifestations.

    c. Diabetes mellitus must be sought and treated.

E. HIDRADENITIS. Simple hidradenitis is a localized dermal-subcutaneous infection involving apocrine and, rarely, eccrine sweat glands. **Hidradenitis suppurativa** is a chronic, indolent disease of the skin and subcutaneous tissues in apocrine gland–bearing areas, principally the axilla, groin, and perineum. The disease occurs in both sexes, but women develop the axillary form of the disease more frequently and men show a greater tendency toward perianal involvement. Hidradenitis appears after puberty; obesity and a genetic tendency to acne are apparent predisposing factors.

    1. Diagnosis. The involved area is diffusely indurated and fibrotic, with multiple intercommunicating sinuses that drain pus. In the acute phase of the disease, *S. aureus* is the most common organism. Chronic cases usually yield *Proteus* or *Pseudomonas*.

    2. Differential diagnosis. Hidradenitis suppurativa is differentiated from furunculosis by skin biopsy. Hidradenitis in the perianal area mimics complex anorectal fistulas. Fistulas have a primary orifice in the anal canal, one or more secondary openings on the perianal skin, and firm tracts connecting the primary and secondary orifices.

    3. Treatment

    a. Unless an abscess is pointing, incision and drainage of individual lesions should be avoided to minimize the formation of draining sinuses. Warm, moist compresses and antibiotics may allow the process to resolve.

    b. Pointing abscesses are incised and drained. Regular cleansing, avoidance of shaving the axillary hair, and discontinuance of topical deodorants and powders may be helpful.

    c. Advanced cases may require excision of *all* affected apocrine-bearing tissue with primary closure or skin grafting.

    d. Perianal hidradenitis may need preliminary diverting colostomy followed by excision of the infected tissue.

    4. Prognosis is good after excision of all affected areas.

F. POSTOPERATIVE WOUND INFECTION. Bacterial contamination of surgical wounds during or immediately after the procedure is a common event. The size of the bacterial inoculum, the pathogenicity of the organisms, and the resistance of the host determine whether infection develops. Diseases (e.g., diabetes) and medication (e.g., immunosuppressants) may compromise host resistance systemically; wound resistance is impaired locally by tissue trauma, devitalized tissue, foreign bodies, and dead space. These problems are minimized by gentle, precise surgical technic. Bacterial contamination is minimized by skin antiseptics and strict surgical asepsis. The value of prophylactic antibiotics is discussed briefly on page 216. Postoperative care must emphasize maintenance of blood volume and oxygenation to preserve the wound's defenses against infection.

In "clean" operations, the incidence of infection is about 1%. In "clean"-contaminated procedures (e.g., biliary or upper GI), wound infection rates of 5%-15% are reported. Heavily contaminated wounds (e.g., perforated colon) may become infected in 20%-30% of cases and are best managed by leaving the skin and subcutaneous fat open for 4-5 days, then approximating the skin with paper tapes if the wound has no signs of infection (delayed primary closure).

1. Diagnosis. Wound infections usually occur in subcutaneous tissues; seldom do they develop deep to the muscle and fascia. Streptococcal and clostridial wound infections cause symptoms and signs as early as 24 hours postoperatively. The majority of infections, those due to staphylococci and gram-negative organisms, become evident 4-10 days after the operation. Occasionally, an infection does not appear until weeks or months have elapsed.

The first sign is fever, and the patient may complain of excessive pain in the wound. Streptococcal cellulitis is evident on inspection, but the wound may not appear grossly inflamed in the other types of infection. The wound is edematous, indurated, and tender; sometimes fluctuance or crepitus is palpable. Subfascial infection is difficult to detect but should be suspected with persistent fever, pain, and localized tenderness.

2. Treatment

a. Streptococcal cellulitis is treated as other cellulitis. It is wise open the wound to ensure that no pus is present.

b. Other infections require opening the wound and allowing it to drain.

c. A culture for aerobes and anaerobes should be obtained. Before the antibiotic era, aerobic streptococci and staphylococci were predominant. After the introduction of penicillin, penicillin-resistant *S. aureus* infections became common. Wound infections are often caused by gram-negative bacteria.

G. NECROTIZING FASCIITIS is a relatively rare, aggressive, invasive infection that has been variously described in the older literature as *acute streptococcal gangrene* and *hospital gangrene*. This infection is characterized by thrombosis of vessels passing from the deep circulation to the skin, producing necrosis of the skin, subcutaneous tissue, and fascia. It is more common in patients with ischemic small vessel disease (e.g., in diabetics).

Most fasciitis is caused by a mixture of bacteria, including group A beta-hemolytic streptococci, anaerobic streptococci, microaerophilic streptococci, *S. aureus,* coliforms, *Bacteroides fragilis,* and *Fusobacterium.*

1. Diagnosis. Puncture wounds, leg ulcers, or perforating injuries of hollow viscera often precede the development of fasciitis. The infection spreads extensively through skin and undermines along fascial planes, causing necrosis of skin, fat, and fascia; muscle and bone remain viable. The appearance in the early stages resembles cellulitis, but edema, hypesthesia, and marked tenderness extend well beyond the erythematous area. Marked edema and hemorrhagic blebs signify death of the skin; fascial necrosis is even more extensive than the cutaneous changes. Crepitus is present if gas-forming organisms are involved. The patient is febrile and toxic. Blood cultures are positive in 10% of patients. Radiographs may show gas in the soft tissues. The operative findings confirm the diagnosis: edematous, dull grey, necrotic fascia and subcutaneous fat. The underlying muscle is usually viable. Thrombi are often visible in penetrating veins.

2. Differential diagnosis

a. Cellulitis, abscess, and phlebitis are usually localized; they are not as rapidly progressive, and there is less systemic toxicity than in fasciitis.

b. Clostridial myositis and gangrene from arterial occlusion are associated with necrosis of muscle.

3. Treatment

a. Correct deficiencies of fluids, electrolytes, and red cell mass; these may be severe.

b. Treat hyperthermia.

c. Obtain aerobic and anaerobic cultures of the wound, do a Gram stain on the wound exudate, and draw blood for the culture.

d. Intravenous antibiotics are begun immediately after obtaining specimens for culture. Initial treatment should be:

(1) Penicillin G, 1.5-4 million units IV every 4 hours.

(2) Clindamycin, 600 mg IV every 8 hours (to cover *S. aureus* and *B. fragilis*).

(3) Gentamicin, 2 mg/kg IV initially, followed by 1.5 mg/kg every 8 hours. Aminoglycloside therapy should be monitored with peak (dose) and trough (dose) serum levels.

e. Surgical debridement and drainage under general or regional anesthesia are mandatory. Excision must extend beyond the fascial involvement. Where necrotic fascia undermines viable skin, longitudinal skin incisions permit debridement of fascia without sacrificing skin. Necrotic muscle is usually not a feature of necrotizing fasciitis.

f. The wound must be inspected repeatedly after operation, and further debridement is performed if necessary.

g. Skin grafts may be placed on the defects after the infection is under control and all necrotic tissue has been removed.

4. Prognosis. The mortality rate is 25%-30%; however, with early recognition and prompt therapy, few patients die of this disease.

H. TETANUS is caused by the neurotoxin of *Clostridium tetani,* which reduces inhibitory activity in the CNS. Tetanus bacilli are ubiquitous in nature and can easily contaminate even minor wounds. Punctures and wounds containing devitalized tissue or foreign bodies provide favorable conditions for the proliferation of these anaerobic organisms. The incubation period for tetanus averages 8 days (1-50 days).

1. Diagnosis is based on a history of injury followed by development of one of the three clinical forms of tetanus. Laboratory tests are of little value.

a. Local tetanus. Persistent, unyielding rigidity of the group of muscles in close proximity to the injury. Symptoms may continue for weeks. It may progress to generalized forms.

b. Generalized tetanus. This is the most common form. Trismus (lockjaw) and spasms of the facial muscles (risus sardonicus) are the initial manifestations in more than 50% of patients. Tonic contractions of the face, neck, back, and abdomen are common; severe spasms of the back muscles may produce opisthotonos. Difficulty swallowing, laryngospasm, and hesitant micturition occur later. Trivial stimuli may elicit gross spasms or seizures. Temperature may rise 2-4° C during these spasms; profuse sweating is common. Tachycardia is a grave sign.

c. Cephalic tetanus. In this unusual form, there is dysfunction of multiple cranial nerves. The incubation period is short, and it develops after otitis media or injuries to the scalp. The prognosis is extremely poor.

2. Prevention. Tetanus is a preventable disease. All persons should be immunized against tetanus, and additional prophylactic measures should be taken when tetanus-prone injuries occur.

a. Previously immunized individuals. If immunized within the past 10 years, give 0.5 ml of adsorbed tetanus toxoid IM. If a tetanus-prone wound occurred more than 24 hours before, give also 250 units of tetanus immune globulin (human) IM and consider penicillin in addition.

b. Individuals not previously immunized.

(1) If tetanus is unlikely because the wound is clean and minor, give 0.5 ml of adsorbed tetanus toxoid IM. The immunization schedule should be completed as follows: second injection 4-6 weeks after the initial one, and a third injection in 6-12 months.

(2) All other wounds require 0.5 ml of adsorbed tetanus toxoid IM plus 250-350 units of tetanus immune globulin (human) IM. Use different syringes and inject at different sites to avoid suppressing the development of active immunity. Consider the use of penicillin. The schedule should be completed as above.

c. Tetanus antitoxin. Equine antitoxin should be used prophylatically only if tetanus immune globulin (human) is not available and only if the possibility of tetanus exceeds the danger of allergic reaction. If the patient is not sensitive to horse serum by history and by testing, give 3000-6000 units of antitoxin IM.

d. Actively immunized patients may not have the usual anamnestic response to tetanus toxoid in the following situations: agammaglobulinemia, exposure to acute doses of radiation, immunosuppressive drugs (including chloramphenicol), and carcinoma of the breast (these patients may not respond to injections of tetanus toxoid in the ipsilateral upper extremity).

e. Debridement and gentle cleansing of the wounds with saline solution or dilute peroxide (use no antiseptics) remove the conditions that favor the growth of tetanus bacilli.

3. Treatment. Tetanus is a true emergency, and therapy should be instituted at once. A team of surgeon, internist, and anesthesiologist provides optimal care.

a. Neutralize the toxin by injecting 3000-6000 units of tetanus immune globulin (human) into the muscle in the region of the wound or further proximal in the extremity. **Do not inject this material intravenously.**

b. Debride the wound about 1 hour after serotherapy. Leave the wound open.

c. Control the muscle spasms and/or seizures by isolating the patient in a dark, quiet room. Diazepam, chlorpromazine, and short-acting barbiturates are used cautiously to avoid respiratory and cardiac depression.

d. IV aqueous penicillin G, 10-20 million units/day in divided doses, may kill the vegetative clostridia and prevent release of neurotoxin. Clindamycin is an alternative in the patient who is allergic to penicillin.

e. Respiratory failure requires intubation and mechanical ventilation.

4. Prognosis. The mortality rate is inversely proportional to the length of the incubation period and directly proportional to the severity of symptoms. Active immunization should be completed in survivors; an attack of tetanus does not confer permanent immunity.

I. OTHER CLOSTRIDIAL INFECTIONS. *C. perfringens (welchii), C. novyi, C. septicum,* and other clostridial species are ubiquitous in soil and in the intestinal tracts of animals and humans. These organisms elaborate toxins that destroy tissue and produce a spectrum of diseases ranging in severity from minor to fulminating. An anaerobic environment is required for these bacteria to proliferate; devitalized tissue, pyogenic infections, and foreign bodies provide suitable conditions.

1. Diagnosis

a. Simple contamination. Infection of superficial necrotic tissue is the least serious of the clostridial infections. The surrounding tissues are healthy, there is no invasion, and there are no systemic symptoms or signs. Debridement of dead tissue is curative. If untreated, it can progress to one of the severe infections listed below.

b. Gas abscess (Welch's abscess) is a localized infection without muscle involvement. There is little pain or systemic toxicity. A foul, brown, seropurulent exudate and gas in tissues some distance from the local infection are characteristic.

c. Anaerobic clostridial cellulitis. This invasive infection remains superficial to the deep fascia but spreads through subcutaneous tissue at an alarming rate. There is little pain and mild to moderate toxicity (compared with myositis). The tissue is edematous, crepitant, and discolored. There may be cutaneous bullae.

d. Clostridial myositis and myonecrosis may be localized or diffuse. The classic diffuse form (gas gangrene) has an acute onset (incubation period <3 days) and a fulminating course. Profound toxemia appears early and progresses to delirium. The wound is severely painful and has shiny edematous skin with bullae and patchy necrosis in some cases. There is a serosanguinous discharge that has a characteristically sweet odor; Gram stain shows a few inflammatory cells and large gram-positive rods. Gas in the tissues is a late finding and may be so finely distributed that it cannot be detected.

Material for Gram stain and culture may be obtained by needle aspiration initially. The results aid in selection of antibiotic therapy prior to definitive surgical treatment.

2. Differential diagnosis

a. The absence of muscle involvement excludes clostridial myositis. The other clostridial infections spare the fascia as well, whereas in necrotizing fasciitis the fascia is necrotic.

b. Other infections can produce gas—e.g., anaerobic-aerobic mixed cellulitis. The differential diagnosis is made by Gram stain of the exudate.

3. Prevention. Clostridial infections are preventable by early debridement of contaminated wounds with devitalized tissue. Prophylactic penicillin is useful, but the emphasis must be on surgical debridement.

4. Treatment

a. Surgical

(1) Radical debridement of all necrotic and damaged tissue is **mandatory.** Tight fascial compartments must be decompressed. Multiple debridements are often required.

(2) Amputation is necessary when there is diffuse muscle necrosis and loss of blood supply to the limb.

(3) Clostridial cellulitis requires aggressive debridement but not amputation. If muscle bleeds well and contracts when stimulated, it should not be excised.

b. Antibiotics. Penicillin G, 20–40 million units in divided doses every 4 hours, is given IV each day. Chloramphenicol and clindamycin are alternatives if penicillin cannot be used.

c. Polyvalent antitoxin. An IV dose of 75,000 units repeated every 6 hours (for a total of four doses) is given only if surgical debridement cannot encompass the infection (e.g., infections in brain, spinal cord, and some abdominal wounds). The effectiveness of this antitoxin is uncertain.

d. Hyperbaric oxygen has value in the treatment of myonecrosis when the affected part cannot be amputated (e.g., perineal or abdominal wounds).

J. SUPPURATIVE (SEPTIC) THROMBOPHLEBITIS is infection in a thrombosed vein and is usually associated with IV catheters (especially in burn patients) or drug abuse. It may be a cause of persistent sepsis in patients with anaerobic pelvic infections. The incidence of septic thrombophlebitis of the subclavian vein has increased since the advent of IV hyperalimentation.

The microorganisms most commonly recovered from burn patients with septic thrombophlebitis are *Klebsiella, S. aureus, Pseudomonas,* and *C. albicans.*

1. Diagnosis. The usual presentation is fever and bacteremia. The diagnosis is established by persistent fever, repeatedly positive blood cultures, and pus within the involved vein on aspiration or incision. Local signs of inflammation are apparent on the extremities but often absent when the subclavian vein is involved.

2. Differential diagnosis. Undrained abscesses, endocarditis, or (rarely) infected arterial catheters can be responsible for fever and positive blood cultures.

3. Complications. Septic shock and death. Extension of septic thrombosis into the great veins of the mediastinum. Bacterial endocarditis. Septic pulmonary emboli.

4. Treatment

a. Antibiotic therapy directed against the organism recovered by blood culture or from the vein.

b. If the diagnosis is suspected, an exploratory venotomy should be done proximal to the venipuncture site. Pus in the vein requires complete excision of the involved vein; the contaminated wound is left open for delayed primary closure or healing by secondary intention.

c. Septic thrombosis of the subclavian or innominate veins or superior vena cava requires anticoagulation and specific antibiotics.

K. INFECTIONS RESULTING FROM DRUG ABUSE. Drug abuse produces a number of challenging atypical infections. The source most often is the skin, but unsterile equipment and contaminated drug mixtures also contribute.

1. Diagnosis. Most of these infections occur on the extremities at sites of IV or extravascular injection. The drug mixtures are often irritating and vasoconstricting, creating a favorable environment for proliferation of bacteria. Various types of infections may occur.

a. Cutaneous and subcutaneous infections vary from simple cellulitis or abscess to necrotizing infections. Large areas of necrosis, multiple abscesses, foul discharge, and gas formation may occur. Suppurative thrombophlebitis is very common.

b. Fascial and subfascial infections. The needle may penetrate the fascia, causing infection in the deep spaces; the external signs of abscess may be absent or minimal.

c. Tetanus. Female addicts are prone to this disease because they more often take drugs by "skin popping" (extravascular injection), and they are less likely to be immunized against tetanus. Inclusion of quinine in the drug mixture creates an anaerobic environment that promotes the growth of tetanus bacilli.

d. Cardiovascular. Infected arteritis and mycotic aneurysms may develop, especially in amphetamine users. Bacterial or fungal endocarditis may occur. *S. aureus,* gram-negative aerobes, and *C. albicans* are common organisms.

e. Pulmonary. Septic pulmonary emboli, empyema, and aspiration pneumonia due to overdose are among the pulmonary infections in these patients.

f. Shared needles may result in parenteral transmission of blood-borne infections, such as hepatitis B and C, malaria, and HIV.

2. Treatment. Bacterial infections in the soft tissues must be incised, pus evacuated, and necrotic tissue debrided. The deep fascial compartments must be opened if the abscess is not discovered more superficially. Antibiotic therapy is advisable. Coexisting endocarditis should be considered if fever does not subside after adequate care of the wound. Involvement of joint spaces should be suspected if soft tissue infections occur nearby—especially in the hand.

L. PILONIDAL SINUS is a chronic infection caused by penetration of a foreign body (hair) into the subcutaneous tissues. The sinus is lined by granulation tissue, and it often leads to a cavity filled with granulation tissue and hair. If the sinus closes temporarily, a pilonidal **cyst** remains in the deeper tissues;

acute exacerbation of the chronic infection produces a pilonidal **abscess.**

   1. Diagnosis. Most pilonidal sinuses are in the posterior midline over the sacrum or sacrococcygeal junction. Acute infection is usually the first manifestation. After spontaneous or surgical drainage, the sinus discharges pus.

   Examination reveals an abscess of one or more sinus tracts. The process can be extensive, with multiple, complex, intercommunicating sinuses over a large area. Aerobic and anaerobic fecal flora can be cultured.

   2. Differential diagnosis

   a. Anorectal fistulas usually open closer to the anus and have a palpable tract extending toward a primary orifice in the anal canal.

   b. Perianal hidradenitis suppurativa may also involve the groin and/or axilla. Pilonidal sinus and hidradenitis usually can be differentiated by clinical examination.

   c. Osteomyelitis of the sacrum is uncommon; lateral radiographs may demonstrate it.

   d. Simple furuncles or even carbuncles are very unusual in this location; a sinus tract with projecting hair is characteristic of pilonidal disease.

   3. Complications. Malignancy arising in chronic pilonidal sinuses has been reported.

   4. Treatment

   a. Drain acute abscesses, usually under local anesthesia. It may be possible to curette the cavity to remove hair and thus accomplish definitive treatment at the same time.

   b. The vast majority of sinus tracts and cysts respond to unroofing, curettage of the contents, and packing. The surrounding hair should be shaved weekly even after healing occurs to avoid recurrence.

   c. In exceptional patients (e.g., those with recurrent sinuses), the involved area can be excised and closed primarily, marsupialized, or left to heal secondarily.

M. ACTINOMYCOSIS. This chronic suppurative and granulomatous disease progresses slowly to form multiple sinuses. The causative organisms are true bacteria. Actinomycetes are gram-positive filamentous organisms. They are strict anaerobes and are found commonly in the pharynx. The head and neck are the most common sites of actinomycosis; about 20% have involvement of the chest, and an equal proportion have abdominal lesions (usually in the cecum and appendix).

1. Diagnosis. There may be no systemic symptoms. Firm, nontender, nodular masses with abscesses and multiple draining sinuses are characteristic. "Sulfur granules"—tiny, yellowish masses that microscopically consist of threads enveloped by dark-staining clubs—appear in the pus. Secondary bacterial infection is common. Pulmonary lesions cause fever, cough, pleuritic pain, and weight loss. The sinuses may eventually penetrate through the chest wall. Abdominal actinomycosis mimics appendicitis or may perforate to form sinuses of the abdominal wall.

2. Treatment. Surgical excision or drainage is required. Actinomycetes usually are sensitive to penicillin (5-20 million units/day) given over many weeks.

N. NOCARDIOSIS. The localized form of nocardiosis resembles actinomycosis. Systemic nocardiosis begins in the lungs and spreads hematogenously to distant sites. It is prone to develop in immunodeficient patients. Surgical drainage and excision of accessible lesions are essential. A sulfonamide (e.g., sulfisoxazole, 6-8 g/day orally) is given for many weeks. Minocycline (200-400 mg/day orally) may be a useful adjunct.

O. THE DIABETIC FOOT. Diabetic patients may present with serious chronic infections in the foot which can result in amputation and death. Diabetic microangiopathy, often associated with peripheral vascular disease, results in inadequate blood supply to the feet. Poor immune response to infection compounds the problem.

1. Diagnosis. The patient may present with a swollen, infected foot or toe. Alternatively, erythema may not be present if there is severe ischemia. The toes and the plantar surfaces of the foot, over the first, second, and fifth metatarsal heads, are the most common areas of infection. A careful vascular examination with measurement of the ankle and brachial blood pressures is important. After control of the infection, an arteriogram to identify a reconstructible vascular lesion should be considered.

2. Complications. Diabetic patients with foot infections should be told at the outset that their limb is in jeopardy. Aggressive medical and surgical therapy is necessary to prevent amputation or at least limit amputation to the lowest possible level.

3. Treatment. Antibiotic therapy should be guided by the Gram stain, culture, and antibiotic sensitivity. Initial coverage of anaerobic and gram-negative organisms is prudent. Areas of moist gangrene should be dried by painting the area with povidone-iodine and placing lamb's wool between the toes. Conservative debridement of nonviable tissue, including tendon and exposed bone, is important. Occult infection frequently tracks much further proximally than suspected by the physical examination. Repeated trips to the operating room to stay ahead of the infection may be necessary. Amputation of the toes and a ray amputation of the fifth metatarsal may be necessary. For more severe infections with pedal pulses detectable by palpation or Doppler ultrasonography, a transmetatarsal amputation may be required. For more proximal infections, a below-knee amputation or even an above-knee amputation may be necessary. All amputation stumps should be left open and revised later once the infection is controlled.

4. Prevention. All diabetic patients should be instructed to inspect and wash their feet daily. Areas between the feet should be dried. Well-padded shoes with a perfect fit should be worn. Walking barefoot, even indoors, should be discouraged. Cuts, abrasions, and blisters are emergencies that should be treated under medical supervision.

V. FUNGAL INFECTIONS

Among the deep mycoses, *Coccidioides* and *Histoplasma* infections are discussed in Chapter 8. **Sporotrichosis** presents as a series of hard, enlarged, nontender nodes along lymphatics draining the site of traumatic inoculation of vegetable matter. Surgical drainage is rarely required, and the disease is self-limiting or responds to antifungal drugs. **Chromomycosis** presents as verrucous cauliflower-like nodes on extremities. Surgical excision and skin grafting may be curative. **Mycetoma** forms deep draining abscesses discharging colored granules, most often on the feet or legs of persons leading a barefoot existence. *Paracoccidioides* infection may result in localized or generalized granulomas in various organs after infection in Central or South America. It may respond to systemic administration of amphotericin B (0.4-0.8 mg/kg/day) or ketoconazole (200-400 mg daily by mouth). **North American blastomycosis** begins as a pulmonary infection but may produce disseminated granulomas, especially in skin, bones, or the genitourinary tract. It may respond to ketoconazole, sometimes with drainage or resection.

In debilitating diseases, addiction, or immunosuppression, opportunistic infections are of surgical concern. ***Candida*** may produce intertrigo, paronychia, vaginitis, or esophagitis. It may also invade, producing endocarditis or renal or pulmonary disease. Ketoconazole orally (200-400 mg/day) or amphotericin B IV is required treatment for candidiasis.

Cryptococcus enters via the lung but often produces meningitis in immunosuppressed patients. The treatment is amphotericin B plus flucytosine. ***Aspergillus* sp.** may proliferate in the immunosuppressed, producing fungus balls in cavities due to other causes or invasive pulmonary granulomas. **Mucormycosis** can occur in debilitated persons, especially with diabetic ketoacidosis. It produces infection in sinuses, lungs, or brain, with aseptic hyphae seen in biopsies. It often requires drainage and resection as well as antifungal drugs.

VI. RABIES

Rabies is a viral encephalitis transmitted to humans through the saliva of animals; left untreated it is fatal. The problem confronting the surgeon is the management of an animal bite.

All bite or scratch wounds should be flushed and cleansed repeatedly with soap and water.

If the responsible animal is a pet, it should be quarantined and observed by a veterinarian. If it dies, the brain must be examined for rabies virus by the Health Department. If the responsible animal is a skunk, bat, fox, coyote, or raccoon, it should be presumed to be rabid. If it can be captured or killed, the brain is examined. Otherwise, the patient should receive the postexposure treatment:

a. Inactivated, diploid cell–grown rabies vaccine in five doses as described by the manufacturer and available through state Health Departments.

b. Tetanus booster dose; consider antimicrobial therapy.

c. The likelihood of a significant exposure to rabies can be discussed with the Consultation Service at Communicable Disease Center, Atlanta, GA (404-329-3311).

d. In cases of severe exposure from probably rabid animals, passive immunization is given: Human rabies immune globulin is administered in a dose of 20 units/kg. Half the dose is infiltrated around the bite wound and the other half is given IM once.

e. Any person receiving rabies vaccine must be observed for possible allergic encephalomyelitis. This occurs rarely with diploid cell vaccine.

Any person at very high risk of rabies exposure, e.g., veterinarians, humane society employees, workers in hyperendemic areas (e.g., rural areas of India or Latin America) should receive preexposure prophylaxis with diploid cell vaccine.

VII. SURGERY AND THE HIV EPIDEMIC

Universal precautions and risk reduction. An estimated 1.5 million Americans are infected with HIV, a retrovirus that is transmitted by (1) sexual intercourse with an infected person, and (2) parenteral exposure to infected blood and body fluids. IV drug users who share needles, individuals who have received transfusions of blood products infected with HIV, and the babies of HIV-infected mothers are at particularly high risk.

There is a risk of nosocomial HIV transmission in the health care setting. The risk of HIV transmission after a hollow needlestick injury is 0.03%. Because HIV is so widespread, all patients should be considered infected and infectious. Universal precautions should be employed when handling blood and body fluids. The underlying assumption of universal precautions is that **blood is a toxic substance.** Blood contact with the skin and mucous membranes of a health care worker is not acceptable. Two pairs of gloves, protective eye wear, water-impermeable gowns, and footwear are standard equipment that should be available in the emergency room and the operating room and on the wards for use in situations when the risk of blood exposure is significant. If a health care worker is exposed to blood or body fluids, he or she should obtain advice and evaluation from a professional with experience in the management of occupational exposure to blood and body fluids.

5

Oncology

Robert S. Warren, M.D.
Patrick S. Swift, M.D.
Alan P. Venook, M.D.

A. STAGING OF CANCER. Staging of malignancies, either clinical or pathologic, is designed to gain information regarding the prognosis of an individual patient, to aid in selecting the type and extent of surgical or medical therapy, and to permit the application of experimental therapeutic protocols to homogeneous cohorts of patients. The most commonly accepted system for staging of cancer is that of the American Joint Committee on Cancer, which has developed a paradigm for classification of solid tumors based on the size and extent of tumor at the primary site (T), the presence and extent of lymph node involvement (N), and the presence of distant metastases (M). This TNM system has been adopted worldwide, although for certain tumors older staging systems remain in common use. For each anatomic site of a primary tumor, early versus advanced disease (T1 versus T4) and minimal versus extensive nodal involvement (N1 versus N3) have been defined, and the relationship between clinical or pathologic stage and clinical outcome has been established. Examples of staging for two common tumors (breast and colorectal) are given in Figures 5-1 and 5-2, respectively.

I. SURGICAL ONCOLOGY

A. SURGERY FOR PRIMARY MALIGNANCIES. Despite advances in our understanding of the mechanisms of carcinogenesis, the development of new antineoplastic agents, and great improvements in the techniques of radiation therapy, surgery remains the mainstay of cancer treatment.

The reader is referred to previous chapters for discussion of the surgical management of malignancies arising in specific tissue sites. Surgery for solid tumors may be undertaken with either palliative or curative intent. Examples of palliative surgery include operation for bowel obstruction, tumorous fistulas, gastrointestinal (GI) hemorrhage, biliary obstruction, and pain produced by tumor growth at a specific site. The magnitude of curative surgical resection and the extent of tumor-free margins which result vary with the anatomic location and size of the primary tumor and take into account its known biologic behavior. For example, intramural extension of colorectal cancer distally rarely exceeds 2 cm, whereas proximal extension of esophageal cancer of more than 5 cm is common. Thus, the optimal surgical therapy of cancer must take into account the biologic and anatomic behavior of the tumor and demands knowledge of therapeutic alternatives to surgery, including antineoplastic drug therapy and radiation therapy. The joint participation of medical oncologists, radiation therapists, and surgical oncologists is critical to the development of effective preoperative and postoperative therapeutic strategies. This chapter highlights important general principles in the multimodality treatment of cancer, including commonly applied regimens of drug and radiation therapy and their complications.

B. SURGERY FOR METASTATIC DISEASE. Patients who have undergone potentially curative resection of a solid tumor are followed on a periodic basis for the development of locally recurrent or metastatic disease. Frequently, specific complaints alert the physician to the presence and site of tumor recurrence. Paradigms exist for the clinical and radiographic follow-up of cancer patients according to the site of primary tumor and its known anatomic pattern of local and distant spread. As an adjunct to physical examination and x-ray studies, the measurement of serum antigens commonly associated with specific cancers has been found useful in the diagnosis of recurrent cancer and in assessing the response to therapy (Table 5-1). None of these, however, is specific for cancer, and many are measurable in patients without malignancy. Thus, their utility in screening the general population is poor, although their use in patients at high risk for developing a particular cancer (e.g., AFP screening for hepatocellular carcinoma in patients with long-standing cirrhosis of the liver, or PSA screening for prostate cancer in elderly males) is under investigation. An elevated tumor marker leads the physician to initiate a work-up for recurrent and metastatic disease with the expectation that some combination of radiation, chemotherapy, or surgery may be of benefit. Although most solid tumors cannot be cured by any modality once distant metastases have developed, certain exceptions to this principle have led surgeons to aggressively treat metastatic disease in carefully selected patients with curative intent, as described below.

    1. Soft tissue sarcoma. These mesenchymal tumors

Text continued on p. 263.

FIGURE 5-1. Staging of breast cancer. (From the American Joint Committee on Cancer: *Manual for staging of cancer, ed 4,* Philadelphia, 1992, JB Lippincott.)

DEFINITION OF TNM

Primary Tumor (T)

Definitions for classifying the primary tumor (T) are the same for clinical and for pathologic classification. The telescoping method of classification can be applied. If the measurement is made by physical examination, the examiner will use the major headings (T1, T2, or T3). If other measurements, such as mammographic or pathologic, are used, the examiner can use the telescoped subsets of T1.

TX   Primary tumor cannot be assessed
T0   No evidence of primary tumor
Tis   Carcinoma *in situ:* intraductal carcinoma, lobular carcinoma in situ, or Paget's disease of the nipple with no tumor
T1   Tumor 2 cm or less in greatest dimension
    T1a   0.5 cm or less in greatest dimension
    T1b   More than 0.5 cm but not more than 1 cm in greatest dimension
    T1c   More than 1 cm but not more than 2 cm in greatest dimension
T2   Tumor more than 2 cm but not more than 5 cm in greatest dimension
T3   Tumor more than 5 cm in greatest dimension

Continued.

T4   Tumor of any size with direct extension to chest wall or skin
  T4a   Extension to chest wall
  T4b   Edema (including peau d'orange) or ulceration of the skin of the breast or satellite skin nodules confined to the same breast
  T4c   Both (T4a and T4b)
  T4d   Inflammatory carcinoma (See the definition of inflammatory carcinoma in the introduction.)

Note: Paget's disease associated with a tumor is classified according to the size of the tumor.

Regional Lymph Nodes (N)

NX   Regional lymph nodes cannot be assessed (e.g., previously removed)
N0   No regional lymph node metastasis
N1   Metastasis to movable ipsilateral axillary lymph node(s)
N2   Metastasis to ipsilateral axillary lymph node(s) fixed to one another or to other structures
N3   Metastasis to ipsilateral internal mammary lymph node(s)

FIGURE 5-1, cont'd. Staging of breast cancer.

DEFINITION OF TNM—cont'd.
Pathologic Classification (pN)

pNX	Regional lymph nodes cannot be assessed (e.g., previously removed, or not removed for pathologic study)
pN0	No regional lymph node metastasis
pN1	Metastasis to movable ipsilateral axillary lymph node(s)
pN1a	Only micrometastasis (none larger than 0.2 cm)
pN1b	Metastasis to lymph node(s), any larger than 0.2 cm
pN1bi	Metastasis in one to three lymph nodes, any more than 0.2 cm and all less than 2 cm in greatest dimension
pN1bii	Metastasis to four or more lymph nodes, any more than 0.2 cm and all less than 2 cm in greatest dimension
pN1biii	Extension of tumor beyond the capsule of a lymph node metastasis less than 2 cm in greatest dimension
pN1biv	Metastasis to a lymph node 2 cm or more in greatest dimension
pN2	Metastasis to ipsilateral axillary lymph nodes that are fixed to one another or to other structures
pN3	Metastasis to ipsilateral internal mammary lymph node(s)

Distant Metastasis (M)

MX Presence of distant metastasis cannot be assessed
M0 No distant metastasis
M1 Distant metastasis (includes metastasis to ipsilateral supraclavicular lymph node(s))

STAGE GROUPING

Stage	T	N	M
Stage 0	Tis	N0	M0
Stage I	T1	N0	M0
Stage IIA	T0	N1	M0
	T1	N1*	M0
	T2	N0	M0
Stage IIB	T2	N1	M0
	T3	N0	M0
Stage IIIA	T0	N2	M0
	T1	N2	M0
	T2	N2	M0
	T3	N1	M0
	T3	N2	M0
Stage IIIB	T4	Any N	M0
	Any T	N3	M0
Stage IV	Any T	Any N	M1

*Note: The prognosis of patients with N1a is similar to that of patients with pN0.

FIGURE 5-2. Staging of colorectal cancer. (From the American Joint Committee on Cancer: *Manual for staging of cancer, ed 4*, Philadelphia, 1992, JB Lippincott.)

DEFINITION OF TNM

The same classification is used for both clinical and pathologic staging.

Primary Tumor (T)

TX   Primary tumor cannot be assessed
T0   No evidence of primary tumor
Tis Carcinoma in situ: intraepithelial or invasion of the lamina propria*
T1   Tumor invades the submucosa
T2   Tumor invades the muscularis propria
T3   Tumor invades through the muscularis propria into the subserosa or into nonperitonealized pericolic or perirectal tissues
T4   Tumor directly invades other organs or structures and/or perforates the visceral peritoneum**

*Note: Tis includes cancer cells confined within the glandular basement membrane (intraepithelial) or lamina propria (intramucosal) with no extension through the muscularis mucosae into the submucosa.
**Note: Direct invasion of other organs or structures includes invasion of other segments of colorectum by way of serosa; for example, invasion of the sigmoid colon by a carcinoma of the cecum.

Regional Lymph Nodes (N)

NX   Regional lymph nodes cannot be assessed
N0   No regional lymph node metastasis

N1   Metastasis in one to three pericolic or perirectal lymph nodes
N2   Metastasis in four or more pericolic or perirectal lymph nodes
N3   Metastasis in any lymph node along the course of a named vascular trunk and/or metastasis to apical node(s) (when marked by the surgeon)

Distant Metastasis (M)

MX   Presence of distant metastasis cannot be assessed
M0   No distant metastasis
M1   Distant metastasis

STAGE GROUPINGS

AJCC/UICC				DUKES
Stage 0	Tis	N0	M0	—
Stage 1	T1	N0	M0	A
	T2	N0	M0	
Stage II	T3	N0	M0	B
	T4	N0	M0	
Stage III	Any T	N1	M0	C
	Any T	N2	M0	
	Any T	N3	M0	
Stage IV	Any T	Any N	M1	—

Note: Dukes B is a composite of better (T3, N0, M0) and worse (T4, N0, M0) prognostic groups, as is Dukes C (Any T, N1, M0 and Any T, N2, N3, M0).

Table 5-1. Tumor markers

Marker	Cancer	Screening	Detect recurrence	Follow response	Elevated in benign disease
Carcinoembryonic antigen	Colon	0	++++	+++	Smokers
	Breast	0	0	++	Pancreatitis
	Unknown primary	0	0	+	Inflammatory bowel disease
CA 125	Ovarian	0	+++	++++	Pregnancy, menstruation
CA 15-3	Breast	0	+++	++	
Alpha-fetoprotein	Hepatocellular carcinoma	++	+++	++++	Hepatic injury or cirrhosis
	Germ cell	+++	++++	++++	
β-HCG (human choriogonadotropin)	Germ cell	++++	++++	++++	Pregnancy
PSA (prostate-specific antigen)	Prostate	++-+++	+++	+++	Prostatitis

+ = ; ++ = ; +++ = ; ++++ = .

may develop within any connective tissue site but most commonly arise in the extremities, the trunk, or the retroperitoneum. The most frequent histologies include liposarcoma, fibrosarcoma, and malignant fibrous histiocytoma. Leiomyosarcoma is most frequently found arising from the smooth muscle of the GI tract or in the retroperitoneum. Although several other histologic types of sarcoma exist, the exact pathologic identity is of considerably less prognostic importance than are tumor size and histologic grade. High-grade tumors are defined as those with poor differentiation, minimal stroma, high vascularity, and >5 mitoses per 10 high power fields. Soft tissue sarcomas of the extremities were once treated primarily by amputation, but limb-sparing wide resection followed by local radiation has yielded equal results in terms of both local recurrence and long-term survival. Lymph node metastasis is exceedingly rare in extremity sarcomas, but pulmonary spread is common with high-grade tumors. These metastatic tumors are rarely responsive to chemotherapy, but selected patients with pulmonary metastases may be treated aggressively with wedge resection of the lung. These need not be limited to patients with solitary metastases, and many thoracic surgeons resect up to 10 metastases with multiple wedge resections. Because preoperative chest CT commonly underestimates the number of lesions found at exploratory thoracotomy, care should be taken in selecting patients for metastasectomy. It is also critical that the tumor at the primary site be controlled. In the case of GI leiomyosarcomas or retroperitoneal sarcomas, isolated metastasis to the liver may occur. In these cases, hepatic metastasectomy should be undertaken again, provided that the primary tumor has been completely resected without evidence of local recurrence.

2. Colorectal carcinoma. The liver is the first site of failure in 70% of patients with recurrent colorectal cancer. Without treatment the average survival in these patients is 9-12 months, and few, if any, are alive at 3 years. Large retrospective as well as prospective noncontrolled studies have indicated that nearly 30% of patients undergoing liver resection for metastatic colorectal cancer may be cured.

Although selection criteria vary among surgeons, generally accepted indications for resection of hepatic metastases include 3 or fewer detectable metastases (which may involve one or both hepatic lobes); the absence of extrahepatic tumor, including portal and celiac lymph nodes; and the ability to withstand major hepatic resection. Preoperative work-up should include chest, abdominal, and pelvic CT, and intraoperative ultrasonography is commonly used to rigorously exclude occult intrahepatic tumor in patients explored for resection. The extent of resection is dictated by the size of the tumors and their relationship to major vascular structures (branches of the portal and hepatic veins). The strategy is to obtain at least a 1-cm tumor-free surgical margin. This may be accomplished by one or more nonanatomic wedge resections, segmentectomies, right or left hepatic lobectomy, or less commonly right or left trisegmentectomy. Because liver regeneration is significantly diminished with aging and in the presence of cirrhosis, major hepatic resection (lobectomy or greater) should be undertaken with great caution in the elderly (>65 years) or in patients with evidence of micronodular cirrhosis or chronic active hepatitis. Recurrence of tumor following hepatic metastasectomy is more common in patients with a Dukes' C primary tumor than in those whose original tumor was classified as Dukes' B. In approximately half of the recurrences, the liver is the initial site. Most of the remainder recur first in the lung. The role of adjuvant chemotherapy following hepatic metastasectomy remains undefined.

Liver resection currently has no demonstrated benefit for isolated metastases from other sites in the GI tract (i.e., esophagus, stomach). However, palliative liver resection of metastatic endocrine tumors of the pancreas should be undertaken when all gross tumor can be removed safely.

Colorectal cancer may also produce solitary metastases to the lung or brain. In carefully selected patients with isolated disease, resection of metastases to these sites yields long-term survival.

3. Ovarian cancer. Metastasis from carcinoma of the ovary commonly involves multiple sites within the peritoneal cavity. This is the only solid tumor for which tumor debulking is of established benefit. The surgical strategy is to remove all gross tumor nodules >1 cm in diameter and routinely requires omentectomy and frequently small bowel resection. This cytoreductive surgery is followed by either systemic or intraperitoneal chemotherapy. Second-look laparotomies are frequently performed with re-resection of otherwise occult recurrent or persistent disease.

4. Lymph node metastases. The spread of a solid tumor to regional nodes occurs in a frequently predictable pattern according to the lymphatic drainage of the primary site. In the absence of gross nodal disease, the benefit of lymphadenectomy in conjunction with resection of a primary tumor in terms of long-term outcome is controversial. In breast cancer, for example, axillary lymphadenectomy is thought to be principally of prognostic rather than therapeutic value. However, in gastric or pancreatic cancer, many experts believe that radical lymphadenectomy at the time of gastrectomy or pancreaticoduodenectomy decreases local recurrence rates and improves disease-free survival. The reader is referred to previous chapters for discussion of the role of lymph node involvement by *recurrent* disease from individual cancers; the role of surgery is most often palliative but may be curative. In general, lymphadenectomy for recurrent squamous carcinoma of the head and neck, urogenital tract, or anus produces the best results. Lymphadenectomy for adenocarcinoma, particularly of the alimentary tract, is not commonly undertaken because recurrent disease of this type is rarely confined to the grossly involved nodes. Rather, chemotherapy and/or radiation therapy is used in this setting.

C. METASTASIS FROM AN OCCULT PRIMARY SITE. Occasionally, cancer of a solid organ may present as a metastatic deposit. This may involve various sites such as lung, brain, or lymph nodes. However, certain patterns of presentation of metastatic tumor from a clinically unknown primary are seen most commonly and merit special consideration.

1. Axillary lymph node. Adenopathy in the axilla which persists beyond 1-2 weeks is almost always pathologic. Physical examination should pay special attention to the skin of the trunk and extremity because malignant melanoma commonly spreads to this site. The diagnosis of carcinoma (versus lymphoma) in an axillary lymph node can usually be made by FNA cytology. Immunohistochemical analysis usually can identify melanoma. If the FNA is nondiagnostic, an incisional biopsy should be performed. In a woman with adenocarcinoma in the axilla, a complete physical examination with careful attention to the breast and bilateral mammograms should be done. ER analysis should be performed, but it should be remembered that ER-negative breast cancers are common in premenopausal women. Lung carcinoma is a common primary site in males and chest radiography should be obtained. If no primary site is identified in a male, most oncologists recommend chemotherapy only in a protocol setting. For women with adenocarcinoma in the axilla and no demonstrable primary site, most experts recommend ipsilateral modified radical mastectomy. Careful sectioning of the breast specimen frequently reveals the primary tumor.

2. Mass in the neck. Evaluation of an isolated lump in the neck should proceed in an orderly fashion according to the site and clinical situation. Anterior cervical adenopathy is common, and commonly benign, especially in the younger patient. A carcinomatous node is frequently hard, nontender, poorly mobile, and >2 cm in diameter. Posterior cervical and supraclavicular masses are more commonly malignant. If lymphoma is not suspected clinically, endoscopy to evaluate the nasopharynx, larynx, and esophagus should be performed. This identifies a primary squamous carcinoma in the majority of patients. Many physicians believe that biopsy should not precede this work-up because neck dissection would customarily accompany definitive surgical treatment of the identified primary. If no primary site is located, an excisional biopsy is performed. If frozen section reveals squamous cancer, a radical neck dissection is carried out.

A neck mass adjacent to the tail of the parotid should undergo a similar work-up, as described above. However, definitive biopsy should include a superficial parotidectomy. The finding of adenocarcinoma in a neck may represent spread from a lung or GI primary in males and occasionally breast cancer in women. In men, a search for a primary site is of questionable utility because no effective therapy is likely to be available outside of a protocol setting.

3. Hepatic metastasis from an unknown primary. Some patients presenting with nonspecific constitutional complaints (fatigue, anorexia, vague abdominal discomfort) are found to have single or multiple solid masses in the liver demonstrated by CT or MRI. Radiographically guided percutaneous biopsy most commonly reveals adenocarcinoma. The distinction between metastatic disease and primary tumor of the liver (hepatocellular carcinoma or cholangiocarcinoma) can usually be made histologically. Chemotherapy for metastatic adenocarcinoma to the liver from an occult primary has yielded disappointing results. Detailed history and physical examination direct successful investigation of the primary site in some patients, but in others the origin of the hepatic tumor remains unknown. Most oncologists recommend colonoscopy to rule out occult colorectal cancer, because this commonly spreads to the liver, and effective surgical as well as drug therapy for both primary and metastatic disease is available for colorectal cancer. Upper GI endoscopy is generally not warranted if the colonoscopy is negative because the yield is very low, and no effective therapy (in an otherwise asymptomatic patient) is available if one finds a carcinoma of the esophagus or stomach. Further work-up should consist of pelvic and chest CT, CEA, and CA 125, and AFP determinations. In the young patient with isolated hepatic metastasis from a primary tumor that remains occult, hepatic resection may be considered. However, few if any patients are cured in this manner.

D. ACUTE ABDOMINAL COMPLAINTS IN THE CANCER PATIENT. Although abdominal pathology common to the general population can complicate the course of treatment in patients with cancer, certain problems merit special consideration.

1. Small bowel obstruction. An adult patient without a history of abdominal surgery who develops signs and symptoms of small bowel obstruction must be considered to have a malignant cause until proven otherwise at laparotomy. For patients who have had a solid malignancy in the past, the development of a small bowel obstruction may herald a recurrence. In either case, laparotomy is undertaken following fluid and electrolyte repletion. Every effort should be made to resect the obstructing tumor. The surgeon should be aware that at least 100 cm of small bowel *plus* a competent ileocecal value (to prevent rapid small bowel transit) are necessary to ensure adequate nutrient absorption. The unresectable tumor may be bypassed, although this may predispose the patient to bacterial overgrowth in the bypassed loop and, depending on the length of the bypassed segment, may result in short bowel syndrome.

Patients with known intraperitoneal tumor recurrence or carcinomatosis may present with small bowel obstruction as a near-terminal event in the course of their disease. Management of such patients must take into account the clinical severity of the obstruction and the expected duration of their survival based upon the extent of tumor involvement with vital organs. Some of these patients may improve sufficiently with nasogastric decompression and IV fluids alone to permit discharge from the hospital. In others, open, laparoscopic or percutaneous gastrostomy in combination with central venous catheter placement for home IV hydration may provide the best palliation, even in those suffering from a complete small bowel obstruction. The aggressiveness of surgical therapy must be tailored to the individual patient.

2. Radiation enteritis. The effect of radiation injury to the small or large bowel may be acute or chronic and occurs most commonly in patients receiving more than 5000 cGy to the abdomen or pelvis. Early manifestations consist of nausea, diarrhea, and hematochezia and result from direct mucosal injury. Abdominal pain and tenderness may form a prominent clinical feature. Treatment is supportive, and symptoms usually resolve within a few weeks after therapy is discontinued. Chronic mucosal injury, particularly in the rectum, may require steroid retention enemas and oral sulfasalazine in a fashion similar to the treatment of chronic ulcerative colitis (see Chapter 12, page 560). A second mechanism of radiation injury to the bowel involves loss of the arteriolar supply to the submucosa and bowel wall, leading to fibrosis and stricture that may develop into small bowel obstruction months to years after the original insult. Radiation-induced strictures pose a surgical challenge. Resection of short segments of small bowel with anastomosis to adjacent radiated small bowel may be complicated by anastomotic leak and abscess or fistula formation. Even minor surgical trauma to radiated small bowel may not heal because of vascular compromise. Bypass of strictured, radiation-injured bowel may lead to blind loop syndrome. Resection of all abnormal bowel frequently results in long-term dependence on home parenteral nutrition.

3. Colonic pseudo-obstruction. Acute dilatation of the colon in the absence of mechanical obstruction, also known as Ogilvie's syndrome, may develop in cancer patients as a consequence of either narcotic analgesics or chemotherapy (typically associated with 5-fluorouracil [5-FU] administration). Clinically, patients develop gaseous distention of the colon, with cecal diameter frequently ≥14 cm. The risk of perforation rises significantly with further dilation. In the setting of chemotherapy administration, severe mucositis of the colon is often present and a toxic megacolon–like clinical picture ensues. Treatment is directed toward preventing perforation. Nasogastric suction and IV hydration are begun. Offending medications are minimized. Colonoscopic decompression is often necessary. If recurrence develops after 2 decompressions, surgical intervention is indicated. Tube cecostomy is often ineffective, and diverting loop ileostomy may be preferable.

4. Neutropenic colitis. Patients who have protracted neutropenia (absolute neutrophil count <500 cells/μl) may develop neutropenic colitis. This phenomenon most commonly occurs in bone-marrow transplant patients and appears to be related to fungal or chemotherapy-induced severe mucositis. Patients present with localized or diffuse peritoneal signs, fever, and signs of ileus. Radiographic findings include small bowel dilatation and air-fluid levels. Surgical mortality in this setting is high. In the absence of perforation, management is expectant, even though the clinical picture of an acute abdomen would warrant exploratory laparotomy when it occurs in a different clinical setting. Broad-spectrum antibiotics, parenteral nutrition, and fluid replacement are the mainstays of therapy. If the neutropenia resolves, the colitis generally improves.

5. Malignant ascites. Peritoneal carcinomatosis, usually as a consequence of ovarian or colorectal carcinoma, may produce severe, tense ascites associated with abdominal pain and pulmonary compromise. The management of symptomatic malignant ascites may be difficult in these debilitated, frequently anorexic and cachectic patients. Repeated paracenteses are effective in the short term, but significant protein loss occurs and the ascitic fluid (always an exudate) rapidly develops. Longer-term palliation may be achieved by placement of a peritoneovenous (P-V) shunt. This device consists of intraperitoneal and IV limbs separated by a one-way valve. The tip of the venous limb is typically passed through the internal jugular or subclavian vein into the right atrium. With each deep inspiration, the intrapleural/peritoneal pressure gradient falls, and fluid flows from the peritoneal cavity into the intravascular space and is ultimately eliminated as urine. This approach is frequently very effective in diminishing respiratory effort and improving patient comfort. Complications include obstruction of the valve by cellular debris and infection. Coagulopathy commonly associated with P-V shunt placement for ascites in patients with liver failure is less of a problem in patients with malignant ascites. The theoretical complication of seeding the lungs with malignant cells from the peritoneal cavity has not been a significant problem. This may be explained in part by the less fertile environment of the pulmonary parenchyma for proliferation of ovarian or colorectal cancer cells. More likely, these patients with advanced malignancy succumb to their intraperitoneal disease before the growth of pulmonary metastases becomes manifest grossly.

II. CHEMOTHERAPY

A. OVERVIEW. Numerous anticancer drugs fall under the category of chemotherapy. These include oral preparations or IV solutions, hormonal agents, biologic modulators, and cytotoxic

Table 5-2. Classification of chemotherapy drugs

Class	Agent	Mechanism of action	Principal toxicity	Disease
Antimetabolites	Methotrexate	Folate antagonist	Mucositis, bone marrow	Breast cancer
	5-Fluorouracil (5-FU)	Incorporation into DNA/RNA DNA/RNA	Mucositis, diarrhea	Head and neck cancer Gastrointestinal cancer
	Cytosine arabinoside	Inhibits DNA/RNA synthesis	Bone marrow	Acute leukemia
Alkylating agents	Cyclophosphamide, ifosfamide, thiotepa	Single-strand alkylation	Bone marrow, hemorrhagic cystitis	Lymphoma, breast cancer
	BCNU, CCNU	Cross-linking DNA	Bone marrow	Lymphoma, brain tumors
	Cisplatin Carboplatin	Cross-linking DNA Cross-linking DNA	Renal, neurotoxicity Bone marrow	Ovarian, testicular, lung, head, and neck tumors

Natural products		Mechanism	Toxicity	Use
	Vincristine	Mitotic inhibitor	Neurotoxicity	Wide range
	Vinblastine	Mitotic inhibitor	Bone marrow	Wide range
	VP-16	Topoisomerase inhibitor	Bone marrow	Leukemia, breast cancer
	Doxorubicin	Intercalation between base pairs	Bone marrow, cardiac	Lymphoma, testicular cancer
	Bleomycin	DNA cleavage	Hypersensitivity, pulmonary fibrosis	
	Mitomycin-C	Cross-linking DNA	Bone marrow	Gastrointestinal cancer

drugs and may or may not have significant systemic side-effects. The choice of a chemotherapeutic agent may be based on theoretical rationale, empiric choice, or solid scientific data supporting a specific therapy for a particular disease.

Chemotherapy drugs are generally categorized by methods of action (e.g., antimetabolites, alkylators). Common chemotherapy drugs and their classification are included in Table 5-2. Drugs in a given category may have very different spectra of activity, toxicity, and dosing. Also included in Table 5-2 are the most common dose-limiting toxicities for each drug, as well as the disease(s) for which each is most commonly used. Not included in the table are agents that are technically chemotherapeutics but do not have the typical side-effect profile. Examples of such drugs are hormonal agents (e.g., tamoxifen, leuprolide). A new class of drugs—biologic response modifiers—are naturally occurring substances that can be bioengineered and delivered in supraphysiologic doses. IFN-α, IL-2, and TNF are examples of such agents.

As the field of oncology has evolved, it has become apparent that combinations of chemotherapy drugs often improve results. These combinations may include multiple chemotherapy drugs with different modes of action and different toxicities, allowing for their coadministration without markedly amplified toxicity. Examples are CAF (cyclophosphamide, Adriamycin [doxorubicin], 5-FU) chemotherapy for breast cancer and CHOP (cyclophosphamide, Adriamycin, vincristine, prednisone) for lymphoma. Chemotherapy drugs may also be used in conjunction with each other based on clinical or laboratory evidence of synergism. One such example is the sequential administration of cisplatin and VP-16. At other times, drugs may be combined because of unique interactions that do not reflect a summation of their individual cytotoxic activities. Two examples of this are 5-FU combined with IFN-α or with leucovorin calcium.

B. CHEMOTHERAPY FOR COMMON CANCERS

1. Breast cancer. Except for women with very small tumors (<1 cm), adjuvant chemotherapy is generally agreed to be appropriate. The precise combination of chemotherapy agents remains a study question, although the choice is governed by prognostic features such as patient age, menopausal status, tumor size, involvement of lymph nodes, and tumor hormone receptor status. Doxorubicin and cyclophosphamide are mainstays in such regimens, although some women might receive only tamoxifen. Women at very high risk for recurrence are considered for high-dose chemotherapy with autologous bone marrow rescue.

2. Colon cancer. The principal agent used to treat colon cancer is 5-FU. In conjunction with levamisole, 5-FU has been shown to improve survival of people with Dukes' C colon cancer following surgical resection. The nature of the drug interaction is uncertain, and, by itself, levamisole has no antitumor activity. The most common combination therapy for colon cancer is 5-FU with leucovorin calcium (folinic acid), which has no cytotoxic activity on its own. It amplifies the activity of 5-FU by interacting with an enzyme in the pharmacologic pathway of 5-FU. 5-FU has also been combined with IFN-α to apparent benefit. All of these combinations may, in the end, be equivalent to giving higher doses of 5-FU alone. Although such therapies may lead to tumor shrinkage, these treatments offer no dramatic survival advantage, and no patients are cured once they have developed metastatic disease.

3. Lung cancer. Although combinations of chemotherapy, particularly cisplatin, are used, no strong evidence exists that the survival of a patient with non–small cell lung cancer can be improved by such treatment. Similar chemotherapies are used to treat patients with small cell lung cancer; those with limited disease at the outset may occasionally be cured, but patients with disseminated small cell lung cancer cannot be cured by chemotherapy.

4. Ovarian cancer. The basis of treatment for ovarian cancer is cisplatin (or carboplatin, a related compound with different toxicity). Women with limited-stage disease may be cured with the combination of surgery and chemotherapy, whereas those with advanced disease may be well-palliated.

5. Testicular cancer. Cisplatin or carboplatin in conjunction with VP-16 is the mainstay of treatment, resulting in cure in most patients.

6. Gastrointestinal cancer. Other than colon cancer, there is no clear evidence that chemotherapy improves the outcome of patients with these malignancies.

7. Lymphoma. About one half of all patients with non-Hodgkin's lymphoma are cured by some combination of chemotherapy (based on cyclophosphamide and doxorubicin) and/or radiation therapy. Patients with Hodgkin's disease do even better.

8. Leukemia. With the use of intensive chemotherapy and

with improving supportive care, patients with acute leukemia have a 53% chance of survival. The mainstays of leukemia chemotherapy are cytosine arabinoside and a doxorubicin-like drug.

9. Bone marrow transplant. Patients with certain diseases (e.g., leukemia, lymphoma) might be more curable if there were no constraints on the dose intensity of chemotherapy that could be used. Although certain chemotherapy toxicities may still be limiting (mucositis, for example), myelosuppression can be circumvented by the use of bone marrow rescue. Bone marrow stem cells, harvested either from an HLA-matched donor or from the patients themselves prior to chemotherapy, may be reinfused following marrow-ablative chemotherapy, enabling the bone marrow to regenerate despite the lethal doses of chemotherapy administered. This aggressive treatment is being tested now in other "chemotherapy-sensitive" tumors such as ovarian cancer and breast cancer.

C. BONE MARROW SUPPORT
1. Colony stimulating factors (G-CSF, GM-CSF). Granulocyte and granulocyte-macrophage colony stimulating factors are naturally occurring peptides that can be administered in supraphysiologic doses. Although the actual FDA-approved indications for these drugs are quite narrow, they are being used with increasing frequency. These agents have been shown to diminish the duration of neutropenia following chemotherapy and therefore may enable the use of higher doses of chemotherapy. They also speed the engraftment of bone marrow following transplantation, leading to less time without neutrophils. Neither of these drugs, however, increases the platelet count, nor have they been shown to be of value when initiated while patients are already neutropenic. Patients taking these drugs need to be monitored closely, and the agents should be continued until the WBC exceeds at least 10,000. Premature cessation of these drugs can lead to dramatic decreases in neutrophil counts. The major toxicity of these agents is a flulike syndrome.

2. Erythropoietin. The major advance from the introduction of erythropoietin has been the diminishing dependency on blood transfusion for patients with chronic diseases and anemia. It is also an adjunct preoperatively for patients wishing to donate autologous blood prior to elective surgery.

III. REGIONAL CANCER THERAPY

The regional delivery of chemotherapy has been explored in an effort to achieve high local drug concentrations while limiting systemic side-effects.

A. HEPATIC ARTERIAL CHEMOTHERAPY. Considerable interest developed in the treatment of isolated hepatic metastases by local delivery of chemotherapeutic agents with the development of the implantable chemotherapy infusion pump. In principle, a pharmacologic advantage exists in the hepatic administration of a drug, such as FUDR, which is nearly completely cleared on first pass through the liver. Such a drug has high hepatic (and tumor) uptake with minimal systemic levels. Arterial delivery takes advantage of the finding that hepatic tumors greater than a few millimeters in diameter derive most of their blood supply from the hepatic artery. In theory, then, such a drug should demonstrate a higher response rate (tumor shrinkage) and fewer systemic side-effects than IV systemic chemotherapy. In the case of unresectable colorectal cancer metastases, this prediction has been tested; indeed, response rates of 50%-65% (>50% reduction in the total volume of hepatic tumor measured radiographically) have been reported by many investigators. This compares with a major response rate of 20%-30% with systemic 5-FU/leucovorin. Further, the systemic side-effects have been minimal. Early studies reported a high frequency of chemical bile duct injury (biliary sclerosis) in such patients, but modulation of the dose and timing of intra-arterial drug administration have nearly eliminated this complication. However, the higher response rate with intra-arterial chemotherapy has yet to be translated into improved survival in these patients, principally because of extrahepatic (pulmonary) recurrence, and hepatic arterial chemotherapy remains an investigational modality.

B. ISOLATED LIMB PERFUSION FOR MELANOMA AND EXTREMITY SARCOMA. Certain patients with malignant melanoma develop multiple recurrent cutaneous or subcutaneous tumors confined to the extremity (satellitosis or in-transit metastases). These patients are commonly treated with infusion of an alkylating agent (melphalan) delivered intra-arterially in a closed circuit in which the venous return from the extremity is diverted through a pump oxygenator and recirculated. The extremity is usually heated to approximately 39° C to enhance melphalan action. In this fashion, transient high drug concentrations in the extremity are achieved with minimal (<10%) leak into the systemic circulation. At the end of the perfusion, the chemotherapy-containing blood is replaced with fresh whole blood prior to removing the arterial and venous cannulas.

Recently, the addition of the cytokine TNF to heated melphalan in limb perfusion has yielded dramatically improved responses (90% complete response), although the durability of this effect remains to be determined. In addition, the combination of melphalan and TNF appears to be very effective in shrinking bulky soft tissue sarcomas of the extremity and may significantly diminish the need for amputation in patients with locally advanced disease.

C. CHEMOEMBOLIZATION. Hepatic arterial devascularization has been used for decades, with varying enthusiasm, in the palliative treatment of unresectable primary hepatocellular carcinoma of the liver. The efficacy of this approach is based upon selective ischemia of the tumor, which derives nearly its entire blood supply from the hepatic artery, whereas the normal liver parenchyma is supplied mainly by the portal vein. In recent years, hepatic arterial ischemia has been accomplished nonoperatively by the percutaneous transarterial embolization of the hepatic artery with absorbable vaso-occlusive material (sterile microfibrillar collagen), which produces effective but transient tumor ischemia. When chemotherapeutic agents are added to the injected collagen (usually mitomycin, cisplatin, and doxorubicin), tumor blood flow is transiently occluded (for days) and these agents, which have little activity when given systemically, now have a marked tumor toxicity. This approach is most commonly used in patients with unresectable hepatoma, with symptomatic metastases from primary neuroendocrine tumors of the pancreas, and with metastatic carcinoid.

D. INTRACAVITARY CHEMOTHERAPY. Occasionally, tumor spread may be confined to a body cavity such as the pleural or peritoneal space. The direct instillation of chemotherapeutic agents may achieve a pharmacokinetic advantage over systemic therapy when the characteristically multiple tumor nodules are ≤3 mm in diameter, because the penetration of drug beyond this depth is poor. In the peritoneal space, large volumes of dilute drug must be employed, usually delivered through a peritoneal dialysis catheter. Postoperative adhesions may limit the distribution of the chemotherapy. The strongest responses to this approach have been seen in ovarian carcinoma refractory to systemic therapy. Cisplatin is the most commonly used agent. In peritoneal mesothelioma, some encouraging results have been reported with a combination of cisplatin and doxorubicin. The results in peritoneal carcinomatosis from GI cancers have been disappointing. Complications of intraperitoneal therapy include fever, infection, pain, ileus, and adhesion formation.

Intrapleural instillation of chemotherapy (most commonly bleomycin) is designed to treat symptomatic malignant pleural effusions. This agent exerts an antineoplastic effect and also leads to sclerosis of the pleura, obliterating the potential space for pleural fluid accumulation. This approach is usually applied to patients with malignant pleural effusions who have failed a trial of tube thoracostomy alone.

IV. RADIATION ONCOLOGY

Radiation has an established role in the curative approach to a number of types of cancer, either as a definitive modality by itself (e.g., Hodgkin's lymphoma, head and neck squamous cell carcinomas, prostate and cervix carcinomas), as an adjunct (adjuvant) to primary surgery (e.g., seminoma, pancreatic carcinoma, primary CNS gliomas, soft tissue sarcomas), or in combination with chemotherapy and surgery (e.g., lung, rectal, anal, and breast carcinomas and pediatric malignancies such as Wilms' tumor, neuroblastoma, and rhabdomyosarcoma). Organ-preservation technics using radiation and chemotherapy with surgery reserved for salvage are under investigation in many sites, including larynx, esophagus, bladder, and rectum. In addition, radiation often is used in a palliative fashion in the course of a cancer patient's illness to reduce symptoms and improve quality of life.

A. DOSE-FRACTIONATION. A typical course of definitive radiation involves daily treatment with a dose (fraction) of radiation delivered to an area of interest (generally the tumor bed plus regional draining lymph nodes), reducing the exposure of as much normal tissue as possible through the use of individually contoured lead-alloy blocks. Small daily fractions reduce the amount of damage to normal tissues by allowing time for these normal tissues to repair some portion of the radiation injury. This repair capacity is lacking to a certain degree in most tumor lines, so that more damage accrues over time in the abnormal than in the normal tissue. The size of the daily dose (measured in centigrams or cGy) is determined by the sensitivity of the cell line as well as the tolerance of the normal structures adjacent to the tumor. Likewise, the total dose delivered is determined by the dose necessary to achieve control of disease, taking into account the dose that normal structures can tolerate. These treatments are delivered daily, or occasionally twice daily (hyperfractionated), for a course of 2-7 weeks. Breaks in the delivery of radiation are undesirable because interruptions allow for tumor repopulation and regrowth, thereby reducing the efficacy of radiation. Ample evidence of this is seen in the negative impact of treatment delays on local tumor control in patients with head and neck or lung malignancies.

Various types of radiation are available for use in cancer therapy. Most commonly, patients are treated with high-energy photons, a type of radiation that is highly penetrating but has a substantial skin-sparing effect. Megavoltage electrons are used to treat superficial areas owing to their limited depth of penetration. In specialized centers around the nation, heavy ions, or charged particles, can deliver very high doses to extremely well-defined areas for tumors in critical locations, such as the base of the skull or along the spinal cord.

B. RADIATION EFFECTS IN NONTUMOR TISSUES. Normal tissue tolerance to radiation is highly variable and depends on a number of factors, including cell type, volume of the organ irradiated, length of time over which the radiation was delivered, prior surgery, prior level of function, administration of concurrent or prior chemotherapy, daily dose size, and total dose delivered. Organs such as the lens of the eye and the spermatocytes sustain damage at doses as low as 50-100 cGy, whereas bone and the brain can tolerate doses as high as 6000 cGy before structural or functional integrity is compromised. Significant liver damage may be expected if the entire liver is irradiated to a dose >3000 cGy, but a small portion of the liver may be treated to doses >6000 cGy without deleterious systemic effect. Likewise, a small portion of lung may be treated to a very high dose without noticeable effect, but treatment of an entire lung with 1800 cGy can result in catastrophic functional loss.

Radiation effects fall into three categories based on their timing. Acute side-effects, seen during the course of radiation or immediately afterward, are a result of the effect of radiation on rapidly cycling cells, such as those of the mucosal lining of the orodigestive tract (mucositis, esophagitis, diarrhea), bone marrow (leukopenia, thrombocytopenia), and skin (erythema, desquamation). These acute effects are generally limited, and most resolve with time after conclusion of the radiation. Subacute effects are those that arise in the weeks to months after completion of therapy. Examples include pneumonitis secondary to delayed damage to Type II pneumocytes and somnolence syndrome due to temporary demyelination in irradiated spine and brain. These effects are less common and are generally self-limited, although they may progress to permanent conditions requiring intervention. Chronic or delayed radiation damage takes months to years to develop and is a function of gradually progressive vascular compromise that may lead to end-organ dysfunction. Radiation enteritis is a classic example which can develop 6 months to many years after radiation has been administered. Other examples of chronic damage include pulmonary fibrosis, osteoradionecrosis, and soft tissue necrosis.

Close preoperative communication between surgeon, radiation oncologist, and medical oncologist is essential to maximal management of the cancer patient. Various surgical considerations can significantly reduce the morbidity of radiation therapy. For example, in the patient with early breast cancer who has decided on breast conservation therapy with lumpectomy and radiation, the location and orientation of the lumpectomy and axillary dissection scars have a major effect on the final cosmetic outcome. Patients whose lumpectomy and axillary dissections are done in continuity are far more likely to have an unsatisfactory result than are those with separate incisions. Placement of metal clips in the lumpectomy site can also guide the radiation oncologist in planning the site to be boosted with higher doses of radiation. In patients with soft tissue sarcomas of the extremities, proper placement and orientation of the incision can significantly reduce the field requiring radiation after wide local excisions, which becomes especially critical in lesions adjacent to joint spaces. Another example is the staging laparotomy in patients with Hodgkin's disease. Placing clips at the splenic hilum after splenectomy and at the sites of any suspicious lymph nodes helps localize the field to be irradiated, and oophoropexy can potentially allow sparing of the ovaries by later blocking the centrally transposed ovaries during radiation. At the time of resection of rectal lesions and other pelvic malignancies as well, the use of an omental or synthetic mesh sling to move the small bowel out of the pelvis may significantly reduce the amount of bowel irradiated at the time of adjuvant chemoradiotherapy. By removing the sensitive intestines from the field of radiation, higher doses of radiation may be administered.

C. BRACHYTHERAPY. Brachytherapy refers to the placement of radioactive sources into tumor sites within the body and is often done under surgical guidance. In patients with soft tissue sarcomas, hollow plastic catheters may be placed into the tumor bed under direct visualization at the time of local excision before closure of the wound. After 5-7 days, radioactive sources are placed into these catheters and left in place for 1-3 days to deliver a high dose of radiation to the areas of greatest risk of persistent disease. Radiation dose drops off precipitously within a few centimeters of the sources, thereby sparing adjacent tissues. This approach is particularly helpful in patients with recurrent disease after prior radiation whose ability to tolerate further external beam radiation therapy is limited. Other sites often treated with brachytherapy include brain gliomas, recurrent head and neck neoplasms, primary tongue and lip cancers, retroperitoneal sarcomas, and cervical and vaginal carcinomas. Discussing the region of interest with the radiation oncologist prior to surgery can ensure that special catheters are prepared and made available for the time of surgery.

D. INTRAOPERATIVE RADIATION THERAPY. Another alternative to standard external beam radiation therapy is the use of intraoperative radiation, an approach that allows the delivery of a very high dose of radiation to the tumor bed after careful removal of all radiosensitive structures from the radiation field. This single dose acts as a boost dose to be augmented either by prior or pursuant external beam radiation. In patients with recurrent or initially unresectable rectal carcinoma, for example, a cone is placed directly over the tumor bed after attempted resection, with care to remove small intestine, ureters, and nerves from the treatment field. Radiation is delivered in the operating suite with the patient under anesthesia using either high-energy electrons with a very limited depth of penetration or orthovoltage photons with a greater depth of penetration. Used in conjunction with external beam radiation, this approach has shown promise in improving local control rates in patients with initially unresectable rectal cancer, completely resected pancreatic cancers, retroperitoneal sarcomas, and recurrent head and neck cancers.

When preoperative planning is done, radiation can best be employed to the benefit of the patient. Surgical considerations can significantly reduce the morbidity of radiation. Likewise, radiation properly used can improve the surgeon's chance of ensuring local control of disease.

V. SUPPORTIVE CARE OF THE CANCER PATIENT

Certain clinical problems are common or even unique to patients undergoing cancer therapy. Their management requires first a high index of suspicion for specific problems in cancer patients and then a reasoned treatment strategy.

A. PARENTERAL NUTRITION. The majority of hospitalized cancer patients demonstrate some degree of PCM. Weight loss, asthenia, anemia, and anorexia are the hallmarks of the syndrome of cancer cachexia. These symptoms may develop in the absence of enteric obstruction and are related to a loss of smell or taste perception or to drug or radiation treatment. Recently, interest has developed in the possible contribution of endogenous host-produced antitumor factors (cytokines) in the syndrome of cancer cachexia, but convincing studies in humans have not been undertaken.

Regardless of the cause of malnutrition in cancer, complication rates in patients undergoing surgery for cancer are clearly higher in the face of PCM (principally due to infections and wound healing abnormalities). Although many trials of preoperative nutritional support have been conducted in such patients, there remains little support for the routine of preoperative TPN in an attempt to reduce the morbidity and mortality of cancer surgery. This may reflect the poor quality of such studies but may also be due to abnormalities in the utilization of protein and energy sources in patients with malignancies. In the absence of reliable data, current recommendations are to provide nutritional support preoperatively to those patients with severe malnutrition (loss >10% of pre-illness weight, albumin <2.5). At least 10 days of preoperative nutritional support is necessary to favorably impact upon surgical outcome. This approach is clearly not an option in patients requiring emergency surgery (e.g., for bleeding or bowel obstruction), but in others, TPN may be administered at home, significantly reducing the cost. Enteral nutrition is preferable to parenteral nutrition if it can be administered safely, because both cost and complications are fewer, and efficacy may be greater. The question of the possible stimulation of tumor growth in the short term is not an important issue in patients ultimately undergoing surgical tumor extirpation. However, in patients with advanced, unresectable disease, the relative benefits of nutritional support may indeed be outweighed by an enhanced proliferation of tumor cells. In the absence of convincing data in this regard, most oncologists limit nutritional support to those malnourished patients for whom potentially effective palliative chemotherapy or radiation therapy exists.

B. METABOLIC COMPLICATIONS OF CANCER OR ITS TREATMENT

1. Hypercalcemia. An elevated serum calcium is common in cancer patients, particularly those with bony metastases from primary tumors of the breast or lung, squamous carcinomas of the head and neck or esophagus, and multiple myeloma. In these patients, osteoclast activity is abnormally high, but ectopic parathyroid hormone (PTH) production can only rarely be demonstrated. Certain host cytokines that are elaborated as part of the host antitumor immunologic response to malignancy may play an important role in osteoclast activation (e.g., transforming growth factor-β, TNF, IL-1, and CSFs). Abnormal PTH production does play a critical role in the severe hypercalcemia of parathyroid carcinoma.

The serum ionized calcium most closely corresponds with signs and symptoms. Early on, these consist of fatigue, weakness, and hyperreflexia but may progress to nausea, vomiting, alterations in mental status, seizures, coma, and death from cardiac arrhythmias. The electrocardiogram in moderate hypercalcemia may demonstrate PR prolongation, shortening of the QT interval, and a widened T wave.

Specific therapy for hypercalcemia varies with severity. Most patients with mild or moderate hypercalcemia (12 mg/dl, corrected for serum albumin) may be managed with IV fluids (250-400 ml/hour) and a loop diuretic (furosemide). Electrolyte abnormalities are corrected, mobilization of bed-ridden patients is attempted, drugs that may elevate calcium levels (e.g., thiazide diuretics) are discontinued, and antitumor therapy, if available, is instituted. For severe or symptomatic hypercalcemia, a variety of additional interventions is available (Table 5-3). High doses of calcitonin (4-8 units/kg given IM every 8-12 hours) inhibit bone resorption, and clinical effects may be evident within 4-8 hours, although tolerance to the hypocalcemic effects generally develops within 48 hours.

Corticosteroids are useful in high doses (prednisone, 50-100 mg daily), especially in patients with steroid-responsive malignancies (breast, lymphoma, multiple myeloma), but require 2-3 days before a hypocalcemic response is seen.

Palmidronate is a biphosphonate that has become the first line of therapy for moderate or severe hypercalcemia. It acts by inhibiting osteoclast-induced bone resorption. A single dose is frequently effective, and an oral form may permit outpatient management of less severe hypercalcemia.

Table 5-3. Management of the hypercalcemia of malignancy

Intervention	Onset of action	Comments
1. Intravenous saline, 200-300 ml/hour; furosemide	Rapid	Use in all patients
2. Corticosteroids— prednisone, 50-100 mg/day	2-3 days	Breast cancer, lymphoma
3. Palmidronate, 30-90 mg IV every 3-7 days	24 hours	Useful in outpatients
4. Calcitonin, 4-8 units IM every 8-12 h	6 hours	Second-line therapy
5. Gallium nitrate, 200 mg/m² daily × 5 days	1-2 days	Hospitalized patients
6. Mithramycin, 20 µg/ kg; may repeat once	12-24 hours	Second-line therapy

Mithramycin as a single dose is a potent hypocalcemic agent whose action begins within 24 hours. However, significant toxicities (renal, hepatic dysfunction, thrombocytopenia) may limit its utility. Gallium nitrate has become the agent of choice in many patients with severe hypercalcemia who fail palmidronate treatment. The hypocalcemic response is seen within 2 days and therapy is usually continued for 5 days, although the maximal effect may occur several days after the drug has been discontinued.

2. Syndrome of inappropriate antidiuretic hormone secretion. Hyponatremia due to SIADH rarely causes symptoms unless the serum sodium falls precipitously. SIADH affects a small percentage of cancer patients, most commonly patients with small cell lung cancer. Other causes of hyponatremia include adrenal insufficiency due to bilateral adrenal metastases, corticosteroid withdrawal, or loss of sodium-containing fluids (vomiting, diarrhea, ascites). Clinical manifestations consist of nausea and anorexia and progress to CNS abnormalities. Treatment consists of discontinuation of contributing medications, institution of specific antitumor therapy, and water restriction (500-1000 ml/day). If these measures are ineffective, demeclocycline (200 mg every 8 hours in the absence of liver or renal disease) can be used to produce a nephrogenic diabetes insipidus. Patients with coma or seizures who are not dehydrated should receive normal saline plus furosemide or hypertonic (3%) saline by intravenous infusion.

3. Tumor lysis syndrome. The treatment of certain rapidly growing tumors such as high-grade lymphoma or leukemia may result in rapid tumor cell death and necrosis, with release of intracellular contents into the circulation. Hyperuricemia may develop as a consequence of metabolism of tumor nucleic acids and may lead to uric acid nephropathy and acute renal failure. Hyperphosphatemia may also ensue and contribute to the renal injury. Hypocalcemia may result from the hyperphosphatemia and induce cardiac dysrhythmias or tetany. Because potassium is predominantly an intracellular ion, hyperkalemia is a frequent concomitant of the tumor lysis syndrome. Treatment of these metabolic abnormalities begins with recognition of patients at risk. Allopurinol (300 mg daily) given at least 3 days prior to the institution of chemotherapy prevents uric acid formation by inhibiting xanthine oxidase activity. Patients are prehydrated with normal saline, and alkalinization of the urine promotes uric acid excretion. Hypocalcemia associated with ECG changes is treated with intravenous calcium gluconate. Hyperkalemia is managed as described in Chapter 2. Acute urinary obstruction from urate calculi may require surgical management. Frequent monitoring of serum electrolytes, uric acid, phosphorus, calcium, and creatinine is important, and hemodialysis may be necessary for renal failure or for a phosphorus level >10 mg/dl.

4. Tumor-associated hypoglycemia. Although unregulated insulin production by islet cell tumors of the pancreas constitutes a common cause of hypoglycemia, many patients who experience this paraneoplastic syndrome are found to have large, bulky sarcomas or hepatocellular carcinoma. Serum insulin levels are low or normal in these latter patients, but other serum factors, termed *NSILA (nonsuppressible insulin-like activities),* frequently can be demonstrated. The NSILA most commonly have been identified as IGF-I and IGF-II and are secreted directly into the circulation by these tumors. Further, a high tumor glucose consumption and a failure in normal glucose homeostasis in such patients may contribute to the hypoglycemia. Symptoms tend to be vague and mild and frequently nocturnal. Acute hypoglycemia is treated by an intravenous dextrose infusion. Long-term control depends upon the resectability of the tumor. Small, frequent feedings may provide relief in patients with mild symptoms. Intermittent glucagon administration may benefit patients for whom antitumor therapy is not available.

Table 5-4. Antiemetic therapy

1. Ondansetron, 0.15 mg/kg every 2-4 hours with or without dexamethasone
2. Dexamethasone, 20 mg IV 30-60 minutes prior to chemotherapy
3. Metoclopramide, 2-3 mg/kg IV before and 1.5 hours after chemotherapy
4. Lorazepam, 0.5-1.0 mg/m^2 PO in combination with metoclopramide

C. NAUSEA. Although many chemotherapeutic agents, particularly cisplatin and cyclophosphamide, can induce nausea and vomiting, other causes of emesis in the cancer patient must be considered. Intestinal obstruction from recurrent GI cancer or from intraperitoneal metastases from extra-abdominal malignancies can usually be excluded in a straightforward fashion. Gastritis or GI dysmotility secondary to medication (e.g., opiates, antibiotics) is frequent in patients undergoing cancer treatment. Chemotherapy-induced emesis typically occurs within 2-3 hours of drug administration, although delayed onset of vomiting (2-3 days after therapy) is a well-recognized pattern.

Improved control of nausea and vomiting has been achieved with the introduction of the serotonin antagonist ondansetron (Table 5-4). When given alone or in combination with dexamethasone, this drug is very effective and exhibits none of the extrapyramidal side-effects characteristic of metoclopramide or compazine.

D. DIARRHEA. Diarrhea can complicate the use of many chemotherapy drugs and is usually self-limited. However, patients receiving 5-FU (either alone or with other agents) can have very severe, life-threatening diarrhea. Once an infectious cause has been ruled out, patients should be managed with bowel rest, replacement fluids, and constipating agents. Octreotide (50-100 μg subcutaneously every 6-8 hours) may speed the resolution of this problem when it is associated with chemotherapy.

E. NEUTROPENIA. Most chemotherapy agents have the potential for causing neutropenia. The onset of neutropenia and its duration depend upon the drug(s) being used and the patient's bone marrow reserve. For example, someone who has had extensive prior chemotherapy or radiation to the pelvis would be expected to suffer more severe neutropenia than an untreated patient. In general, patients who have not suffered complications do not receive prophylactic antibiotics unless they have been treated for leukemia or lymphoma. Even though many patients become neutropenic (with an absolute neutrophil count <500), the majority do not have febrile episodes or apparent infections.

A patient with a fever associated with neutropenia needs to be treated with antibiotics after appropriate cultures and evaluation for source of infections have been completed. This evaluation should include a thorough physical examination, with emphasis on IV sites and the perirectal region, although a digital rectal examination should not be done in a neutropenic patient. The choice of antibiotics depends on the clinical suspicion for site of origin. When no source is apparent, a third-generation cephalosporin with or without an aminoglycoside is usually adequate. A suspected bowel source might be covered with metronidazole, or a potential line infection might be treated with agents to which *S. aureus* is sensitive.

F. SUPERIOR VENA CAVA SYNDROME. In the past, obstruction of the superior vena cava by a malignant tumor was considered an oncologic emergency, requiring immediate radiation therapy to prevent life-threatening complications. Indeed, when cardiac failure, cerebral edema, or airway compromise is present, urgent treatment is indicated. However, the majority of patients present with a slowly developing syndrome in which significant collateralization has had time to develop. Frequently, a diagnosis of malignancy has not been made, and initial efforts are directed at obtaining histologic confirmation of cancer. Carcinoma of the lung (either squamous cell or small cell) is most common; lymphoma represents the cause in about 15% of patients. In patients not requiring emergency treatment, chemotherapy is effective in both small cell lung cancer and lymphoma. Anticoagulation is generally not used owing to the risk of cerebral bleeding.

G. SPINAL CORD COMPRESSION. Vertebral metastasis, typically from carcinoma of the breast, lung, or prostate, may erode into the epidural space and produce compression of the spinal cord. Patients typically present with pain but may progress rapidly to develop sensory loss, weakness, and autonomic dysfunction. The recognition of early signs and symptoms in patients at risk for spinal cord compression is the key to effective therapy. MRI has replaced myelography in many centers as the diagnostic study of choice. Therapy consists of IV corticosteroids (e.g., dexamethasone, 10 mg IV followed

Table 5-5. Commonly used analgesics*

Agent	Dose	Duration	Comments
Oral agent			
Aspirin	650-1000 mg	4-6 hr	Inhibits platelet function for lifetime of platelet
Acetaminophen	650-1000 mg	4-6 hr	No platelet dysfunction Hepatic toxicity
Ibuprofen	200-800 mg	4-6 hr	Reversible platelet dysfunction
Codeine	32-65 mg	4-6 hr	Used in combination with acetaminophen
Oxycodone	5-10 mg	2-4 hr	Used in combination with aspirin (Percodan) or acetaminophen (Percocet)
Methadone	5-20 mg	6-8 hr	Long t1/2; requires 2-3 doses to achieve therapeutic levels
Levorphanol	2-4 mg	4-6 hr	Good oral potency; long half-life
Parenteral agent (IM)			
Ketorolac	30-60 mg loading dose, then 15-30 mg q4-6h	4-6 hr	Only parenteral nonsteroidal anti-inflammatory antipyretic analgesic
Meperidine	50-100 mg	3-4 hr	
Morphine	5-10 mg	4-6 hr	Standard for comparison of other analgesics
Hydromorphone	1-2 mg	4-6 hr	
Oxymorphone	1-2 mg	4-6 hr	Rectal suppository form available

*Agents are listed in order of increasing potency and under the most frequently used route of administration. Consult product information for precautions, adverse reactions and dosing options.

by 2 mg IV every 6 hours) to diminish cord edema, followed by vertebral radiation. Surgery is usually limited to patients with recurrence after radiation or those for whom a tissue diagnosis is necessary. Decompressive laminectomy may be performed if initial radiation is ineffective. The short-term outcome in those patients in which a diagnosis can be made *before* paralysis develops is quite good.

H. PAIN IN THE CANCER PATIENT. Cancer pain is frequently multifactorial. Direct tumor erosion into bony structures, distention of the hepatic capsule, inflammation of the parietal pleura or peritoneum, or involvement of splanchnic or peripheral nerves may produce pain that is either intermittent or constant and of varying severity. Cancer therapy can also be a source of pain (e.g., chemotherapy-induced mucositis, postoperative wound pain, or radiation-induced nerve injury). Occasionally, pain management involves the direct instillation of anesthetic agents (e.g., celiac sympathetic block by injection of 6% phenol in patients with pancreatic cancer, intercostal nerve block, continuous epidural anesthesia) or surgical intervention (cordotomy). Most commonly, cancer pain is treated with oral or parenteral analgesics. Non-narcotic agents are used first, and narcotic analgesic agents with increasing potency (and side-effects) are progressively added as more or longer-acting analgesia is required. Table 5-5 provides a list of frequently used drugs in the control of cancer pain. Other medicines may be given as adjuvants to analgesics such as phenothiazines, tricyclic antidepressants, and antihistamines. The reader should be familiar with the pharmacology, drug interactions, and side-effects of these agents prior to use.

6

Endocrine Surgery

Orlo H. Clark

I. THYROID

A. THYROID FUNCTION

1. Physiology. The human thyroid gland consists of two functionally separate but structurally intermixed populations of endocrine cells: the **follicular cells,** which concentrate iodide, synthesize thyroglobulin, and secrete the thyroid hormones T_4 and triiodothyronine T_3; and the **parafollicular cells** (C cells), which synthesize, store, and secrete calcitonin.

Iodide is absorbed from the GI tract, actively trapped by the follicular cells, oxidized, and combined with tyrosine in thyroglobulin to form monoiodotyrosine (MIT) and DIT. MIT and DIT are coupled to form the active hormones T_4 and T_3, which are stored in the colloid until released into the bloodstream.

Circulating T_4, the primary secretory product of the thyroid, and T_3, most of which arises from conversion of T_4 to T_3 in the liver, are bound to plasma proteins, chiefly to TBC and to a lesser degree to TBPA. Free T_3 and T_4 concentration are responsible for the physiologic effects of thyroid hormones.

Under normal conditions, the hypothalamus secretes TRH, which stimulates the anterior pituitary to secrete TSH. The secretion of T_4 and T_3 is regulated by a feedback mechanism that involves the hypothalamus and pituitary. An increase in circulating free thyroid hormone levels inhibits the pituitary's production of TSH, whereas a decrease stimulates TSH production.

Calcitonin inhibits bone resorption and acts in conjunction with PTH to protect against fluctuations in ionized calcium levels in the blood. PTH increases serum calcium levels while calcitonin lowers them.

2. Thyroid function tests

a. TSH (RIA). (Normal: μU/ml; varies with laboratory.) This test measures TSH in the serum by radioimmunoassay. A new, highly sensitive test for TSH now makes this test the best and most cost effective test for determining whether a person is euthyroid, hypothyroid (high), or hyperthyroid (low). Serum TSH concentrations are also low in secondary hypothyroidism (pituitary hypothyroidism) and tertiary (hypothalamic) hypothyroidism.

b. T_4. (Normal: 5.3-14.5 μg/dl). This test measures total thyroxine by CPB or displacement (T_4D) or by radioimmunoassay (RIA) and is unaffected by exogenous iodides. Measurements of T_4 are influenced by altered thyroxine binding. Thus, increased levels are found in pregnancy and women taking birth control pills; decreased levels occur in patients receiving anabolic steroids or androgens, and in patients with liver disease and nephrosis. Salicylates, sulfonamides, and phenytoin also lower T_4 (CPB) levels.

Analysis of serum T_4 levels is an excellent, simple screening test for hyperthyroidism or hypothyroidism and is 90% accurate in diagnosing these conditions. It is most often used in conjunction with a test to determine binding to TBG and expressed as an index (see Section 2d).

c. T_3 (RIA). (Normal: 60-190 ng/dl; varies with laboratory.) This test measures total circulating T_3 by radioimmunoassay. It is unaltered by iodide and is increased in hyperthyroidism, T_3 toxicosis, and in patients with stimulated thyroid glands. It decreases with fasting, advancing age, in severe systemic illness, and after corticosteroid administration. T_3 (RIA) is very useful if T_4 levels are at the upper limit of normal or the patient has symptoms or signs of thyrotoxicosis.

d. Radioactive T_3 uptake of red cells or resin (T_3RU). (Normal: varies with laboratory.) This test indirectly measures the concentration of unsaturated TBG. When thyroxin-binding proteins in the blood increase, the proportion of free or unbound thyroxine decreases. When used with T_4, T_3RU corrects for an abnormal concentration of serum proteins. T_3RU values generally parallel the serum T_4 level; i.e., they are increased in hyperthyroidism and decreased in hypothyroidism. During pregnancy or in women taking birth control pills, however, T_4 levels are falsely high owing to increased TBG, while T_3RU levels are low. In contrast, low concentrations of T_4 and high T_3RU levels are found in patients receiving phenytoin, salicylates, phenylbutazone, anticoagulants, cortisone, androgens, anabolic steroids, or large doses of penicillin, and in patients with nephrosis or severe liver disease.

3. Thyroid scanning. Several scanning technics are used.

a. Radioiodine scan is useful in determining whether thyroid nodules are single or multiple and whether they are functioning (warm or hot) or nonfunctioning (cold). Hot nodules may cause hyperthyroidism but are rarely malignant, whereas approximately 20% of cold solitary nodules are malignant. After total thyroidectomy, radioiodine scanning is useful for documenting metastatic papillary or follicular carcinoma.

b. Radioiodine uptake. The normal uptake of radioactive iodine is 10%-30% at 24 hours. [123]I has replaced ^{131}I because of its lower radiation hazard. The thyroidal uptake of radioactive iodine is increased in hyperthyroidism, glandular hormone depletion, iodine depletion, and conditions of excessive hormonal losses. Uptake is low in primary and secondary hypothyroidism, conditions of increased dietary or medicinal iodine (including contrast media), and patients receiving exogenous thyroid hormone. Uptake is also low or absent in patients with subacute thyroiditis because of an increased release of thyroid hormone from the thyroid gland.

c. Technetium-99 rectilinear scanning is more sensitive than radioiodine in detecting small nodules. The vascularity of a nodule may be estimated by this technic, but no differentiation as to malignant potential is made between hypo- or hyperfunctioning thyroid nodules.

4. Percutaneous aspiration biopsy cytology. Percutaneous needle biopsy is the most efficient and cost-effective method of determining whether a thyroid nodule is benign, suspicious, or malignant. It requires an experienced cytologist for interpretation. Ninety-nine percent of malignant, 20% of suspicious, and <5% of benign thyroid nodules have cancer by permanent pathology. Biopsy has minimal risk, can diagnose nonneoplastic thyroid conditions such as infections and thyroiditis, and can determine the type of cancer such as medullary.

5. Serologic tests. Antibodies against human thyroglobulin and against subcellular thyroid components are found in high titers in patients with Hashimoto's disease, but not in patients with dyshormonogenic or iodine-deficient goiters. Low titers of antithyroglobulin and antimicrosomal antibodies are observed in about 60% of patients with Graves' disease. Serum thyroglobulin levels, as determined by radioimmunoassay, are useful in the posttreatment follow-up of patients with differentiated thyroid cancer; such patients with elevated thyroglobulin levels often have metastatic thyroid cancer.

6. Other tests

a. TSH response to TRH (200 μg IV) is useful in diagnosing subclinical primary hypothyroidism (the TSH response to TRH is increased) and subclinical hyperthyroidism (the TSH response to TRH is decreased or absent).

b. T_3 suppression test (75-100 μg of T_3 daily for 10 days) helps determine whether the thyroid gland or a thyroid nodule is functioning autonomously. After T_3 is given, the thyroid ^{123}I uptake decreases to less than half its initial value in normal individuals but not in patients with hyperthyroidism.

c. Serum cholesterol levels (normal: 150-240 mg/dl) are often elevated in severe hypothyroidism and low in hyperthyroidism.

d. A relative *lymphocytosis* and *monocytosis,* with normal or slightly low total leukocyte count, are characteristic blood findings in hyperthyroidism.

e. Human thyroid-stimulating immunoglobulins (TSI) and thyroid-blocking immunoglobulins (TBI) have been found in the plasma of patients with Graves' disease and hypothyroidism, respectively; they correlate well with the early uptake of radioiodine by the thyroid and have replaced long-acting thyroid stimulator (LATS).

B. HYPERTHYROIDISM is due to excess circulating thyroid hormone. Diffuse toxic goiter (Graves' disease) and toxic nodular goiter (Plummer's disease) account for most cases. There is a variety of other (rare) causes, including subacute thyroiditis, factitious hyperthyroidism due to taking thyroid hormone creating new thyroid, molar pregnancy, functioning thyroid neoplasms, TSH-secreting pituitary tumor, and struma overii.

Graves' disease appears to be an autoimmune disease. Increased levels of TSI are found in many of these patients. Hyperthyroidism is six times more common in women than in men. A few patients with hyperthyroidism have normal serum T_4 levels, normal radioiodine uptakes, and normal protein binding, and are toxic due to increased serum T_3 levels (T_3 toxicosis).

1. Diagnosis. Virtually every organ system is affected by hyperthyroidism. The clinical manifestations may be subtle or marked, and they tend to exacerbate and remit. Many cases are easily diagnosed on the basis of symptoms and signs, but others (mild or apathetic hyperthyroidism) are recognized with difficulty. Graves' disease usually causes more severe hyperthyroidism than does toxic nodular goiter.

a. Symptoms. Nervousness; irritability; sweating and heat intolerance; palpitations; muscular weakness and increased fatigue; increased frequency of bowel movements; polyuria; menstrual irregularities and infertility; eye irritation; weight loss (despite an increased appetite).

b. Signs. Staring appearance; warm, thin, moist skin; fine hair or alopecia; goiter; tachycardia or atrial fibrillation; weight loss; shortened Achilles' reflex time. Extrathyroidal manifestations are almost exclusively limited to Graves' disease: exophthalmos; pretibial myxedema; vitiligo; onycholysis (longitudinal striation and flattening of nails); thyroid acropachy (clubbing of digits); gynecomastia.

c. Laboratory tests. TSH is low; T_4 and T_3 levels are increased; radioactive iodine uptake is usually increased; T_3RU is increased; TSH response to TRH is absent; thyroidal radioactive iodine uptake does not suppress with exogenous T_3 administration; hypercalciuria and occasional hypercalcemia; blood cholesterol level may be low.

2. Differential diagnosis. Anxiety neurosis, heart disease, anemia, cirrhosis, and pheochromocytoma may be difficult to distinguish from hyperthyroidism. Tachycardia at rest, a goiter, increased serum T_4, low TSH, and increased radioactive iodine uptake make the diagnosis of hyperthyroidism a certainty.

3. Complications

a. Hyperthyroid crisis (thyroid storm) is characterized by fever and exaggerated thyrotoxic manifestations involving the cardiovascular, gastrointestinal, and central nervous systems. Coma and jaundice may occur. Storm is usually precipitated by physical stress (e.g., surgery, infection, trauma).

Treatment must begin immediately and includes: (1) Diagnosis and treatment of any underlying illness. (2) General support measures: oxygen, sedatives, IV fluids, and corticosteroids (hydrocortisone 300 mg parenterally daily). (3) Sodium iodide USP 1-2 gm IV every 8 hours. (4) High doses of the antithyroid drug (propylthiouracil 300 mg) given orally or by nasogastric tube every 6 hours. (5) Propranolol 1-2 mg IV (total dose 2-10 mg) controls cardiac and psychomotor abnormalities within 10 minutes; its effect lasts for 3-4 hours.

b. Severe exophthalmos. (1) Ocular manifestations of Graves' disease may be mild or severe. The mild form is due to hyperactivity of the sympathetic nervous system, and the severe type is due to infiltration of the retroorbital tissues. The infiltrative form is uncommon. Progressive ophthalmopathy occurs more frequently, is more severe in men than women, and is usually bilateral. Patients usually improve when euthyroid, but the course is unpredictable. (2) *Symptoms and signs:* edema of orbital contents and periorbital tissues; chemosis (protrusion of edematous, injected scleral conjunctiva); excessive lacrimation; photophobia; protrusion of eyes (exophthalmos); paresis or paralysis of ocular muscles causing diplopia, squint, loss of convergence; visual loss. (3) *Treatment* depends upon the severity of ophthalmopathy (ophthalmologic consultation is recommended); maintain the patient in a euthyroid state; protect the eyes from light and dust with dark glasses and eyeshades; elevate head of the bed; methylcellulose eyedrops; corticosteroids (60 mg prednisone) for several weeks; retroorbital radiation; lateral tarsorraphy or retroorbital surgical decompression. (4) In patients with *severe* or *progressive* exophthalmos, subtotal thyroidectomy should be delayed until the eyes have stabilized.

4. Treatment. Hyperthyroidism may be treated by antithyroid drugs, radioactive iodine therapy, or subtotal thyroidectomy. The choice of treatment depends upon the patient's age and the size and consistency of the goiter.

a. Antithyroid drugs. Reliable patients with mild hyperthyroidism and small diffuse goiters are good candidates for antithyroid medications. (1) Use PTU, 100-300 mg orally every 6 hours, or methimazole (Tapazole), 10-30 mg orally every 8 hours. (2) About 30% of patients will remain euthyroid if the drug is discontinued after 18 months. (3) Severely toxic patients should be started on these antithyroid drugs as well as on the β-adrenergic blocking agent propranolol, 5 mg initially and then up to 40 mg orally 4 times daily, before other forms of definitive therapy are instituted.

Patients receiving PTU or Tapazole should be warned to discontinue these medications and see their doctor immediately if they develop a sore throat or fever, because granulocytopenia and fatal agranulocytosis may develop. If the leukocyte count falls <4500 or if there are <45% granulocytes, the drug should be discontinued.

b. Radioiodine (^{131}*I)* is the treatment of choice for recurrent hyperthyroidism, poor risk patients, and patients >45 years of age with diffuse thyroid enlargement. The treatment is effective and avoids an operation. Radioiodine should not be used in children or in pregnant women because of the radiation hazard; it should not be used in a toxic patient with a nonfunctioning nodule within the hyperfunctioning gland because the nodule may be malignant. Nearly all patients treated with radioiodine eventually become hypothyroid.

c. Subtotal thyroidectomy is the recommended form of treatment in: (1) patients with very large goiters, especially if multinodular or with low radioiodine uptake; (2) children or pregnant women; (3) patients with a thyroid nodule that may be malignant; (4) psychologically or mentally incompetent patients in whom long-term follow-up will be difficult to obtain. Advantages are the rapid return to the euthyroid state and a lower incidence of hypothyroidism than can be achieved with radioiodine treatment.

Preparation for surgery includes administration of an antithyroid drug until the patient becomes euthyroid. 10-15 days before operation potassium iodide or Lugol's solution (3 drops orally, twice daily) are started and given in conjunction with PTU until the time of operation. Propranolol (5-40 mg orally, 4 times daily) used to prepare severely toxic patients for operation should be continued for about 4 days after thyroidectomy because circulating levels of thyroid hormone remain elevated for several days after subtotal resections of the gland. Propranolol should not be used in patients with asthma or congestive heart failure because of the risk of precipitating bronchospasm or heart failure.

The mortality rate of subtotal thyroidectomy is <0.1%. Permanent injuries to the parathyroid glands or to the recurrent laryngeal nerves occur in <2% of cases. Recurrent hyperthyroidism develops in about 5% and hypothyroidism in about 15% of patients. Most patients can be discharged within 1 or 2 days of surgical treatment.

5. Prognosis. Untreated thyrotoxicosis causes progressive and profound catabolic disturbances and cardiac damage resulting in death by thyroid storm, heart failure, or cachexia. Any patient with hyperthyroidism may eventually become hypothyroid; therefore yearly thyroid function tests are advisable.

C. HYPOTHYROIDISM. The clinical manifestations of hypothyroidism may be subtle, and the diagnosis is often overlooked.

1. Diagnosis

a. Symptoms. Weakness; intolerance to cold; dry skin; alopecia; menometrorrhagia; constipation; periorbital swelling. There may be a history of previous treatment for hyperthyroidism or family history of goiter.

b. Signs. Rough, dry skin; yellow pallor; coarse hair; hoarse voice; some patients become comatose (myxedema coma).

c. Laboratory tests. In primary hypothyroidism, serum T_4 is low and TSH levels are increased; the response of TSH to TRH is increased. In secondary (pituitary) and tertiary (hypothalamic) hypothyroidism, serum T_4 and TSH levels are low. Elevated blood cholesterol, hyponatremia, hypoxemia, and CO_2 retention are present when the hypothyroidism is severe.

2. Treatment

a. Myxedema coma. Five hundred micrograms of thyroxine IV should be given immediately, followed by 100 μg of T_4 daily. Hydrocortisone (100 μg IV every 8 hours) should also be given in this life-threatening condition.

b. Patients with severe hypothyroidism and heart disease without coma should, in contrast, be started on very low doses of L-sodium thyroxine (25 μg orally, daily). The dose is increased by 25 μg every 2 weeks until euthyroidism is achieved. ECGs and myocardial enzymes should be obtained before the initial dose, and before each increase because hypothyroidism itself may cause elevated myocardial enzyme levels.

D. NONTOXIC NODULAR GOITER is a compensatory response to inadequate production of thyroid hormones. It may stem from a congenital defect (dyshormonogenesis); it also occurs in people living in endemic (iodine-poor) regions, or it may result from prolonged exposure to goitrogenic foods or drugs. If not treated, the goiter may become multinodular. The incidence of carcinoma in multinodular goiters is approximately 1%.

The *symptoms* are awareness of a neck mass, dyspnea, or dysphagia. T_4, T_3, TSH and T_3RU measurements are usually normal but radioiodine uptake and TSH levels may be slightly increased.

Differential diagnosis includes physiologic enlargement of the thyroid during puberty or pregnancy, inflammatory thyroid disease, hyperthyroidism, and thyroid tumors.

Most small diffuse goiters and some larger nodular goiters decrease in size in response to administration of thyroid hormone. Indications for removal of nontoxic nodular goiter are: suspicion or cytologic examination suspicious or diagnostic of malignancy; history of radiation to the head or neck; pressure symptoms; substernal extension; progressive enlargement; cosmetic deformity; familial thyroid cancer.

E. INFLAMMATORY THYROID DISEASE (THYROIDITIS)
may result in acute, subacute, or chronic thyroiditis. These conditions are of surgical importance because they sometimes are confused with thyroid cancer and occasionally require emergent surgery.

1. Acute suppurative thyroiditis is rare; it is characterized by the sudden onset of severe neck pain, dysphagia, and fever and usually follows an upper respiratory illness. The diagnosis is made by needle aspiration and treatment is surgical drainage. A fistula from the pyriform sinus should be suspected in children or in recurrent cases.

2. Subacute thyroiditis may be **silent** (asymptomatic) or cause pain, swelling, generalized weakness, malaise, and weight loss. The erythrocyte sedimentation rate and serum gamma globulin are almost always elevated, and radioiodine uptake is low or absent. Serum T_4 levels may be increased. Salicylates and steroids effectively relieve the symptoms. This disease is self-limited, and thyroid function returns to normal. The acute symptoms last about 10 days to 1 month.

3. Hashimoto's (chronic lymphocytic) thyroiditis is believed to be an autoimmune phenomenon. Patients have high levels of antimicrosomal and antithyroglobulin antibodies. About 25% become hypothyroid. This thyroiditis occurs almost exclusively in women and is characterized by a firm diffusely enlarged, nontender thyroid gland. *Treatment* is with thyroid hormone. Operation is indicated only if a malignant tumor is suspected or if local pressure symptoms are severe. Surgical division of the isthmus provides dramatic relief of pressure symptoms. Percutaneous fine-needle biopsy helps clarify the nature of suspicious nodules.

4. Riedel's thyroiditis is a rare form of chronic thyroiditis. It appears as a hard, woody mass with tracheal compression and infiltration into the adjacent muscles, thus making it difficult to differentiate clinically from anaplastic thyroid cancer. It is sometimes associated with retroperitoneal fibrosis. Patients are usually hypothyroid. Surgical treatment is necessary to relieve tracheal or esophageal obstruction or to rule out carcinoma.

F. THYROID TUMORS. Most benign or malignant thyroid tumors occur in euthyroid patients who are symptomatic. Solitary nodules are more likely to be malignant (5%-35%) than are multinodular glands (1%-5%). Cold thyroid nodules may be malignant, whereas functioning nodules are rarely malignant. Thyroid cysts are rarely malignant and can be accurately diagnosed by echography. Although thyroid disease and thyroid malignancy are more common in women, a solitary nodule is more likely to be a cancer in a man. About 50% of solitary cold thyroid nodules in children are malignant. Exposure to ionizing radiation in infancy or childhood doubles the possibility of a nodule being malignant. Percutaneous aspiration biopsy helps distinguish benign from malignant nodules.

G. BENIGN TUMORS. Benign thyroid nodules are follicular adenomas, involutionary nodules, cysts, or localized thyroiditis. Adenomas are firm, nontender, discrete, encapsulated, and slowly growing; they may compress the adjacent thyroid or other structures. The major reasons for removal are a suspicion of malignancy, local symptoms (pain, dysphagia), functional overactivity producing hyperthyroidism, or cosmetic disfigurement.

H. ECTOPIC THYROID. The thyroid develops from a pharyngeal outpocketing that migrates caudally. Aberrant development of migration may result in agenesis of one or both lobes of the thyroid; a lingual thyroid protruding from the base of the tongue; thyroglossal ducts (midline cysts) located anywhere from the foramen cecum of the tongue to the thyroid; or thyroid rests. In 70% or more of patients with a lingual thyroid, this is the only thyroid tissue present and removal results in hypothyroidism. About 1% of thyroglossal duct cysts contain thyroid cancer; cysts are removed for diagnostic, infectious, or cosmetic reasons. Thyroid rests are situated in the midline and are benign, whereas laterally located thyroid tissue in lymph nodes (lateral aberrant thyroid) is metastatic differentiated carcinoma in most cases.

I. THYROID CARCINOMA. There are two major types of primary malignant thyroid tumor: differentiated (papillary, mixed papillary and follicular, follicular, Hürthle cell, medullary) and undifferentiated. Lymphoma and sarcoma are in another category of lesions that occur occasionally.

Cancers of lung, breast, and kidney may metastasize to the thyroid, but metastatic lesions are rarely solitary, and the primary tumor is usually apparent.

1. Differentiated carcinoma

a. Papillary adenocarcinoma accounts for 85% of all thyroid malignancies. It tends to occur in young adults. This lesion grows slowly and spreads via the intra- and extrathyroidal lymphatics, so that involvement of the contralateral thyroid lobe and ipsilateral thyroid lymph nodes occurs in 30%-85% of patients. Growth is stimulated by TSH. Mixed papillary-follicular thyroid carcinoma is classified with papillary carcinoma and has a similar favorable prognosis.

b. Follicular carcinoma. Approximately 10% of malignant thyroid tumors are follicular. The patients are older than those with papillary cancer. Clinically, the lesion is rubbery or soft, smooth, nontender, and encapsulated; it spreads via the bloodstream to bone, lungs, or other sites.

c. Hürthle cell carcinoma accounts for about 3% of malignant thyroid tumors. It arises from the follicle cell and spreads via the lymphatics to lungs, bone, and other sites. It makes thyroglobulin but usually does not take up radioactive iodine.

d. Medullary carcinoma accounts for 3% of malignant thyroid tumors. It arises from the C cells (calcitonin cells or parafollicular cells). It may occur sporadically or in association with hyperparathyroidism, pheochromocytoma, ganglioneuromatosis, and neurofibromatosis (Sipple's syndrome or type II multiple endocrine adenomatosis). Premedullary carcinoma (a premalignant condition) has been diagnosed in family members of patients with Sipple's syndrome by documenting increased serum calcitonin levels in response to provocative testing with calcium or pentagastrin. Medullary carcinoma is more aggressive than papillary or follicular carcinoma and metastasizes early via lymphatics. It does not usually take up radioiodine.

2. Undifferentiated carcinomas

2. Undifferentiated carcinomas include small cell, giant cell, spindle cell, and squamous cell types. They occur principally in elderly women and comprise 3% of thyroid malignancies. They grow and invade rapidly and are rarely curable. In contrast to differentiated tumors, they often cause symptoms in the neck. Cervical lymphadenopathy and pulmonary metastases are common. These tumors do not take up radioiodine.

3. Diagnosis

3. Diagnosis. Most thyroid cancers are diagnosed by aspiration biopsy cytology. Some patients with familial medullary cancer are diagnosed by increased basal or stimulated calcitonin levels.

4. Treatment

a. Cold solitary thyroid nodules should be removed by total lobectomy. If papillary or follicular cancer is diagnosed, total or near-total thyroidectomy is advised, preserving parathyroid function.

If lymph node metastases are present, a conservative neck dissection preserving the sternocleidomastoid muscle and spinal accessory nerve is performed. Bilateral cervical node involvement requires bilateral neck dissections delaying done side to the jugular vein after an interval of 6 weeks.

For patients with follicular and papillary carcinomas >1.5 cm, T_3 is given postoperatively (75 μg orally daily) for 3 months, and a low iodine diet is prescribed. T_3 is then discontinued and after 12 days a radioiodine total body scan is performed. Possible persistent tumor revealed by scan is ablated with a therapeutic dose of radioiodine. The patient is then treated with suppressive doses of L-sodium thyroxine, 0.2-0.3 mg orally daily.

Determination of serum thyroglobulin levels is useful after total thyroidectomy. If thyroglobulin levels increase, residual thyroid cancer is present.

b. Medullary carcinoma is treated by total thyroidectomy, a thorough central neck dissection, and prophylactic neck dissection on the side of the lesion. Calcitonin and CEA levels are useful for monitoring recurrence.

c. Undifferentiated thyroid tumors are rarely curable and often inoperable. Thyroidectomy when possible is advocated before or after chemotherapy (usually doxorubicin) and external radiation therapy.

4. Prognosis.

Average survival rates after treatment of various forms of thyroid cancer are shown in Table 6-1. The prognosis is better in women and in patients under age 60 years. Locally invasive tumors have a more ominous prognosis than tumors that have metastasized to regional lymph nodes. Medullary carcinoma is more aggressive than papillary or follicular carcinoma, although the clinical course is variable. Most

Table 6-1. Survival rates (%) after treatment for thyroid cancer

Years	Papillary	Follicular	Undifferentiated
10	81	58	11
20	61	48	8

patients with undifferentiated thyroid tumors are dead within a year of diagnosis.

II. PARATHYROID

A. HYPERPARATHYROIDISM is the excessive secretion of PTH. It may be **primary,** caused by adenoma (85%), double adenoma (4%), hyperplasia (12%), or cancer of the parathyroids (1%); **secondary,** due to diseases that lower plasma concentrations of ionized calcium; **tertiary,** a consequence of secondary hyperparathyroidism (hyperplastic glands fail to regress in the presence of hypercalcemia); or **ectopic** (pseudo) hyperparathyroidism, due to secretion of PTH or PTH-like polypeptides by nonparathyroid tumors. Serum calcium levels are elevated in most patients with primary and clinically significant secondary hyperparathyroidism.

B. PRIMARY HYPERPARATHYROIDISM is unusual in children; it is most common in women between the ages of 30 and 60. Most cases are sporadic, but it may also be associated with multiple endocrine adenomatosis (type 1 and 2) and familial hyperparathyroidism. Most patients with familial hyperparathyroidism have hyperplasia.

   1. Diagnosis is made by documenting hypercalcemia and increased PTH levels or by eliminating other causes of hypercalcemia and carefully evaluating the clinical picture and laboratory tests.

   a. Symptoms and signs. No symptoms: hypercalcemia detected on routine screening tests. Nonspecific symptoms: polydipsia, weight loss, muscular weakness and pain, lethargy, depression, anorexia, constipation. Other: nephrolithiasis, nephrocalcinosis, hypertension, peptic ulcer disease, pancreatitis, gout or pseudogout; clinically evident osteitis fibrosa cystica is now distinctly uncommon. Parathyroid adenomas are palpable in only 4% of patients; carcinomas are palpable in 50%. Band keratopathy occurs in approximately 10% of patients with hypercalcemia (including hyperparathyroidism); it is best seen with a slit lamp.

   b. Laboratory tests. The classic biochemical abnormalities in primary hyperparathyroidism are hypercalcemia, hypophosphatemia, hyperchloremia, hypercalciuria, and increased serum PTH levels. However, one or more of these tests may be normal in an individual patient.

The chloride-to-phosphate ratio in the serum is usually >33 in patients with hyperparathyroidism who have not been vomiting and are not in renal failure. The ratio is <33 in patients with hypercalcemia from other causes.

Other tests: alkaline phosphatase (increased), blood pH (decreased), serum uric acid (increased), nephrogenous cyclic AMP (increased), serum magnesium (decreased), tubular reabsorption of phosphate (<80 in 80% of patients). Renal function (BUN, creatinine), serum electrophoresis, sedimentation rate, hemoglobin, hematocrit, 24-hour urinary calcium level, and urinalysis help to rule out other causes of hypercalcemia. Increased urinary deoxypyridinoline cross-link levels document increased bone turnover.

Special tests may be required in patients with renal stones and suspected normocalcemic hyperparathyroidism. Since hypoalbuminemia, impaired renal function, excessive dietary phosphate intake, acute pancreatitis, and magnesium or vitamin D deficiency may decrease serum calcium concentration, these conditions should be considered and corrected if possible. The ionized calcium should be measured; sometimes it is increased when total calcium is normal. A trial of thiazide diuretics, which decrease urinary calcium excretion and "unmask" hypercalcemia, is useful.

c. Radiographs. Subperiosteal resorption or osteitis fibrosa cystica (bone cysts) are found in about 10% of cases, and osteoporosis is even more common. Subperiosteal resorption is best seen on the radial aspect of the index finger; it is rare unless the alkaline phosphatase is increased. Dual photon bone densitometry detects bone loss. Abdominal radiographs may reveal renal or pancreatic calcifications. Intravenous urogram and chest radiograph may help exclude other causes of hypercalcemia.

2. Differential diagnosis

a. Malignancy (breast, multiple myeloma, metastatic cancer, leukemia, PTH-like hormone-secreting tumors of the lung, kidney, or other organs) is the most common cause of hypercalcemia in hospitalized patients. Bone pain, a lung or renal lesion, increased sedimentation rate, hematuria, proteinuria, a low serum chloride level, normal phosphorus level, and increased alkaline phosphatase levels without subperiosteal resorption all suggest malignant disease.

b. Hyperparathyroidism is the second most common cause of hypercalcemia; it occurs in about 1 in every 1000 patients. Hyperparathyroidism and malignancy account for 90% of cases of hypercalcuria.

c. Other causes of real or apparent hypercalcemia: laboratory error, venous stasis due to a tight tourniquet, immobilization, idiopathic hypercalcemia of infancy, hyperthyroidism, hypothyroidism, thiazide diuretics, milk-alkali syndrome, sarcoidosis, vitamin D or A overdosage, Paget's disease, Addison's disease, dysproteinemias, and benign familial hypocalciuric hypercalcemia.

3. Complications. Patients with untreated hyperparathyroidism have a higher death rate from cardiovascular and malignant disease. Untreated hyperparathyroidism may result in renal failure, hypertension, mental depression, or hypercalcemic crisis. Renal failure, once established, is sometimes progressive despite successful parathyroidectomy, emphasizing the importance of early diagnosis and treatment.

Hypercalcemic crisis. Symptoms include nausea and vomiting, drowsiness, stupor, weakness, or coma. Treatment includes: (a) Hydration with saline, up to 2 liters IV in 3 hours, and 8 liters/day. (b) Diuresis with furosemide (Lasix), 40-100 mg over 4-6 hours. **Do not use** thiazide diuretics. (c) Correct electrolyte abnormalities (hypokalemia, hypomagnesemia, hypophosphatemia). (d) Avoid immobilization. (e) If patients fail to respond, give hydrocortisone 200 mg IV daily, or calcitonin 0.5-5 MRC units/kg/hour IV, or mithramycin 25 µg/kg IV, or etidronate 7.5 mg/kg/day IV for 3 consecutive days. Corticosteroids are effective in patients with vitamin D intoxication, sarcoidosis, and Addison's disease, but they are effective in only 50% of patients with hypercalcemia of malignancy and in 10% of those with hyperparathyroidism. Dialysis is rarely required.

4. Treatment. Operation is the treatment of choice for primary hyperparathyroidism. It should be performed only after the diagnosis is firmly established. At operation, all 4 parathyroids should be identified. 80% of patients have 4 glands, 15% have 5 or more, and 5% have fewer than 4. If an adenoma is present, it is removed. If there is hyperplasia of all 4 glands, 1 gland should be subtotally resected and the others removed completely.

Experienced surgeons successfully identify and remove the hypersecreting gland(s) in >95% of patients. The hyperparathyroidism disappears rapidly.

Transient hypoparathyroidism with hypocalcemia and hypomagnesemia causes perioral numbness and positive

Chvostek and Trousseau signs. This condition most often develops about 48 hours after operation in patients with generalized decalcification of the skeleton, or in patients treated by subtotal parathyroidectomy. See page 305 for treatment of hypoparathyroidism.

C. SECONDARY-TERTIARY HYPERPARATHYROIDISM.

Secondary hyperparathyroidism occurs most often in patients with renal failure, but it may stem from any situation that results in low plasma concentrations of ionized calcium. Hypocalcemia causes stimulation of PTH secretion, and if the stimulation is prolonged, chief cell hyperplasia results. In secondary hyperparathyroidism due to renal failure, the serum phosphorus is usually high, whereas with malabsorption, osteomalacia, or rickets, phosphorus is normal or low.

The clinical manifestations of secondary hyperparathyroidism include bone pain, pruritus, metastatic calcification including tumoral calcinosis and, rarely, calciphylaxis. **Treatment**—the majority of patients with secondary hyperparathyroidism may be treated medically: Lower serum phosphate levels by the administration of aluminum carbonate or hydroxide gel 30 ml, 3 times daily with meals; increase the calcium concentration in the dialysis solution (this decreases serum PTH levels); prescribe 1,25-dihydroxyvitamin D.

Indications for subtotal parathyroidectomy in patients with secondary hyperparathyroidism are severe bone pain and progressive osteitis fibrosa cystica, a calcium-phosphate product of 70 or greater, metastatic calcification, severe pruritus, and calciphylaxis. Dramatic and rapid improvement of these conditions usually follows surgical treatment. Patients with aluminum bone disease and mild hyperparathyroidism should not be treated surgically.

Occasionally, a patient with secondary hyperparathyroidism develops parathyroid hyperplasia that behaves autonomously. This is tertiary hyperparathyroidism. It appears in patients on chronic hemodialysis or follows renal transplantation. In most cases of secondary hyperparathyroidism, serum calcium returns to normal within 6 months of renal transplantation. Subtotal parathyroidectomy is occasionally indicated.

D. HYPOPARATHYROIDISM.

Parathyroid insufficiency is most commonly a complication of thyroidectomy. Permanent hypoparathyroidism is unusual after parathyroidectomy, although transient hypocalcemia due to "hungry bones" is not uncommon in young patients with elevated serum alkaline phosphatase.

1. Diagnosis

a. Symptoms and signs. (1) Postoperative hypoparathyroidism: latent tetany (paresthesias, positive Chvostek or Trousseau signs), anxiety, depression, muscle cramps, carpopedal spasm, laryngeal stridor, convulsions, papilledema. (2) Idiopathic hypoparathyroidism: malformation of the nails, poor dentition, thin dry hair, congestive heart failure. (3) Chronic hypoparathyroidism of any cause: cataracts, convulsive disorders, intestinal dysfunction, malabsorption, anxiety, chorea, paralysis agitans, retarded physical development, and mental deterioration; these manifestations are related to both the degree and duration of hypocalcemia.

b. Laboratory tests. Hypocalcemia, hyperphosphatemia, low or absent PTH and urinary phosphate, high tubular resorption of phosphate, low urinary calcium and systemic alkalosis. Serum alkaline phosphatase, BUN, and creatinine levels are normal. The Q-T interval of the ECG may be prolonged.

c. Radiographs. Calcification of the basal ganglia, arteries, and external ear may be present.

2. Differential diagnosis.

A history of thyroid or parathyroid surgery is most important. Tetany may develop from the alkalosis of hyperventilation. Tetany after parathyroid operations may result from hypomagnesemia; this possibility should be considered in symptomatic patients who do not respond to calcium supplementation. Patients with renal failure also have hyperphosphatemia and hypocalcemia, but renal function tests are abnormal, PTH levels are increased, and these patients are acidotic, not alkalotic. Hypocalcemia occurs in rickets and osteomalacia due to vitamin D deficiency or resistance, renal tubular dysfunction, or malabsorption. These conditions are implicated by a careful history revealing lack of exposure to sunshine (chronic invalidism), pancreatitis, or steatorrhea.

3. Treatment.

The goals of therapy are to bring the patient out of tetany, to increase serum calcium concentration, and to lower serum phosphate to prevent metastatic calcification.

a. Emergency treatment of postoperative tetany

(1) Reassure the anxious patient to avoid hyperventilation. Have the patient breathe into a bag if necessary.

(2) Obtain a blood sample for calcium, phosphorus, and magnesium concentrations.

(3) If patient is very symptomatic, give calcium chloride or calcium gluconate, 10-20 ml of 10% solution **slowly** IV,

until tetany disappears. (Rapid infusion of calcium may cause a cardiac arrest, especially in patients receiving digitalis.) Avoid extravasation because these solutions cause tissue necrosis.

(4) 10-50 ml of 10% calcium chloride may then be added to 1 L of saline or 5% dextrose solution and administered slowly IV. Adjust infusion rate so that symptoms are controlled and serum calcium levels remain normal.

(5) If the hypocalcemia and tetany are severe, vitamin D therapy (Rocaltrol 0.25-2.0 μg daily) may be necessary. Thyroid function should be assessed and appropriately treated, because vitamin D is more effective in euthyroid than in hypothyroid patients.

b. Maintenance therapy

(1) Once tetany is controlled, change from IV calcium to an oral calcium preparation. Use calcium glubionate (Neo-Calglucon) 30 ml orally three times daily; or calcium carbonate 250 mg/tab, 1 or 2 tabs four times daily; or calcium lactate 2-4 g orally three times daily; or calcium gluconate 8 g orally three times daily.

(2) Begin a high calcium, low phosphorus diet.

(3) Vitamin D: Calcitriol (Rocaltrol, 1,25-dihydroxycholecalciferol, 0.25-1 μg/day) has replaced other forms of vitamin D for acute management of hypocalcemia, because of its rapid onset and short duration of action. It is effective in patients with renal failure.

(4) Aluminum hydroxide with magnesium hydroxide or magnesium trisilicate, 15 ml (or 20.5 g tablets) three times daily with meals, reduces serum phosphorus levels.

4. Prognosis. The chronic management of hypoparathyroid patients may be difficult because the difference between the controlling and intoxicating dose of vitamin D is often small. Episodes of hypercalcemia in treated patients may occur after months or even years of good control, and therefore serum calcium and phosphorus should be determined periodically.

E. PSEUDOHYPOPARATHYROIDISM AND PSEUDOPSEUDOHYPOPARATHYROIDISM

1. Pseudohypoparathyroidism is characterized by hypocalcemia, hyperphosphatemia, and variable somatic and skeletal abnormalities including a round face, a short thick body, shortened metacarpal and metatarsal bones, mental deficiency, and radiographic evidence of soft tissue and cerebral calcification. It is inherited as an X-linked autosomal trait.

These patients have abnormal guanyl nucleotide regulatory proteins and an end-organ resistance to parathyroid hormone. PTH levels are increased and parathyroid glands are normal or hyperplastic, whereas in hypoparathyroidism, parathyroid tissue is lacking or defective and serum PTH levels are absent or low. Some patients also have hypothyroidism or ovarian dysfunction. Treatment is similar to that described for hypoparathyroidism. Smaller doses of vitamin D usually are effective, and resistance to vitamin D is uncommon.

2. Patients with **pseudopseudohypoparathyroidism** resemble those with pseudohypoparathyroidism in body habitus, chondrodystrophy, and subcutaneous calcifications, but they have normal serum calcium and phosphorus levels.

III. ADRENALS

The adrenal glands are composed of an outer cortex and inner medulla which are distinct from one another in their origin and function. Increased adrenal hormone secretion may be due to hyperplastic or neoplastic change; the clinical manifestations depend upon the type and amount of adrenal secretion. Decreased hormone production may result from hypoplasia, atrophy, destruction, or surgical removal.

A. PHYSIOLOGY. The adrenal cortex is essential to life. It has a major role in intermediary metabolism and in resistance of the body to stress and a subsidiary role in sexual development and function. ACTH secreted by the pituitary regulates the secretion of cortisol, corticosterone, androgens, and possibly estrogens and has a trophic effect upon the adrenal cortex. It also has a minor effect on aldosterone secretion. Corticotropin-releasing factor from the hypothalamus and the plasma-free cortisol level regulate ACTH secretion.

There are 3 major types of adrenocortical hormones.

1. Glucocorticoids. *Cortisol and related steroids* (a) Play a vital role in response to stress. (b) Promote the catabolism of protein and formation of glucose (gluconeogenesis), and inhibit tissue utilization of glucose, thereby increasing blood sugar. (c) Encourage deposition and redistribution of body fat (high levels cause lipolysis, hyperlipidemia, and hypercholesterolemia). (d) Have a weak aldosterone effect (decrease urinary excretion of sodium and increase potassium and hydrogen excretion, but unlike aldosterone, they increase water excretion). (e) Increase the number of red cells and neutrophils and decrease the number of eosinophils and lymphocytes in the blood.

2. Mineralocorticoids. Aldosterone is the most potent endogenous salt-retaining steroid. It causes retention of sodium and excretion of potassium and hydrogen ions, and it also helps to regulate extracellular fluid volume and blood pressure. Several mechanisms control aldosterone secretion: (a) Renin-angiotensin system (volume depletion increases and volume expansion suppresses). (b) Serum potassium level (hyperkalemia increases and hypokalemia decreases). (c) ACTH (increases). (d) Serum sodium concentration (hyponatremia increases and hypernatremia decreases).

3. Sex hormones. The normal adrenal cortex secretes small amounts of testosterone as well as a number of less potent androgenic substances including 17-ketosteroids (17-KS), dehydroepiandrosterone (DHEA), etiocholanolone, androsterone, and the 11-oxy-derivatives. Excess androgens and estrogens may be produced by adrenocortical tumors (usually carcinoma) or hyperplasia.

B. PRIMARY HYPERALDOSTERONISM. In this syndrome, excessive secretion of aldosterone independent of renin-angiotensin and ACTH regulation causes sodium retention, potassium depletion, and hypertension in nonedematous patients. It accounts for 1% of all cases of hypertension. Primary hyperaldosteronism is twice as common in women as in men. The adrenal lesion is an adenoma in 75%, bilateral nodular hyperplasia in 25%, and carcinoma rarely. Patients with atypical clinical syndromes are more likely to have bilateral hyperplasia or carcinoma.

In **secondary hyperaldosteronism,** aldosterone secretion is increased in response to overactivity of the renin-angiotensin system. Plasma renin levels are invariably increased in these cases, whereas they are low in patients with primary hyperaldosteronism.

1. Diagnosis

a. Symptoms and signs. Hypertension, usually persistent and mild; headache, muscle weakness, polydipsia, nocturnal polyuria; edema usually.

b. Laboratory tests. Hypokalemic alkalosis, normal or elevated serum sodium, decreased serum chloride and magnesium. Plasma aldosterone levels are elevated and plasma renin levels are low; low sodium diets and diuretics must be discontinued before these tests are obtained. The following suggests primary hyperaldosteronism: inappropriately high urinary potassium ($>$30-40 mEq/L) despite hypokalemia. Correction of hypokalemia after 100 mg of spironolactone (Aldactone) four times daily for 3 days (a dose that does not raise serum potassium in normal subjects). Urinary excretion of $>$20 μg of aldosterone daily in a sodium and potassium repleted patient. Low plasma renin level despite at least 4 hours of ambulation while on a low sodium diet, in a patient who also has elevated aldosterone levels while on a high sodium diet (2 g sodium per meal for 3 days).

c. Other tests. ECG may show the changes of hypokalemia and chronic hypertension. Adrenal scan with CT scan, 19-iodocholesterol, or selective adrenal vein catheterization may localize a small adrenal tumor.

2. Differential diagnosis. Primary hyperaldosteronism (high aldosterone, low renin) should be considered in any hypertensive patient with muscular weakness or hypokalemia. Diuretic drugs are the most common cause of hypokalemia; their effects may persist for several weeks after discontinuation.

Secondary hyperaldosteronism (high aldosterone, high renin), with or without hypertension, may occur with renal or renovascular disease, cirrhosis, congestive heart failure, renin-secreting tumors, Bartter's syndrome, orthostatic hypotension, diabetes mellitus, or contraceptive steroid therapy.

3. Complications of primary hyperaldosteronism are related to prolonged hypertension and hypokalemia. Hypertension leads to cardiac and renal dysfunction, and hypokalemia increases the risk of developing cardiac arrhythmias, especially in patients taking digitalis.

4. Treatment

a. Medical. Spironolactone is the choice for patients with adrenocortical hyperplasia and in preparation of patients with adrenocortical adenomas for operation. Amelioride, the potassium-sparing medication, is also effective.

b. Surgical. Preparation: The potassium depletion should be corrected by prescribing a low-sodium diet with potassium supplements (8 g potassium chloride daily) and giving spironolactone.

Adrenalectomy is usually performed for adrenocortical adenomas through a posterior incision. Hyperplasia is usually treated medically but occasionally patients with adenomatous hyperplasia are treated by unilateral adrenalectomy.

Postoperative care: Glucocorticoids are rarely required if only 1 gland is removed. Transient postoperative aldosterone deficiency is treated by saline IV initially, then liberal sodium intake orally. Fludrocortisone (50-100 µg/day orally) may be needed for about 1 month.

5. Prognosis. The response to removal of an adenoma is excellent, although blood pressure may not fall for weeks or months. Surgical treatment of hyperplasia is less successful, and some degree of hypertension usually remains. Overall, about 70% of patients with primary hyperaldosteronism become normotensive and normokalemic, and the hypertension is improved in others after operation.

C. HYPERADRENOCORTICISM. Increased secretion of cortisol may be classified as Cushing's disease or syndrome. **Cushing's disease** signifies pituitary hypothalamic-dependent ACTH excess, which causes bilateral adrenocortical hyperplasia. **Cushing's syndrome** refers to hypercortisolism of any origin (administration of exogenous corticosteroids, steroid-producing adrenal adenoma or cancer, adrenal rest tumor of the gonads, or tumors of nonendocrine or endocrine tissues which elaborate on ACTH-like polypeptide).

In patients with primary cortisol-secreting adrenal tumors, hypothalamic CRF and pituitary ACTH are suppressed, and the uninvolved adrenal is atrophic. In patients with adrenal rest tumors, both adrenals and ACTH production are suppressed, whereas patients with ectopic or pituitary ACTH-producing neoplasms have bilateral adrenal hyperplasia.

Cushing's syndrome is three times more common in women than in men, and it occurs most often in patients between 20 and 40 years of age. Most cases of hyperadrenocorticism are due to administration of exogenous corticosteroids. Of the remaining cases, about 70% are due to hypothalamic or pituitary disorders, 10% are caused by ectopic ACTH-producing tumors, and 20% are due to adrenal neoplasms. Approximately 75% of the adrenal tumors are benign; malignant tumors are more common in children. About 98% of tumors are unilateral.

1. Diagnosis and differential diagnosis

a. Symptoms and signs. Gradual or fulminant onset. Change in menstrual cycle, often progressing to amenorrhea. Virilization (hirsutism, balding) in women if androgens are among the hormones secreted excessively. Weight gain, lassitude, muscular weakness, psychiatric disturbance, polyuria, hypertension, easy bruisability, edema, "buffalo hump," purple striae. Pituitary tumors and ectopic ACTH-secreting tumors usually also secrete melanotropins (MSH), which increase skin pigmentation, obesity, and growth retardation in children. The rapid onset of hypercortisolism with hypokalemic alkalosis, hypertension, and edema suggests an ectopic ACTH-producing tumor.

   b. Laboratory tests. These tests are performed sequentially to confirm the diagnosis of Cushing's syndrome and to identify the cause.
   (1) *Plasma cortisol levels* are normally highest upon awakening (5-30 μg/dl at 8 AM) and at lowest (<10 μg/dl) at bedtime. This circadian rhythm is lost in Cushing's disease.
   (2) *Low-dose dexamethasone suppression test:* 1 mg of dexamethasone is given at 11 PM, and plasma cortisol is measured at 8 AM the next day. If the cortisol is not suppressed (<5 μg/dl), the next test is required.
   (3) *Urinary free cortisol excretion* (normal: 80-400 μg/day) is elevated in virtually all patients with Cushing's syndrome. If this value is high in a patient whose plasma cortisol did not suppress in test (2), the diagnosis of Cushing's syndrome is confirmed.
   (4) Cause of Cushing's syndrome is sought by plasma *ACTH assay* and the *high-dose dexamethasone suppression test* (dexamethasone 8 mg orally over 24 hours, then urinary 17-hydroxycorticosteroids [17-OHCS] are measured for 24 hours). (a) High ACTH, no 17-OHCS suppression: ectopic source of ACTH. (b) Low ACTH, no 17-OHCS suppression: adrenal tumor. (c) Normal to high ACTH, 17-OHCS suppression: Cushing's **disease.**
   (5) *Metapyrone test* is sometimes helpful. Metapyrone blocks conversion of 11-deoxycortisol compounds to cortisol; normal subjects and some with Cushing's disease respond by producing more ACTH, which is reflected in increased urinary excretion of 17-OHCS. Patients with adrenal neoplasms or ectopic ACTH syndrome do not show this response.

   c. Other tests. CT scan, NP 59 iodocholesterol scan, and occasionally angiography are used to localize adrenal tumors. MRI scans and selective catheterization of the petrosal veins for ACTH bilaterally may identify a pituitary tumor.

   2. Complications of the hormone excess are those of diabetes mellitus, hypertension, and severe weakness.

   3. Treatment
   a. Medical therapy with metapyrone, aminoglutethimide, or o,p'DDD (a derivative of DDT) controls Cushing's

syndrome in a few patients, but side-effects and escape from control are common. o,p′DDD is useful for treatment of unresectable adrenocortical carcinoma.

b. Cushing's disease can be treated by *radiation* to the pituitary; a clinical response may take 18 months, however, and recurrences are frequent. *Transsphenoidal hypophysectomy* with resection of the adenoma is the preferred method of treatment.

c. Adrenalectomy is the treatment of choice for Cushing's syndrome and for some patients with recurrent Cushing's disease or ACTH-secreting nonpituitary tumors.

Preparation: Electrolyte disorders (especially hypokalemia) must be corrected and diabetes mellitus should be controlled. Exogenous corticosteroids must be provided postoperatively (see below).

Operation: Unilateral adrenalectomy is performed for adenoma or carcinoma; total adrenalectomy is recommended for bilateral hyperplasia. A posterior approach is recommended if the tumor is <4 cm in diameter.

Postoperative care: Cortisol hemisuccinate is given IV initially (100 mg every 8 hours). After total adrenalectomy, permanent replacement therapy is necessary (cortisol 30 mg daily orally, 20 mg in morning and 10 g in afternoon); fludrocortisone 0.1 mg/day orally provides mineralocorticoid. After unilateral adrenalectomy, the dose of cortisol is tapered to physiologic levels (30 mg/day orally) and further reduced gradually over several months; alternate-day treatment minimizes inhibition of endogenous ACTH.

Postoperative complications may develop in patients with Cushing's syndrome: wound infection, wound dehiscence, bleeding, peptic ulcer, and pulmonary problems.

4. Prognosis. Nelson's syndrome occurs in 15% of patients after total bilateral adrenalectomy; it is due to excessive pituitary secretion of ACTH. Hyperpigmentation, headaches, exophthalmos, and an enlarged sella turcica (occasionally leading to blindness) secondary to a pituitary tumor are present. It may be prevented by irradiation of the pituitary before adrenalectomy.

Hypoadrenocorticism and panhypopituitarism are chronic complications of total adrenalectomy or pituitary ablation, respectively. The prognosis of adrenocortical carcinoma is poor, but for benign lesions is excellent.

D. VIRILIZING AND FEMINIZING CONDITIONS
1. Virilizing conditions

a. Congenital adrenal hyperplasia (adrenogenital syndrome) is due to deficient steroidogenesis; as a result of abnormally low cortisol production, ACTH is increased, and the adrenals are stimulated to secrete androgens. If this occurs during fetal development, female infants have ambiguous genitalia (pseudohermaphroditism) and males have macrogenitosomia. The condition may become apparent during childhood or adult life as well. Treatment consists of replacement with glucocorticoids and mineralocorticoids.

b. Cushing's syndrome may include virilizing manifestations if androgens are secreted excessively.

c. Enzymatic blockers (metapyrone, o,p'DDD) may cause virilization.

d. Androgen-secreting tumors. The adrenal cortex ordinarily secretes the 17-KS, androstenedione and estrone, and only small amounts of androgens and estrogens; the gonads primarily secrete the 17-OHCS, testosterone, and estradiol. Thus, high 17-KS levels in a masculinized female generally suggests an adrenal source, and elevated 17-OHCS with normal or only slightly increased urinary 17-KS suggest gonadal origin.

2. Feminizing tumors of the adrenal are rare. They produce tender gynecomastia and testicular atrophy in the male, and sexual precocity (breast development, uterine bleeding, pubic and axillary hair, and advanced bone age) in prepubital females. 90% are due to adrenocortical carcinomas.

E. PHEOCHROMOCYTOMA are rare catecholamine-producing tumors that arise from chromaffin cells in the adrenal medulla or elsewhere in the sympathetic nervous system in the abdomen, thorax, pelvis, neck, or urinary bladder. They are characterized by excessive production, storage, and release of epinephrine and norepinephrine. These tumors account for 0.1%-0.2% of all patients with hypertension. 10% of pheochromocytomas are malignant, 10% are bilateral, and 90% occur in the adrenal or periadrenal area.

1. Diagnosis
a. Symptoms and signs depend upon the amount and type of catecholamines secreted. (1) Sustained or paroxysmal hypertension. (2) Development of hypertension during anesthetic induction or operative procedures. (3) Paradoxical increases in blood pressure when treated with catecholamine-

releasing antihypertensive agents (e.g., guanethidine, methyldopa). (4) Excessive perspiration, pallor, flushing, palpitations, chest pain, trembling, weakness, anxiety, nausea; fever of unknown origin occasionally. (5) Patients with neurocutaneous syndromes (café-au-lait spots, neurofibromatosis, Von Hippel-Lindau's disease, Sturge-Weber disease, tuberous sclerosis, Sipple's syndrome) have an increased incidence of pheochromocytoma. Sipple's syndrome, or MEA II, includes medullary carcinoma of the thyroid, hyperparathyroidism, neurofibromatosis, and ganglioneuromatosis.

b. Laboratory tests

(1) Test urine for metabolites of catecholamines—e.g., VMA, normetanephrine, and metanephrine. One or more of these screening tests is positive in >90% of patients. Spurious elevations of VMA occur with coffee, tea, chocolate, vanilla extract, and bananas. Drugs such as glycerol guaiacolate, chlorpromazine, and nalidixic acid also increase urinary VMA. Normetanephrine and metanephrine are falsely increased by methyldopa (Aldomet).

(2) If the screening test is positive, measure urinary free epinephrine and norepinephrine. These values may be falsely elevated by methyldopa, sympathomimetic nasal sprays, quinidine, vitamin preparations, tetracyclines and other fluorescent compounds, and acute stress.

(3) Blood and urine glucose levels are often elevated.

(4) Provocative tests are potentially dangerous and rarely necessary. If other tests are equivocal, the glucagon test is the safest method of stimulation, and phentolamine (Regitine) is the best method of suppression.

c. Radiographs.

CT or MRI scans are best for localizing pheochromocytomas situated in the adrenal glands and MIBG scanning is best for localizing extraadrenal pheochromocytomas. MIBG scanning has also been used as a screening test of patients at high risk of developing medullary adrenal hyperplasia or recurrent pheochromocytoma.

2. Differential diagnosis includes all causes of hypertension, hyperthyroidism, carcinoid syndrome, and intracranial lesions causing psychologic disturbances.

When epinephrine constitutes 20% or more of the total catecholamine secretion, the tumor is either in the adrenal medulla or the organ of Zucherkandl; norepinephrine-secreting tumors may be found in the adrenal or in other sites anywhere from neck to pelvis. Malignant chromaffin tumors are more likely to produce catecholamine precursors than are benign pheochromocytomas.

3. Complications include the consequences of hypertension. Pheochromocytomas occasionally bleed or infarct, resulting in hypotension or death.

4. Treatment

a. Preparation with pharmacologic agents and by restoration of blood volume is essential. (1) The α-adrenergic blocking agent phenoxybenzamine (Dibenzyline) should be given in doses of 10-80 mg every 12 hours, for at least 10-12 days and longer if cardiomyopathy is suspected. Phentolamine (Regitine) is a shorter-acting α-blocker, but Dibenzyline is generally preferred because of its longer duration of action, better hypertensive control, and fewer side-effects. (2) Propranolol, a beta blocker, is used only for the treatment of arrhythmias and should never be given before Dibenzyline, as it may precipitate a hypertensive crisis.

b. Operation. (1) Careful intraoperative monitoring (central venous pressure, arterial pressure, ECG) is vital. (2) The patient should be well-anesthetized and thoroughly α-blocked. Nitroprusside (3 μg/kg/min) or IV phentolamine (10 mg in 1 dl saline) is used to treat intraoperative hypertension. (3) An anterior abdominal approach is recommended because tumors may be multiple or ectopic, although if all localization tests suggest a unilateral tumor, a posterior or lateral approach is acceptable in patients at low risk for multiple tumors. Before the adrenal is excised, blood volume should be carefully replaced to avoid hypotension once the source of excessive catecholamines is removed.

5. Prognosis. If all tumor has been successfully removed, urinary catecholamines should return to normal in 1 week. Periodic evaluation thereafter is recommended, especially in young patients and in those with familial syndromes, because additional pheochromocytomas may develop. In patients with malignant disease, chronic administration of phenoxybenzamine and propranolol is helpful.

7

Head and Neck

Thomas A. Tami

I. TRAUMA TO THE NECK*

A. PENETRATING TRAUMA. All penetrating wounds of the neck are potentially serious because of the large number of vital structures in this relatively small space.

1. Diagnosis

a. Symptoms and signs depend on the structures that are injured: **Larynx and trachea**— hoarseness, dyspnea, stridor, subcutaneous emphysema. **Blood vessels**—hematoma, external bleeding, shock. Neurologic deficit may result from injury to the carotid artery. **Pharynx and esophagus**— no symptoms initially; later dysphagia, hematemesis, and infection in the neck or mediastinum. **Cervical spine and spinal cord**— see Chapters 17 and 18. **Nerves** – Mirror examination of the larynx (Figure 7-1) shows recurrent laryngeal nerve injury. Cranial nerves, phrenic nerves, and the cervical and brachial plexuses may be injured. **Salivary glands**—leakage of saliva. Associated head and thoracic injuries must be sought in all penetrating wounds of the neck.

b. Radiographs of the soft tissues and the cervical spine are essential. **Arteriography** is required for suspected vascular injuries at the base of the neck or above the angle of the jaw. Esophagram is useful for detection of pharyngeal and esophageal injury. CT scan is especially good in laryngeal injuries.

2. Treatment

a. General measures. An **airway** must be established by oropharyngeal, nasopharyngeal, or orotracheal intubation (see Chapter 3). Tracheostomy (Figure 7-2) should **not** be attempted by inexperienced physicians in emergencies; **crico-**

---

*Injuries to the cervical spine and spinal cord are covered in Chapters 17 and 18. Injuries to the scalp, face, and maxillofacial bones are discussed in Chapter 15. Injuries to the head are covered in Chapter 17.

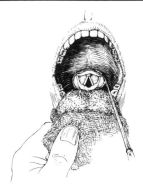

FIGURE 7-1. Indirect mirror examination of the larynx and adjacent structures.

thyrotomy (placement of a tube through the cricothyroid membrane) is more rapid and safer in desperate situations.

Do not attempt to pass a nasogastric tube in the emergency room because coughing and gagging cause further bleeding. Treat shock (see Chapter 1).

b. Surgical exploration of the neck, in the operating room and under general anesthesia, is usually required if the platysma has been penetrated. In some centers, operation is not performed in the absence of a hematoma, bruit, airway obstruction, or radiographic evidence of vascular esophageal injury. The management of these injuries depends upon the zone of the neck involved (Fig. 7-3). Zone II injuries can be safely observed if there are no major indications for exploration, as noted above. On the other hand, injuries in zone I or III mandate immediate arteriography (either carotid arteriography or a formal aortic arch study). A generous oblique incision along the anterior border of the sternocleidomastoid muscle gives good exposure and can be extended if necessary.

Laryngeal and **tracheal** injuries are sutured; laryngeal stenting is not usually recommended, but a tracheotomy for airway control is usually necessary. Major **arterial** injuries may require sternotomy to gain proximal control. Management is discussed in Chapter 11.

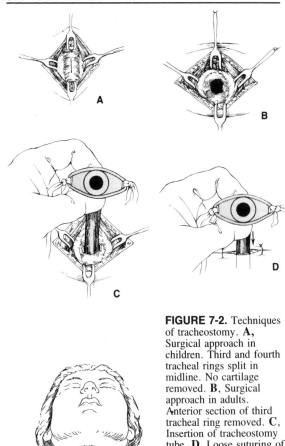

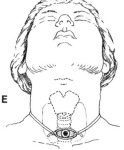

FIGURE 7-2. Techniques of tracheostomy. **A,** Surgical approach in children. Third and fourth tracheal rings split in midline. No cartilage removed. **B,** Surgical approach in adults. Anterior section of third tracheal ring removed. **C,** Insertion of tracheostomy tube. **D,** Loose suturing of both ends of wound. **E,** Tube tied in place. **Note:** Use endotracheal intubation or cricothyrotomy in emergencies.

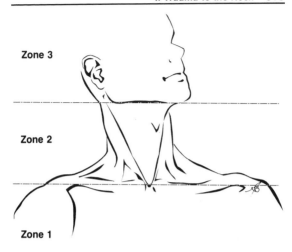

FIGURE 7-3. The three surgical zones of the neck are shown above. The nature of the diagnostic evaluation and planned surgical intervention varies among these zones.

Injuries to the internal jugular or other **veins** are treated by ligation. Keep the patient's head lowered to avoid **air embolism** until the vein is controlled.

Esophageal perforations and hypopharyngeal injuries are repaired with absorbable suture, and external drainage of the sutured area is provided. Systemic antibiotics are required. Parenteral or tube feeding for 7-10 days is advisable.

Nerve injuries are repaired if possible. The great auricular nerve provides a suitable graft to bridge extensively damaged motor nerves.

Salivary gland injuries are debrided and closed. Major ducts can be repaired with fine silk sutures over a small Silastic catheter. Associated injury of the facial nerve in the parotid gland should be identified and repaired. A postoperative salivary fistula usually resolves with the use of a pressure dressing and local wound care, but this may occasionally require surgical excision of the involved gland.

3. Prognosis. The mortality rate depends on the extent of damage and the structures injured. The overall mortality rate is about 5%.

B. BLUNT TRAUMA to the neck may involve any of the structures discussed above, but vertebral and spinal injuries (Chapters 17 and 18) and fracture of the larynx are especially frequent.

C. FRACTURE OF THE LARYNX. The thyroid cartilage is usually fractured; in severe cases, the cricoid cartilage, hyoid bone, and tracheal rings can be fractured and the arytenoid cartilages dislocated.

1. Diagnosis

a. Symptoms and signs. Pain, swelling, hoarseness, hemoptysis, airway obstruction (dyspnea, stridor), ecchymosis, loss of palpable laryngeal landmarks, and subcutaneous emphysema. Direct laryngoscopy (Figure 7-4) or mirror laryngoscopy reveals mucosal lacerations and blood in the larynx.

b. Radiographic findings. Fracture of the larynx is diagnosed on clinical grounds but radiographs may show dislocation of laryngeal structures, narrowing of the airway, and edema and emphysema of the soft tissues. High-resolution CT scanning is essential for confirming the diagnosis.

2. Treatment. Maintain the **airway.** Orotracheal intubation may be impossible and tracheotomy may be life-saving. Operative treatment is preceded by CT, followed by direct laryngoscopy to fully assess the injury. Open laryngotomy is performed, mucosal lacerations are sutured, and the laryngeal fractures are reduced and fixed with nonabsorbable sutures, wires, or microplates. Although the use of various airway stents is controversial, they are generally avoided.

3. Prognosis. Laryngeal stenosis and voice disturbances can result if fractures are not recognized and repaired.

II. EPISTAXIS (NASAL BLEEDING)

Epistaxis can result from erosion of a superficial blood vessel of **Kiesselbach's plexus** in the mucosa overlying the cartilaginous nasal septum **(anterior epistaxis)** or can be caused by disruption of blood vessels in the posterior nasal vault, usually a terminal branch of the internal maxillary artery **(posterior epistaxis)**. Trauma (external or digital) and inflammation (infection or allergy) are common causes. Other

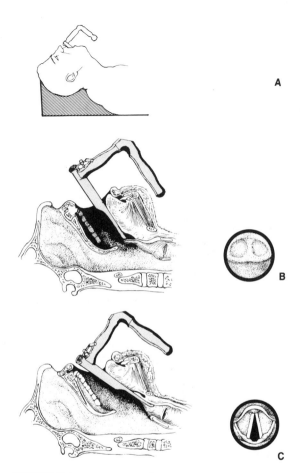

FIGURE 7-4. Laryngoscopy. **A,** Position of patient for direct laryngoscopy. **B,** Standard distal lighting laryngoscope being introduced. Tip of laryngoscope in vallecula. *At right,* interior surface of epiglottis and vallecula as seen with the laryngoscope in the position shown at left. **C,** Tip of laryngoscope within larynx. *At right,* direct view within larynx as seen with tip of laryngoscope in the position at left.

diseases associated with epistaxis include nasal or sinus neoplasms, acute infectious diseases of childhood, hypertension, arteriosclerosis, and coagulation defects. Owing to the varying presentations and treatments of these two entities, they are considered separately.

A. ANTERIOR EPISTAXIS

1. Diagnosis. Anterior epistaxis is most common in young patients. The bleeding site is almost invariably at the anterior end of the cartilaginous nasal septum, an area that is readily accessible for control of bleeding. A history of trauma, either external or digital, can often be obtained. Physical examination usually reveals the bleeding site in this region, allowing relatively easy access. Typically, compression of the external nose with the fingers results in temporary control, whereas this is usually not the case in the more serious posterior epistaxis. Nasal septal deviation can often be a contributing factor by producing turbulent airflow and mucosal drying of the nasal septum.

2. Treatment. The patient should sit upright and lean forward to avoid swallowing or aspirating blood. In most cases, the bleeding site can be readily identified and cauterized. Topical 4% cocaine or a lidocaine/Neo-Synephrine mixture is helpful in obtaining anesthesia and vasoconstriction prior to applying silver nitrate, electrocautery, or some other hemostatic technic. A head light or head mirror is invaluable in this situation to facilitate the use of both hands in the treatment process. Suction is also very important to clear blood clots and to allow easy identification of the bleeding site. Occasionally, local hemostatic measures are inadequate and nasal packing is required. In these instances, an anterior pack using up to 6 feet of ½-inch petrolatum-coated gauze is necessary. This technic, if performed properly, is usually quite effective in controlling bleeding. Anterior packing can usually be safely removed in 24 to 72 hours.

B. POSTERIOR EPISTAXIS

1. Diagnosis. Unlike anterior epistaxis, posterior epistaxis usually affects an older population. The bleeding site is in the posterior nasal cavity, usually the lateral nasal wall. The bleeding is usually brisk, and the precise bleeding site is usually not identifiable. Attempts at nasal compression do not result in cessation of the epistaxis, but rather cause the blood to flow down the nasopharynx into the mouth or around the posterior choana and into the opposite nasal passage. Systemic manifestations of severe blood loss such as hypotension and shock may be present.

2. Treatment. The patient should sit upright and lean forward to minimize aspiration and swallowing of blood. Good illumination (head mirror or headlight) and suction are imperative. A posterior pack usually is required for bleeding from the nasopharynx or the posterior choana.

The traditional posterior nasal pack is the **gauze three-string pack.** Three strings (braided O silk) are sewn through the center of a rolled 4 × 4-inch gauze sponge. The nose and nasopharynx are anesthetized as for anterior epistaxis. A soft red rubber catheter is inserted through the nostril, and the tip is withdrawn through the mouth. Two strings are tied to the oral end of the catheter; the nasal end of the catheter is then pulled, bringing the two strings through the mouth and nasopharynx and out the nose. The gauze is then manipulated into the nasopharynx, taking care not to roll the uvula up into the nasopharynx. The third string is cut short at the level of the incisor teeth and allowed to dangle in the pharynx. It is used for later removal of the pack. The anterior nasal cavity is then packed as described for anterior epistaxis. The two nasal strings are tied over a bolster at the anterior nares.

A 12 or 14 Fr **Foley catheter** with a 30-cc balloon is also an effective device that can be used in place of this traditional pack. The catheter is inserted into the nose, the tip is positioned in the nasopharynx, and the balloon is inflated with water until the soft palate bulges slightly. Anterior traction on the catheter provides compression at the posterior choana as well as a "backstop" for anterior packing. The catheter is then secured with an umbilical clamp over a bolster at the anterior nares.

Commercially available balloon catheters are now available to treat epistaxis. These packs are equipped with both an anterior and a posterior balloon. The catheter is advanced along the floor of the nose until the posterior balloon is well into the nasopharynx. After the posterior balloon is inflated with water or saline, it is pulled anteriorly until it becomes firmly impacted into the posterior nasal choana. At this point, the anterior balloon is inflated, creating a tight seal of the nasal cavity. These devices are usually effective for short-term control of nasal bleeding.

With any pack, the patient must be followed closely to detect potential complications of nasal packs, including recurrent bleeding, otitis media, pressure necrosis of the skin of the anterior nares, sinusitis, or toxic shock syndrome. Patients with posterior nasal packs require hospitalization and close monitoring. Pulse oximetry is vital to detect O_2 desaturation, which can accompany the placement of these packs. Persistent or recurrent bleeding may require replacement of the pack under general anesthesia. Arterial ligation or arteriographic embolization is necessary in some cases of persistent bleeding.

III. INFECTIONS

A. ACUTE EXTERNAL OTITIS is a diffuse infection of the skin of the external ear canal. It often is a secondary infection of eczematoid or seborrheic dermatitis aggravated by scratching. Foreign bodies (cotton swabs, water) causing local trauma are common causes. Gram-positive and gram-negative bacteria and, infrequently, fungi may be cultured.

1. Diagnosis. Itching, pain, and discharge are the usual symptoms. There is pain with motion of the pinna. Erythema and edema of the skin of the canal are seen; occasionally the canal is occluded completely, producing hearing loss. Fever and regional lymphadenopathy indicate more severe infection.

2. Differential diagnosis. Myringitis bullosa is identified by typical blebs. Acute otitis media is usually associated with a normal external auditory canal; in cases of acute otitis media with perforation, however, it may be difficult to distinguish the 2 conditions if edema obscures the tympanic membrane.

3. Treatment. The canal should be cleansed with suction or fine cotton applicators, and cotton wicks medicated with topical antibiotic-steroid combinations (e.g., neomycin-polymyxin, bacitracin-hydrocortisone) or Burow's solution (aluminum acetate) should be inserted for 24 hours. Systemic antibiotics (penicillin, cephalosporin, erythromycin) may be required for severe infections. Analgesics often are necessary. *"Malignant" external otitis* is a term used to describe osteomyelitis of the temporal bone and skull base usually occurring in elderly diabetics. This life-threatening condition is usually due to *Pseudomonas aeruginosa* and requires intensive treatment with high-dose IV antibiotic therapy.

4. Prognosis. External otitis may be refractory to treatment and recurrences are frequent. Malignant external otitis is often fatal.

B. ACUTE SUPPURATIVE OTITIS MEDIA. Acute infection of the middle ear is most common in children, often in association with upper respiratory infections. *Streptococcus pneumoniae, Moraxella catarrhalis,* and *Haemophilus influenzae* are the most common offending organisms.

1. Diagnosis. Pain, fever, hearing loss, and a full feeling in the ear are the usual symptoms. Purulent discharge indicates spontaneous perforation. The tympanic membrane at first is hyperemic and retracted; later it is red, dull, swollen, and bulging, as evidenced by loss of visible landmarks. Leukocytosis is common.

2. Differential diagnosis. External otitis (see above). Pain in the ear (reflex otalgia) may be associated with pharyngitis, laryngitis, dental disease, subacute thyroiditis, tumors of the pharynx, larynx, and hypopharynx, or temporomandibular joint disease; there are no acute inflammatory changes in the ear canal or tympanic membrane in these conditions.

3. Complications include perforation of the tympanic membrane, acute mastoiditis, labyrinthitis, meningitis, and facial nerve paralysis.

4. Treatment. Systemic antibiotics (oral penicillin, cephalosporin, or trimethoprim/sulfamethoxazole in adults, and ampicillin or amoxicillin in children) must be given for 10 days; topical antibiotics may be effective in cases of perforation. Analgesics and nasal decongestants are also often helpful. Myringotomy is indicated if the infection does not resolve promptly or if middle ear culture is required, such as for immunocompromised hosts. Myringotomy is most safely accomplished in the anterior portion of the tympanic membrane.

Frequent recurrent episodes of acute otitis media may require insertion of ventilating tubes, tonsillectomy and adenoidectomy, or adenoidectomy alone. Antibiotic prophylaxis is also often used to prevent multiple recurrent infections.

5. Prognosis. With rare exceptions, acute otitis media resolves if treatment is begun promptly. After the acute infection clears, fluid may persist in the middle ear for up to several weeks; follow-up examination is necessary to prevent chronic hearing loss.

C. SEROUS OTITIS MEDIA. Serous fluid in the middle ear causes a full feeling in the ear and conductive hearing loss. The middle ear is completely filled with fluid or a fluid level is seen behind the tympanic membrane. Antibiotics and decongestants usually resolve the problem, but refractory cases require tonsillectomy, adenoidectomy, myringotomy, and placement of drainage tubes.

Evaluation and treatment of nasal allergy are also often effective. Adults who present with unilateral serous otitis media must be carefully examined to exclude the possibility of a tumor in the nasopharynx causing Eustachian tube obstruction.

D. ACUTE MASTOIDITIS is a complication of acute otitis media associated with necrosis of the bony cellular structures of the mastoid, usually in the second or third week of the infection. Headache, fever, mastoid tenderness, and postauricular swelling are indications of mastoiditis. CT scanning reveals opacification of the mastoid air cells and destruction of bony trabeculae leading to coalescent abscesses. Culture should be obtained from spontaneous drainage or via myringotomy.

Treatment must be started to prevent serious complications of labyrinthitis, meningitis, intracranial abscess, lateral sinus thrombosis, or facial nerve paralysis. Myringotomy is essential if spontaneous perforation and drainage have not occurred. IV antibiotic therapy should be started while awaiting culture results. Early cases may resolve completely. Simple mastoidectomy is required for bony involvement or persistence of drainage.

E. ACUTE SINUSITIS. Pyogenic infection of any of the paranasal sinuses (frontal, ethmoid, sphenoid, maxillary) usually follows an upper respiratory infection, a dental infection, or nasal allergies.

1. Diagnosis. Local pain, tenderness, swelling over the involved sinus, nasal congestion, and purulent nasal discharge are common manifestations. Pain is usually greater during the day. Frontal sinus infection causes pain and swelling in the medial roof of the orbit. The pain of ethmoid sinusitis is medial to and behind the eye and is aggravated by eye motion.

Sphenoid sinusitis typically presents as pain localized to the vertex of the skull. Maxillary sinusitis causes infraorbital or tooth pain. Fever and systemic symptoms vary with the severity of the infection. Leukocytosis is common, and culture typically reveals *Streptococcus pneumoniae, Moraxella catarrhalis,* or *Haemophilus influenzae* as the infecting organism. Plain sinus radiographs are effective in diagnosing frontal and maxillary sinusitis, but the ethmoids and sphenoid are poorly visualized. Direct coronal CT is superior to plain sinus radiography for evaluating all of the paranasal sinuses.

2. Differential diagnosis. Acute dental infection causes tender swelling lower in the cheek and greater tenderness to percussion of the involved tooth than does maxillary sinusitis.

Migraine or other headache syndromes can often be confused with sinusitis.

3. Complications. Chronic sinusitis is the most common complication and is often due to inadequate treatment of the acute condition. Frontal and ethmoid sinusitis can lead to intracranial infection (meningitis and abscesses), osteomyelitis of the frontal bone, orbital cellulitis, and orbital abscess. Sphenoid sinusitis is commonly associated with meningitis. All acute sinus infections can lead to cavernous sinus thrombosis.

4. Treatment

a. Medical treatment is sufficient for most patients. Systemic antibiotics, oral decongestants and 0.25%-0.5% phenylephrine are given for 3 weeks, and local heat usually gives prompt relief of pain. Mild infections can be managed on an outpatient basis. More severe infections (especially frontal and ethmoid) or those associated with complications require hospitalization and large doses of parenteral antibiotics.

b. Surgical treatment of persistent infection or complications is often necessary when medical therapy has failed to arrest or reverse the infectious process. Irrigation of the maxillary sinus through either the inferior meatus or the canine fossa, incision and drainage of an orbital abscess, trephine of a frontal sinus, and definitive sinusotomy are among the surgical procedures used in some cases.

F. CHRONIC SINUSITIS often produces few symptoms other than postnasal drainage, a nonproductive cough, and nasal and sinus pressure and congestion. Nasal obstruction and purulent rhinorrhea may also occur. Occasionally, an intracranial complication may be the presenting symptom. CT scanning of the paranasal sinuses is invaluable in establishing the diagnosis.

Systemic antibiotic treatment, based on culture and antibiotic sensitivity tests if possible, followed by drainage procedures such as maxillary sinus irrigations, may occasionally clear a chronic infection. In contradistinction to acute sinusitis, *Staphylococcus aureus* and anaerobic bacteria play a larger and more important role in the pathogenesis of chronic sinusitis. Endoscopic surgical procedures to improve drainage and aeration of the affected sinus may often be effective in managing this condition; however, when they are ineffective, external surgical procedures should be considered.

G. ACUTE PURULENT SIALADENITIS is an infection of the major salivary glands and ducts by pyogenic bacteria. It usually follows obstruction of the duct by stricture, calculi, or mucous plugs; the submaxillary glands are especially prone to infection from these causes. Decreased production of saliva in debilitated dehydrated patients can also result in acute sialadenitis, particularly of the parotid glands.

1. Diagnosis. Unilateral pain, swelling, tenderness, fever, and sometimes septicemia are symptoms of this disease. Pus may be expressed from the duct orifice by pressure on the gland. There is leukocytosis and radiographs may reveal calculi. Mumps, cervical adenitis, and infection of cervical fascial spaces must be differentiated.

2. Complications include extension of infection into the deep fascial spaces of the neck.

3. Treatment in the early stages (before abscess formation) is with antibiotics, hydration, local heat, and sialogogues such as lemon drops to increase the flow of saliva. Antibacterial coverage should include *Staphylococcus aureus* and oral flora. Antibiotic sensitivity tests from cultures of the salivary secretion may alter later treatment. If resolution does not occur in 4-6 days, abscess formation may require external incision and drainage. Recurrent episodes of acute sialadenitis can be an indication for surgical removal of the involved gland.

4. Prognosis is generally good, but in the severely debilitated elderly patient a very poor prognosis can be expected if treatment is not vigorously instituted.

H. CHRONIC SIALADENITIS. Recurrent infections by pyogenic bacteria cause repeated swelling, destruction, and scarring of ducts and acini with resultant ductal dilation. The patient complains of recurrent pain and swelling, especially with meals, but has no systemic symptoms. The gland is enlarged and tender, and the secretions are tenacious or purulent. Radiographs may show calculi, and sialography (injection of contrast medium through the duct orifice) often reveals strictures and dilation of the duct.

Dilation of the ducts, antibiotics for acute episodes, intraoral extraction of calculi, meatotomy, and hydration may relieve symptoms. Total excision of the involved gland is indicated if prolonged medial therapy is ineffective.

I. SIALOLITHIASIS. Salivary calculi occur most frequently in the submaxillary gland and duct (Wharton's duct). About 75% are radiopaque.

Obstruction of duct by calculi frequently causes swelling of the involved gland with eating. Infections can occur. Glandular enlargement with a stone in the duct is diagnostic. Stones may be palpated or demonstrated by radiography.

Complications of calculi include acute and chronic secondary infection.

Slitting the orifice or excision of the papilla often permits complete removal of small stones near the duct orifice. Larger stones in the terminal third of Stensen's duct and terminal two thirds of Wharton's duct may be removed intraorally by incising through buccal mucosa into the duct; there is no need to repair the duct. Symptomatic stones in the proximal third of Wharton's duct or in the submaxillary gland should be removed by total external excision of the submaxillary gland.

J. PERITONSILLAR ABSCESS is a complication of acute tonsillitis that occurs when infection extends into the fascial space between the tonsillar capsule and the pharyngeal constrictor muscles. Culture usually shows streptococci, staphylococci, or a mixture of anaerobic flora.

1. Diagnosis
a. Symptoms. Sudden unilateral increase in pain, progressive dysphagia, and trismus a few days after the onset of ordinary tonsillitis.

b. Signs. Asymmetric swelling of the pharynx and tonsils with fullness of the anterior pillar and soft palate on the affected side and deviation of the uvula to the opposite side. There is often cervical adenitis.

2. Differential diagnosis includes tonsillar abscess or
neoplasm, retropharyngeal abscess, and deep neck abscess (parapharyngeal abscess). If typical signs of peritonsillar abscess are accompanied by swelling at the angle of the jaw with obliteration of this bony landmark, then parapharyngeal abscess must be strongly suspected and ruled out.

3. Treatment. Attention to nutrition and hydration, oral
or parenteral antibiotics, analgesics, and warm saline throat irrigations can occasionally produce resolution if started within the first 1-2 days of the infection. When an abscess forms, intraoral incision and drainage or needle aspiration is required. This is done with the patient sitting and leaning forward; minimal topical anesthesia should be used, and care should be taken to avoid both injury to the deeper vascular structures and aspiration. Peritonsillar abscess can be an indication for tonsillectomy if recurrent or if associated with recurrent tonsillitis.

K. RETROPHARYNGEAL ABSCESS occurs in the fascial space between the posterior pharyngeal wall and the prevertebral fascia and usually results from suppurative lymphadenitis.

Because the retropharyngeal lymph nodes are prominent in infants and children, this disease is more common in children than in adults.

1. Diagnosis. Symptoms include fever, pain, dysphagia, and, at times, difficulty breathing. Examination reveals cervical adenitis with swelling and even fluctuance of the posterior pharyngeal wall. Torticollis can occasionally be a prominent feature. A lateral soft-tissue radiograph of the neck shows widening of the retropharyngeal space.

2. Differential diagnosis. Tuberculous involvement of the cervical spine, trauma, foreign body, tonsillitis, adenoiditis, and peritonsillar abscess.

3. Complications. Airway obstruction, spread of infection to other fascial spaces of the neck, erosion of blood vessels, and aspiration of abscess content.

4. Treatment. Intravenous antibiotics in conjunction with drainage (either intraoral or extraoral) are imperative. The induction of anesthesia is best accomplished in the Trendelenburg position to avoid potential aspiration. The surgeon must always be prepared to do a tracheotomy if necessary.

L. PARAPHARYNGEAL ABSCESS is an infection of the potential space bounded by the pharyngeal constrictor muscles medially and the superficial layer of the deep cervical fascia laterally. This space contains the carotid sheath and extends from the base of the skull to the superior mediastinum. The source of infection is usually tonsillitis, peritonsillitis, or dental abscess.

1. Diagnosis. Pain, fever, dysphagia, and trismus with diffuse swelling in the neck are the usual symptoms. The lateral wall of the pharynx is swollen, with displacement of the tonsil and lateral wall medially; later there is brawny swelling of the neck behind and below the angle of the jaw. The differential diagnosis includes infection of the neck spaces, cervical adenitis, tuberculous adenitis, tonsillitis, neoplasm, and branchial cysts.

2. Complications can be very severe, including airway obstruction due to edema of the neck and larynx, extension of the infection into the mediastinum, involvement of carotid sheath structures with hemorrhage or septic jugular vein thrombosis, and meningitis or intracranial abscess.

3. Treatment. If an abscess is present, IV antibiotics should be combined with external surgical drainage. In cases of impending airway compromise, preliminary tracheotomy should be considered. External incision and drainage at the angle of the jaw should be done with blunt dissection deep to the deep cervical fascia. The intraoral approach to the lateral pharyngeal space is not advised because of the proximity of vital vascular structures.

4. Prognosis is good when adequate treatment is provided and complications are avoided. When complications occur, the prognosis is often poor.

M. LUDWIG'S ANGINA is a pyogenic infection of the sublingual and submandibular spaces of the floor of the mouth and upper neck.

1. Diagnosis. Patients have pain on moving the tongue and swallowing and swelling of the floor of the mouth and submental area. Motion of the tongue and mandible is limited, and the tongue is elevated to the roof of the mouth, causing airway obstruction at times. Leukocytosis is usually present. CT scanning is helpful in defining abscesses collections; however, the physical findings are usually diagnostic. Radiographs are not helpful unless they show dental infection or salivary calculi. Differential diagnosis includes sialadenitis, dental abscess, and neoplasm of the tongue or floor of mouth.

2. Complications. Rapidly developing airway obstruction requiring emergency tracheostomy.

3. Treatment. High-dose antibiotics, analgesics, and hydration are important, and external incision and drainage may be necessary. The fascial spaces above and below the mylohyoid muscle must be opened by blunt dissection. Airway management must always remain a primary concern.

4. Prognosis is good if airway obstruction is avoided and therapy is instituted in a timely manner.

N. ACUTE CERVICAL LYMPHADENITIS is the most common infection in the neck of children and adults. Usually it is secondary to infection in the scalp, facial skin, ear, or nasal or oral cavity.

1. Diagnosis. The symptoms vary in severity from mild enlargement of the lymph nodes to marked enlargement with pain, tenderness, fever, and symptoms of systemic sepsis. Enlarged tender nodes in the posterior triangle suggest primary infection in the scalp or nasopharynx. Adenitis in the anterior triangle results from infection in the mouth, pharynx, or face. The differential diagnosis includes infected branchial cleft cyst, infectious mononucleosis, salivary gland infection, and neoplasm. CT is a valuable tool for evaluating abscess or necrotic centers within infected nodes.

2. Treatment. Antibiotic therapy is often effective, but incision and drainage are needed if the nodes suppurate. Superficial abscesses may be drained by sharp dissection, but deep abscesses are more safely entered by blunt dissection after the skin and platysma are incised. Needle aspiration is also often an effective technique for managing and diagnosing this condition.

O. TUBERCULOSIS

1. Cervical tuberculous lymphadenitis. Tuberculosis of the cervical lymph nodes may result from tuberculosis of the gums, tonsils, or distant sites (e.g., lungs). Painless swelling is the initial symptom, followed by sinus formation and drainage if left untreated. The upper cervical nodes are often affected first, with the lower nodes becoming invalued later. Multiple matted, firm nodes and draining sinuses can also be noted. Mycobacteria can often be identified if fine-needle aspiration is performed. Even when the organism is not identified initially, evidence of granuloma is often seen, allowing medical therapy to be instituted while culture results are pending. In arrested cases, calcification is seen by radiography. Antituberculous chemotherapy (see Chapter 4) usually results in resolution of this problem; however, in cases of persistent or enlarging masses despite therapy, surgical excision is necessary.

2. Laryngeal tuberculosis is an unusual complication of pulmonary tuberculosis. Hoarseness, pain, and dysphagia are the symptoms. Inflammation usually affects the posterior half of the glottic area, although any part of the larynx and epiglottis can be involved. Differential diagnosis includes carcinoma, syphilis, and other granulomatous diseases. Treatment with antituberculous drugs usually results in rapid resolution of this problem, although the pulmonary tuberculosis is more significant in determining prognosis.

IV. FOREIGN BODIES OF THE NOSE AND EAR*

A. FOREIGN BODIES OF THE NOSE are a common problem that physicians often take too lightly. Although many na-

---

*Foreign bodies of the tracheobronchial tree are covered in Chapter 9.

Small, hard objects are extracted with a small blunt hook or dull ring curette which is carefully passed beyond the foreign body and withdrawn. A suction tip retrieves some objects. Only in the most unusual circumstances is it necessary to surgically enlarge the bony ear canal or approach the canal through a mastoid incision.

4. Prognosis. With care almost all foreign bodies are satisfactorily removed. Middle ear damage is uncommon.

V. TRACHEAL STENOSIS

Tracheal stenosis is most commonly caused by cicatrix at the site of tracheal mucosal ulceration from pressure by the balloon cuff on an endotracheal or tracheostomy tube. It can also occur at the site of tracheostomy if excessive tracheal cartilage is removed. External trauma and complications of surgery for neoplasms or tracheoesophageal fistula can produce stenosis. Partial asymptomatic obstructions can become severe rapidly and cause death if only a small amount of tracheal edema is added to the stenosis.

Dyspnea, stridor, and difficulty clearing secretions develop 10-40 days after extubation. Narrowing of the tracheal air shadow is seen on lateral radiographs of the neck or CT scans. Laryngoscopy and bronchoscopy differentiate tracheal stenosis from other (laryngeal or pharyngeal) causes of obstruction. Pulmonary function studies are consistent with upper airway obstruction. Late onset of dyspnea and stridor may be confused with asthma.

Tracheal stenosis due to endotracheal and tracheostomy tubes is preventable. Tracheal tubes with cuffs designed to minimize pressure necrosis (large volume, low pressure cuffs and others) are available. Pressure in the cuff should be minimized, using just enough to produce a seal or even allow a small leak. The tube should remain in place with the cuff inflated for the least time possible. Tube and cuff should be of nonreactive tissue implantable material.

Thin stenotic webs can be stretched with dilators or excised with a laser. Unfortunately, symptomatic stenosis often does not respond and surgical resection with end-to-end anastomosis is required. If the distal trachea is mobilized and the larynx is released by division of the suprahyoid muscles, as much as 3 cm of trachea can be resected and repaired primarily. Results are generally good.

VI. NEOPLASMS

A. BENIGN NEOPLASMS OF THE ORAL CAVITY

1. Warts, verrucae, and papillomas form folded ridges of epithelium over a scant connective tissue and vascular stalk. They are usually solitary and either sessile or pedunculated, and are excised under local or topical anesthesia.

2. Leukoplakia is a premalignant lesion that is common in heavy smokers. Whitish plaques appear on the oral mucosa; thickened fissured areas are more suspicious of malignancy than thin, soft, smooth patches. Lichen planus often resembles leukoplakia.

Correction of sources of chronic irritation (jagged teeth, ill-fitting dentures, and tobacco) may reverse the leukoplakic process. Small patches may be excised completely. Larger areas require close observation and multiple biopsies at frequent intervals when areas of malignancy are suspected. Patients with extensive oral leukoplakia should always be encouraged to stop smoking.

3. Hemangiomas are purplish and **lymphangiomas** are pale. Either may be capillary, cavernous, or mixed. The diagnosis is made by inspection and palpation, **not** by biopsy. If there is no functional disability, observation is preferred because those tumors may resolve spontaneously. Surgical excision can be done if there is a good chance of total excision with safety. Sclerosing agents have also been used with varying success.

4. Median rhomboid glossitis is not a neoplasm but it resembles one. It is a congenital developmental defect caused by improper fusion of the anterior two thirds and the posterior third of the tongue. Biopsy is unnecessary and no treatment is required.

5. Torus palatinus also is not a neoplasm; it is a mucosa-covered exostosis in the midline of the hard palate. It is usually asymptomatic and needs no treatment unless it interferes with the fitting of an upper denture. The overlying mucosa can be elevated and the bony protrusion excised with a chisel and rongeur or dental burr. The overlying mucosa may be traumatized by hot or rough food, producing a painful ulcer that might be mistaken for neoplasm. The ulcer usually heals in 7-10 days.

B. SQUAMOUS CELL CARCINOMA accounts for 95% of malignancies of the oral cavity; adenocarcinoma, melanoma, and sarcomas the remainder.

1. Diagnosis. Pain is the usual presenting symptom. Advanced lesions cause bleeding, airway obstruction, and interference with swallowing and speech. Typically the cancer is an indurated ulcer, often best appreciated on bimanual palpation (Figure 7-5). The presence of suspicious nodes in the neck should be noted (Figure 7-6). Biopsy is mandatory to make the diagnosis. Bony involvement should be determined by radiograph or CT scan of the mandible, palate, and sinuses. Distant metastases are sought by obtaining chest and other radiographs and isotope scans as appropriate.

The differential diagnosis includes chronic granulomatous diseases, trauma, benign neoplasms, aphthous stomatitis, and other infectious lesions.

2. Treatment. Oral cancer should be managed by a team of specialists including a surgeon, radiation therapist, and chemotherapist. Generally, treatment depends on the size and location of the tumor, the presence of invasion into bone, and the presence of regional or distant metastases.

Tumors of the oral cavity <2 cm can be treated adequately with either primary surgical or radiation therapy. Larger tumors, tumors involving the mandible, and those with metastases to the cervical lymph nodes generally require combination therapy (surgery and radiation). When cervical nodes are involved with metastasis, radical neck dissection is generally performed.

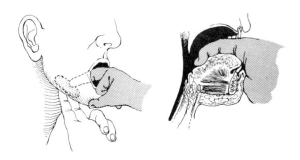

FIGURE 7-5. Manual palpation of the structure of the floor of the mouth.

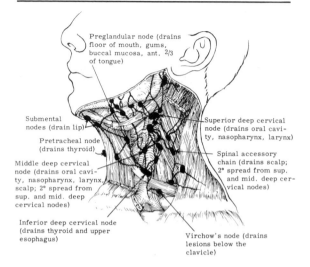

FIGURE 7-6. Lymphatic drainage in the neck (left lateral view) (modified after Richards).

3. Prognosis. Small tumors (<2 cm in diameter) without cervical metastasis have a 70%-80% 5-year survival rate. Larger tumors, especially with cervical metastasis, have a correspondingly poorer prognosis.

C. BENIGN NEOPLASMS OF NOSE AND SINUSES

1. Papilloma is common in the skin of the nasal vestibule and is easily excised. Squamous papillomas arising in the nasal chamber or paranasal sinuses present greater problems (inverting papilloma). They do not metastasize but can invade and erode vital structures locally, causing proptosis, diplopia, blindness, meningitis, and death. A 5%-10% rate of malignant degeneration has been reported in inverting papilloma.

Nasal obstruction (usually unilateral) and the presence of an irregular, meaty polypoid mass filling the nasal chamber lead to the diagnosis. Papillomas may be mistaken for inflammatory or allergic nasal polyps or carcinoma. CT or MRI scans show size and location of these tumors as well as bony involvement.

Intranasal excision is inadequate treatment for these lesions. Lateral rhinotomy with complete removal of the papilloma is necessary to prevent extension and recurrence. Often the nasal sinuses, the lateral nasal wall, and at times the orbital contents must be removed. Growth through the cribriform plate or extension into the pterygomaxillary fossa is a cause of failure. Radiation therapy has been used postoperatively and for recurrence with indifferent success.

2. Osteomas occur chiefly in the frontal and ethmoid sinuses. They are usually asymptomatic incidental findings on radiography. Obstruction of the nasofrontal duct may lead to stasis and infection, and extension into the orbit may produce diplopia and proptosis. No treatment is necessary if asymptomatic. Excision is by external frontoethmoid sinusotomy.

3. Ossifying fibroma is a fibrous tumor containing bony spicules in varying amounts. They most commonly arise in the maxillary sinus and upper jaw, grow slowly, and produce symptoms by encroachment on neighboring structures. The treatment is surgical excision, which must be extensive if the palate and orbit are involved.

4. Nasal polyps are nonneoplastic lesions, usually bilateral, and usually associated with allergies. The polyps are smooth, pale, and boggy in appearance. Intranasal excision followed by control of associated allergy and infection is the preferred treatment.

D. MALIGNANT NEOPLASMS OF NOSE AND SINUSES.
Squamous cell carcinoma is the most common malignancy in the nose and paranasal sinuses; adenocarcinoma, sarcoma, and lymphoma also occur.

Nasal obstruction, epistaxis, postnasal drainage, and pain in the forehead, face, or teeth are the symptoms. A meaty friable nasal mass, swelling of the cheek, signs of orbital invasion, and cranial nerve paresthesia and hypesthesia are seen. Bony involvement is shown on radiographs. Infection, foreign body, and benign neoplasms must be differentiated.

Radical excision is the treatment of choice. Unresectable lesions are managed by a drainage procedure and radiation therapy. Radical neck dissection is added if cervical nodes become involved in otherwise favorable cases.

The 5-year survival rate is about 50%.

E. BENIGN NEOPLASMS OF THE JAW
1. Adamantinoma (amelobastoma) is a tumor of the enamel organ epithelium of a tooth. It occurs more often in

the mandible and grows slowly, causing a painless swelling of the bone. Radiographs often show cystic features of the tumor. Biopsy makes the diagnosis. Small tumors can be excised. Large tumors may require extensive resection of the mandible with reconstruction.

2. Giant cell tumors of the mandible and maxilla are similar to giant cell tumors of bone elsewhere in the body. Although usually benign, malignant varieties occur. It is histologically indistinguishable from the brown tumor of hyperparathyroidism. Treatment is by excision.

F. PRIMARY MALIGNANT TUMORS are rare in the jaw.

G. BENIGN NEOPLASMS OF THE NASOPHARYNX

1. Juvenile fibroma (juvenile nasopharyngeal angiofibroma) occurs most often in adolescent males. They arise in or near the vault of the nasopharynx and can reach considerable size. Histologically, the tumor is composed of vascular connective tissue.

Juvenile fibroma causes nasal obstruction (unilateral or bilateral), epistaxis, headache, otalgia, and deafness. Bleeding can be severe. A friable, bleeding mass is visible intranasally or with indirect mirror examination. Serous otitis media occurs with auditory tube obstruction. Radiography shows a soft tissue mass in the nasopharynx, and CT and MRI scan may show extension into maxillary sinus, sphenoid sinuses, and pterygomaxillary space. Biopsy should not be done unless complete hospital surgical facilities are available.

Surgical excision is the treatment of choice. Hemorrhage during operation can be severe, and blood products must be available. Preliminary ligation or embolization of the internal maxillary artery can usually decrease operative blood loss.

Recurrence results from incomplete excision. Improved surgical approaches have decreased the incidence of recurrence. Spontaneous involution often occurs with increasing age.

H. MALIGNANT NEOPLASMS OF THE NASOPHARYNX

1. Squamous cell carcinoma (transitional cell carcinoma, lymphoepithelioma) commonly arises in Rosenmuller's fossa. Histologically, the cells may be so anaplastic as to make it difficult to determine their type, and lymphoid tissue is abundant. It is a common disease in Chinese people.

Symptoms are nasal obstruction, epistaxis, cervical mass, hearing loss, and visual disturbances. Mirror examination shows a friable mass. One half of patients have a palpable cervical mass at first examination. Any of the cranial nerves can be involved. Radiography and CT may show erosion of the bone in the base of the skull. Intracranial extension can occur through the foramina of the base of the skull without any erosion of bone or cranial nerve involvement. CT or MRI is valuable to determine the size of the tumor. Complications include intracranial extension and cervical and distant metastases as well as hemorrhage.

External radiation therapy is the treatment of choice for both the primary tumor and the cervical metastasis. Radical neck dissection is done infrequently because it does not remove the first level of lymph node metastasis (retropharyngeal nodes). Absence of cranial nerve involvement and cervical adenopathy improves the outlook.

2. Squamous cell carcinoma of the tonsil causes a sticking sensation in the throat, pain, otalgia, interference with swallowing, and trismus. A foul, ulcerated mass in the tonsil often spreads to pillars, tongue, and palate. Cervical nodes may be involved. Lymphomas and granulomas must be distinguished.

Radiation therapy is preferred for smaller lesions; however, radical surgical excision is combined with radiation for more extensive tumors.

I. BENIGN NEOPLASMS OF THE LARYNX AND HYPOPHARYNX. Polyps, papillomas, vocal nodules, and leukoplakia on the vocal cords produce hoarseness. Mucosal cysts in the vallecula are usually asymptomatic. Fibroma, neurofibroma (neurilemmoma), and lipoma in the hypopharyngeal wall can cause dysphagia. The diagnosis is made by indirect mirror examination or by direct laryngoscopy and biopsy. Small tumors are treated by local excision, but large tumors may require external laryngotomy for removal. Microsurgery and the CO_2 laser enable laryngologists to excise lesions with less destruction of normal tissue.

J. MALIGNANT NEOPLASMS OF THE LARYNX AND HYPOPHARYNX. Nearly all laryngeal malignancies are squamous cell carcinomas. About 60% arise on the vocal cords and the others occur in the laryngeal ventricles, false cords, aryepiglottic folds, epiglottis, arytenoid, and subglottic areas. Hypopharyngeal cancer arises in the pyriform sinuses, pharyngeal walls, and postcricoid area.

1. Diagnosis
a. Symptoms. Hoarseness is the chief symptom of vocal cord tumors. Minor throat discomfort, sometimes referred

to the ear, or a mild cough may be the only early manifestations. Voice change, stridor, and dyspnea occur later with enlargement in the larynx.

b. Signs. Fullness beneath the mucosa, a mass, or ulceration is seen. Biopsy should be done. Cervical metastases may be palpable.

c. Radiographs. CT scans and MRI help determine size and extent of tumors, especially in the ventricle and subglottic areas, which are difficult to see.

2. Differential diagnosis. Chronic laryngitis, leukoplakia, tuberculosis, syphilis, contact ulcer, and granuloma are differentiated by biopsy and specific tests for these diseases.

3. Complications. Airway obstruction, hemorrhage, dysphagia, and effects of distant metastasis.

4. Treatment. Very small (2 mm) **vocal cord tumors** can be removed endoscopically with forceps and electrocoagulation of the base or by laser. Tumors confined to the vocal cord (T1) can be treated by external radiation therapy or in some cases by laser excision. Larger lesions of the vocal cord extending either superiorly or inferiorly usually necessitate surgery and radiation combined. Radical neck dissection depends on the size and site of the tumor and is often included for advanced-stage disease.

K. BENIGN NEOPLASMS OF THE SALIVARY GLANDS.
Most neoplasms of the salivary glands are benign.

1. Benign mixed tumor (pleomorphic adenoma) is the most common benign lesion. The parotid gland is the usual site. The tumor causes slowly progressive painless swelling, and a firm nontender mass is the only finding. Biopsy should **not** be done to avoid seeding tumor into uninvolved tissue. The differential diagnosis includes sialolithiasis and sialadenitis, which are usually evident because of diffuse and fluctuating enlargement of the gland; radiography rules out sialolithiasis and, if necessary, a retrograde sialogram demonstrates sialadenitis. Preauricular lymph nodes are more mobile than parotid tumors; hyperplastic nodes within the gland usually become smaller with time. Malignant salivary tumors grow faster, are tender, and may cause paresis of the facial nerve.

Benign mixed tumor of the superficial lobe of the parotid gland should be treated by superficial lobectomy with preservation of the facial nerve; local excision or enucleation gives rise to recurrence because the tumor sends projections through the capsule. Lesions arising in the deep lobe are more difficult to remove without injury to the facial nerve, but every attempt should be made to do so. Mixed tumors of the submaxillary gland are managed by total excision of the gland with care to protect the marginal mandibular branch of the facial nerve and the lingual and hypoglossal nerves.

2. Papillary cystadenoma lymphomatosum (Warthin's tumor) occurs in the parotid gland and is bilateral in 10% of patients. They cause painless enlargement, often in the inferior pole of the superficial lobe. Lobectomy with preservation of the facial nerve is the treatment.

L. MALIGNANT TUMORS OF THE SALIVARY GLANDS

may be clinically indistinguishable from benign tumors presenting as a firm mass in the gland. Rapid growth, pain, tenderness, and facial nerve involvement suggest malignancy. Definitive diagnosis depends on microscopic examination of the excised tumor specimen. Biopsy is indicated only in rare salivary gland tumors that are inoperable and highly suspicious of malignancy.

1. Squamous cell carcinoma of ductal origin in the salivary gland spreads rapidly and has a poor prognosis. Wide surgical excision with sacrifice of the facial nerve and radical neck dissection is usually necessary. Radiation therapy is an adjunct to surgery in some cases and is used alone in others.

2. Adenoid cystic carcinomas (cylindroma) occur in the major or minor salivary glands of young adults. They grow slowly and spread by direct extension, along nerve sheaths, to regional nodes, and via the blood stream. Wide excision followed by radiation therapy is the treatment of choice. Although every attempt is made to preserve the facial nerve, sacrifice of involved branches is occasionally unavoidable. This tumor is characterized by its tendency to recur locally or distally 10-15 years or more after primary treatment.

3. Mucoepidermoid tumors are carcinomas that can be either low grade or high grade. Low-grade tumors are characterized by slow local growth and rare cervical or distant metastasis. Wide local excision via a parotidectomy is usually adequate therapy. On the other hand, high-grade tumors are typically aggressive locally, with a much higher rate of regional metastasis. Parotidectomy is often combined with radical neck dissection and/or postoperative radiation therapy to prevent recurrence.

M. NEOPLASMS OF BLOOD VESSELS

1. Chemodectoma (carotid body tumor) is a rare, slowly growing tumor arising in paraganglionic tissue at the carotid bifurcation. A mass in the neck is the only early symptom; pain and dysphagia occur later. The mass is fixed to the carotid bifurcation, and arteriography shows a vascular soft tissue lesion at this site. Small tumors are excised easily; larger ones may require resection and reconstruction of the carotid artery. The prognosis is good.

2. Glomus jugulare arises from the jugular bulb and extends upward into the middle ear, where it can be seen as a pink or blue mass behind the tympanic membrane. Tinnitus and weakness of cranial nerves that exit through the jugular foramen are the symptoms. Arteriography, CT scan, and jugular venography are needed for thorough evaluation. Total excision is usually possible if approached by an experienced team of skull base surgeons.

8

Breast

William H. Goodson, III

I. EVALUATION OF BREAST DISEASE

The initial evaluation of breast disease is always designed to answer one question: does the patient have breast cancer? Therefore, the initial evaluation of breast problems is the same until the question of malignancy has been resolved.

A. ANATOMIC CONSIDERATIONS. The glandular tissue of the breast consists of 15-20 segments arranged radially around the nipple. Each segment drains into a single duct which has a dilated portion directly behind the areola: this retroareolar, dilated duct is soft, except during lactation when it is distended. Each of the 15-20 ducts empties through a single opening in the nipple. Most of the glandular tissue is in the upper outer quadrant or directly behind the areola. There is less tissue in the upper inner and lower outer quadrants, and a minimal amount in the lower inner quadrant. Accessory breast tissue may arise anywhere along the "milk line," which extends from the anterior axillary fold down to the groin. About 60% of women have discernible lumps in their breasts, so soft lumps that are distributed uniformly throughout the breast can be considered "normal." Usually, one breast is slightly larger than the other.

B. HISTORY

1. Lump or mass. Note when and how the mass was detected and whether its size changes with the menstrual cycle.

2. Pain is a common complaint. Breast cancer is not usually painful, but there are exceptions, and one should not assume that painful lesions are always benign. The most common type of pain is due to stretching associated with premenstrual engorgement of the breast: it is usually bilateral and diffuse. Severe pain may radiate to the underside of the arm or the lateral chest wall. Localized pain requires careful evaluation. It may indicate a deep abscess, an area of trauma or, rarely, malignancy. Very rarely, cervical root pain may radiate to the breast.

3. Discharge from the nipple. Usually, a discharge from the nipple is clear, but it may be bloody, green, or brown. Over 80% of premenopausal women have some discharge if the nipple is manipulated; therefore, determine whether the discharge is spontaneous or elicited only by manipulation. Eighty percent of patients with bloody nipple discharge have either benign intraductal papillomas or ductal ectasia; malignancy is responsible for some of the remainder. It is rare to find malignant cells by cytologic examination of the nipple discharge unless a cancer is located in the duct immediately adjacent to the nipple, and this is uncommon. Determine which duct is producing the discharge by applying finger pressure systematically around the areola. The position where pressure causes discharge is recorded as though the areola were the face of a clock.

4. Risk factors. One out of nine women in the United States develops breast cancer assuming a life span of 110 years. The risk is slightly increased if there is a first-degree relative (mother, sister, aunt) with postmenopausal breast cancer. A marked increase is not seen unless the first-degree relative has had bilateral breast cancer, premenopausal breast cancer, or bilateral premenopausal breast cancer. An increased risk of breast cancer is also associated with menarche before 11 or after 14 years of age, first pregnancy after age 30 years, late menopause, and obesity. Birth control pills are not associated with increased risk of breast cancer in older women or women who have had a full-term pregnancy, but use of oral contraceptives by teenagers may be associated with an increased risk of breast cancer. Exogenous estrogens used for hormone replacement at the time of menopause also carry no demonstrated risk. Women who have had surgical removal of the ovaries before menopause seem to have a decreased risk; if they take replacement estrogen, the risk of breast cancer returns to that of the general population.

5. Other history. Whether or not the patient is or has been recently pregnant is important because pregnancy may obscure masses. The time of the last menstrual period should be noted; a recent change in menstrual cycle suggests general hormonal changes, with secondary effects in the breasts. Was the mass present previously? (see Section IIA3). What was the pathologic diagnosis of any previously biopsied mass? What, if any, medications are being used? Are there any systemic symptoms (bone pain, weight loss, etc.)?

C. PHYSICAL EXAMINATION is about 70% accurate in diagnosing cancer of the breast. Normal physical findings change cyclically because the breast retains fluid under the influence of monthly hormonal fluctuations. Fluid retention is maximal just before menstruation begins and tapers off rapidly as menstruation ends. Optimal examination is obtained approximately 7-14 days after the beginning of the menstrual period because fluid retention is least pronounced at this time. Breast examination in the pregnant patient may be extremely difficult because of breast growth and distention.

1. The patient should be examined in both the sitting and supine positions. **While the patient is sitting,** inspect the breasts for symmetry (Figure 8-1**A**). Evaluate the skin of the breast for dimpling while the patient leans forward, while she raises her arms above her head (Figure 8-1**B**), or while she flexes the pectoralis muscles by pushing the hands against the hips (Figure 8-1**C**). Check for nipple inversion. If it is present, inquire for how long, because recent nipple inversion suggests possible deep malignancy. Examine and record the status of the axillary and supraclavicular nodes (Figures 8-1**D** and **E**) both in malignancy and in benign disease for future reference. The nipple and the area directly behind the areola are the most easily palpated when the patient is sitting. The nipple is usually firm, but the tissue behind the areola is soft and loose.

2. The patient is then examined in the **supine position** (Figure 8-1**F**). Because the majority of breast tissue is located in the upper outer quadrant, examination is facilitated by elevating the patient's arm and placing her hand behind her head; this maneuver flattens the breast and displaces it medially.

3. Examination should be performed in a **uniform fashion** in every patient. Begin palpating one portion of the breast and proceed according to a systematic pattern that covers all areas from clavicle to inframammary crease and sternum to latissimus dorsi muscle. Verticle or horizontal row patterns are more efficient than circular or radial patterns. Use a combination of finger palpation and gentle rotatory motion of the examining hand on the skin. Moistening the skin with rubbing alcohol may allow the detection of more subtle lumps when gliding the hand over the skin.

4. If there is uncertainty whether a mass exists, the patient should be **reexamined** at frequent intervals (perhaps at different times during her menstrual cycle) until the matter is resolved. Sometimes, areas of thickening "soften" if a mild diuretic is given to eliminate fluid engorgement before a midcycle examination (e.g., hydrochlorothiazide, 25 mg twice daily, orally for 3-5 days). If a mass is no longer palpable after di-

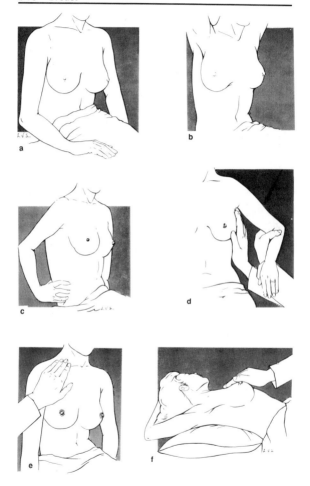

FIGURE 8-1. Inspection of breasts.

uretics, it may be assumed that the mass was not solid tissue. Conversely, elimination of the surrounding engorgement sometimes makes a cancer more prominent.

5. All women should have a yearly breast examination by a trained health provider. Women are also encouraged to examine their own breasts once a month. The system of **self-examination** is similar to that described above for routine physical examination. Begin with inspection while sitting or standing before a mirror, then careful palpation. The patient palpates each breast with the contralateral hand; the arm should be elevated as in examination by the physician.

6. Benign lesions tend to be soft, well-circumscribed, and easily moveable within the surrounding breast tissue; frequently, they have a regular, round or elliptical shape. Small, early breast cancers also may have these characteristics. Classic signs of breast cancer, such as large, hard, irregular masses, edema of overlying skin, fixation to skin or underlying structures, enlargement of superficial veins, or ulceration, reflect the extremes of advanced disease.

7. Even the best physical examination cannot determine the **histologic diagnosis** of any lump in the breast. It can define the presence or absence of a lump and its consistency, moveability, firmness, and approximate size. The only way to obtain a pathologic diagnosis, however, is by some type of sampling technic that provides tissue for pathologic study. All other diagnostic methods are based on inference and are subject to error.

D. LABORATORY TESTS. Routine laboratory tests are of little worth in the evaluation of breast disease except in patients with advanced cancer.

E. RADIOGRAPHY
   1. Mammography. The typical malignant lesion has a stellate appearance and irregular borders; frequently, it contains clustered, spiculated microcalcifications. Benign lesions are well-circumscribed and have round edges; if calcifications are present, they are round and less likely to be clustered. Mammography is about 90% accurate in determining whether a lesion is malignant or benign. Unfortunately, mammograms are less accurate in patients with dense breast tissue because the mammogram depends upon the contrast of a dense lesion against surrounding radiolucent fat. Young women often have radiographically dense breasts, and mammography in this age group has a relatively high rate of false-negatives. **A negative**

mammogram does not rule out cancer, especially in a young woman. The dose of radiation varies with the technic used (e.g., 0.5 cGy/picture for xeromammograms and magnification films, 0.1 cGy/film for routine films, and 0.05 cGy/film for low-dose screen films).

2. Ultrasonography is useful only to determine whether a mass seen on a mammogram is a cyst or a solid lesion.

F. SPECIAL PROCEDURES

1. Aspiration may be performed for two reasons: to drain cysts and to obtain material for cytologic study.

a. Aspiration of cysts. Many acutely painful, tender, noninflamed lesions are cysts. They are aspirated readily with a 22-ga needle attached to a 20-ml syringe. The mass is immobilized with one hand and the skin is cleansed before aspiration; local anesthesia is not used. If the aspirated fluid is yellow or green, if there is no blood in it, and if the mass disappears entirely after aspiration, one may assume that the cyst is benign. If **any** of these criteria are not met, there is a higher risk of breast cancer and biopsy should be performed. The breast is reexamined in 4-6 weeks to see that a presumably benign cyst has not refilled. Many experts believe that a mass can be safely aspirated a second time, but a third recurrence warrants a biopsy. Cytologic examination is not usually done unless the cyst has refilled.

b. Solid lesions are aspirated to obtain material for cytologic study. (1) A 22-ga needle and a 10-ml syringe are used and the skin is cleansed. It is not desirable to attempt to anesthetize the lesion, because that causes more pain than the aspiration process. Aspiration is uncomfortable during the time that negative pressure is applied (<60 seconds). (2) The needle is inserted through the skin into the middle of the mass. One hand is used to draw back on the syringe. Holding the syringe and needle as a unit with one hand and immobilizing the breast mass with the other, the needle is passed through the mass multiple times (at least 20-25). Several pistol-grip holders are available, and they facilitate manipulation of the syringe and needle. (3) Suction is released while the needle point is still under the patient's skin. The entire assembly is withdrawn from the skin. Be careful not to push the specimen from the needle nor to pull it into the syringe while the needle is being withdrawn. (4) The air in the syringe is used to push the aspirated material onto a glass slide and a second slide is used to make a smear. One slide is allowed to dry in air and the other is immediately placed in alcohol fixative. (5) The slides must be interpreted by a cytopathologist trained in evaluating breast aspirates. Material from malignant lesions typically shows very large pleomorphic cells with prominent nucleoli, and individual malignant cells with intact cytoplasm are frequently encountered. Aspirations from benign lesions have small, regularly shaped nuclei without prominent nucleoli. Single cells are often seen with fibroadenomas, but they are usually only "bare" nuclei (without cytoplasm). (6) When correlated with physical examination and mammography, results of fine-needle aspiration cytology approach 99% accuracy for both malignant and benign lesions.

2. Biopsy. Immediate frozen section diagnosis of a biopsy followed by immediate mastectomy if cancer is found offers no survival advantage to the patient; moreover, this approach imposes unnecessary stress and precludes patient participation in decisions about her own care. An interval of 4 weeks may elapse between biopsy and initiation of definitive treatment without adverse effects on patient survival.

a. Routine biopsy. Optimally, biopsy is done under local anesthesia (e.g., 1% lidocaine with epinephrine). For extremely anxious patients, mild sedation (e.g., diazepam 10 mg IM) may be appropriate. The breast is almost insensitive to cutting, but it is extremely sensitive to stretching and pressure. Therefore, very little local anesthetic is required except in the area of small blood vessels, because they and their accompanying nerves are quite sensitive. Because of the heat it produces and the current that passes through tissue, electrocoagulation is painful and should be applied sparingly. The wound is closed with a subcuticular absorbable suture and paper tapes on the skin; drainage is contraindicated.

b. Needle localization biopsy. When a suspicious lesion is seen on mammogram but cannot be palpated, it may be biopsied with needle localization technic. Using the mammogram as a guide, a needle is placed in the lesion in the breast. A second mammogram is taken to confirm correct positioning of the needle. Methylene blue (0.1 ml) is injected through the needle to stain the lesion and the surrounding tissue. The needle may be left in the breast or replaced with a hooked wire. The wire is less likely to be dislodged. The shaft of the needle or the wire is used as a guide to locate and remove stained tissue. A radiograph of the specimen is obtained to make certain that the mammographic lesion is present in the excised tissue and the specimen is then submitted to the pathologist. Needle localization technics are also used under local anesthesia.

II. BENIGN DISEASES OF THE FEMALE BREAST

A. FIBROCYSTIC CONDITION is the most common cause of a mass in the breast. The incidence reaches a peak between 35 and 40 years of age and tapers after the menopause. Fibrocystic condition is a large diagnostic category that encompasses many clinical and histologic diagnoses such as metaplasia, cystic disease, duct ectasia, epithelial duct hyperplasia, fibrosis, sclerosing adenosis, and chronic inflammation.

1. Diagnosis

a. Symptoms. (1) Pain or discomfort in the breast occurring or worsening just before the menses. (2) One or more masses, usually painful, which fluctuate in size and sensitivity during the menstrual cycle. Masses may disappear and reappear at the same or new sites.

b. Signs. (1) Multiple masses, thickened areas, and nodularity bilaterally, most marked in the upper outer quadrants. (2) Masses are often tender. (3) Lesions change in number, size, and tenderness during the menstrual cycle. Examination should be repeated at different phases of the menstrual cycle or through several menstrual cycles.

c. Radiographs. Mammography is discussed on page 349.

2. Treatment

a. A dominant solid mass, a mass that does not disappear cyclically, or a cystic mass that does not meet the criteria described in the section on aspiration of cysts must be distinguished from malignancy by biopsy (or, in selected cases, by needle aspiration cytology).

b. Premenstrual pain may be alleviated by avoidance of salt late in the cycle and during the first few days of menstruation. In more severe cases, diuretics may be used intermittently (e.g., hydrochlorothiazide, 25-50 mg twice daily, orally for the 5 days before expected menstruation each month); potassium intake should be supplemented by fruits and other potassium-rich sources.

c. "Lumpiness" of the breasts may be reduced in some patients by elimination of caffeine (coffee, tea, cola beverages, headache medications, etc.) from the diet. However, some women consume large amounts of caffeine and still have no breast disease, whereas others with severe dysplasia obtain no benefit from elimination of caffeine.

d. Oral contraceptives need not be discontinued in most patients.

e. Danazol, a synthetic androgen, is reserved for severe cases. The usual dose is 100-400 mg/day. Side-effects include mild masculinization, voice changes, weight gain, acne, and male hair distribution. Side effects may not be reversible.

3. Prognosis. Pathologists should provide or be asked to describe the specific features of fibrocystic condition found in any biopsy. There is no increased risk of subsequent breast cancer in women with adenosis, apocrine metaplasia, cysts, duct ectasia, fibrosis, mild hyperplasia, periductal mastitis, and squamous metaplasia. There is only a slightly increased risk with moderate hyperplasia or papilloma with a fibrovascular core. There is a moderately increased risk in women whose biopsy shows atypical ductal or lobular hyperplasia: between 15% and 20% of women with atypical hyperplasia develop invasive breast cancer in the 25 years following biopsy. The cancer may arise anywhere in either breast so wide excision of an atypical lesion does not prevent future development of malignancy. Additional surgery is not usually recommended for mammary dysplasia, but a patient whose biopsy indicates increased risk of malignancy should be followed by regular breast evaluation.

B. FIBROADENOMA is the second most common cause of a breast lump. The peak incidence of fibroadenomas is between 20 and 25 years of age. Fibroadenomas are rare after menopause. They may grow rapidly during pregnancy.

1. Diagnosis. Fibroadenoma is usually asymptomatic and is discovered accidentally. Fibroadenomas are multiple in 10%-15% of cases. The tumor is firm, rubbery, nontender, spherical, discrete, and "slippable" (so easily moveable that it slips away from examining fingers).

The primary concern is to distinguish between fibroadenomas and cancer. It is necessary either to excise the tumor or to confirm the diagnosis with fine-needle aspiration. The major risk if a fibroadenoma is not excised is that it will grow and become painful, especially during pregnancy. It is unusual to find cancer invading a fibroadenoma, and extremely rare (no more than 1 in 1000) to find a cancer actually originating in a fibroadenoma (most are in situ cancers). Because the risk of cancer arising in any breast is at least one in 18, the chance of cancer in a fibroadenoma is less than the risk of cancer in the entire breast.

2. Treatment. The preferred treatment for a small fibroadenoma is excision under local anesthesia. In young patients with small lesions, the diagnosis can be made by fine-needle aspiration if the patient does not want to undergo excisional biopsy. Larger fibroadenomas (>2 cm) should be removed because they may cause pain and because they may grow further.

C. INTRADUCTAL PAPILLOMA is a benign tumor that grows as a small (1-5 mm) "polyp" within a large duct of the breast. It typically causes symptoms by blocking the duct at the skin level of the nipple. Secretions accumulate behind this obstruction; when there is enough pressure to force secretions beyond the papilloma, there is discharge associated with bleeding because of microscopic damage to the papilloma. The epithelium of a papilloma is well-differentiated and does not have immediate malignant potential. However, long-standing papillomas sometimes seem to degenerate into malignancies in a way similar to adenomatous polyps of the colon. Multiple papillomas should not be confused with papillomatosis, which is actually an epithelial hyperplastic lesion of mammary dysplasia.

1. Diagnosis. The usual presentation is bloody nipple discharge. Most papillomas are too small and too soft to be palpated, but occasionally a large (1-2 cm) intraductal papilloma can be palpated. Small lesions are localized by fingertip pressure at successive points around the areola, observing for discharge from a single orifice.

2. Treatment is excision of the tumor. Through a circumareolar incision, identify the dilated duct and excise a small portion of the dermis from the underside of the nipple to ensure complete excision of the papilloma. All of the tumor and dilated duct tissue are then excised. The tumor may extend several centimeters through subdivisions of the duct into the breast lobule.

D. GALACTORRHEA is persistent milky discharge from the nipple. Such a discharge may persist long after cessation of nursing, particularly if the patient stimulates her nipple by checking to see whether a discharge is still present. A woman who has not been nursing a child also may develop a discharge from the nipple if it is stimulated on a regular basis. Pharmacologic agents (e.g., chlorpromazine and oral contraceptives) may contribute to the discharge. A pituitary adenoma producing high levels of prolactin is another cause of galactorrhea.

Treatment. Stimulation of the breast should be avoided. Drugs should be discontinued if they are suspect. If prolactin levels are elevated, a pituitary adenoma should be sought.

E. DERMATITIS OF THE NIPPLE may occur in women of childbearing age.

1. Diagnosis. The first procedure always is to rule out Paget's disease (ductal carcinoma arising in epithelial rests in the skin of the nipple) by nipple biopsy. The nipple is infiltrated with 1% lidocaine with epinephrine, and a small (1-2 mm) wide wedge of skin is excised from the lesion in the nipple. No sutures are used, and the skin of the nipple is approximated with wound closure tapes to avoid the discomfort of suture removal.

2. Treatment. Only after benign biopsy results have been obtained, dermatitis may be treated with topical steroids. Paget's disease may respond to initial treatment with steroids, so a biopsy is essential before beginning any treatment. After the skin lesion has cleared, intermittent topical steroids are often needed to prevent recurrence.

F. SUPERFICIAL PHLEBITIS is a spontaneous painful inflammation of subcutaneous veins. Pain may be quite severe. The breast should be thoroughly evaluated, including mammograms, to look for underlying malignancy. Treatment is symptomatic, with warm compresses and analgesics as needed. Any masses associated with the dilated superficial vein(s) must be biopsied. Overlying skin may retract as inflammation subsides, raising the suspicion of carcinoma, but the long linear retraction and the history are typical of phlebitis.

G. BREAST ABSCESSES are most often associated with pregnancy and lactation.

1. Diagnosis. Abscesses are inflamed, tender masses. Biopsy is required to distinguish a simple abscess from inflammatory carcinoma or an abscess caused by invasive carcinoma.

2. Treatment. Particularly in women who are either pregnant or nursing, there is a tendency to underestimate the extent of breast abscesses; therefore, it is advisable to use a general anesthetic for draining all but the most superficial of these lesions. It is not usually desirable to open a large breast abscess with a single long incision; make two small separate incisions and pass a soft rubber drain into the abscess with the ends projecting out through the two incisions. This method ensures adequate drainage with minimal subsequent deformity. Tissues should be obtained for biopsy.

H. FAT NECROSIS is secondary to previous trauma, but often the patient does not remember the inciting injury. The lesion is a hard, irregular mass, sometimes with retraction of overlying skin. Treatment is excision to confirm the diagnosis because the physical examination and mammography frequently suggest malignancy.

I. MASTALGIA. About 70% of breast pain cannot be placed in one of the above categories. Unusual causes of breast pain include referred pain from cervical radiculitis, lateral thoracic nerve syndrome, and failure to support the breast adequately during strenuous physical activity.

J. PREMATURE THELARCHY is the most common cause of breast lumps in prepubertal girls.

1. Diagnosis. Determine whether the patient is entering puberty by looking for other secondary sex characteristics such as axillary and pubic hair or maturation of genital skin. Determine at what age the mother and female siblings entered puberty. If the patient has other signs of puberty in the absence of a familial tendency toward early puberty, an endocrine evaluation is indicated.

2. Treatment. Surgical treatment is rarely necessary for a breast lump in a prepubertal female because the lump usually represents the entire anlage of the breast and because malignancy is extremely rare in this age group. There are fewer than 100 cases of breast cancer reported in the world literature in females under age 20; half of these were rapidly growing anaplastic lesions leading to death in 2 years, and the other half were unusual secretory adenocarcinomas with excellent survival rates.

III. MALIGNANT DISEASES OF THE BREAST

A. INVASIVE CARCINOMA (DUCTAL OR LOBULAR) accounts for 85% of breast cancer. Many histologic types of invasive carcinoma have been described (e.g., scirrhous, comedo, medullary, tubular), but these distinctions are not important in selecting treatment.

1. Diagnosis
a. Symptoms. (1) Breast cancer is usually a painless lump, but a painful lesion also may be cancer. (2) Nipple discharge is uncommonly associated with cancer. (3) Erythema, hardness, asymmetry, and nipple inversion reflect advanced disease. (4) Symptoms remote from the breast, such as dyspnea, bone pain, weight loss, etc., may indicate metastatic disease.

b. Signs. Early breast cancers frequently have physical characteristics similar to benign lesions. They may be soft, well-circumscribed, easily moveable within the surrounding tissue, and frequently have a round or elliptical shape. More advanced tumors present with large, hard, firm, irregular masses, edema of the overlying skin (peau d'orange), fixation to the skin or underlying structures, enlarged superficial veins, or other forms of skin invasion such as ulceration.

c. Laboratory tests. There are no abnormalities in localized disease. Elevated serum alkaline phosphate may reflect hepatic or bone metastases. If bilirubin, alkaline phosphatase, lactic dehydrogenase, and SGOT are all normal, liver metastases are essentially excluded. Hypercalcemia may occur with advanced malignancy.

d. Radiographic findings. Mammography may suggest whether or not a specific lesion is malignant. It cannot, however, be used as the sole basis for further treatment. Chest radiograph is obtained routinely if breast cancer is suspected. Other radiographs and radionuclide scans (e.g., bone or liver scan) are not routinely obtained in patients with early lesions. Advanced disease or suspected metastases are reasons for ordering these tests. The most common sites for metastases of breast cancer are lungs, bone, liver, and brain; ovary and pancreas are less common targets.

e. Special tests. (1) **Fine needle aspiration** may be used to diagnose malignancy. If cancer is suspected on the basis of physical examination, mammography, or the patient's history and a needle aspiration does not show cancer, one should proceed directly to biopsy. (2) **Biopsy.** Histologic section of an excised portion of a tumor is the most certain method to distinguish cancer from other disease, but even this diagnostic modality has a small but definable chance of error (approximately 1%). (3) **Estrogen and progesterone receptors,** when possible, should be obtained on all tumor specimens at the time of biopsy. Tissue must be placed in liquid nitrogen within 15 minutes; otherwise a low reading is obtained. Values >10 ftm/mg cytosol protein are considered positive. (4) Estimates of proliferative rate such as S-phase from flow cytometry or direct measurement are desirable information, if available.

f. Staging. Histologic staging based on the TNM system should be used for all patients. T0 is carcinoma in situ; T1 is invasive cancer <2 cm; T2 is a primary between 2 and 5 cm; T3 is a primary >5 cm; T4 is a primary that is invading skin or chest wall. N and M refer to the status of lymph nodes and whether there are distant metastases. Because physical examination of lymph nodes is only about 70% accurate (both false-positive and false-negative), lymph nodes should be removed for histologic evaluation in all patients with pervasive cancer (see Figure 8-2).

g. Histologic characterization. Favorable prognosis is associated with a well-differentiated tumor showing gland formation and rare mitosis. Poor prognosis is associated with any of the following: undifferentiated tumor, blood vessel, lymphatic or perineural invasion; diffusely invasive tumor margins; perinodal invasion of fat in the axillary specimen; high number of mitotic figures.

2. Treatment. The following are established principles in treatment of breast cancer: (1) Breast cancer has an essentially fixed rate of recurrence for 15-20 years after initial treatment. This is in marked contrast to most other cancers, for which 5-year survival can be considered a "cure." This is most easily

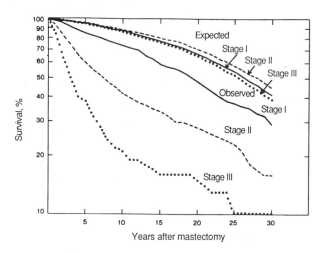

FIGURE 8-2. Comparison of expected and observed survival curves for patients in pathological stages I, II, and III. (From Ferguson DJ, et al: *JAMA* 248:1337.)

shown when a survival curve is drawn on a semi-log graph (Figure 8-2). (2) Cancer spreads by both vascular and lymphatic routes. Disseminated disease can recur even if excised lymph nodes were free of tumor. (3) Breast cancer is multicentric; a second primary can be found in at least 30% of mastectomy specimens; but it is clear that many of these second cancers do not grow. Two thirds of these cancers are in segments of the breast remote from the original tumor. In some series, 30% of patients with invasive cancer have direct involvement of the nipple with cancer (thus, efforts to "bank" the nipple for use in future reconstructive plastic surgery carry a high risk of transplanting the tumor). Surprisingly, these multicentric second cancers are only rarely a problem when breast conservation treatment is used. (4) Although more lymph nodes are removed, radical mastectomy does not improve survival over modified radical mastectomy. (5) Gross tumor must be removed surgically. When radiation alone is used to treat gross tumor there is failure of radiation treatment and/or a local recurrence rate as high as 60% within 6 months. (6) Adjuvant radiation therapy after mastectomy does not improve survival, but it does reduce the early incidence of local recurrence. (7) Axillary dissection of clinically uninvolved nodes at the time of mastectomy or partial mastectomy does not affect survival; however, it is the best index of extent of disease (Table 8-1).

   a. Surgical treatment. Modified radical mastectomy is the traditional treatment of early invasive breast cancer. The total breast is removed, along with the segment of overlying skin which includes the nipple, the skin over the mass, and the incision from the previous biopsy, if present. Axillary dissection is performed in continuity with the mastectomy.

   Complications of surgical treatment include significant edema of the arm (5%), some loss of range of motion in the arm (25%), occasional phantom pain (30%), and a small incidence of operative complications, such as slough of skin flap and wound infection.

   For some patients who have mastectomy, an external prosthesis that maintains the form of the breast under clothing is adequate. Other patients benefit greatly from plastic surgical procedures to reform the breast mound. The breast mass is restored with a silicone gel prosthesis implanted beneath the pectoral muscles. Extra skin may be supplied with a latissimus dorsi or rectus-abdominal myocutaneous flap, or local skin can be stretched with a tissue expander. It is best to defer reconstruction until after adjuvant therapy has been completed in the case of stage II lesions. Local recurrence can be detected in

Table 8-1. Staging of breast cancer

		Approximate 10-year survival*
Stage I	Tumor <2 cm diameter; negative nodes on histology; no evidence of distant metastases	85%
Stage II	Tumor 2-5 cm diameter with or without positive nodes; or tumor <2 cm diameter with positive nodes on histology	60%
Stage III	Any tumor with fixed lymph nodes and/or supraclavicular or infraclavicular lymph nodes; or tumor >5 cm with or without nodes; or tumor fixed to skin or muscle with any node status	35%†
Stage IV	Any tumor or node status with distant metastases	<5%

*Approximate averages for comparison purposes because actual numbers vary between published series.
†Stage III with negative nodes may have >60% 10-year survival.

spite of a prosthesis, and radiation therapy can be given over and through a prosthesis (for dose purposes, a silicon gel implant is similar to water or tissue density).

b. Partial mastectomy and radiation therapy. Breast conservation is a good alternative for patients with early breast cancer. There is no decrease in survival and only a slight increase in local recurrence. Breast conservation is not advised for extensive or multicentric cancer. The location of the cancer or the size of the cancer relative to the size of the breast may be a relative contraindication to breast conservation; but the medical decision should be based on whether the cancer is reasonably excised, not whether the surgeon judges the cosmetic result better or worse than mastectomy with reconstruction. Adequate surgical excision is very important and local recurrence rates are three times higher after simple lumpectomy than after partial mastectomy with wide margins.

Partial mastectomy is usually combined with axillary dissection. The *axillary dissection* should be thorough enough to determine if nodes are positive but not so extensive as to cause unnecessary morbidity. Arm edema is four times more common after removal of level III lymph nodes (medial to pectoralis minor muscle) and stripping of the axillary vein. Adequate staging information is obtained by removing nodes behind and lateral to the pectoralis minor muscle (level I and level II) with less morbidity.

If partial mastectomy and radiation therapy are chosen, external radiation is usually given to the whole breast in a dose of 4500-5000 cGy, 5 days a week over 5-6 weeks. Larger fractions lead to more complications, such as rib fractures. Lower doses give less effective control of tumor. After radiation of the entire breast a boost is frequently given to the area of the tumor. This is usually done with an external electron beam, although iridium needles, which are implanted into the area of the tumor can be used. The local boost usually increases the dose by a minimum of 2000 cGy.

Complications of radiation therapy include arm edema (5%), symptomatic pneumonitis (10%), radiographic evidence of fibrosis of the underlying lung (40%), rib fractures (5%), and potential effects of radiation scatter to the chest, upper abdomen, contralateral breast, and neck (e.g., possible carcinogenesis).

c. Follow-up includes examination at least every 3 months for the first year. Thereafter, patients should be followed at 6-month intervals for at least a total of 5 years. Chest radiographs should be obtained every 6 months for the first year and yearly thereafter. Contralateral mammograms should be repeated yearly. If the breast involved has not been removed but treated with only local resection, a new baseline mammogram should be obtained 4 months following surgery or radiation. New complaints such as pain, masses, respiratory symptoms, and so on should receive immediate evaluation. The yield of routine follow-up blood studies (CBC, alkaline phosphatase, CEA, etc.) is low, but so is their cost.

Equally as important as the various medical and surgical therapies of breast cancer is emotional support of the patient. Not only is life threatened, but because of the high social importance placed on the breast, there is also a great impact on self-image. Patients, even those who choose to retain the breast, need careful counsel and support. They need reassurance that their value as employees, family members, and sexual partners is not diminished.

d. Adjuvant therapy. (1) **Chemotherapy** is beneficial for premenopausal or perimenopausal women who have one or more nodes involved with tumor. The most commonly employed regimens are cyclophosphamide and 5-fluorouracil and either methotrexate or doxorubicin (Adriamycin) [CMF]. These drugs are given for 6-12 months and prolong survival. Vincristine or prednisone may be added to either of these regimens for treatment of advanced stage II and III lesions; these agents are more toxic, but the potential benefit is greater because the patient population is at higher risk. Chemotherapy has some benefit in postmenopausal women, but the increment of survival is much less striking. Complications of chemotherapy are leukopenia, anemia, hair loss, sterility, amenorrhea, nausea, and malaise; there is also a slight risk of inducing leukemia. Chemotherapy has also been advocated for all premenopausal node-negative patients, but the relative value of this indication is not uniformly agreed upon. (2) **Radiation therapy** after mastectomy does not improve survival. When used after mastectomy, it significantly increases the risk of arm edema. It should be reserved for those patients who have a high risk of local recurrence, as when tumor is known to have been left on the chest wall or when many axillary lymph nodes contain tumor. (3) **Hormone manipulation** has long been used for the treatment of disseminated disease. The estrogen-blocking agent tamoxifen (10 mg twice daily) increases 10-year survival in patients who have positive axillary lymph nodes and estrogen receptor-positive tumors. Tamoxifen has also been advocated for node-negative patients and is being considered for chemoprevention of breast cancer in high-risk women. Megestrol acetate, a potent progestin, also is beneficial to the treatment of advanced breast cancer.

e. Palliative treatment. (1) **Hormone manipulation.** Ablative procedures (that remove hormone sources) such as oophorectomy, adrenalectomy, and hypophysectomy are beneficial for about 30% of premenopausal or perimenopausal patients. Approximately 60% of postmenopausal patients respond to the administration of either diethylstilbestrol or androgens. There is no satisfactory explanation of why premenopausal and perimenopausal patients benefit from removal of estrogen, whereas postmenopausal patients benefit from the addition of estrogens. The presence or absence of estrogen receptors is now used to help predict the response to endocrine therapy. Most patients with postmenopausal cancer are estrogen and progesterone receptor-positive and patients who are estrogen receptor-positive are more likely to respond to hormonal manipulation. These patients can be treated either by ablative surgery or the drugs tamoxifen (which blocks the effects of estro-

9

Pulmonary System

Scot H. Merrick

I. GENERAL PRINCIPLES

A. DIAGNOSTIC AND THERAPEUTIC PROCEDURES

1. Thoracentesis. This procedure is most commonly performed for inflammatory and malignant conditions of the pleura or lung. It is diagnostic in approximately 75% of cases.

a. Preparation of the patient. The site of the tap is selected by radiography, sonography, CT scan, or physical examination. An accumulation of approximately 500 ml of fluid is necessary before it becomes visible on standard chest films (blunting of the costophrenic angle). With free-flowing effusions, the site of aspiration is usually the seventh or eighth intercostal space in the posterior axillary line. The most frequent error is choosing an interspace level that is too low. Pneumonia, atelectasis, trauma, and phrenic nerve paresis (seen in malignant lesions of the lung) may result in a loss of lung volume and/or elevation of the diaphragm. In these situations, selection of a higher intercostal space is advisable. The patient is placed in a comfortable sitting position, leaning slightly forward on a padded stand or supported by an attendant. Premedication with diazepam or Midazolam is optional. The skin of the chest wall is prepared with antiseptic and draped.

b. Technic of the tap. Aseptic technic must be used throughout. The chest wall is anesthetized with 5 to 20 ml of 1% lidocaine through a 22-ga needle, making sure the skin, rib, periosteum, and parietal pleura are infiltrated. Thoracentesis is virtually painless if this is done properly. A thoracentesis kit, which contains a large syringe, a one-way valve, an introducing needle, a soft catheter with multiple side holes, tubing, and a collection bag, is used to maximize drainage and to minimize lung injury and introduction of air. With firm, steady pressure, the introducing needle is advanced into the pleural space. In order to avoid injury to the intercostal nerve and vessels, the needle is passed through the chest wall at the lower margin of the intercostal space, over the rib. Complications are rare but include hemorrhage and pneumothorax. Multiple thoracenteses may result in loculation of pleural fluid, which may be very difficult to drain completely.

c. Volume of fluid removed at one sitting depends upon circumstances. A total of 2000 ml can often be gradually evacuated at one sitting from a large effusion. If the patient complains of a feeling of tightness in the chest, cough, palpitation, fatigue, faintness, or other untoward symptoms, the aspiration should be slowed or discontinued until another occasion. Removal of volumes in excess of 2000 ml has been associated with unilateral pulmonary edema ("reexpansion" edema), which is thought to be the result of increased capillary permeability from a reperfusion injury.

d. Laboratory examination of pleural fluid may include one or more of the following: total volume, odor, color, turbidity, viscosity, coagulability, specific gravity, smear for Gram stain and acid-fast stain, total and differential blood cell count, protein, amylase, LDH, pH, aerobic, anaerobic, and acid-fast cultures, and cytologic study for neoplastic cells. In general, a *transudative* effusion has an LDH level less than 200 μ, a pleural fluid/serum LDH ratio less than 0.6, and a pleural fluid/serum protein level less than 0.5. *Exudative* effusions are characterized by LDH and protein levels in excess of these values.

2. Tube thoracostomy. Close drainage of the pleural spaces is obtained by tube thoracostomy. Chest tubes are used routinely after thoracostomy, and they are required in the management of traumatic or spontaneous pneumothorax, hemothorax, recurrent pleural effusions, and empyema.

Three technics of tube thoracostomy are commonly used. The chest tube can be passed percutaneously over a trocar after a small incision in the skin. This technic is most effective with a small tube (No. 12, 16) in the elective setting for pneumothorax. The second method is to insert the tube through an opening made in the chest wall with a hemostat, after incision of the skin with a scalpel. This method allows insertion of a finger into the pleural space to be certain that the pleural cavity, not the abdomen, has been entered and also to ensure that adhesions of the lung to the pleura do not result in damage to the lung when the tube is inserted. The third method is to insert a small pigtail catheter under CT or ultrasound guidance. This is most suitable for smaller loculated collections.

The tube should be clamped during insertion. Prior to connection to water seal drainage, a sample of fluid may be taken for analysis. The tube should then be secured to the chest wall with a simple stitch. Care of chest tube is described on page 371.

3. Bronchoscopy. Flexible fiberoptic bronchoscopes are used routinely in the elective setting to examine the tracheobronchial tree and to perform biopsies, brushings, and washing of abnormal areas for diagnosis. This procedure requires only topical anesthesia and is easily performed. Massive hemoptysis and tracheobronchial foreign bodies may require the use of a rigid bronchoscope. This procedure usually requires general anesthesia.

4. Cervical mediastinoscopy is performed by passing a short endoscope along the pretracheal space into the upper mediastinum through a small transverse incision just above the suprasternal notch, using general anesthesia. Biopsy of mediastinal nodes and masses is possible as far down as the carina and upper mainstem bronchi. This procedure has been used as a routine part of the preoperative staging of lung cancer. Many advocate a selective approach, based on the finding of nodes or masses greater than 1.5 cm in size on CT or MRI scans. Several nonsurgical thoracic diseases of the antero/superior mediastinum, such as lymphoma and sarcoid, may require substantial tissue for diagnosis, which can be achieved with this approach. Complications are infrequent and include hemorrhage (0.3%), pneumothorax, and injury to the laryngeal nerve and esophagus.

5. Anterior mediastinoscopy (Chamberlain procedure) is performed by a small incision over the left third costosternal cartilage. The medial head of the third rib and cartilage is resected in order to expose the aortopulmonary window. This is the frequent site of nodal metastases from left upper lobe lung cancers and is inaccessible by cervical mediastinoscopy. A short endoscope is then placed into the aortopulmonary area to sample lymph nodes. CT or MRI should indicate enlarged lymph nodes in this area before anterior mediastinoscopy is performed.

6. Scalene node biopsy. Anterior scalene and paratracheal nodes may be excised for diagnostic purposes if they are enlarged. Mediastinoscopy has replaced biopsy of clinically uninvolved scalene nodes as a staging procedure because the diagnostic yield is low.

7. Percutaneous needle biopsy. Many lung and mediastinal masses can be biopsied or aspirated percutaneously under fluoroscopic or CT guidance in order to obtain tissue for diagnosis. Pneumothorax may occur in 2% to 10% of patients, and air embolism is rare but usually fatal.

8. Thoracoscopy. Through an incision similar to that used for tube thoracostomy, a videothoracoscope is inserted into the pleural space. This is usually performed under general anesthesia, using a double-lumen endotracheal tube to allow collapse of the lung on that side. Biopsy and stapling instruments can be inserted through separate incisions, providing for generous samples of the lung, pleura, or mediastinum. This technic has replaced thoracotomy for lung biopsy and is particularly useful in patients with undiagnosed diffuse interstitial lung infiltrates.

9. Thoracotomy. This is a major surgical procedure in which the pleural cavity is opened under direct vision by an incision in an intercostal space for both diagnostic and therapeutic procedures. Exploratory thoracotomy may occasionally be indicated when intrathoracic pathology is present and noninvasive means of diagnosis are unsuccessful. Thoracotomy is most often performed as a therapeutic procedure. Examples include drainage of a loculated empyema, resection of a mediastinal mass, and pulmonary resection for lung cancer (most common). Types of resection include wedge resection, segmentectomy, lobectomy, sleeve lobectomy, pneumonectomy, and sleeve pneumonectomy. The exact procedure is determined by the pathologic process.

B. PREOPERATIVE AND POSTOPERATIVE CARE

1. Preoperative evaluation. It is necessary to evaluate patients for their ability to withstand thoracotomy, particularly if pulmonary resection is planned. All major organ systems and in particular the pulmonary system must be evaluated for reserve function. Tests of pulmonary function and preparation of the patient with chronic respiratory disease are discussed in Chapter 2.

2. Postoperative care. The immediate objective of management after thoracic surgery or trauma is complete expansion and normal function of the lung, without residual air or fluid collections in the chest.

a. Position and ambulation. (1) The patient should be placed in a semisitting position as soon as tolerated. This makes breathing and coughing more efficient. (2) Pneumonectomy patients should lay alternately on the back and on the operated side. If such a patient is placed on his normal side, severe respiratory embarrassment may result. (3) Ambulation should be started as soon as possible postoperatively. Breathing and other exercises to mobilize the shoulder girdle and thoracic cage should be taught preoperatively and encouraged throughout the convalescent period.

b. Prevention of atelectasis. See Chapter 2.

c. Pain relief. The dosage of narcotics given parenterally to thoracic patients should be individualized. Pain relief sufficient to make coughing bearable is essential, but depression of respiration and cough reflex must be minimized. Barbiturates can be used for sedation to reduce the need for narcotics. Supplementary methods for obtaining pain relief include intercostal nerve blocks and epidural or intrapleural catheters for local delivery of analgesics. Epidural morphine may provide dramatic analgesia but can be accompanied by significant respiratory depression. Careful monitoring is essential.

d. Ventilatory assistance. See Chapter 2.

e. Management of chest tubes. One or more chest tubes for postoperative drainage of fluid and air are usually placed through the intercostal spaces prior to thoracotomy closure. Tubes are rarely used when pneumonectomy has been performed. Continuous functioning of these tubes is essential to ensure full lung expansion and obliteration of pleural space. Tubes should be attached at the operating table to gentle suction with water seal incorporated into the system. Modern versions of the three-bottle suction system are available in disposable plastic form.

When an air leak from the lung is present, suction should be adjusted to the chest catheter to produce continuous bubbling is seen in the water seal chamber. For large air leaks, it may be necessary to increase the pleural suction up to 40 cm of water or more, in order to pull the lung out to the chest wall and seal the leak. Chest tubes are removed from 24-48 hours after air has stopped leaking, pleural fluid has stopped draining, or the tubes are no longer functioning.

Alveolar air leaks may continue for days and occasionally weeks after segmental resection or lobectomy. These usually seal if tube drainage and constant suction are properly maintained. If an undrained air space of significant size persists, a tube should be placed to obliterate the space. If not, empyema or restricted lung may result. Small, sterile air pockets usually resorb completely without drainage; supplemental oxygen may hasten reabsorption by replacing alveolar nitrogen.

C. COMPLICATIONS. Wound infection and bleeding are uncommon complications after elective thoracic operations, and blood transfusions are seldom required. Complications specific to thoracic surgery are as follows:

1. Atelectasis and pneumonia are frequent after thoracic surgery; they can be minimized if appropriate measures, such as nasotracheal suctioning and incentive spirometry, are taken (see Chapter 2). Reduction of functional residual capacity, impaired tracheobronchial ciliary action, and underlying obstructive lung disease play a significant role in these complications.

2. Chest fluid and empyema. Fluid or blood occasionally accumulates in the chest in spite of tube drainage. Small amounts of sterile fluid and blood resorb without incident. Fluid of sufficient volume to be apparent on radiography should usually be removed as completely as possible by thoracentesis, and cultures should be obtained. If the fluid is infected (empyema), complete evacuation by tube thoracostomy is usually indicated. A loculated empyema often requires precise localization with ultrasonography or CT scan before tube insertion. Systemic antibiotics are administered empirically, then altered as necessary when sensitivity studies are known. Complete removal of air and fluid from the chest and full expansion of the lung preoperatively are the most important means of preventing empyema.

3. Bronchopleural fistula occurs when an air leak from a bronchial stump into the pleural space develops. This complication occurs in approximately 2% of patients and may or may not be associated with an empyema. The fistula usually opens within the first 1-2 weeks after pulmonary resection and is manifest by fever, productive cough, and an air-fluid level on chest radiography. Many close with prolonged closed tube drainage. Bronchoscopic plugging of segmental or subsegmental bronchi may be successful in some patients. Others require open drainage by a short chest tube or rib resection. Rarely, transpericardial closure of the bronchial stump or muscle flap coverage of the fistula via thoracotomy is required.

4. Atrial arrhythmias. Supraventricular arrhythmias, especially atrial fibrillation, occur in up to 20%-30% of patients undergoing thoracotomy. Prophylactic use of appropriate antiarrhythmic drugs is appropriate in some circumstances, but in most patients arrhythmias may be treated as they develop.

5. Gastric dilation. Gastroduodenal ileus is common after thoracotomy. A dilated stomach should be looked for postoperatively, both by physical examination and on the postoperative chest radiograph. If present, it should be treated with nasogastric suction until resolution occurs.

6. Pulmonary insufficiency. Persistent failure of oxygenation and/or ventilation may occur in some patients following thoracotomy, especially if a significant amount of lung tissue was resected. Severe pain, atelectasis, pneumonia, and aspiration are contributing factors, but in most patients obstructive lung disease and emphysema are the primary causes. Aggressive pulmonary toilet, antibiotics, bronchodilators, and mechanical ventilation are usually needed.

7. Myocardial infarction. Although this complication is not specific to thoracic operations, it is the most common cause of operative mortality. Because most patients undergoing pulmonary resection for lung cancer are older and heavy smokers, a careful cardiac history should be elicited preoperatively. This topic is covered in Chapter 2.

II. TRAUMA

Mechanisms of chest injury include penetrating trauma, such as stab wounds; blunt trauma, such as occurs in motor vehicle accidents; blast injury; and electrical injury. Injury to other intrathoracic and extrathoracic organs often occurs along with chest wall and pulmonary injury, but these are not dealt with in this section.

A. RIB FRACTURES. Direct violence is the usual cause of rib fractures, but pathologic fractures may occur with minimal force at sites of metastatic malignancy or bone disease. Flail chest is paradoxical in and out movement with respiration of a segment of chest wall isolated by multiple rib fractures. Ventilation is severely impaired in these patients. An important component of respiratory distress in flail chest is the underlying lung contusion.

Pain sharply localized to the fracture site and aggravated by breathing and other motions of the rib cage is typical. Tenderness and limitation of respiratory motion on the injured side are often present. Severe injury may be complicated by subcutaneous emphysema, pneumothorax, and hemothorax (see below). The above findings are diagnostic of rib fracture, even if chest radiographs with detailed views of the rib do not demonstrate the fracture.

Fractured ribs over the spleen or liver should raise the

question of associated injuries to these organs. Fracture of the first or second rib denotes severe trauma, and the possibility of associated major vascular injury should be considered and ruled out by angiography. A direct correlation exists between the number of ribs fractured and both associated injuries and death.

Treatment. All patients with flail chest, young patients with multiple rib fractures, and elderly patients with any rib fractures must be hospitalized. Serial blood gas determinations and continuous measurement of oxygen saturation are essential.

The pain of uncomplicated rib fracture is best controlled by oral or parenteral analgesics, intercostal nerve block, or epidural catheter. Localized strapping with tape or belts should be avoided owing to limitations of chest wall motion resulting in atelectasis or pneumonia.

Severe thoracic trauma with multiple fractures and flail chest requires immediate intubation with a cuffed endotracheal tube. If this is not available, the patient should be placed flail side down to stabilize the segment. Several weeks of positive-pressure ventilation may be necessary before the chest wall becomes stabilized. Tracheostomy is done if chest wall stabilization has not occurred after 2 or 3 weeks. A tracheostomy tube with a low-pressure cuff controlled by a pilot balloon is preferred. Intensive pulmonary care is required (see Chapter 2). Operative stabilization of a flail segment is required occasionally.

B. STERNAL FRACTURE is caused by severe direct trauma such as a steering wheel injury and may be present in 5%-10% of all thoracic injuries. Multiple rib fractures and other injuries are usually also present. Contusion of the heart is not uncommon. Severe precordial pain and dyspnea are chief symptoms, and arrhythmias are the most common sign. Crepitus and deformity of the sternum may be present.

Often, the only treatment required is rest in the sitting position and pain relief with narcotics or intercostal nerve block for associated rib fractures. If the chest wall is excessively mobile, internal stabilization by controlled mechanical ventilation is the usual treatment. This must be continued for days or weeks until the chest wall stabilizes. Occasionally operative fixation may be indicated.

C. TRAUMATIC RUPTURE OF THE TRACHEA OR BRONCHI. Severe crushing trauma to the chest may cause injury to the trachea or major bronchi. Bronchial rupture, usually with

1-2 cm of the carina, occurs about four times as often as tracheal tear. Tracheobronchial injuries are often overlooked.

Symptoms and signs include dyspnea, subcutaneous emphysema, cyanosis, pain, hemoptysis, shock, cough, pneumothorax, extensive atelectasis, and hemothorax. Chest films and bronchoscopy are indicated. The diagnosis may be overlooked until weeks or months after the injury, when the patient presents with recurrent atelectasis or bronchiectasis from a bronchial stricture.

Treatment is closure of the bronchial tear with suture if the patient's other injuries do not contraindicate thoracotomy. Emergency operation is usually required to relieve airway obstruction or to correct uncontrollable air leak, tracheobronchial hemorrhage, or rapidly advancing mediastinal emphysema. Chronic stricture with obstruction due to delayed treatment requires bronchoplastic surgery. The distal lung, although collapsed, is often functional when reexpanded. Pulmonary resection should therefore be reserved for cases of irreversible damage to the lung parenchyma, airways, or vascular structures.

D. LUNG INJURY. Pulmonary contusion results from blunt or penetrating trauma. Rupture of alveoli, extravasation of blood, and transudation of fluid into the injured area lead to airway obstruction and atelectasis. Copious bloody secretions, chest pain, and evidence of respiratory distress develop 12-24 hours after the injury. Regular chest radiographs frequently underestimate the severity of the injury, showing opacification of variable amounts of parenchyma. Chest CT scans are more accurate. Intensive pulmonary care is required. Avoidance of fluid overload is critical.

Pulmonary laceration is usually caused by penetrating injury, including fragments of fractured ribs. Pneumothorax and hemothorax are treated as outlined below. These measures usually succeed in expanding the lung out to the pleural surface where it adheres, and the laceration heals.

E. HEMOTHORAX. In 90% of cases the source of blood in the pleural space after trauma is systemic vessels in the chest wall, diaphragm, or mediastinum. Bleeding from the pulmonary parenchyma tends to be self-limited. Continued bleeding usually is of systemic origin. Several liters of blood may accumulate in the thorax. In 75% of patients, the blood remains fluid.

Symptoms are related to the chest injury, either penetrating or blunt. Shock may be present with large amounts of blood loss. Chest radiography is confirmatory.

Treatment is directed toward immediate replacement of blood loss and closed pleural drainage by large-bore tube thoracostomy. Autotransfusion should be considered if bleeding is brisk. Other general supportive measures are also instituted. If marked hemorrhage continues or recurs (as indicated by reappearance of shock or continued loss of 100-200 ml or more of blood every hour through the thoracostomy tube), operation should be considered. Most such persistent bleeding is from systemic vessels, most commonly the intercostal vessels. Only 10%-20% of patients require operation. Hemopneumothorax is common. Early placement of large-bore chest tubes through both the upper anterior and lower posterolateral chest wall may be necessary to achieve complete evacuation of air and blood and full lung expansion. Some cases require special studies such as arteriography for definitive diagnosis.

F. TRAUMATIC PNEUMOTHORAX. Air may enter the pleural space from an open sucking wound in the chest wall or more commonly an air leak in an injured lung. It can also be caused by injury to major airways or the esophagus.

1. Sucking wounds of the thorax must be closed immediately with a bulky occlusive dressing of petrolatum gauze held in place by adhesive tape or a bandage encircling the chest. Open pneumothorax causes marked to-and-fro shifting of the mediastinum during respiration (mediastinal flutter), which must be promptly controlled to prevent respiratory and circulatory failure. Surgical closure of the wound in the chest wall is carried out as soon as the patient's condition permits. Meanwhile, air is evacuated from the chest (see below).

2. Closed pneumothorax is caused by air leak from the lung, tracheobronchial tree, or esophagus. It may result from either a penetrating chest wound or blunt injury. Treatment is described in this chapter.

G. SUBCUTANEOUS AND MEDIASTINAL EMPHYSEMA occurs when air leaking from an injured tracheobronchial tree, lung, or esophagus dissects into the mediastinum and subcutaneous tissues. In advanced cases, emphysema extends from head to foot and produces an alarming degree of swelling and crepitation, especially of the head, neck, and scrotum. Air in the tissues causes little harm and as a rule requires no specific treatment.

Attention should be directed toward correction of the underlying cause. Pneumothorax frequently accompanies mediastinal emphysema and should be treated with tube thoracostomy.

Mediastinal emphysema on rare occasions produces sufficient tension to threaten life; if dyspnea, cyanosis, tachycardia, and shock progress in spite of other measures, tracheostomy or cervical mediastinotomy are indicated to decompress the tissue under tension.

H. AIR EMBOLISM is a highly lethal problem occurring in 4% of major thoracic trauma cases. Rib fracture or penetrating injury results in a fistula between the bronchus and pulmonary vein. With positive airway pressure (Valsalva or intubation), air is forced into the systemic circulation, causing focal neurologic deficits or cardiovascular collapse. Fundoscopic examination shows air in the retinal capillaries. Stable patients are treated by stapling of the lacerated lung; emergency thoracotomy and clamping of the hilum may salvage 50% of unstable patients.

I. EMPYEMA. Traumatic violation of the pleural space may result in bacterial contamination, resulting in empyema.

J. PNEUMONIA. Atelectasis, pneumonia, and possibly respiratory failure may develop after chest wall or lung injury. The likelihood of these problems depends on a balance of the severity of injury, degree of proper management, and individual pulmonary reserve.

III. TRACHEOBRONCHIAL FOREIGN BODY

Infants, children, and intoxicated, anesthetized, or unconscious individuals are most likely to aspirate foreign bodies. Coughing, choking, and cyanosis may occur immediately after inhalation but often subside for a variable period. Depending upon the size, nature, and site of lodgment of the foreign body, later findings may include cough, wheezing, atelectasis, and pulmonary infection. Unless the foreign body is radiopaque, radiographic evidence is indirect: obstructive emphysema, atelectasis, or pneumonitis. Intermittent findings of this nature, especially in children, are highly suggestive of foreign body. Rigid bronchoscopy should be performed and removal of the foreign body attempted. If it is successful, inflammatory reaction usually subsides promptly. If it is unsuccessful, thoracotomy and bronchotomy or resection is necessary. Foreign bodies in the tracheobronchial tree should always be removed because prolonged retention usually leads to bronchiectasis or abscess formation requiring pulmonary resection.

IV. DISEASES OF THE CHEST WALL

A. DEFORMITIES. Pectus excavatum (funnel breast) is a congenital malformation characterized by depression of the sternum below the sternomanubrial junction, with symmetric inward bending of the costal cartilages. It may be familial but is most often sporadic in incidence. It is more common in patients with congenital heart disease or Marfan's syndrome. As the infant develops, kyphoscoliosis may also occur. Severe degrees of pectus excavatum very rarely impair pulmonary and/or cardiac functions. Usually, the only disturbance is cosmetic. Operative treatment may be indicated for either reason and entails resection of the deformed costal cartilages with sparing of the perichondrium and elevation of the sternum. Operation before the age of 5 years is technically easier and spares the child the psychological trauma of the deformity.

Pectus carinatum (pigeon breast) is a related but much less common deformity than pectus excavatum. The sternum is elevated by outward bending of the costal cartilages. This is strictly a cosmetic problem. Operative treatment is performed by resection of the abnormal costal cartilages, and depression and stabilization of the sternum to the level of the anterior chest wall.

B. TUMORS of the chest wall may arise from the soft tissues or bony structures and include primary neoplasms, metastatic neoplasms, and neoplasms that invade by direct extension (e.g., primary lung carcinoma). Primary neoplasms are uncommon, and about half are malignant. Pain and mass effect are the salient clinical features. Chondrosarcoma, fibrosarcoma, and plasmacytoma are the most common malignant tumors, and chondroma and fibrous dysplasia are the most common benign lesions. Males are affected twice as often as females. Radiographic findings may be characteristic, and CT scans are essential in planning resection. Accurate histologic diagnosis, usually by a generous incisional biopsy, is critical to treatment. Benign lesions are cured with local excision, whereas malignant lesions respond best to a multidisciplinary approach based on histopathology.

Metastatic chest wall tumors are uncommonly treated by surgical means because widespread disease is usually present. Tumors of the genitourinary tract, thyroid, and colon and soft tissue sarcomas are particularly likely to spread to the chest wall. Tumors that directly invade the chest wall are most commonly lung cancers. If the lung cancer is otherwise resectable, concomitant chest wall resection with a 2-cm margin is indicated, and prognosis is not adversely affected.

V. DISEASES OF THE PLEURA

Pleural problems may result from inflammation, infection, neoplasm, and altered fluid dynamics.

A. SYMPTOMS AND SIGNS. Pleuritic pain is chest pain associated with inspiration and expiration. Pleuritic pain arises in the parietal pleura or diaphragm. The visceral pleura contains no pain fibers. Respiratory excursion may be limited on the affected side. Acute inflammation is associated with tenderness in the intercostal spaces. A friction rub may be audible. If pleural effusion develops, pleuritic pain and friction rub lessens, tactile fremitus to the spoken voice diminishes, and dullness to percussion is present. Breath sounds may be exaggerated or bronchial in the area of effusion. Dyspnea may occur with large effusions.

B. PLEURAL EFFUSION. Fluid in the pleural space occurs most commonly in congestive heart failure, pneumonia of both bacterial and viral origin, malignant diseases, pancreatitis, pulmonary embolism, cirrhosis with ascites, gastrointestinal diseases, and collagen vascular disease.

Hydrothorax is a serous effusion, either a transudate or exudate depending on the specific gravity, protein content, LDH content, and cell count of the fluid. Pyothorax is synonymous with empyema and is discussed below. Hemothorax is blood in the pleural space, and chylothorax is the accumulation of chyle.

Pleural effusions may be categorized as resulting directly from diseases of the mediastinum, lungs, or chest wall, or indirectly from systemic diseases or diseases affecting distant organ systems. Transudates occur most commonly in congestive heart failure; renal disease, cirrhosis, sarcoidosis, and myxedema are other causes. The specific gravity is less than 1.016 and the protein count is less than 3 g/dl. Exudates have a higher specific gravity and protein count and occur most commonly with malignancy (lung or breast), infections, collagen vascular disease, trauma, and pulmonary embolism. Bloody effusions (>10,000 RBC/ml) occur most commonly in malignancy, trauma, and pulmonary embolism. Fat droplets with low protein levels are characteristic of chylothorax.

Primary or metastatic malignancy of the lung or pleura can

cause pleural effusions. Diagnosis is made by serologic examination of pleural fluid and/or by pleural biopsy. Bronchogenic carcinoma and metastatic breast carcinoma are the most common causes of malignant effusion.

Treatment must be individualized based on life expectancy, extent of disability from the effusion, and the tumor sensitivity to radiation or chemotherapy. Treatment options include repeated thoracentesis, tube thoracostomy with or without pleural sclerosis using doxycycline or talc, thoracostomy with drainage and pleurodesis, and finally hormonal, chemotherapy, or radiation therapy. The prognosis is poor.

C. EMPYEMA is a suppurative pleural exudate. The pleural space becomes infected by one of the following:
1. Direct spread from a pneumonic focus
2. Lymphatic spread
3. Iatrogenic contamination as a result of operation, thoracentesis, or tube thoracostomy
4. Extension from below the diaphragm
5. Hematogenous infection
6. Ruptured thoracic viscus
7. Lung abscess
8. Generalized sepsis

Causative organisms include aerobic and anaerobic bacteria, fungi, and the tubercle bacillus. The AIDS epidemic has added a new immunosuppressed patient population with pleural infections due to unusual causes. Approximately 50% of empyemas are secondary to complications of pneumonia.

1. Acute and transitional empyemas

a. Diagnosis of acute empyema is seldom difficult. A predisposing condition is usually apparent. Findings related primarily to the empyema consist of chest pain, cough, malaise, fever, and leukocytosis. Large acute effusion may be associated with considerable toxicity and dyspnea. Physical examination discloses signs of pleural fluid. More accurate localization is provided by chest films, CT scan, or ultrasonography. If air is seen in the empyema cavity on radiography, it can generally be assumed that a bronchopleural fistula has developed, although occasionally gas-producing organisms may be the cause. Thoracentesis is done promptly to obtain material for smears, cultures, and antibiotic sensitivity studies. Bronchoscopy should always be considered to rule out endobronchial tumor or foreign body.

b. Treatment. The principles of treatment in empyema are early evacuation of all fluid and purulent exudate to achieve complete lung expansion, and eradication of the infecting organisms by adequate drainage, antibiotic therapy, and supportive measures. Thoracentesis may be used for diagnosis and for localization of the optimal site for chest tube drainage. Rarely, repeated aspiration by thoracentesis may be used for therapy in smaller, more serous collections or in pediatric patients. Tube thoracostomy, however, is usually the treatment of choice. If the exudate is thick or large in volume, adequate chest tube drainage should be provided. Although tube thoracostomy is the mainstay of treatment, even acute empyema may loculate early (especially with *Staphylococcus aureus*) or form septations (transitional). Many of these patients benefit from instillation of fibrinolytic enzymes (e.g., streptokinase) through the chest tube or thoracoscopy, to break down the loculations and promote complete drainage. If these methods fail, thoracotomy and open evacuation may be necessary.

c. Prognosis. Postpneumonic empyema usually subsides promptly when treatment is begun early. Empyema due to other causes is often more complicated and the prognosis less satisfactory. When closed methods of management fail, treatment must be along the lines described below. Successful treatment should result in full expansion of the lung.

2. Chronic empyema is an established abscess of the pleural space, usually beginning 4–6 weeks following the acute illness. As an empyema becomes chronic, fibroblasts and capillaries infiltrate the pleura, which thickens and adheres firmly around the encapsulated exudate. There may be a history of recent acute empyema, or chronic empyema may exist for years in a latent or intermittently symptomatic state.

Empyemas become chronic for the following reasons:
1. Delay in diagnosis or inadequate treatment of the acute stage
2. Bronchopleural fistula
3. Specific infections such as tuberculosis or actinomycosis
4. Retained foreign body
5. Osteomyelitis of a rib
6. Disease of the lung preventing expansion
7. Underlying malignant neoplasm
8. Immunosuppression

a. Diagnosis. Cough and recurrent fever are usually the principal complaints. When some form of suppurative lung disease is associated with the empyema, the cough is usually productive of frankly purulent and sometimes foul-smelling sputum. Chest pain, clubbing of the fingers, chronic malaise, dyspnea, anorexia, and weight loss may occur. Draining sinuses are occasionally present. Physical examination discloses signs of chest fluid or thickened pleura. Respiratory excursions are usually limited on the affected side, sometimes accompanied by contraction of the thoracic cage. These changes are usually readily apparent on radiography.

Thoracentesis is performed to obtain material for examination of smears and cultures for pyogenic and acid-fast organisms.

b. Treatment. Anemia, malnutrition, and debility due to chronic sepsis should be corrected. Systemic antibiotic therapy is usually indicated as an adjunct to drainage or other local treatment.

The specific method of local drainage requires judgment and attention to individual detail in each case. If the exudate is relatively thin and the pleura not markedly thickened, closed drainage by tube thoracostomy may be effective. However, chronic empyema frequently requires open drainage. This is accomplished under local or general anesthesia by resection of a small segment of rib over the lower portion of the cavity. A generous biopsy specimen of the wall of the empyema cavity should be obtained for culture and pathology. A large tube is inserted and is shortened gradually as the cavity slowly heals, which may require many weeks or even months.

Large or complex cavities, such as postpneumonectomy cavities associated with bronchopleural fistula, are well managed by the Eloesser flap method to provide chronic open drainage.

A well-drained residual cavity, such as a postpneumonectomy empyema space, may occasionally be sterilized using the closed Claggett method. Patients in whom infection has been controlled by antibiotics or drainage may be suitable candidates for decortication, in which thickened pleura is excised to permit full expansion of the lung. Expansion is carefully maintained postoperatively by closed tube drainage. Decortication combined with pulmonary resection is the treatment of choice in selected cases of bronchopleural fistula, bronchiectasis, lung abscess, and other disorders in which the underlying lung is severely damaged.

A final form of treatment is resection of the empyema cavity. This is indicated for small, well-developed empyema cavities. The advantage of this technic is that the entire cavity may be removed en bloc without spillage of the infected material.

3. Tuberculous empyema, much less common since the advent of antituberculosis drugs, is always a complex management problem. Bronchopleural fistula and secondary infection are frequently present. The proper timing and selection of therapeutic procedures require experience and judgment. Consideration must be given to the systemic reaction of the patient, the extent of the tuberculosis, and the response to specific chemotherapy.

Tuberculous empyema (without secondary infection) may respond to general supportive measures, appropriate antibiotics and closed drainage by repeated thoracentesis or tube thoracostomy. Closed drainage is always used in order to minimize secondary pyogenic infection.

Mixed infections of the pleura with tuberculosis, usually associated with bronchopleural fistula, may occasionally respond to intensive treatment along the same lines combined with appropriate antibiotic agents. In these cases, decortication with or without resection is more often required.

Rarely some cases of chronic empyema or tuberculous empyema may progress to form a *fibrothorax*. In this condition, the lung is entrapped by a thick, rigid layer of fibrous tissue. Significant restrictive lung disease may follow and may respond dramatically to decortication.

D. NEOPLASMS OF THE PLEURA. Primary tumors of the pleura are very rare. The majority of pleural tumors are metastatic, with carcinoma of the lung and breast and lymphoma accounting for 75% of cases. Benign primary tumors such as lipomas, endotheliomas, and cysts do occur but are very rare. The most common and clinically important primary pleural neoplasms are mesotheliomas. Chest films, chest CT scans, cytologic analysis of pleural fluid, and pleural biopsy should lead to a diagnosis in most patients with pleural tumors.

The most frequent primary pleural neoplasm is mesothelioma. Both benign and malignant forms exist, but the malignant form is far more common. Benign mesothelioma is localized tumor that arises from the visceral pleura in approximately 70% of cases. Half of the time, this tumor is asymptomatic. In approximately 20% of cases, a paraneoplastic syndrome such as hypertrophic pulmonary osteoarthropathy or hypoglycemia exists. The treatment is surgical resection, which cures approximately 90% of patients.

Malignant mesothelioma may develop at the site of pleural injury from a number of causes. The inhalation of asbestos fibers, especially crocidolite, is carcinogenic and is associated with the development of disease in 5%-7% of patients. A latent period of 20-40 years between the time of exposure and the development of disease is not uncommon. The chief complaint is usually pleural pain, but large size may be attained without any symptoms. Malaise, weakness, cough, dyspnea, weight loss, and fever are also common. Physical and radiologic signs are pleural fluid and thickening.

Histologically, mesotheliomas are classified with soft tissue sarcomas, although a number of types are described (epithelial, sarcomatoid, transitional). The distinction between the epithelial type (most common) and metastatic adenocarcinoma is often difficult. Chest radiographs and CT scan are critical for both diagnosis and staging. Cytologic diagnosis from pleural fluid is frequently inadequate; usually only hyperplastic mesothelial cells are retrieved. Needle biopsy of the pleura is equally unrewarding for lack of sufficiently cellular material; seeding of the biopsy tract with tumor is a recognized problem. Thoracoscopy or thoracotomy is often required to obtain sufficient material for analysis. Hematogenous dissemination is present in about 50% of patients, but these metastases are usually clinically silent, and death generally results from complications arising from the primary lesion. At present, the treatment of malignant pleural mesothelioma is only palliative. Conservative strategies include chemical pleurodesis for control of pleural effusions. Aggressive radiation and/or chemotherapy has some success in controlling symptoms, but no survival benefit has been documented. Similarly, radical pleurectomy and extrapleural pneumonectomy have not been shown to significantly alter survival, which averages 8-12 months.

VI. DISEASES OF THE LUNG

A. LUNG ABSCESS. The causes of lung abscesses are (1) aspiration of infected material or foreign body (50%), (2) necrotizing pneumonia (20%), (3) septic embolus or infection of a pulmonary infarct, (4) bronchial obstruction by tumor, (5) infection of a cyst or bulla, (6) extension of bronchiectasis into the parenchyma, (7) penetrating chest trauma, and (8) transdiaphragmatic extension of infection, such as a subphrenic or amebic abscess. When a lung abscess develops in childhood, a foreign body should be suspected, whereas in older age groups, bronchial obstruction by cancer should be considered.

1. Diagnosis

a. Symptoms. A history of alcoholism, IV drug abuse, or immunosuppression is often present. There may be a latent period of several days or weeks during which only malaise and fever are noted. Cough, pleuritic pain, chills, and fever occur as the process develops. Within a few days, the patient may suddenly cough up a large among of foul, purulent sputum, usually blood-streaked or frankly bloody. Copious malodorous sputum associated with the debility of long-standing infection is typical of chronic abscess.

b. Laboratory tests. Leukocytosis and anemia are usually consistent with severe infection. Sputum shows infection and may disclose the cause, such as tuberculosis or neoplasm.

c. Radiographs. Early chest radiographs often show only an area of consolidation; cavitation with fluid level and surrounding pneumonitis is seen later. CT scans are useful to reveal the location, extent, and early evidence of cavitation. It may also reveal neoplasm or multiple abscesses.

d. Bronchoscopy is usually indicated to rule out an obstructing bronchial lesion such as carcinoma or foreign body and to ascertain the degree of internal drainage, and may be therapeutic.

2. Complications

include brain abscess, massive hemoptysis, amyloidosis, and pyopneumothorax. Rupture of the abscess into the pleural space may produce tension pneumothorax or localized empyema. There may be sudden onset of pleural pain, dyspnea, and occasionally shock. This can be a surgical emergency requiring immediate tube thoracostomy.

3. Medical treatment.

In acute abscess, antibiotics are the mainstay of treatment to minimize lung destruction and eradicate the infection. The majority of lung abscesses are either staphylococcal or streptococcal. More than 90% of acute lung abscesses respond favorably to intensive antibiotic therapy. The response of chronic abscesses is less satisfactory, but antibiotics usually reduce the pulmonary infection to a significant degree. Adjuvant supportive therapy includes postural drainage, bronchoscopic aspiration to promote drainage, and adequate nutrition. Hospital mortality for lung abscess is now approximately 5%.

4. Surgical treatment

a. Acute abscess. Medical measures should be given a thorough trial before surgery is considered. Evidence of satisfactory progress includes decrease in cough, sputum, fever, and toxicity and radiologic evidence of diminishing pulmonary infiltration and/or cavitation. If improvement has not occurred or if progress is arrested after 3-6 weeks, surgical treatment may be warranted. The condition of the patient may make resection unwise, and simple palliative drainage is indicated. This may be accomplished by closed tube thoracostomy, pigtail catheter insertion by interventional radiology, or rib resection. Massive hemoptysis can usually be controlled by angiographic embolization.

b. Chronic abscess that is unresponsive to medical management usually requires resection of the involved segment or lobe. Preoperatively, infection should be vigorously treated by antibiotics, postural drainage, and general supportive therapy. Bronchoscopy and chest CT scans should be obtained to explore the possibility of foreign body or neoplasm. In very poor risk patients, tube thoracostomy or interventional radiology drainage may be appropriate.

B. BRONCHIECTASIS is a disorder characterized by tubular or saccular dilatation and chronic infection of the distal bronchial tree. Most cases are secondary to focal pneumonitis occurring in childhood during an attack of pertussis, measles, scarlet fever, or other infection. Obstruction of the bronchi by foreign body is an occasional cause. The basal segments of the lower lobes, the lingula, and the right middle lobe are the usual sites of bronchiectasis. Bronchiectasis has markedly diminished in incidence since the introduction of antimicrobial agents for bacteria and tuberculosis.

1. Diagnosis

a. Symptoms and signs. Chronic cough productive of much purulent sputum, more marked on arising in the morning, and recurrent attacks of pulmonary infection, often dating back to childhood, with fever, malaise, and increased cough and sputum, are characteristic. Hemoptysis occurs at some time in about half of cases and may be severe.

Coarse, moist rales are audible over the involved segments. Bronchial breathing and other chest findings are related to the extent of parenchymal involvement. Clubbing and hypertrophic pulmonary osteoarthropathy occur in severe cases.

b. Laboratory tests. Bacteriologic studies of the sputum always reveal mixed infection, usually predominantly streptococci and staphylococci. Acid-fast infection should be ruled out.

c. Radiographs. Plain films of the chest usually show increased bronchial markings and a variable degree of peribronchial infiltration, but changes may be minimal or absent. High-resolution CT scans show dilated distal bronchi and have replaced bronchography.

d. Bronchoscopy should be performed to obtain uncontaminated material for culture, to localize infected segments, and to rule out neoplasm or foreign body.

2. Treatment. Postural drainage, antibiotics, and treatment of underlying conditions (e.g., sinusitis) are important. Bronchodilators and expectorants may assist in clearing secretions. Good nutrition and ample rest are essential.

Pulmonary resection is performed in rare patients who have disease limited to one lobe and who do not respond to medical therapy.

C. PULMONARY SEQUESTRATION is a developmental anomaly of the lung in which a bud of lung tissue fails to communicate with the tracheobronchial tree. Two types are recognized: intralobar, which is completely surrounded by normal lung, and extralobar, in which the abnormal tissue is surrounded by a separate pleural lining. The former is more common, usually presenting in children or young adults as a lower lobe lung abscess with cough and fever. The latter is associated with other congenital anomalies, and most patients present with respiratory insufficiency in the neonatal period. Surgery is necessary for both types, and care must be taken to identify the arterial blood supply to the sequestration, which is usually from the thoracic or abdominal aorta.

D. TUBERCULOSIS. The incidence of this disease has been increasing over the past 5 years as a result of the AIDS epidemic. Early tuberculosis is usually asymptomatic and is detected on routine chest radiography. Characteristic symptoms of advanced disease include cough, weight loss, night sweats, hemoptysis, and pleuritic pain.

The skin test with intermediate strength PPD is positive (>10 mm of induration after 48-72 hours) in >90% of patients with active disease. Culture of sputum, gastric aspirate, or pleural fluid (which may take 3 to 6 weeks for growth) or biopsies of pleura or lung prove the diagnosis.

Antituberculosis chemotherapy is effective in most cases (see Chapter 4). Surgical treatment is indicated for patients with an uncertain diagnosis, failure to respond to chemotherapy, destroyed lung, persistent bronchopleural fistula, intractable hemorrhage, tuberculous bronchiectasis, atypical mycobacterial infections, or surgical complications. Pulmonary resection is the surgical method of choice, but lesser procedures (decortication, drainage of empyema) are sometimes useful. Operative mortality rate for resection is 1%-10%, depending on the extent of the procedure.

E. FUNGAL AND PARASITIC INFESTATIONS

1. Histoplasmosis is a systemic infection caused by the fungus *Histoplasma capsulatum* and is usually manifested by a benign transient pneumonia. The organism is worldwide in distribution, but it is particularly prevalent in central United States, Mexico, Central and South America, northern Europe, and Australia. Histoplasmosis in its chronic form may be associated with nodular pulmonary densities (which may be difficult to distinguish from primary lung carcinoma), apical cavities, bronchiectasis, empyema, or pneumothorax.

Most (90%) patients who inhale *H. capsulatum* spores remain asymptomatic, although some develop a flulike illness. The diagnosis is based on radiographic findings, serologic and skin tests, and cultures of sputum, exudates, or tissues. The clinical picture resembles chronic tuberculosis, from which it may be differentiated by cultures and skin tests. The differentiation is sometimes made difficult by the fact that many patients have both diseases. Involvement of the mediastinal lymph nodes may produce *fibrosing mediastinitis*, which can be a cause of superior vena cava syndrome. Disseminated histoplasmosis is frequently fatal and fortunately rare and is seen most commonly in immunosuppressed patients.

Medical **treatment** consists of itraconazole or amphotericin B. The former is administered orally and is very effective for mild disease. The latter is now reserved for life-threatening cases. Surgical excision is performed for diagnosis in patients with solitary pulmonary nodules or for treatment of large cavitary lesions.

2. Coccidioidomycosis, also known as valley fever, is caused by *Coccidioides immitis,* which is endemic in certain regions of the southwestern United States, Mexico, and Central and South America. The highly infectious organisms (arthrospores) are carried on wind-borne dust and inhaled. Even very brief exposure may produce the disease, and persons traveling through endemic areas may become infected.

About 60% of infections occur without symptoms and are detected only by the conversion of the coccidioidin skin reaction from negative to positive. Clinical manifestations in overt cases usually suggest a respiratory infection and include fever, cough, erythema nodosum, and pleuritic pain. Radiography of the lungs during the primary disease, which may last a few weeks, shows patchy soft infiltration; as this clears, residual nodules or thin-walled cavities with little surrounding infiltration may persist in 5% of patients. In the acute stage, the organisms may be found in sputum cultures. The coccidioidin skin test usually becomes positive after 10-14 days and remains positive for years. The primary infection progresses to the granulomatous stage in 0.2% of cases, and approximately 1% develop disseminated disease (particularly meningitis).

Treatment of mild cases is with itraconazole, although at least 3 months of therapy is needed for effective control. Amphotericin B should be given for chronic cavitary disease or for dissemination. Surgical excision of a nodule or resection of an involved lobe is needed occasionally.

3. Echinococcus (hydatid) cyst of the lung is the larval stage of the dog tapeworm, *Echinococcus granulosis*. Human infection occurs from ingestion of material contaminated with dog feces containing tapeworm eggs, which hatch in the intestine; the larval embryos then penetrate the bowel wall and disseminate via the bloodstream. The larvae may come to rest and develop into hydatid cysts in any part of the body, but the liver (70%) (see Chapter 12) and lungs (20%) are most commonly affected.

Hydatid cyst of the lung may be asymptomatic but usually causes productive cough, minor hemoptysis, chest pain, and fever by local pressure or by rupture with secondary infection. Radiography shows a characteristic sharply defined round or oval density in the lung field. A small crescent of air is sometimes seen between the cyst and the surrounding lung and is pathognomonic. A ruptured, infected cyst has the appearance of a lung abscess. Hydatid cysts are usually solitary but may be multiple. They grow slowly and occasionally reach 15 cm or more in diameter. They are most commonly confused with neoplasm or lung abscess.

Because of the risk of cyst rupture resulting in aspiration or dissemination of disease, all hydatid cysts should be removed surgically if the patient's general condition permits. Unresectable lesions should be treated with mebendazole.

F. PNEUMOTHORAX refers to air or gas in the pleural space. This may originate from rupture of the respiratory system (trachea, bronchi, alveoli), esophagus, or chest wall or may be generated by microorganisms in the pleural space. Pneumothorax may be classified as spontaneous, traumatic, or iatrogenic, depending on the cause. Spontaneous pneumothorax also occurs from barotrauma, commonly in the intensive care setting in patients being ventilated with positive end-expiratory pressure. These patients frequently have underlying chronic obstructive pulmonary disease. Patients with AIDS may develop a particularly refractory spontaneous pneumothorax due to a necrotizing *Pneumocystis* pneumonia. Endometriosis and malignancy are rare causes.

Symptoms are usually acute and are characterized by chest pain, cough, and dyspnea. Physical signs are proportional to the extent of pneumothorax and consist of hyperresonance and diminished to absent breath sounds on the involved side. Diagnosis is confirmed by chest radiography.

Simple pneumothorax is air in the pleural space which equilibrates and stabilizes. **Tension pneumothorax** develops when air progressively accumulates in the pleural space. This usually occurs from a lung leak that acts as a one-way valve, allowing air into but not out of the pleural space. Complete collapse of the lung occurs rapidly, positive pressure develops in the pleural space, and the mediastinal structures shift to the opposite side as intrapleural pressure rises. When positive pressure rises above 15 to 20 cm H_2O in the pleural space, venous return to the heart is impeded and circulatory collapse results. Physical signs include marked dyspnea, cyanosis, shift of the trachea and the apical impulse of the heart to the opposite side, and tympany to percussion and absent breath sounds on the involved side. It may be necessary to begin treatment promptly without waiting for radiography of the chest.

1. Treatment

a. A small pneumothorax (<25% collapse) absorbs completely within a few weeks unless the air leak in the lung continues. The patient need not be at bed rest during this period, but his activity should be limited. Supplemental oxygen may hasten the reabsorption of a pneumothorax by replacing alveolar nitrogen. More rapid expansion can be accomplished by aspiration, preferably with a small plastic catheter, usually through the second interspace anteriorly.

b. Large pneumothorax (>25% collapse) should be treated by tube thoracostomy to expand the lung rapidly and thereby reduce morbidity. Constant suction (-25 cm of water) is applied to the tube, and immediate expansion of the lung usually occurs. Once the lung shows full expansion on radiography and the air leak has ceased for 24 hours, the tube or catheter is removed. The entire process of expansion usually requires 3-5 days.

c. Tension pneumothorax. When tension pneumothorax occurs, a needle should be inserted into the chest through the second or third interspace anteriorly. Air rushes out under pressure and relieves the tension. Treatment thereafter is the same as for spontaneous pneumothorax.

d. Recurrent pneumothorax, either ipsilateral or contralateral, occurs in approximately 20% of cases. If two or more episodes have occurred on one side, the incidence of subsequent episodes rises and further treatment is necessary. Pleural symphysis can be attempted by instillation of sclerosing agents into the pleural cavity without thoracotomy. If this is not successful, thoracoscopy should be considered to excise or staple the blebs and create a pleural symphysis, preferably by pleural abrasion.

G. BENIGN NEOPLASMS OF THE LUNG. Overall, benign tumors represent up to 15% of solitary lesions of the lung, but in nonsmokers represent up to 60% of isolated pulmonary nodules (coin lesions).

1. Hamartoma is the most common benign pulmonary neoplasm (8% of all coin lesions). It is an embryologic remnant consisting largely of cartilage containing variable quantities of epithelial, adipose, or muscular tissue. Men are afflicted more commonly than women, and >80% are asymptomatic. These tumors are usually found in the periphery of the lung; radiographically, their borders are lobulated and sharp and speckled calcifications may be seen, giving the appearance of "popcorn." Wedge resection is performed for diagnosis and therapy; the prognosis is excellent.

2. Other benign tumors are rare and include tumors of epithelial origin (e.g., papilloma, polyps), of mesodermal origin (hemangioma, arteriovenous fistulas, lipomas), and of unknown origin (granuloma, plasma cell tumor). Careful bronchoscopy, fine-needle biopsy, CT, and MRI may provide useful information in the evaluation of these tumors.

H. PRIMARY CARCINOMA OF THE LUNG has consistently been the most common cause of death from cancer in men and since 1985 has surpassed breast cancer as the most common cause of death from cancer in women. Approximately 170,000 new cases of lung cancer were diagnosed in 1992, with 146,000 deaths. The peak incidence is between the ages of 50 and 70 years. Cigarette smoking is the most important causative factor and is present in 90% of cases. Asbestos and other industrial materials are causative as well.

1. Pathologic types

a. Epidermoid (squamous cell) carcinomas comprise 25%-35% of lung tumors. About one third arise in the periphery and two thirds near the hilus. Variable histologic differentiation of these tumors is common; some are well differentiated and others poorly so. Squamous cell carcinomas tend to grow slowly and spread to regional and mediastinal lymphatics prior to hematogenous dissemination.

b. Adenocarcinomas once accounted for about 15% of all lung cancers, but recent epidemiologic data suggest that this is changing dramatically, with recent reports showing that up to 30% of lung cancers are adenocarcinomas; 75% are peripheral and 25% are central. Some that arise in the periphery appear to originate in previous scars. Scar carcinomas (adeno) tend to have a less malignant nature. The more centrally located adenocarcinomas tend to be more malignant than epidermoid cancers and less malignant than small cell cancers.

c. Bronchoalveolar carcinoma is a primary tumor of the lung arising within alveoli and terminal bronchioles and spreading along the surface of the airways to involve other parts of the lung. Compared with bronchogenic carcinoma, bronchoalveolar tumors are less likely to be associated with smoking or chronic lung disease and appear to be a variant of adenocarcinoma. The incidence is approximately 3%-5%. It tends to have a more favorable prognosis and is the only tumor that spreads endobronchially.

d. Undifferentiated small cell (oat cell) carcinomas are highly malignant. About 15%-20% of malignant tumors are of this type; most (80%) arise centrally. These tumors may secrete endocrine hormones and frequently account for paraneoplastic syndromes. The majority of patients have metastatic disease at the time of presentation.

e. Undifferentiated large cell carcinomas are less malignant than oat cell cancers. About 3%-5% of tumors fit into this category.

f. Bronchial adenomas are low-grade malignant tumors; about 15% metastasize. Bronchial carcinoid is the most common type (85%); this is a neuroendocrine neoplasm that occurs twice as often in women. The majority arise in mainstem or lobar bronchi. This tumor is capable of secreting many hormones, although serotonin is the most common.

g. Papillary carcinomas, sarcomas, and hemangiopericytomas are rare, nonbronchogenic malignant tumors of the lung.

2. Diagnosis

a. Symptoms and signs. About 20% of lung cancers are asymptomatic when diagnosed by routine chest radiography or, rarely, sputum cytology. About 85% of asymptomatic lung nodules in smokers over the age of 50 years prove to be malignant. A changing pattern of cough, hemoptysis, chest pain, dyspnea, or weight loss may occur. Pneumonia, localized wheeze, or atelectasis due to bronchial obstruction may be the presenting symptoms, particularly for bronchial carcinoids. Pleuritic pain and pleural effusion may occur. A serous effusion is often caused by lymphatic obstruction, whereas a bloody effusion usually indicates direct pleura extension of the tumor.

A large variety of extrathoracic manifestations may occur even in the absence of metastases. These paraneoplastic syndromes include endocrine and metabolic disorders, vascular and hematologic effects (e.g., thrombophlebitis), connective tissue disorders (e.g., dermatomyositis), and neuromyopathies.

Pancoast's syndrome is a consequence of a tumor in the superior pulmonary sulcus. It consists of pain, weakness of the arm, and Horner's syndrome (ptosis, miosis, enophthalmos, and decreased sweating on the involved side).

Mediastinal spread may cause hoarseness from involvement of the left recurrent laryngeal nerve, diaphragmatic paralysis from phrenic nerve involvement, and superior vena caval obstruction. Hematogenous spread may cause alterations in mental status (brain) or musculoskeletal pain (bone). Metastases to the adrenal glands or liver are usually asymptomatic.

b. Laboratory tests. Sputum cytology is positive in <50% of cases, but this percentage may be improved by repeated specimens or postbronchoscopy specimens from washings or biopsies.

c. Radiographs. Chest films may show a mass in the periphery or in the hilum. Signs of extension may be present. Most peripheral lesions have irregular, indistinct margins. CT scans may be particularly helpful in clinical staging, by assessing the size and location of the primary tumor, mediastinal adenopathy, direct extension of the tumor into the mediastinum or chest wall, and distant metastases, especially adrenal and liver. Head and bone scans should be obtained selectively.

d. Special tests. Bronchoscopy, mediastinoscopy, thoracentesis, percutaneous biopsy, and aspiration cytologies are directed at confirming the diagnosis of lung cancer and assessing its resectability or spread.

Table 9-1. New international staging system for lung cancer: TNM definitions

Primary tumor (T)

TX   Tumor proven by the presence of malignant cells in bronchopulmonary secretions but not visualized by roentgenography or bronchoscopy, or any tumor that cannot be assessed as in a retreatment staging.

T0   No evidence of primary tumor.

TIS   Carcinoma in situ.

T1   A tumor that is 3 cm or less in greatest dimension, surrounded by lung or visceral pleura, and without evidence of invasion proximal to a lobar bronchus at bronchoscopy.*

T2   A tumor greater than 3 cm in greatest dimension, or a tumor of any size that either invades the visceral pleura or has associated atelectasis or obstructive pneumonitis extending to the hilar region. At bronchoscopy, the proximal extent of demonstrable tumor must be within a lobar bronchus or at least 2 cm distal to the carina. Any associated atelectasis or obstructive pneumonitis must involve less than an entire lung.

T3   A tumor of any size with direct extension into the chest wall (including superior sulcus tumors), diaphragm, or the mediastinal pleura or pericardium without involving the heart, great vessels, trachea, esophagus, vertebral body, or a tumor in the main bronchus within 2 cm of the carina without involving the carina.

T4   A tumor of any size with invasion of the mediastinum or involving heart, great vessels, trachea, esophagus, vertebral body, or carina or with presence of malignant pleural effusion.†

Nodal involvement (N)

N0   No demonstrable metastasis to regional lymph nodes.

N1   Metastasis to lymph nodes in the peribronchial or the ipsilateral hilar region, or both, including direct extension.

N2   Metastasis to ipsilateral mediastinal lymph nodes and subcarinal lymph nodes.

N3   Metastasis to contralateral mediastinal lymph nodes, contralateral hilar lymph nodes, or ipsilateral or contralateral scalene or supraclavicular lymph nodes.

Distant metastasis (M)

M0   No (known) distant metastasis.

M1   Distant metastasis present—specify site(s).

---

*The uncommon superficial tumor of any size whose invasive component is limited to the bronchial wall and may extend proximal to the main bronchus is classified as T1.

†Most pleural effusions associated with lung cancer are due to tumor. There are, however, some few patients in whom cytopathologic examination of pleural fluid (on more than one specimen) is negative for tumor and the fluid is nonbloody and is not an exudate. When these elements and clinical judgment dictate that the effusion is not related to the tumor, the cases should be staged T1, T2, or T3, with effusion being excluded as a staging element.

From Mountain CF: *Surg Clin North Am,* 67(5), 1987.

3. Staging. Lung cancer spreads via lymphatics to hilar, paratracheal, supraclavicular, or abdominal nodes. Direct invasion may involve the pericardium or chest wall. Hematogenous metastases commonly affect brain, liver, adrenal, and bones. Preoperative staging of the tumor is imperative for assessing therapeutic options and prognosis. The most common classification is the TMN system for staging tumors. This has recently been revised for lung cancer and is outlined in Tables 9-1 and 9-2. Staging is critical for forming a treatment plan and for prognosis.

4. Treatment protocols recognize two types of lung cancer, non–small cell and small cell. The primary approach and essentially the only curative approach to **non–small cell tumors** is surgical. Radiation therapy and chemotherapy are used as adjuncts. The biologic behavior of **small cell carcinoma** is such that in most cases, it is a disseminated problem at the time of presentation. Surgery therefore is usually not the primary approach, but it may have a role in early-stage disease. The primary approach to small cell carcinoma is combination chemotherapy and radiation. A 70%-90% remission rate and a 15% long-term survival (possible cures) can be expected with stages I to III. Remission rates are about 30% and long-term survival rate is poor for disseminated disease.

Cure rates for non–small cell carcinoma are determined primarily by stage of disease, although histopathology also has some influence. Once tumor spreads to the mediastinal lymph

Table 9-2. New international staging system for lung cancer: stage grouping

Occult carcinoma	TNM		
	TX	**N0**	**M0**
	Carcinoma in situ		
Stage 0			
Stage I	T1	N0	M0
	T2	N0	M0
Stage II	T1	N1	M0
	T2	N1	M0
Stage IIIa	T3	N0	M0
	T1-3	N2	M0
Stage IIIb	Any T	N3	M0
	T4	Any N	M0
Stage IV	Any T	Any N	M1

From Mountain CF: *Surg Clin North Am,* 67(5), 1987.

nodes (N2 disease), 5-year survivals fall significantly, to about 20%-30%.

Two thirds of patients with lung cancer are incurable when the diagnosis is made. Signs of incurability include metastases outside the thorax, metastases to paratracheal nodes or contralateral hilar nodes, malignant pleural effusion, recurrent laryngeal nerve palsy, superior vena cava syndrome, and involvement of the main pulmonary artery. These problems reflect stages IIIb and IV.

Features that do not categorically indicate incurability, but that carry an unfavorable prognosis include involvement of the chest wall, Pancoast's syndrome, tumor visible bronchoscopically within 2 cm of the carina, oat cell tumor, and phrenic nerve involvement.

The patient's medical condition, especially pulmonary function, may contraindicate surgery. An FEV_1 of 1 L or less or resting hypercarbia is a predictor of high risk for pulmonary resection. Patients who are likely to be curable should have staging chest CT scans followed by careful bronchoscopy. Cervical mediastinoscopy to confirm malignant nodal involvement should be done in patients with mediastinal adenopathy >1 cm in diameter which is located in the subcarinal or paratracheal areas by CT scan. Anterior mediastinoscopy (Chamberlain procedure) can be done in patients with adenopathy in the aortopulmonary window, usually associated with left upper lobe primary carcinomas.

About 5%-10% of patients are found to be incurable at operation despite thorough preoperative evaluation. The remainder are treated by pulmonary resection: segmental resection, wedge resection, lobectomy if possible, bilobectomy, sleeve resection, or pneumonectomy if necessary.

Radiation therapy is used for palliation or occasionally as a preoperative adjunct (e.g., in Pancoast's syndrome). Postoperative radiation therapy is recommended for patients with stage III or IIIa disease, to reduce the incidence of local recurrence. Adjuvant chemotherapy may prolong disease-free survival for stage II and II patients. Preoperative radiation with chemotherapy ("neoadjuvant" therapy) may improve resectability rates for advanced tumors (IIIa, IIIb), and the impact on survival is under investigation.

5. Prognosis. Ninety-five percent of patients are dead within 2 years if surgery is not done. The operative mortality rate depends upon age, general condition, and extent of resection; less than 5% of patients aged 40-60 years die after major pulmonary resection. The 5-year survival rate is increased to

60%-80% after lobectomy for stage I carcinoma. Because two thirds of patients are not candidates for operation, the overall survival rate from lung cancer is approximately 10%. However, asymptomatic patients who are operated on solely on the basis of an abnormal radiographic finding with stage I carcinoma have a 5-year survival rate of 80%. This illustrates the importance of routine chest radiography. The prognosis is less favorable if lymph node involvement or blood vessel invasion has occurred. Epidermoid and bronchoalveolar carcinomas are generally considered to have a better prognosis than other cell types; however, it should be emphasized that the single most important prognostic factor is lymph node status.

I. METASTATIC TUMORS. The lungs are the most frequent site of metastases from nearly all organs. Carcinoma of the colon, kidney, breast, testis, uterus, head and neck, and ovary, as well as sarcomas and melanomas, are especially prone to metastasize to the lungs. More than 80% of patients are asymptomatic; typically, peripheral lung nodules are found on screening chest films obtained during follow-up of the original tumor. Surgical resection may be beneficial if the primary tumor is under control, there is no evidence for spread outside the lungs, and resection will not severely compromise lung function. CT scans of both lungs should be done to exclude bilateral metastases. Survival has been shown to correlate with the disease-free interval, number of metastatic lesions, tumor histology, and tumor doubling time. It is important to bear in mind that a pulmonary lesion may be primary instead of metastatic in a patient with a history of cancer elsewhere.

The 5-year survival rate after resection of solitary pulmonary metastases is approximately 25%-40%. Resection is still considered palliative; most patients die of local recurrence or systemic spread of the primary lesion.

J. SOLITARY PULMONARY NODULES. Coin lesions are peripheral, discrete lesions that usually appear on routine radiographs in asymptomatic patients. The lesions may be benign or neoplastic. The incidence of malignancy increases with age (15% <40 years old, 75% >70 years old).

Smoking history, cough, hemoptysis, weight loss, and hypertrophic osteoarthropathy are suggestive of malignancy. Granulomatous disease is unlikely if skin tests are negative. Sputum cytology proves the diagnosis of malignancy in 5%-20% of cases. Concentric or laminated calcification and documented absence of growth for 1 year are strong radiographic indications of benignity.

The differential diagnosis includes granulomas, hamartomas, primary lung cancer, metastatic tumors, and vascular malformations. Patients in whom malignancy cannot be excluded should be managed by surgical excision for diagnosis and treatment. The 5-year survival rate for removal of a malignant coin lesion is as high as 90%, and operative mortality rate is 1%.

VII. MEDIASTINUM

A. MEDIASTINAL MASSES. The mediastinum consists of all structures between the two pleural cavities and is bounded superiorly by the thoracic inlet and inferiorly by the diaphragm. The mediastinum has been divided into anterior, middle, and posterior compartments, each having a predilection for certain diseases (Table 9-3).

1. Diagnosis. About half of mediastinal tumors are discovered on routine chest radiography, and the majority of these are asymptomatic. Specific symptoms and signs depend upon the size, location, and nature of the tumor. Cough, chest pain, and dyspnea are among the commonest complaints. Many tumors produce systemic syndromes as the result of hormone secretion. For example, excessive ACTH production by mediastinal carcinoids can produce Cushing's disease, and mediastinal pheochromocytoma may produce hypertension. In addition, thymomas have a poorly understood association with myasthenia gravis, red cell aplasia, and collagen vascular disorders.

Table 9-3. Distribution of tumors and other mass lesions in the mediastinum

All parts of mediastinum: Lymph node lesions, bronchogenic cysts

Middle mediastinum: Teratoma, thymoma, parathyroid adenoma, aneurysms, lipoma, myxoma, goiter

Anterior mediastinum: Teratoma, lymphangiomas, angiomas, pericardial cysts

Posterior mediastinum: Neurogenic tumors, pheochromocytoma, aneurysms, enterogenous cysts, spinal lesions, hiatus hernia

Physical signs are frequently absent or minimal. The following are of particular interest when present and suggest malignancy: cervical or generalized lymphadenopathy; venous congestion in the head, neck, and upper extremities (superior vena caval or innominate vein obstruction); hoarseness (recurrent nerve palsy); Horner's syndrome (involvement of the cervical sympathetic nerves); and elevation of the diaphragm (phrenic nerve paralysis). Approximately 30% of mediastinal masses are malignant; when this is suspected, a careful search should be made for evidence of primary or metastatic neoplasms outside the mediastinum.

Laboratory tests include chest films, CT or MRI scan, and if a vascular lesion is suspected, angiography. Blood and bone marrow studies for blood dyscrasias are indicated if a lymphoma is suspected. Numerous mediastinal tumor markers have been reported, but only alpha-fetoprotein (nonseminomatous germ cell tumors) and human chorionic gonadotropin (teratomas) are clinically useful. Sputum smears, cultures, and cytologic studies may be indicated. Thyroid scan is diagnostic in substernal goiter. Bronchoscopy and esophagoscopy are useful in some cases. Mediastinoscopy should not be done in potentially curable cases. Direct needle biopsy or aspiration cytology of the mediastinal mass by percutaneous needle or limited anterior thoracostomy may occasionally be feasible in order to establish the diagnosis in an accessible but obviously inoperable tumor, or a lymphoma to be treated with radiation therapy or chemotherapy. Open direct incisional biopsy may be indicated to clarify the specific cell types in lymphoma in order to plan chemotherapy or radiation therapy options.

CT or MRI scans may be misleading when attempting to determine respectability; benign and malignant lesions may be removable even when these scans suggest invasion of vascular or nervous structures.

2. Treatment. The majority of mediastinal masses require thoracotomy or median sternotomy for positive diagnosis and definitive treatment. In most cases nothing is to be gained by delay of exploration when an operable lesion cannot be ruled out. Even benign, asymptomatic lesions should rarely be treated expectantly, because serious complications such as obstruction of vital structures, infection, rupture, or hemorrhage are not uncommon. Some benign lesions can also undergo malignant degeneration.

B. COMMON MEDIASTINAL TUMORS

1. Mediastinal goiter. In 50% of cases, the disease is asymptomatic and is detected by routine chest films; in the remainder, symptoms include dyspnea, cough, pain, and dysphagia. Approximately 10% of patients have hyperthyroidism. The cervical portion of the thyroid is readily demonstrated by radiography. Some degree of tracheal (and possibly esophageal) deviation and compression is typically present. The rounded, homogeneous density in the mediastinum is continuous above with the cervical shadow, and on fluoroscopy the mass is usually seen to move upward with swallowing. Findings on chest CT scan are characteristic, consisting of a nonhomogeneous mass with distinct borders containing coarse calcifications. Prolonged enhancement of the mass after injection of iodinated contrast is typical. If functioning thyroid tissue is present in a mediastinal goiter, the diagnosis can be confirmed by thyroid scan. Superior mediastinal masses consistent with thyroid origin should be examined by radioisotope scanning.

Histologically, intrathoracic thyroid tumors are usually multinodular goiters. Follicular adenoma may be present on occasion, and approximately 3%-5% contain occult carcinoma. Mediastinal goiter should be approached through the usual thyroidectomy incision except in the rare instance (e.g., posterior mediastinal goiter) in which a combined thoracic (median sternotomy) and cervical approach may be required.

2. Bronchogenic and enteric cysts represent embryologic remnants of the respiratory and alimentary tracts, respectively. Bronchogenic cysts are the most common, are lined with respiratory epithelium, and may contain smooth muscle and cartilage in the wall. They are most often found within the pulmonary parenchyma or in the parahilar or right paratracheal regions. Enteric cysts are usually closely associated with the esophagus or are actually intramural and are lined by squamous, gastric, or intestinal epithelium. They are sometimes referred to as alimentary tract duplications.

Bronchogenic cysts usually become symptomatic only in adult life, if at all, whereas 75% of enteric cysts are diagnosed in the first year of life because of such serious complications as peptic ulceration, perforation into a bronchus or pleural cavity, or hemorrhage. The symptoms of both types of cysts depend primarily on their size and location and on the presence of infection. Chest pain, cough, wheezing, and slight dysphagia are the commonest complaints. By radiography, bronchogenic cysts are ovoid, smooth in outline, and homogeneous in density except when a bronchial fistula exists, in which case an air-fluid level can be seen. They are usually located near the midline and, because of their close relation to the trachea, bronchi, and esophagus, may be seen on fluoroscopy to move up and down with respiration or swallowing.

The treatment of these cysts is surgical removal.

3. Thymoma and myasthenia gravis. Several neoplastic conditions may involve the thymus gland, including thymoma, thymic carcinoma, and carcinoid. Of these, thymoma is by far the most common. Thymomas comprise 10%-20% of all mediastinal tumors. Fifty percent of patients are asymptomatic. The histologic differentiation of benign from malignant variants of thymoma is difficult or impossible. About 25% of these lesions break through their capsule and invade locally or implant on neighboring surfaces; in this sense they are "malignant." Lymphogenous or hematogenous metastases are quite rare. Roentgenographically, the benign tumor is round or oval and sharply delineated from the surrounding tissue. Its typical location is anterior to the aortic arch and the base of the heart.

Thymoma occurs in about 15% of patients with myasthenia gravis, and various estimates indicate that 20%-50% of patients with thymoma have myasthenia gravis. In the past, the occurrence of myasthenia in patients with a thymoma was thought to have a negative impact on survival. With improvement in drug therapy and plasmapheresis, this is no longer true. In young women, the removal of a nonneoplastic thymus gland is associated with an increased remission rate in myasthenia gravis. Thymomas should be removed because 25% are locally invasive. Total thymectomy (median sternotomy) is indicated in most patients with myasthenia gravis whether or not a tumor is present; patients with a nonthymomatous gland respond best.

4. Teratomas. The term *teratoma* indicates that a tumor is composed of tissues derived from all three germ layers and that all those tissues are foreign to the organ in which they are found. They are most frequently seen in persons between the ages of 20 and 40 years. About 33% are asymptomatic; the remainder cause cough, chest pain, dyspnea, or other pressure symptoms. About 20% are malignant. Dermoid cyst is a type of benign, unilocular teratoma containing sebaceous material and hair and lined by squamous epithelium and dermal appendages. Teratomas are homogeneous, discrete, round, and smooth unless local invasion has occurred. Typically, chest CT scans show a cystic structure that may contain calcium, bone, and fat.

Treatment is by excision, which is curative in benign lesions. The prognosis of malignant teratoma is **very poor,**

as most patients die within 2 years after diagnosis. Chemotherapy may prolong survival.

5. Lymphoma is the most frequent cause of a mediastinal mass. The majority of mediastinal lymphomas are found in the anterior and middle compartments, arising from nodal tissue as a part of systemic disease; in 10% of patients, the disease is confined to the mediastinum. The commonest symptoms are cough, pain, dyspnea, wheezing, hoarseness, weight loss, fatigue, and fever. Peripheral lymphadenopathy or splenomegaly may be present. The mediastinal tumor consists of involved lymph nodes, usually in the anterior or middle mediastinum. Hodgkin's lymphoma, lymphoblastic lymphoma, and diffuse large-cell non-Hodgkin's lymphoma account for 90% of primary mediastinal lymphomas. Adequate histologic sampling of lymphomas may be critical, as the tumor biology and response to therapy vary according to the type of lymphoma. Radiation therapy and chemotherapy are the primary treatment modalities.

6. Neurogenic tumors are tumors arising from intercostal nerve sheaths (neurilemmoma, neurofibroma), autonomic ganglia (ganglioneuroma, ganglioneuroblastoma), or paraganglionic nervous system (chemodectoma, pheochromocytoma). They account for 20% to 25% of all mediastinal tumors in adults and 50% of mediastinal tumors in children. Nearly all are found in the posterior mediastinum; neurofibroma and neurilemmoma are the most common types. The malignancy rate is 1%-4% in adults and 50% in children.

Neurogenic tumors are usually asymptomatic. Hormone secretion by ganglioneuromas (VIP) and pheochromocytomas (catecholamines) can produce watery diarrhea and hypertension, respectively. Chest radiographs characteristically show a round, homogeneous mass with distinct borders in the posterior mediastinum. Rib or vertebral erosion may occur. Approximately 10% extend into the intervertebral foramen, resulting in the "dumbbell" lesion.

Treatment is by excision. It is important to perform myelography or CT preoperatively if intraspinal extension is suspected because the surgical approach may be different in these cases.

C. MEDIASTINITIS. Acute or chronic mediastinitis usually occurs as a complication of some other primary disorder such as dental or oropharyngeal infection (Ludwig's angina), esophageal perforation, tracheobronchial perforation, trauma, or esophageal leak following intrathoracic surgical anastomosis, or as a complication of some other interventions, such as median sternotomy for cardiac surgery. Chest pain, fever, leukocytosis, and malaise are common symptoms, and the patient may appear quite toxic. Chest CT scans should be obtained promptly to define the location and extent of infection and to provide a baseline for therapeutic response.

Management of mediastinitis is varied and should be directed toward the underlying cause. Esophageal or tracheobronchial perforations should be promptly treated surgically with primary repair and mediastinal drainage. Acute mediastinitis secondary to oropharyngeal infection may simply require debridement and drainage of either one or both pleural cavities. Supportive therapy such as IV antibiotics, nasogastric suctioning, and total parenteral nutrition may be critical.

Anterior mediastinal infection after cardiac surgical procedures occurs in approximately 2% of patients and may be treated with sternal debridement and closure over irrigation catheters for antibiotic instillation. Most recently, muscular flaps (latissimus dorsi, pectoralis major, and rectus abdominis muscles) have significantly improved the prognosis after serious mediastinal infections following cardiac surgery.

10

Heart and Great Vessels

Fraser Keith

The surgical management of diseases of the heart and great vessels requires application of general surgical principles, a knowledge of special diagnostic techniques (ECG, echocardiography, radionuclide scanning, MRI, and CT imaging, cardiac catheterization, and angiography) as well as familiarity with the technology of extracorporeal circulation.

The ability to assess adequacy of cardiac function, peripheral perfusion, and gas exchange is crucial. This requires a thorough and systematic evaluation of multiple systems including cerebral function (mental status), pulmonary function (ventilation, arterial blood gases), renal function (urine output, serum/urine electrolytes, osmolarity, creatinine, BUN), hepatic function (bilirubin, AST, ALT, coagulation factors), and extremity perfusion (pulses, skin color/temperature). These clinical observations must then be integrated with the various hemodynamic indices (systemic/pulmonary artery pressure, central venous and pulmonary artery wedge pressure, cardiac output, arterial and mixed venous O_2 saturations) in order to determine whether cardiac function is satisfying tissue needs.

The technology of **extracorporeal circulation** enables blood flow to be temporarily diverted from its normal pathways in the body and directed instead through externally positioned mechanical devices (pumps, oxygenators, heat exchangers, dialysis/ultrafiltration membranes). Specially trained individuals—perfusionists—operate these devices, but all surgical and anesthesia personnel should be familiar with the scientific principles. Despite improvements in technology, extracorporeal circulation has numerous deleterious effects (activation of the coagulation, fibrinolytic, and complement cascades; platelet aggregation; and neutrophil activation) that result from contact of blood with the artificial surfaces and limit the duration of safe use. Continuous systemic anticoagulation, usually with heparin, is essential during extracorporeal circulation to prevent clotting. The adequacy of anticoagulation must be checked periodically by simple tests (ACT, heparin level) and additional anticoagulant provided to meet target values. Once extracorporeal circulation is discontinued, systemic anticoagulation must be reversed (protamine neutralizes heparin) to achieve satisfactory hemostasis.

Cardiopulmonary bypass is the most frequently used form of extracorporeal circulation. The patient's venous blood is continuously drained by gravity through large-bore cannulas inserted into the venae cavae or right atrium. When cardiopulmonary bypass is described as *full* or *complete,* all of the venous blood returning from the body is diverted away from the right ventricle and lungs. Rarely, situations occur in which it is advantageous to divert only part of the venous blood (*partial* cardiopulmonary bypass). Oxygen is added and carbon dioxide is removed from the diverted venous blood by an oxygenator (bubble or membrane). The blood must then be pumped continuously back into the patient's arterial system through another large-bore cannula inserted into the ascending aorta or other suitable site. A blood reservoir is usually incorporated into the circuit so that transient changes in venous return can be accommodated without affecting pump flows. Anticoagulated blood in the surgical field can be aspirated, filtered to remove any particulate matter, and then added back to the reservoir in the perfusion circuit. Elaborate precautions are taken to prevent inadvertent pumping of air into the patient's arterial system, which could result in serious injury or death. Cardiopulmonary bypass can also be used to control a patient's systemic temperature and take advantage of the reduced oxygen demand and hence blood flow requirements at low temperatures. Short periods of circulatory arrest (<60 minutes) are well tolerated at very low body temperatures (<20°C) and may be necessary to facilitate repair of congenital heart defects or in aortic surgery. A successful operative result depends not only upon good visualization and precise repair but also upon meticulous attention to perioperative myocardial preservation. Intraoperatively, there are many situations in which it is advantageous to temporarily stop coronary blood flow. The coronary circulation can be isolated from the rest of the body by clamping the ascending aorta. To prevent myocardial ischemic injury while coronary circulation is stopped, the coronary arteries or veins are intermittently perfused with one of several different chemical cardioplegia solutions. This results in diastolic arrest of the heart and a reduction of the myocardial oxygen requirements to less than 10% of that required in the beating and ejecting state. Heart function can be preserved successfully for several hours, enabling repair of even the most complex cardiac problems.

I. TRAUMA

A. PENETRATING INJURY OF THE HEART. Penetrating cardiac injuries are most commonly caused by a knife, bullet, or ice-pick but may also include iatrogenic injuries from pacemaker wires and angiographic catheters. Pericardial lacerations are usually included. The immediate life-threatening problems are cardiac tamponade and hypovolemia from blood loss into the pleural space. Other potential problems are myocardial ischemia/infarction resulting from epicardial coronary artery injuries, acute valvular insufficiency caused by disruption of intracardiac valves, and intracardiac shunts from injuries to the interatrial or interventricular septa.

1. Diagnosis. The history and physical examination provide clues to the possibility of a penetrating cardiac or great vessel injury. Often the victim can recall the exact weapon used and the direction of the attack, and this information, coupled with the various entrance and exit wounds; should lead the physician to suspect the correct diagnosis.

a. Symptoms. Pain in the vicinity of the wound, dyspnea, altered consciousness (may result from low cardiac output, hypoxemia, or air embolism).

b. Signs. Hypotension, distended neck veins (may become visible only during restoration of intravascular volume), diminished heart sounds, paradoxical pulse (>10-15 mm Hg discrepancy between measured systolic blood pressure during inspiration and expiration), diminished breath sounds, oliguria, cool extremities, weak peripheral pulses.

c. Laboratory tests. No specific laboratory tests are diagnostic. Hemoglobin and hematocrit are usually normal. ABGs may show metabolic acidosis.

d. Chest radiography. A widened mediastinal contour and/or a pleural effusion is usually present. Metallic FB fragments may occasionally be visible.

e. ECG. Sinus tachycardia, low voltage (pericardial effusion), localized ST-segment elevations (coronary artery injury).

f. Echocardiogram. Echocardiography has the potential to be quite useful but is seldom done in the emergency room trauma patient because of lack of trained personnel and equipment. In the operating room, after control of the bleeding site, it may be helpful to assess ventricular function, valve competence, or intracardiac shunts. In the catheterization laboratory or operating room following iatrogenic perforation, echocardiography may show whether there is continued intrapericardial bleeding and help guide the placement of drainage catheters or determine the need for operative repair.

f. Cardiac catheterization. Catheterization is almost never required acutely. Later it may be helpful to assess coronary anatomy, valve function, and intracardiac shunts.

2. Differential diagnosis. Isolated or combined injuries to adjacent structures including the great vessels, lungs, tracheobronchial tree, esophagus, chest wall, and diaphragm must be considered.

3. Natural history. Low cardiac output secondary to either acute cardiac tamponade or hypovolemia is immediately life-threatening, and many of these patients die at the accident scene or en route to the hospital. Late complications include ventricular dysfunction from myocardial infarction, valvular insufficiency, and intracardiac shunts. Systemic or pulmonary embolization of bullets or other foreign body fragments can occur, but infection at the site of the cardiac injury is extremely uncommon.

4. Treatment

a. Resuscitation. Several peripheral large-bore IV lines should be placed and intravascular volume rapidly restored with crystalloid solutions and blood (type-specific or O neg if necessary). A central venous line provides another IV site for fluid administration as well as for monitoring venous pressure. Other components of advanced life support may also be necessary. Pericardiocentesis may occasionally help confirm the diagnosis of cardiac tamponade as well as allow temporary stabilization prior to more definitive treatment.

b. Operative management. Thoracotomy may be required in the emergency department to control bleeding and relieve cardiac tamponade in unstable trauma patients. The traditional left anterior thoracotomy incision in the fourth intercostal space provides rapid access to the pericardium, the left lung, the descending thoracic aorta, and the anterior aspects of the right and left ventricles. It can also be extended across the sternum and into the right side to provide access to the right atrium and right lung. Lacerations of the right or left ventricle

can usually be controlled with finger pressure and then either
sutured or stapled. Direct injuries of small coronary arteries and
most coronary veins can be safely sutured even if occlusion of
the vessel results. However, injuries to proximal major coronary arteries (LAD, RCA, Cx) should ideally be repaired using cardiopulmonary bypass and conventional coronary artery
surgery techniques to preserve myocardial function. Significant
valvular injuries should ideally be repaired during the initial
surgery. The majority of iatrogenic right atrial and right ventricular perforations seal spontaneously and do not require thoracotomy for control. Pericardial drainage may be provided by
percutaneous catheters or by subxiphoid pericardial window.

5. Prognosis. Most patients die at the site of the injury.
Among the survivors the prognosis depends upon the extent of
injury and the duration of low cardiac output. Gunshot wounds
are more likely to be fatal than stab wounds. Hospital survivors frequently have ECG abnormalities (40% have ventricular ectopy), but most regain full functional capacity.

B. BLUNT INJURY OF THE HEART. Blunt cardiac injury often results from direct compression of the chest against a steering wheel or other object. The heart may be either contused or
lacerated.

1. Diagnosis
a. Symptoms. Chest pain, dyspnea, altered consciousness.

b. Signs. Hypotension, weak peripheral pulses, distended neck veins, cool extremities. A paradoxical pulse is an
important finding.

c. Laboratory tests. CPK-MB enzymes are elevated on
serial measurement.

d. Chest radiography. The chest radiograph may show
a widened mediastinum and rib or sternal fractures.

e. ECG. The ECG may be normal or may show a variety of abnormalities, including myocardial ischemia (ST-
segment elevation, T-wave inversions) or infarction (Q waves).
Ventricular ectopy and other dysrhythmias may also be present.

f. Echocardiogram. The echocardiogram is useful in
showing regional wall motion abnormalities (hypokinesia, aki-
nesia, or dyskinesia) and is quite specific. It may also demonstrate valvular insufficiency or pericardial effusion.

g. Cardiac catheterization/angiography. Cardiac
catheterization is almost never performed to diagnose blunt

cardiac injury. Aortography, however, is essential to exclude aortic disruption.

2. Differential diagnosis. The differential diagnosis includes myocardial ischemia/infarction due to preexisting coronary disease, and injuries to adjacent structures including the lungs, diaphragm, great vessels, chest wall, and esophagus.

3. Natural history. The complications include ventricular dysfunction from extensive myocardial contusion, dysrhythmias, cardiac tamponade, valvular insufficiency, and organ dysfunction secondary to poor cardiac function.

4. Treatment

a. Medical. Patients with clinical evidence of myocardial contusion (ECG, elevated enzymes, dysrhythmias) but no hemodynamic compromise should be monitored and treated as for acute myocardial infarction. If the patient is hemodynamically unstable, an echocardiogram may provide crucial information as to whether cardiac tamponade or ventricular dysfunction is responsible. Patients with cardiac tamponade may be temporarily stabilized by periocardiocentesis prior to definitive surgical treatment.

b. Operative management. A left anterior thoracotomy in the fourth intercostal space provides rapid access to the pericardium for decompression, and the incision may be extended across the sternum to facilitate repair of disruptions of the venae cavae and right atrium. An alternate approach via midline sternotomy is also feasible.

5. Prognosis. The prognosis depends upon the extent of myocardial contusion and associated injuries (e.g., head, pulmonary, vascular, abdominal, skeletal).

C. PENETRATING INJURY OF THE GREAT VESSELS.
Penetrating wounds of the great vessels (aorta, brachiocephalic arteries, main pulmonary artery) have the same causes as those of the heart (e.g., knives, bullets), and also result in bleeding into the pleural space, mediastinum, or pericardium. The presenting clinical manifestation is usually low cardiac output from either hypovolemia or cardiac tamponade. A careful history and physical examination provide the clues to the correct diagnosis.

1. Diagnosis

a. Symptoms. Pain in the vicinity of the wound, dyspnea, altered consciousness.

b. Signs. Hypotension, diminished peripheral pulses, distended neck veins, diminished heart sounds, paradoxical pulse, diminished breath sounds, oliguria, cool extremities.

c. Laboratory tests. No specific laboratory tests are diagnostic. Hemoglobin and hematocrit are normal. ABGs may show metabolic acidosis.

d. Chest radiography. A widened mediastinum and/or pleural effusion is present. There may also be displacement of trachea, mainstem bronchi, and esophagus. Metallic FB fragments may occasionally be seen.

e. ECG. Sinus tachycardia, low voltage (pericardial effusion).

f. Echocardiogram. Echocardiography is seldom available, although it might be helpful in diagnosing a pericardial effusion or excluding significant valvular or ventricular dysfunction in an unstable patient.

g. Cardiac catheterization/angiography. Cardiac catheterization is almost never required. Aortography is helpful in disclosing the site of vascular injury.

2. Differential diagnosis. Injuries to adjacent structures including the heart, lungs, tracheobronchial tree, esophagus, chest wall, and diaphragm must all be considered.

3. Natural history. Death results from hemorrhage or organ dysfunction resulting from prolonged low cardiac output. Infection at the site of vascular injury is rare.

4. Treatment

a. Resuscitation. Similar to that for penetrating cardiac injury. If cardiac tamponade is suspected clinically, pericardiocentesis may help to confirm the diagnosis and stabilize the patient prior to definitive surgical treatment. Large-bore chest tubes should be inserted if a hemothorax or pneumothorax is suspected clinically or by radiography. Persistent chest tube output or hemodynamic instability is an indication for thoracotomy.

b. Operative management. An anterior thoracotomy through the fourth intercostal space provides sufficient access to both pleural spaces, the pericardium, and the anterior mediastinum to deal with most emergency situations. If the patient is stable enough to undergo angiographic studies, the surgical approach can be modified accordingly.

5. Prognosis. Most patients die of exsanguination at the site of injury. The prognosis among those who reach the emergency department depends upon the extent of the injury and the duration of low cardiac output. Gunshot wounds to the great vessels are much more likely to be fatal than are knife wounds.

D. BLUNT INJURY OF THE GREAT VESSELS. Disruption (transection) of the great vessels commonly follows sudden, severe deceleration injuries such as occur in high-speed automobile/motorcycle accidents or falls from heights and is the most common cause of immediate death following such accidents. The mechanism of death in such cases is free rupture into the pleural space and exsanguination. Those who do survive to reach the emergency department are at risk for rupture over the next few hours. The usual site of disruption is the descending thoracic aorta just beyond the origin of the left subclavian artery, but the ascending aorta, brachiocephalic artery, and aortic arch may ocassionally be involved. This injury can also occur in the absence of any other major trauma, and its lethal potential warrants consideration and exclusion in every case.

1. Diagnosis

a. Symptoms. Chest pain, dyspnea, altered consciousness.

b. Signs. There are no specific signs. Pulse and blood pressure differentials between the two arms or between the arms and legs are suggestive. A systolic murmur may be audible over the precordium or posteriorly between the scapulas. Palpable rib or sternal fractures indicate severe trauma to the torso and should raise suspicion. Diminished breath sounds suggest effusion or pulmonary contusion. If the diagnosis of aortic disruption is confirmed, it is extremely important to document neurologic function (extremity sensory and motor function, deep tendon reflexes, and anal sphincter tone) prior to any therapeutic interventions.

c. Laboratory tests. No specific laboratory tests are diagnostic. Hemoglobin and hematocrit are usually normal.

d. Chest radiography. The cardinal finding on AP chest radiograph is mediastinal widening, often combined with deviation of the trachea, left mainstem bronchus, or esophagus, blurring of the aortic silhouette, or presence of a pleural cap. A pleural effusion, pulmonary contusion, and skeletal injuries including fractures of the ribs, sternum, and scapula are also commonly present.

e. ECG. The ECG is usually normal unless concomitant myocardial injury has occurred.

f. Echocardiogram. Echocardiography is seldom available in the emergency department on short notice, but this may change if new and sensitive imaging techniques can be developed.

g. Cardiac catheterization. Aortography remains the standard diagnostic test. In the acute setting CT and MRI techniques have not proved to be as sensitive or specific.

2. Differential diagnosis. The differential diagnosis includes injury to the heart, lungs, tracheobronchial tree, esophagus, chest wall, and diaphragm. Mediastinal hematomas can occur in the absence of serious thoracic visceral injury.

3. Natural history. In the majority of patients, death occurs from rupture and exsanguination into the pleural or pericardial space. A small number of patients with either unrecognized injury or contraindications to urgent operative repair ultimately develop chronic false aneurysms.

4. Treatment. Treatment involves resuscitation from shock and control of immediately life-threatening problems (active bleeding, airway compromise, ventilatory failure, hypoxemia). After the patient is stabilized, diagnostic aortography should be performed. If there are no contraindications (life-threatening cardiac, pulmonary, or CNS problems), urgent operative repair is performed. Lesions involving the ascending aorta, brachiocephalic artery, and aortic arch are repaired on cardiopulmonary bypass through a median sternotomy. The more typical descending aortic transection is best approached through a left posterolateral thoracotomy. A variety of surgical techniques all appear to have equivalent risks, and none has emerged as uniformly superior. The simplest involves clamping the aorta above and below the site of injury and either repairing the transection primarily or inserting a short segment of a Dacron tube graft to bridge the gap between the transected ends. The incidence of paraplegia and renal failure increases with the duration of aortic clamping.

5. Prognosis. Prognosis depends upon the extent of other injuries, particularly to the head. Most survivors do not have long-term sequelae. A small percentage, 5% to 10%, experience acute renal failure or infarction of the spinal cord and paraplegia as a result of poor perfusion of the distal aortic segment during the operation.

II. THORACIC AORTA

A. ANEURYSM. Aneurysms of the thoracic aorta are most commonly degenerative and are often associated with atherosclerosis. Other causes include syphillis, generalized disorders of connective tissue (Marfan's syndrome, cystic medial necrosis), and trauma. Any aortic segment may be involved from the level of the aortic sinuses to the diaphragm. Aneurysms are described as saccular when only a localized portion of the aortic circumference is dilated and fusiform when dilatation is more generalized. Like their counterparts in the abdomen, thoracic aortic aneurysms continue to enlarge and eventually cause symptoms as a result of their size and proximity to adjacent structures (tracheobronchial tree, vertebral column, chest wall, lung, esophagus) or as a result of rupture into the pericardium, mediastinum, or pleural space.

1. Diagnosis
a. Symptoms. Aortic aneurysms may be asymptomatic, an incidental finding on routine chest radiography. If the aneurysm involves the aortic sinuses or ascending aorta, the aortic valve may be incompetent with symptoms of heart failure (fatigue, dyspnea, fluid retention). Arch aneurysms can cause hoarseness due to tension on the left recurrent laryngeal nerve. Cough and hemoptysis result from tracheobronchial compression or erosion into the lung. Expansion against the vertebral column, sternum, or chest wall can produce localized pain.

b. Signs. There are few specific signs. Careful examination may reveal evidence of a generalized connective tissue disorder (asthenic habitus, arachnodactyly, joint/skin laxity, dislocated lenses, peripheral aneurysms). Signs of aortic insufficiency (e.g., diastolic murmur, widened pulse pressure, bounding peripheral pulses) should also be carefully sought. Paralysis of the left vocal cord indicates recurrent nerve involvement.

c. Laboratory tests. Serologic tests for syphilis should be performed routinely.

d. Chest radiography. PA, lateral, and oblique views show widening and elongation of the aortic contour. Enlargement of the cardiac silhouette (left ventricle) and pulmonary edema suggest aortic insufficiency or some other cause of left ventricular dysfunction. The trachea, main bronchi, and esophagus may be displaced by the aneurysm, and if airway compression is severe atelectasis or consolidation of the lung may also be present.

e. ECG. The ECG is nonspecific and usually not particularly helpful.

f. Echocardiogram. Two-dimensional imaging techniques provide good visualization of the ascending and descending thoracic aorta but have not been as good for the transverse arch. The echocardiogram also allows assessment of valvular function and ventricular wall motion.

g. Cardiac catheterization/angiography. Aortography defines the extent of the aneurysm as well as the origin of the major arch vessels and is extremely useful in planning surgery. Because myocardial ischemia/infarction is a major source of perioperative morbidity and mortality in these patients, assessment of the coronary arteries and left ventricular function should be performed preoperatively. Coronary angiography is performed routinely on every adult patient undergoing elective surgery on the ascending aorta or arch and selectively, based on the results of noninvasive stress myocardial perfusion imaging, for those undergoing elective surgery on the descending aorta.

h. CT/MRI scanning. Both techniques are capable of defining the extent of aneurysmal dilatation as well as allowing quantitative measurements of aneurysmal dimensions on a serial basis. This information can be extremely useful in selecting the appropriate timing for initial aortic surgery or as a check on the remaining aortic segments afterward. CT/MRI is also helpful in excluding other sources of mediastinal abnormalities on plane chest radiographs such as tumors or cysts.

2. Differential diagnosis. The differential diagnosis includes other causes of aortic insufficiency and mediastinal abnormalities (tumors or cysts).

3. Natural history. The major complication is rupture with exsanguination. Approximately 50% of patients with thoracic aneurysms die as a result of rupture within a few years of diagnosis. Patients with ascending aortic aneurysms and aortic insufficiency may also die of progressive heart failure.

4. Treatment. Medical management is purely supportive and does not reverse the progressive arterial dilatation. Nevertheless, many of these patients are elderly and have other associated life-threatening/limiting diseases (e.g., coronary artery disease, cerebrovascular disease, COPD, cancer) of which they eventually die. Thus the decision for operative management must include assessment of the risk of the operative procedure, the likelihood of aneurysmal rupture, and the natural history of the patient's other diseases. Indications for surgery are progressive aortic insufficiency, symptomatic aneurysms (chest pain, cough, hoarseness, dysphagia), progressive enlargement on CT/MRI (threshold about 5 to 6 cm diameter), or rupture.

a. Ascending aorta. The aorta is exposed via a median sternotomy, and cardiopulmonary bypass is required. The aneurysmal segment is replaced with an appropriately sized Dacron tube graft. Significant aortic insufficiency is usually treated by aortic valve replacement with a prosthetic valve. If aneurysmal dilatation of the sinus portion of the ascending aorta is present, reimplantation or bypass of the coronary arteries is performed.

b. Transverse arch. A variety of exposures is available, and cardiopulmonary bypass is usually required. The aneurysms present a formidable challenge in order to preserve both myocardial and cerebral function during repair. More recently approaches employing profound systemic hypothermia (20°C) and total circulatory arrest have been used. Again the basic principle has been to replace the aneurysmal segment with a Dacron tube graft and reimplant an "island" of the aorta containing the origins of the brachiocephalic vessels.

c. Descending aorta. The descending aorta is exposed via a posterolateral thoracotomy. Extensive aneurysms may require more than one intercostal incision. The aortic segment to be replaced is usually excluded by clamps and repaired with a Dacron tube graft. In spite of considerable reasearch, the optimal method of protecting the spinal cord and other viscera during the period of aortic clamping is not known, and the incidence of postoperative paraplegia remains 5%-10%. Some surgeons attempt to maintain flow to the distal aorta with partial cardiopulmonary bypass or a temporary shunt placed between the proximal and distal aorta.

5. Prognosis. The operative and long-term results are influenced by the urgency of the procedure, the site of the aneurysm, and concomitant disease (e.g., ventricular dysfunction, coronary artery disease, cerebrovascular disease, COPD). All patients require life-long medical follow-up with periodic chest radiography/CT/MRI to detect and treat aneurysmal dilatation in other aortic segments.

B. DISSECTION. Aortic dissection is a condition in which a hematoma within the wall of the vessel separates the layers of the media for a varying length and circumference. The hematoma is thought to arise as a result of a tear(s) in the intima and then to propagate proximally and distally with the pulsatile flow of blood. Aortic dissections are classified according to their chronicity and whether or not the ascending aorta is involved. Acute dissections, usually considered to be those less than 2 weeks old, are the most common catastrophic aortic disease, surpassing even ruptured abdominal aortic aneurysms in incidence. Overall the disease is more common in men, but no gender predilection is evident among patients less than 40 years of age. Interestingly, 50% of the women under 40 years of age are also pregnant at the time. The incidence is highest between the ages of 45 and 70 and is greater among those with connective tissue disorders (Marfan's syndrome, cystic medial necrosis), coarctation of the aorta, and congenital aortic valve stenosis. A history of hypertension may be present in as many as 80% to 90% of patients.

1. Diagnosis

a. Symptoms. The cardinal symptom is sudden, severe chest pain that often radiates to the back. This may be accompanied by neurologic symptoms (e.g., paraplegia, hemiparesis, visual disturbances, slurred speech), abdominal pain, or leg numbness resulting from compromised blood flow to the brain, spinal cord, viscera, or extremities. Aortic insufficiency and impending cardiac tamponade result in severe dyspnea.

b. Signs. Hypotension, pulmonary edema, pleural effusion, diminished heart sounds, pulse and blood pressure differentials between the extremities, aortic insufficiency murmur, oliguria, and signs of reduced peripheral perfusion may be present. Careful evaluation of any neurologic deficit is essential.

c. Laboratory tests. No specific laboratory tests are diagnostic. Hemoglobin and hematocrit are usually normal. ABGs may show metabolic acidosis if cardiac output is low or visceral hypoperfusion occurs.

d. Chest radiography. The chest radiograph almost always shows a widened mediastinum. Oblique and lateral views may help to differentiate ascending from descending aortic dissections. Pleural effusions, a widened cardiac silhouette, and pulmonary edema may also be present.

e. ECG. The ECG helps to distinguish acute dissection from acute myocardial infarction. However, if the ascending aorta is dissected proximally into the sinuses of Valsalva, myocardial ischemia/infarction may result from compromise of the coronary arteries. LVH is consistent with the increased incidence of hypertension in these patients.

f. Echocardiogram. Transesophageal echocardiography is both sensitive and specific for aortic dissection and is the first-line diagnostic test at some institutions. Besides precise diagnosis and localization, it provides valuable information about pericardial effusions, competence of the aortic valve, and ventricular function.

g. Cardiac catheterization/angiography. A CT scan or aortogram is the primary tool for diagnosis at some institutions. Aortography or selective angiography may also be used to visualize the major brachiocephalic, visceral, and extremity vessels for their sites of origin or evidence of compromise. Coronary angiography is not routinely performed in patients with acute dissections but can be useful in planning treatment for those with chronic dissections or whenever clinical suspicion exists of co-existing coronary artery disease.

h. CT/MRI. In addition to their role in diagnosis, CT/MRI techniques can be used to follow patients with chronic dissections or those who have undergone surgery.

2. Differential diagnosis. The main differential diagnosis includes other causes of sudden chest pain such as acute myocardial infarction, pulmonary embolus, and perforated viscus. Occasional patients present with loss of extremity pulse and are misdiagnosed initially as having an embolus or acute thrombosis. For patients who present with asymptomatic mediastinal abnormalities, the differential diagnosis includes atherosclerotic or post-traumatic aneurysms, tumors, and cysts.

3. Natural history. The major complication is death from rupture. The mortality among medically treated patients with acute proximal aortic dissections may be as high as 40% at 24 hours and 80% at 2 weeks. Other causes of early morbidity and mortality include cardiac tamponade, heart failure from acute aortic insufficiency, myocardial ischemia/infarction, cerebral/spinal cord infarction, mesenteric ischemia/infarction, and extremity ischemia. The risk of early rupture is much lower among medically treated patients with acute dissections distal to the aortic arch. Patients who survive the acute stage are at a similar risk for the development of long-term problems of aortic expansion, rupture, valvular insufficiency, and heart failure as those with degenerative aneurysms in similar aortic segments.

4. Treatment. Management decisions are usually based upon the onset (acute versus chronic), whether the ascending aorta is dissected or not, and the presence and severity of associated injuries or diseases (e.g., stroke, myocardial infarction, mesenteric infarction, COPD, cancer). Most chronic dissections are managed like aortic aneurysms at the same location (see Aortic Aneurysm in this chapter) and operated on when they become symptomatic or are observed to expand to a critical point. In most institutions the decision regarding initial operative management of acute dissections depends upon whether the ascending aorta is involved. Involvement of the ascending aorta identifies a subset of patients with a particularly dismal early prognosis on medical management, and unless there are compelling contraindications all of these patients should have emergent operative repair. Patients with dissections in the arch or distal aorta are usually treated medically (antihypertensive plus negative inotropic therapy) and operated on if they remain symptomatic or develop evidence of impending rupture (progressive mediastinal widening, anemia, bloody pleural effusion).

a. Ascending aorta. The principles of repair of acute ascending aortic dissections are to replace the dissected tubular portion with a Dacron tube graft, preserve the sinus portion, resuspend the aortic valve commissures to create a competent aortic valve or replace the valve with a prosthesis, and redirect blood flow into the "true" lumen at the level of the brachiocephalic vessels or arch. If the origins of the coronary arteries are involved in the dissection, they are repaired or bypassed. For chronic ascending aortic dissections replacement of the entire ascending aorta with a composite Dacron graft and prosthetic aortic valve is usually necessary. The origins of the left and right coronary arteries are anastomosed to the side of the prosthetic graft. Profound hypothermia and circulatory arrest may simplify performance of the distal aortic anastomosis and is essential if a partial or total replacement of the arch is required.

b. Descending aorta. Dissections involving the descending thoracic aorta are approached through a left thoracotomy. Similar principles of replacing the most dilated portion of the aorta and redirecting distal blood flow with a Dacron tube graft are followed. In chronic dissections it may not be possible to totally redirect all of the distal blood flow through the "true" lumen, as major visceral vessels may now originate from the "false" lumen. Once again the best method of intraoperative protection of the spinal cord and viscera is controversial, and no one technique has proven to be superior.

5. Prognosis. The operative mortality for both acute and chronic dissections has decreased with improved surgical techniques and averages 5%-15%. The current surgical techniques reliably prevent premature death from aortic rupture, cardiac tamponade, or acute aortic insufficiency. Operations on the descending thoracic aorta are still accompanied by a 5%-10% risk of spinal cord infarction and acute renal failure. Long-term follow-up studies indicate that up to one third of patients require further operative treatment and emphasize the importance of careful medical surveillance and blood pressure control.

III. PERICARDIUM

A. PERICARDITIS. Pericarditis is an inflammation of the parietal and visceral layers of the pericardium. The outer portion of the myocardium may be involved as well. Causes includes infection (TB, bacterial, or viral), trauma including cardiac surgery, myocardial infarction, malignancy, radiation, uremia, lupus or other systemic collagen-vascular disease, and the largest group—idiopathic. For most this is a relatively benign disease that is treated medically. Surgical management may be required for initial diagnosis of pericarditis if the cause is obscure and for definitive treatment of infectious pericarditis. More commonly surgical treatment is required for the complications of pericarditis such as recurrent/persistent effusion and pericardial constriction.

1. Diagnosis.

a. Symptoms. The most common presenting symptom is chest pain, which may be pleuritic in nature. Patients with chronic pericardial constriction can present in occult heart failure with fatigue, exertional dyspnea, and fluid retention, particularly ascites.

b. Signs. A triphasic pericardial friction rub is classically present in acute pericarditis. The intensity of the rub may vary with time and the patient's position. The rub may be absent if a significant effusion is present. Hypotension and other signs of low cardiac output may be present. A paradoxical pulse may be observed if the size of the effusion is sufficient to interfere with ventricular filling. Impending cardiac tamponade or constrictive physiology is associated with an elevated jugular venous pressure. Kussmaul's sign (increased jugular venous pressure with inspiration rather than the normal decrease) is consistent with constrictive pericarditis because the cyclic variations in intrapleural pressures are not transmitted to the heart by the thickened pericardium. Other manifestations include hepatomegaly, ascites and peripheral edema.

c. Laboratory tests. The TB skin test is usually positive in cases of tuberculous pericarditis. In purulent pericarditis the organisms can be cultured from the pericardial fluid/pericardium. However, even in fairly convincing cases of viral pericarditis, viral cultures of pericardial fluid/pericardium are frequently negative. Cytology and/or histology is usually positive if malignant pericardial involvement is present. The white blood cell count and erythrocyte sedimentation rate are commonly elevated in acute pericarditis. There may be hyperbilirubinemia and hypoalbuminemia plus other evidence of protein-losing enteropathy in cases of constrictive pericarditis.

d. Chest radiography. The cardiac silhouette often assumes a widened or globular (water bottle) appearance if a significant effusion is present. Careful examination may reveal pericardial calcifications in up to half of the patients with constrictive pericarditis.

e. ECG. Atrial arrhythmias and nonspecific ST-T wave changes are fairly common. The voltage is usually reduced in the presence of significant effusions or constriction.

f. Echocardiography. Echocardiography is extremely sensitive in diagnosing pericardial effusion. It can also show compression of the atria and right ventricle in cases of impending cardiac tamponade. It may be particularly helpful in distinguishing restrictive cardiomyopathy from constrictive pericarditis and provides valuable data concerning venticular and valvular function.

g. Cardiac catheterization. Hemodynamic measurements (particularly diastolic pressure measurements) are a mainstay of diagnosing pericardial disease. Right atrial pressure is elevated in almost all cases. In cardiac tamponade the y descent in the right atrial pressure disappears and the x descent is often exaggerated. In constrictive pericarditis the diastolic pressure in the right ventricle exhibits a characteristic dip and rapid plateau with a very small a wave.

h. CT/MRI. CT/MRI scans may reveal the primary tumor or evidence of pleuropericardial spread in malignant cases. Pericardial thickening is seen in over 80% of patients with constrictive pericarditis.

2. Differential diagnosis. If the onset of pericarditis is acute, it may be difficult to distinguish from acute myocardial ischemia/infarction. Other potential considerations include pneumonia, pulmonary infarction, pleuritis, and chest wall or upper GI causes of pain. Constrictive pericarditis can be mistaken for hepatic or GI disorders and restrictive cardiomyopathy.

3. Natural history. Rapid accumulation of a pericardial effusion can lead to cardiac tamponade and organ dysfunction secondary to low cardiac output. Prompt recognition and treatment with pericardiocentesis or pericardial window is lifesaving in these cases. Some patients with initially idiopathic effusive, post-traumatic, or infectious pericarditis go on to develop fibrous pericardial scarring and constrictive pericarditis. The cause of constrictive pericarditis is unclear in the majority, however. Long-standing cases can result in cardiac cachexia as a result of poor cardiac output and protein loss or malabsorption through the GI tract.

4. Treatment

a. Medical. The medical treatment of acute pericarditis consists of bedrest during the acute stages, analgesics for pain, and therapy directed against the specific causative factors. Occasionally steroids and nonsteroidal antiinflammatory agents are used. Relapse may occur in up to 10% of those with an idiopathic cause.

b. Surgical. Tamponade with severe hemodynamic compromise is best treated with immediate subxiphoid pericardiocentesis followed later by a more definitive pericardial window or excision. Purulent pericarditis requires pericardiotomy through either a subxiphoid or anterior thoracotomy followed by prolonged tube drainage. Therapeutic options for relapsing acute pericarditis include formation of a subxiphoid or pleuropericardial window and pericardiectomy. Pericardiectomy with complete decortication of both ventricles is the only satisfactory treatment for constrictive pericarditis and can be a very challenging operation. Multiple layers or sheets of fibrous tissue separated by loculated fluid must be carefully removed from the epicardium while avoiding injury to the epicardial coronary arteries, the phrenic nerves, the pulmonary artery, and the right ventricle.

5. Prognosis. Most patients with relapsing pericarditis have a good prognosis following creation of a pericardial window and do not suffer recurrences or develop constrictive pericarditis. Following pericardiectomy for constrictive pericarditis, about 75% of the survivors have a good result. The remainder continue to be symptomatic from either technically incomplete pericardial resections or intrinsic myocardial disease (atrophy, fibrosis). The operative mortality rate is approximately 10%.

IV. ARRHYTHMIAS

A. HEART BLOCK. Cardiac conduction disturbances include defective impulse formation (sinoatrial node dysfunction, sick sinus syndrome) and delay or interruption of impulse propagation (heart block). Symptoms are due to low cardiac output secondary to bradycardia, asystole, or escape tachyarrhythmias. The most common cause of heart block is degeneration of the specialized conductive tissue of the heart. Other causes are myocardial infarction or ischemia secondary to coronary artery disease, cardiomyopathy, drug effects, operative injury, and congenital defects.

1. Diagnosis

a. Symptoms. Common symptoms are dizziness, syncope, fatigue, palpitations, and dyspnea. Prolonged cerebral hypoperfusion may occasionally result in a seizure (Stokes-Adams attack).

b. Signs. Bradycardia, depressed mental status, and, less commonly, heart failure are present.

c. Laboratory tests. Serum electrolytes including magnesium should be checked on all patients. Both hyperkalemia and hypermagnesemia are associated with conduction blocks. In addition, patients who are receiving digitalis or other antiarrhythmic drug should have the appropriate levels measured.

d. Chest radiography. Usually noncontributory. If a transvenous or epicardial pacemaker lead has previously been placed, the lead should be carefully checked for breaks in continuity.

e. ECG. The standard ECG is diagnostic. Sometimes ambulatory ECG monitoring may be required to detect rhythm abnormalities in patients with intermittent symptoms. Long sinus pauses, complete heart block, or high-degree first- or second-degree heart block, atrial fibrillation with slow ventricular response, and various bundle branch blocks may be seen.

2. Differential diagnosis. Asymptomatic resting sinus bradycardia is a normal finding among trained atheletes. Often the differential diagnosis is between vasovagal syncope, an abnormally sensitive carotid sinus, a primary seizure disorder, or cerebrovascular disease affecting the vertebral-basilar system.

3. Natural history. Sudden death may occur from asystole, but more commonly it is from escape ventricular tachycardia or fibrillation. Prolonged periods of low cardiac output

may also result in cerebrovascular injury and visceral organ damage.

4. Treatment

a. Medical. Bradycardia in the setting of drug toxicity, electrolyte imbalance, or myocardial infarction is initially treated medically. Temporary placement of a transvenous pacemaker may be required at times until the acute process has resolved.

b. Surgical. Irreversible causes of heart block which are either symptomatic or associated with a short-term poor prognosis from bradyarrhythmias are best treated by implantation of a permanent pacemaker. The technology of both pacemaker leads and electronic circuitry contained within the pacemaker generator is now extremely sophisticated. Most leads are positioned transvenously in either the right atrium, the right ventricle, or both. Epicardial leads are available for patients with congenital heart defects or tricuspid valve prostheses that preclude transvenous placement. The most remarkable advances have been made in sensing technology. The current systems are capable of sensing not only electrical activity within the heart (p waves, QRS complex) but also physical activity, respiratory muscle activity, and venous blood temperature. Through complex electronic algorithms the heart rate can be more closely matched to metabolic demands. For all their electronic complexity, most modern pacemaker generators are remarkably compact and are positioned unobtrusively in subcutaneous pockets in the subclavicular or epigastric region.

5. Prognosis. Before pacemakers became available the 1-year survival rate for patients with complete heart block was only 50%. Current permanent transvenous systems can be implanted with extremely low operative risk even in debilitated, elderly patients and result in good palliation of symptoms as well as prolongation of life. The current lithium battery technology limits the life-span of the unit to about 3-5 years, but replacement is usually quite simple. The incidence of displacement of transvenous leads is about 5% (less with leads that are actually screwed into the myocardium), and displacement usually occurs within 48 hours of lead placement. Late complications of infection, lead fracture, pacemaker generator extrusion, and electronic component failure are rare.

V. CORONARY ARTERY DISEASE

Coronary artery disease is an all-encompassing term describing pathologic conditions that affect the coronary arteries. Congenital coronary artery anomalies are rare and consist mainly of anomalous origin of the coronary arteries from the pulmonary artery or arteriovenous fistulas. Acquired coronary artery disease includes trauma, aortitis, and other inflammatory arteritides and by far the most significant cause, atherosclerosis. Coronary atherosclerosis is a chronic disease that focally affects the epicardial vessels and is manifest by progressive luminal narrowing, which restricts blood flow. The disease is also characterized by sudden deterioration as a result of plaque rupture, intramural hemorrhage, or thrombosis. Episodic vasospasm may also be a feature in some patients. The sequelae of coronary artery disease are myocardial ischemia/infarction, ventricular dysfunction, and arrhythmias. In North America coronary artery disease is the leading cause of death among adults and one of the major sources of health care costs.

Epidemiologic studies have identified hyperlipidemia (hypercholesterolemia), hypertension, advanced age, male gender, cigarette smoking, and a family history of premature coronary artery disease as risk factors. The clinical classifications of coronary artery disease are based upon the severity of chest pain or ischemia equivalent (e.g., asymptomatic, stable angina, unstable angina, postinfarction angina) and the angiographic extent of the disease (single-, double-, or triple-vessel or left main coronary disease).

1. Diagnosis

a. Symptoms. Chest pain, dyspnea, fatigue, palpitations, syncope.

b. Signs. The signs are those of associated conditions or the sequelae of myocardial ischemia. An S_3, pulmonary rales, or mitral insufficiency murmur may be present, particularly during ischemia, indicative of ventricular dysfunction. Signs of low cardiac output (hypotension, poor peripheral perfusion) and congestion (peripheral edema, pulmonary rales) may be present during acute myocardial infarction or late as a result of ischemic cardiomyopathy. In certain pathologic hyperlipidemic states, signs such as arcus senilus, xanthelasma, or tendon xanthomas may be seen. A careful search for other sites of vascular disease should be performed (carotid bruits, blood pressure or pulse differentials between the arms, diminished or absent peripheral pulses, aneurysmal dilatation of the abdominal aorta or peripheral arteries).

c. Laboratory tests. Hypercholesterolemia or an abnormal lipoprotein pattern may be present. These abnormalities are particularly important to identify so that appropriate dietary and pharmacologic therapy can be instituted.

d. Chest radiography. The chest radiograph is usually noncontributory. The cardiac silhouette may be enlarged if there is a left ventricular aneurysm, significant ischemic mitral insufficiency, or ischemic cardiomyopathy. Pulmonary edema is suggestive of left ventricular dysfunction or mitral insufficiency.

e. ECG. No characteristic changes occur on the resting ECG, and it is often normal. In some patients prior transmural myocardial infarction is manifest as Q waves. Nonspecific ST-segment and T-wave abnormalities are also fairly common. ECGs performed during episodes of subendocardial ischemia may show ST-segment depression or T-wave inversion, which then reverts to normal following resolution of the ischemic episode. During episodes of transmural myocardial ischemia (acute myocardial infarction, Prinzmetal's angina) the ST-segments are characteristically elevated in the leads corresponding to the distribution of the involved coronary artery. The diagnostic sensitivity of the ECG for coronary artery disease can be enhanced by stress testing (procedures that increase the myocardial oxygen demand by exercise- or pacing-induced tachycardia). Stress tests can be accompanied by radionuclide scans to determine regional perfusion (thallium) or ventricular function (technetium-labeled red blood cells). In patients who cannot exercise persantine-induced stress combined with thallium perfusion imaging can be used. Stress testing also provides information about the amount of myocardium that is in jeopardy, which is important in terms of both prognosis and treatment.

f. Echocardiography. In the absence of prior myocardial injury or acute ischemia, the echocardiogram is normal. The characteristic feature of coronary artery disease is a regional wall motion abnormality (absence of systolic thickening or shortening). Stress testing using regional wall motion is also a sensitive test for myocardial ischemia. Function of the remaining portions of the left ventricle and mitral valve provide further important prognostic information.

g. Cardiac catheterization. Coronary angiography documents both the extent and severity of coronary artery disease. Images of the obstructive lesion in multiple planes are obtained, and both the length and extent of reduction in luminal diameter are important physiologically. A focal 50% reduction in luminal diameter is equivalent to a 75% reduction in cross-sectional area and constitutes a hemodynamically significant lesion. Luminal diameter reduction of 70% or more usually exceeds the normal compensatory vasodilatory ability of the distal coronary circulation and is termed "critical" because resting coronary blood flow may be insufficient. Ventriculography adds important information about regional contractility and mitral valve function.

h. Radionuclide studies. Three types of studies are commonly performed. Areas of recent myocardial infarction may be detected with pyrophosphate scanning. Technetium-labeled red blood cells are used for studies of global right and left ventricular function. Finally, thallium, an isotope that is distributed to the myocardium in proportion to blood flow and avidly taken up by viable myocardium, is used for perfusion and viability studies. The hallmark of myocardial ischemia is a defect on thallium scanning which is present during exercise or persantine stress and disappears completely during rest.

2. Differential diagnosis. The differential diagnosis includes other causes of chest pain such as pericarditis, aortic dissection, pneumonia, pulmonary infarction, pleuritis, esophageal diseases, and chest wall, and upper GI problems.

3. Natural history. The major life-threatening complications associated with coronary artery disease are myocardial infarction, ventricular dysfunction, and ventricular arrhythmias. Acute myocardial infarction with necrosis or dysfunction involving more than 40% of the left ventricle results in cardiogenic shock. Other acute mechanical complications of myocardial infarction include rupture of the free wall with cardiac tamponade, mitral insufficiency, and ventricular septal defect. Ventricular aneurysms usually occur somewhat later.

4. Treatment. There is an ever-expanding variety of treatments for coronary artery disease. Currently, pharmacologic management, PTCA, and CABG constitute the mainstays. On the horizon are drugs that may help to "dissolve" atherosclerotic plaques and angiographic catheters that can mechanically remove them.

a. Pharmacologic treatment. The goal of pharmacologic management is to reduce myocardial oxygen demands (nitrates, beta-blockers), prevent vasospasm (calcium channel blockers), and reduce thrombosis (aspirin, heparin). Attention should also be focused on correcting "reversible" risk factors such as hypertension, hyperlipidemia, and cigarette smoking.

The principles of pharmacologic management are applicable to all patients with coronary artery disease, and for some patients drug therapy may be all that is required to relieve symptoms and prevent premature death.

b. PTCA. Coronary angioplasty was originally applied to patients with single-vessel coronary artery and severe symptoms, but the indications have expanded to include selected patients with double- and triple-vessel disease. Primary success, defined by reduction in lesion severity or residual stenosis, is achieved in the majority of patients (80%-90%). Acute vessel closure leading to death, myocardial infarction, or need for emergency coronary artery bypass surgery occurs in less than 5% of patients. Angioplasty is extremely effective in restoring vessel patency in patients with acute myocardial infarction. It is attractive to both patients and cardiologists because of the shortened hospital stay and lack of surgery-related morbidity. The tendency for restenosis is the Achilles' heel of angioplasty, however, averaging about 30% overall within the first few months. Clinical trials are underway to determine the long-term effects of angioplasty on survival and cardiovascular morbidity.

c. Coronary artery bypass grafting. CABG is indicated in patients with severe angina or life-threatening myocardial ischemia for which PTCA is either not possible (chronic total occlusions) or not advisable (multiple lesions, complex or lengthy lesions). In several large clinical trials CABG has been shown to be superior to medical management in terms of symptom relief and long-term survival (left main coronary, triple-vessel, double-vessel including proximal left anterior descending disease), and the benefit seems to be particularly great in those patients who have associated left ventricular dysfunction. In fact, no modern study has shown a disadvantage for surgically treated patients.

5. Prognosis. The operative risk for patients undergoing CABG depends upon the urgency of the operation (emergent, urgent, elective), the extent of ventricular dysfunction, the age of the patient, and the severity of co-morbid diseases (e.g., renal failure, COPD). These risk factors tends to interact in a multiplicative rather than additive fashion so that although the baseline risk is approximately 1%-2%, it rapidly escalates as more risk factors are present. Nevertheless, it is extremely difficult to deny anyone CABG on the basis of operative risk because the risk of medical management is usually much greater. Long-term follow-up studies have shown an incidence of recurrent angina or need for reoperation of about 5% of patients per year. The cause is usually progression of disease in the native coronary circulation or atherosclerosis of the saphenous vein grafts). The incidence of saphenous vein graft atherosclerosis increases between 5 and 10 years postoperatively so that by 10 years approximately one third are patent, one third are patent but diseased, and one third are occluded. Reoperative CABG is technically more difficult, and the operative mortality is approximately double that for primary surgery. CABG using arterial conduits (mammary arteries, right gastroepiploic artery) has been associated with superior long-term graft patency, patient survival, and a reduced incidence of late coronary reoperations. Most surgeons now routinely use at least one mammary artery bypass graft whenever longevity is an issue.

A. CORONARY ARTERY BYPASS GRAFTING. The indications for isolated CABG have already been discussed. CABG may also be performed during the course of surgery for another cardiac problem (e.g., valve, aneurysm, VSD) without much additional operative risk. The goal of the procedure is to revascularize viable heart muscle as completely as possible by performing bypass grafts to all major epicardial coronary arteries (1.5 mm or greater in diameter) that are affected by proximal hemodynamically significant stenoses (>50%). Occasionally endarterectomy may enable revascularization of a myocardial segment supplied by an otherwise diffusely diseased, nongraftable coronary artery. CABG is performed in several stages. In the first, segments of saphenous vein (greater or lesser system), internal mammary artery(ies), or other appropriate bypass conduits are "harvested" from the patient. Next the patient's heart is exposed, arterial and venous cannulas are placed, and total cardiopulmonary bypass is initiated. The aorta is cross-clamped and the heart is arrested with cardioplegia. The sequence of bypass grafting is based upon individual surgeon preference; usually the mammary artery grafts are the last ones to be performed. The aortic cross-clamp is removed once all of the distal graft to coronary artery bypasses have been completed and coronary artery flow is restored with normokalemic blood. When the heart has recovered satisfactorily, the patient is weaned from cardiopulmonary bypass and the cannulas are removed. The incisions are closed and the patient is then transferred to an intensive care unit for hemodynamic monitoring for the next 24-48 hours.

B. LEFT VENTRICULAR ANEURYSMECTOMY. Left ventricular aneurysms are discrete areas of full-thickness scar which appear dyskinetic on ventriculography (bulge during systole and get smaller during diastole). Aneurysmal segments present a volume load to the left ventricle (that lost into the aneurysm during ventricular systole) with the need for both compensatory dilatation and hypertrophy of adjacent normal segments. The function of these segments may deteriorate with time, producing the clinical picture of congestive heart failure. Aneurysms most commonly follow an acute proximal occlusion of a major coronary artery (LAD, RCA), that previously had minimal collateral blood supply. A variable portion of the interventricular septum is frequently involved as well. Up to 50% contain mural thrombus, and the endocardial border between normal myocardium and scar can also be the source for reentrant ventricular tachycardias. In older retrospective and autopsy studies following acute myocardial infarction, the incidence was 10%-15%. More recently, the incidence appears to be decreasing, perhaps reflecting more frequent use of acute thrombolysis or PTCA or better post–myocardial infarction care. Rare causes of aneurysms include trauma and congenital heart defects. Most patients with isolated left ventricular aneurysms are managed medically (digoxin, diuretics, vasodilators, antiarrhythmics, anticoagulants) and referred for surgical treatment only if there is intractable heart failure, ventricular tachycardia, recurrent thromboemboli, or myocardial ischemia. Rarely, an otherwise asymptomatic aneurysm is resected during the course of coronary artery bypass or valvular surgery in order to preserve ventricular function. Pseudoaneurysms are localized myocardial ruptures contained by the pericardium or mediastinal structures. Unlike true left ventricular aneurysms, pseudoaneurysms have a propensity for rupture and almost all require surgical management. They can follow endocarditis, trauma, or myocardial infarction and occasionally appear as a complication of previous cardiac surgery.

Patients with recurrent ventricular tachycardia and left ventricular aneurysms require careful preoperative and intraoperative electrophysiologic mapping to locate the site(s) of the reentrant pathway(s). The ventricular arrhythmias are induced and mapped during normothermic cardiopulmonary bypass. The endocardial sites of earliest ventricular activation are then removed by either endocardial stripping or cryoablation. If concomitant coronary artery bypass grafts or valve procedures are required, the aorta is cross-clamped and hypothermic cardioplegia is administered. The fibrous margins around the resected aneurysm may be reapproximated or closed with a prosthetic/pericardial patch. Great care must be taken to avoid embolization from mural thrombi or air during the procedure. In uncomplicated cases the operative mortality is approximately 5% and long-term survival is 80% at 4 years. The risk factors are advanced age, emergent presentation, extent of coronary artery disease, left ventricular dysfunction, and organ failure (renal, hepatic, pulmonary). Among several institutions the operative mortality for electrophysiologically guided resections in patients with recurrent ventricular tachycardia is 0%-20%, and 40% of patients are still inducible at follow-up electrophysiologic testing. The operative risk factors are much the same for this group. In the future such patients may be more appropriate candidates for radiofrequency catheter ablation, an AICD device, or cardiac transplantation.

C. POSTINFARCTION VENTRICULAR RUPTURE (VSD).

In postmortem studies of patients dying after a recent acute myocardial infarction, the incidence of ventricular rupture is approximately 8%-10%. In many of these cases the extent of the original infarct was large enough to have precluded survival even with conventional revascularization and repair techniques. A small number (1%-2%), however, had VSDs with less extensive myocardial infarcts and were potentially salvageable. The usual clinical presentation is acute onset of shock or heart failure 4 to 12 days after the onset of the myocardial infarction. Survival with medical therapy is poor. The right-to-left shunt impairs systemic cardiac output, and the right ventricle fails owing to volume overload. There is usually a rapid progression to multisystem organ failure (pulmonary, renal, hepatic). The mortality rates are 24% after 24 hours, 65% after 2 weeks, and 81% after 2 months, and only 7% of patients survive 1 year after the development of a postinfarction VSD. The pathophysiology is similar to that for left ventricular aneurysm, and postinfarction hypertension may be a risk factor. On physical examination a holosystolic murmur is audible along the left sternal border. Two thirds of patients have a palpable thrill. The diagnosis is confirmed at the bedside with a Swan-Ganz catheter or in the catheterization laboratory by demonstrating a step-up in venous oxygen saturation within the right ventricle. Coronary angiography shows an acute occlusion of the left anterior descending, right coronary, or posterior descending coronary artery. Unless the patient has a trivial VSD or is at prohibitive risk for surgical correction (advanced age, debility, irreversible organ failure) an intraaortic balloon pump should be inserted and the patient expeditiously transported to the operating room.

The surgical technique involves direct visualization of the septal defect, usually from the left ventricular side of the septum, with prosthetic/pericardial patch closure on cardiopulmonary bypass. Coronary artery bypasses and valve repair/replacement procedures are performed during aortic cross-clamping and hypothermic cardioplegic arrest. The operative mortality is 20%-50% and depends upon left ventricular function and extent of preoperative organ dysfunction. Long-term survival among operative survivors is generally excellent.

VI. VALVULAR HEART DISEASE

A. AORTIC STENOSIS. Aortic stenosis is a chronic valvular condition characterized by progressive obstruction of the left ventricular outflow with compensatory left ventricular hypertrophy. Death ultimately results from left ventricular failure or arrhythmia. The disease can be classified according to the presence or absence of symptoms (angina, syncope, dyspnea) or the extent of reduction in cross-sectional area. Patients with systolic pressure gradients greater than 60 mm Hg between the left ventricle and ascending aorta or calculated aortic valve area of 0.7 cm^2 or less (normal 3 to 4 cm^2) are considered to have severe aortic stenosis. Even in adult patients the most common cause is congenital deformity of the valve with degenerative changes leading to leaflet fibrosis and calcification, which then progressively narrow the valve orifice. Other less frequent causes include rheumatic fever, prosthetic valve thrombosis or degeneration, and senile calcification of the aortic valve.

1. Diagnosis

a. Symptoms. The classic symptoms of angina (subendocardial ischemia), syncope (baroreceptor dysfunction), and dyspnea (left ventricular dysfunction) usually appear late in the course of the disease. Patients are also likely to become more symptomatic if they develop atrial fibrillation or lose the atrial contribution to filling of their noncompliant hypertrophied left ventricle.

b. Signs. Delayed upstroke of the carotid pulses and diminished pulse volume are usually present. A systolic ejection murmur is commonly heard best in the right parasternal area over the second interspace. There may be an associated thrill, which is virtually diagnostic. The murmur is usually transmitted to the carotids. The left ventricular apical impulse is prominent but is not displaced laterally until late in the course of the disease.

c. Laboratory tests. No laboratory tests contribute to the diagnosis.

d. Chest radiography. The left heart border and apex appear prominent, but overall cardiac size is usually normal unless there is concomitant aortic or mitral valve insufficiency. The ascending aorta may be enlarged by post-stenotic dilatation.

e. ECG. Left ventricular hypertrophy or a strain pattern is invariably present.

f. Echocardiogram. Transthoracic or transesophageal echocardiography combined with Doppler flow velocity assessment are diagnostic and provide a very useful means for serial assessment in patients with mild to moderate aortic stenosis.

g. Cardiac catheterization. The main findings are a pressure gradient between the left ventricle and the aorta during systole and an elevated left ventricular end-diastolic pressure. The valve area is determined from the Gorlin formula using calculated values for the aortic flow and the mean systolic gradient. Cardiac output and left ventricular end-diastolic volume are usually normal. In aortic stenosis there is an inverse relationship between the left ventricular ejection fraction and wall stress so that a depressed ejection fraction by itself does not necessarily indicate left ventricular systolic dysfunction. Coronary angiography should be performed routinely in patients over 40 years of age or with risk factors for coronary artery disease.

2. Differential diagnosis. Other causes of left ventricular outflow obstruction including IHSS and tumors. Angina and syncope require evaluation to exclude significant coronary or cerebrovascular disease.

3. Natural history. The main complications are sudden death, congestive heart failure, and endocarditis. The average survival after the onset of angina or syncope is less than 5 years, and symptoms of heart failure (e.g., dyspnea, orthopnea, edema) portend an even worse prognosis.

4. Treatment

a. Medical. Medical management of aortic stenosis is unsatisfactory. Many of the strategies used for control of angina or heart failure (nitrates, digoxin, vasodilators, diuretics) can exacerbate the physiologic abnormalities in aortic stenosis and must be used with extreme caution. Aortic balloon valvuloplasty has not proven to be as useful as hoped and is now reserved solely for patients who are not deemed candidates for aortic valve replacement owing to their advanced age or debility.

b. Surgical. Valve replacement (porcine bioprosthesis, mechanical prosthesis, or homograft) is the preferred treatment for most patients who either have symptomatic aortic stenosis or demonstrate progressive left ventricular dysfunction on follow-up. Coexisting coronary artery disease, carotid disease, or mitral valve disease can be treated simultaneously without much additional risk of mortality or morbidity.

5. Prognosis. The operative mortality averages 2% to 8% in most recent series and depends upon the patient's age, extent of ventricular dysfunction, and comorbidity (e.g., pulmonary, renal). Long-term survival is good (80% to 85% at 5 years), and most patients are asymptomatic. The left ventricular ejection fraction and hypertrophy also improve with relief of the valvular obstruction.

B. AORTIC INSUFFICIENCY. Aortic insufficiency can be an acute or chronic disease. In acute aortic insufficiency the clinical manifestations are those of low cardiac output combined with elevated left ventricular end-diastolic filling pressures. The effective forward cardiac output is reduced by the regurgitant flow across the valve as well as by early closure of the mitral valve as left ventricular diastolic pressure exceeds left atrial pressure. The main causes of acute aortic insufficiency are acute ascending aortic dissection and endocarditis. Rarely, trauma may result in acute aortic insufficiency, and patients with previous prosthetic aortic valves may present with leaflet tears or mechanical dysfunction. In chronic aortic insufficiency the compensatory mechanisms of left ventricular dilatation and hypertrophy are capable of maintaining resting cardiac output and left ventricular end-diastolic pressure in the normal range until very late in the course of the disease. Causes of chronic aortic insufficiency can also be divided into those affecting the valve leaflets or aortic annulus, such as rheumatic fever, myxoid degeneration, Marfan's syndrome, Ehlers-Danlos syndrome, anklyosing spondilitis, annulo-aortic ectasia, chronic ascending aortic dissection or aneurysm, and syphilitic aortitis.

1. Diagnosis

a. Symptoms. In chronic aortic insufficiency the severity of symptoms is not necessarily indicative of the severity of the disease, and symptoms may be either mild or absent even in the presence of advanced left ventricular dysfunction. Inadequate cardiac output usually presents as easy fatigability or reduced exercise tolerance. Elevated left ventricular end-diastolic pressure results in dyspnea, orthopnea, and paroxysmal nocturnal dyspnea.

b. Signs. A multitude of eponymic signs are associated with chronic aortic insufficiency. Most are in some way related to the wide pulse pressure and rapid diastolic run-off that characterizes this disease. The diastolic murmur is usually described as being of high pitch or musical quality. It may be best heard along the sternal border if the patient leans forward and holds his breath at end-expiration. The murmur may be difficult to hear in acute aortic insufficiency or if there is early equilibration of aortic and left ventricular diastolic pressure. The left ventricular apical impulse is both prominent and displaced laterally.

c. Laboratory tests. If endocarditis is suspected, it is extremely important to get several sets of blood cultures from different sites before beginning antibiotic therapy. Otherwise, no specific tests are helpful for diagnosis.

d. Chest radiography. Left ventricular enlargement always accompanies chronic aortic insufficiency. Dilatation of the ascending aorta may also be present. In acute aortic insufficiency the radiographic findings may be limited to pulmonary congestion or edema.

e. ECG. Left ventricular hypertrophy or strain. In endocarditis, prolongation of the PR interval or the development of more advanced heart block suggests annular involvement by the infection.

f. Echocardiography. Transthoracic or transesophageal echocardiography is diagnostic and Doppler flow velocity maps or contours permit assessment of the severity of the regurgitation. The echocardiogram may provide insight into the mechanism by visualization of intimal flaps (dissection) or vegetations (endocarditis). In addition, echocardiography is extremely valuable for following patients with aortic insufficiency for evidence of progressive left ventricular dilatation or dysfunction (indications for surgical repair).

g. Cardiac catheterization. Contrast aortography performed with a catheter in the ascending aorta has been the mainstay for diagnosis and quantification of the severity of aortic insufficiency. The degree of opacification of the left ventricular cavity and the rapidity with which the contrast is cleared from the left ventricle is graded from mild (1+) to severe (4+) aortic insufficiency. The resting left ventricular end-diastolic pressure, ejection fraction, and cardiac output are usually normal despite the greatly increased end-diastolic volume. Coronary angiography is performed routinely in patients over 40 years of age or in those with risk factors for coronary artery disease.

2. Differential diagnosis. Chronic aortic insufficiency rarely presents a problem in terms of differential diagnosis. Chronic biventricular volume overload resulting from peripheral AV shunts or left ventricular volume overload from systemic–to–pulmonary artery shunts can produce many of the clinical manifestations of chronic aortic insufficiency but should be readily discernible on the basis of others. Acute aortic insufficiency with cardiogenic shock may sometimes be hard to differentiate from acute pulmonary embolism with right ventricular failure or acute myocardial infarction with severe left ventricular dysfunction ($>$40% of the left ventricle involved) or myocardial rupture with VSD.

3. Natural history. Patients with hemodynamically significant acute aortic insufficiency die quickly of the combined effects of low cardiac output and poor perfusion of the coronary and other visceral circulations and hypoxemia caused by intractable pulmonary edema. The clinical course in chronic aortic insufficiency is protracted, and patients may not experience significant symptoms until late in their disease. Left ventricular dysfunction manifested by low ejection fraction ($<$50%) and high end-diastolic volume ($>$90 ml/m^2) is associated with high operative mortality and a greater chance of a poor long-term functional result. Death in these cases occurs secondary to heart failure.

4. Treatment

a. Medical. Medical treatment for acute aortic insufficiency is applicable only to those patients without clinically significant heart failure or those who are at prohibitive risk for valve replacement. Antibiotic therapy is guided by the results of blood or tissue cultures in cases of endocarditis. It is neither necessary nor always possible to complete a prescribed course of antibiotic treatment before valve replacement. With careful monitoring, vasodilators and diuretics may improve gas exchange, effective cardiac output, and organ blood flow. Heart rates that are slightly above normal are desirable to decrease the diastolic time interval and the amount of regurgitant flow. Vasodilators and diuretics have a more definite role in the management of patients with chronic aortic insufficiency where they may improve symptoms and delay the progression of the disease. Careful follow-up and early referral for valve replacement are essential to prevent irreversible left ventricular dysfunction.

b. Surgical. Valve replacement (porcine bioprosthesis, mechanical prosthesis, or homograft) is the preferred surgical treatment for most patients. Clinical experience with aortic valve repair techniques is increasing, and ultimately valve repair may assume a major role. All patients with hemodynamically significant acute aortic insufficiency should undergo urgent valve replacement unless there are compelling contraindications (e.g., recent major intracranial hemorrhage, coma, severe chronic debility). In chronic aortic insufficiency, valve replacement should be performed in symptomatic patients (NYHA classes 3 and 4) and in asymptomatic or mildly symptomatic patients (NYHA classes 1 and 2) when progressive left ventricular enlargement or decrease in ejection fraction on serial follow-up is present.

5. Prognosis. The operative mortality for aortic valve repair/replacement in acute aortic insufficiency is 5% to 10% and depends upon the patient's age, left ventricular function, and degree of preoperative visceral organ dysfunction. The average operative mortality for chronic aortic insufficiency in most institutions is 4% to 6% and is affected by the same variables. Long-term survival and functional results have been generally good, particularly among younger patients and those with preserved left ventricular function.

C. MITRAL STENOSIS. Mitral stenosis is most commonly seen in adults as a late sequela (>20 years) of acute rheumatic fever. The process of valvular inflammation and repair characteristically results in leaflet fusion at the commissures, leaflet thickening and calcification, and variable amounts of retraction and scarring of the chordae tendineae and papillary muscles. Fortunately this disease has become less common in developed countries with better systems of health care and prompt treatment of streptococcal infections. Nevertheless, among developing third-world countries it remains a significant problem. Rare causes also include degenerative mitral valve/annular calcification seen among the elderly, prosthetic valve thrombosis or degeneration, congenital deformity (association with hypoplasia of the left ventricle, aortic valve, or aorta), carcinoid syndrome, systemic lupus erythematosus, and rheumatoid arthritis. The pathophysiology of mitral stenosis is progressive narrowing of the mitral valve orifice, which creates a diastolic pressure gradient between the left atrium and left ventricle. The left atrial pressure is increased and the atrium dilates. Although cardiac output at rest is normal, with exercise, cardiac output is limited by the concomitant increase in left atrial pressure. This gives rise to the two most frequent symptoms of mitral stenosis—dyspnea and fatigue. Patients also experience worsened symptoms when they develop atrial fibrillation or lose the atrial contribution to ventricular filling. Left ventricular function is generally preserved and left ventricular volumes and pressures are normal. Right ventricular and pulmonary artery pressures are increased on the basis of both the increased left atrial pressure and vascular reactivity. Some patients may even develop systemic levels of pulmonary hypertension, but this is unusual. Other common manifestations include atrial fibrillation and right ventricular dysfunction (hepatomegaly, peripheral edema, ascites, tricuspid insufficiency). Atrial fibrillation and intracardiac stasis are important risk factors for the development of left atrial thrombus with its attendant propensity for peripheral embolization.

1. Diagnosis

a. Symptoms. A history of rheumatic fever is present in half of the patients with presumed rheumatic mitral stenosis. The classic symptoms are dyspnea, orthopnea, and fatigue. Patients rarely experience symptoms as a result of displacement of the left main bronchus or esophagus by a dilated left atrium. Enlargement of the left pulmonary artery may cause hoarseness by pressure on the left recurrent laryngeal nerve.

b. Signs. Typically the patients appear thin and cachetic, with "ruddy" cheeks (mitral fascies) and often peripheral cyanosis. The jugular venous pressure is elevated with volume overload or tricuspid insufficiency. Rales at the lung bases, hepatomegaly, and peripheral edema may often be present. A prominent right ventricular heave is suggestive of right ventricular enlargement or pulmonary hypertension. The classic auscultatory findings are an increased intensity of S_1 and P_2, an opening snap, and a low frequency diastolic rumbling murmur. Atrial fibrillation is also a common finding.

c. Laboratory tests. No specific laboratory tests aid in diagnosis.

d. Chest radiography. Enlargement of the left atrium is most often apparent in the lateral view or as a retrocardiac double density on the PA view. The left ventricle is not enlarged unless there is associated mitral insufficiency or aortic valve disease. Enlargement of the superior pulmonary veins and peripheral Kerley B lines are common.

e. ECG. Atrial fibrillation develops at some point in all patients. Patients in sinus rhythm may show a biphasic P wave as evidence of atrial enlargement. Right axis deviation and right ventricular hypertrophy are also commonly present.

f. Echocardiography. Transthoracic or transesophageal echocardiography is diagnostic and may render cardiac catheterization unnecessary for some patients. They provide extremely detailed anatomic information about the extent of valve deformity as well as important physiologic data in terms of the pressure gradient and valve area. Echocardiography is also helpful in evaluating the status of the aortic valve, tricuspid valve, and overall ventricular function.

g. Cardiac catheterization. The gradient across the mitral valve can be determined by simultaneous pressure measurements from the left atrium (transatrial puncture) and left ventricle or estimated from the simultaneous pulmonary wedge pressure tracing. The valve area is then calculated from a measured cardiac output (thermodilution or Fick) by means of the Gorlin formula. The normal mitral valve area is 3 cm^2/m^2 of body surface area. Mitral stenosis becomes significant at a valve area of less than 1 cm^2/m^2 and severe at about 0.6 cm^2/m^2. Coronary angiography is performed routinely in patients over the age of 40 years and in those with risk factors for coronary artery disease.

2. Differential diagnosis. Left atrial myxoma, a primary cardiac tumor, may mimic many of the clinical findings of rheumatic mitral stenosis. This diagnosis should be suspected if symptoms are episodic or positional in nature.

3. Natural history. Systemic emboli (over 50% cerebral) are a major source of morbidity and mortality among patients with mitral stenosis. The incidence among medically treated patients may be as high as 15%-30%, particularly those with atrial fibrillation. Patients may also succumb of respiratory failure or low cardiac output during an acute medical illness or stress such as pneumonia. Bacterial endocarditis is also a long-term risk, and appropriate antibiotic prophylaxis prior to any invasive procedures is mandatory. In the final stages of untreated disease, secondary organ failure (hepatic, renal) may be present.

4. Treatment

a. Medical. The medical management consists of diuretics to prevent fluid overload and digoxin to control the ventricular rate in patients with atrial fibrillation. Long-term oral anticoagulation with sodium warfarin should be administered to all patients with atrial fibrillation and to any patient with left atrial thrombus or a history of systemic emboli. Recently, transatrial balloon catheter techniques have been developed for dilatation of stenotic mitral valves. The ultimate utility of this nonsurgical technique awaits further trials.

b. Surgical. The indications for operative management of mitral stenosis are moderate to severe symptoms (NYHA classes 3 and 4), onset of atrial fibrillation, worsening pulmonary hypertension, systemic embolization, and endocarditis. Closed mitral commissurotomy (blind dilatation of the mitral valve via the left atrium or ventricle without cardiopulmonary bypass) has largely been supplanted by more precise techniques performed while the patient is supported on cardiopulmonary bypass. Under direct vision the commissures are opened, the valve leaflets and annulus are debrided of calcium and scar, and the subvalvular structures are mobilized. The extent of calcification and deformity may limit the ability to restore the valve function, and valve replacement (porcine bioprosthesis or mechanical prosthesis) may be required.

5. Prognosis. The operative mortality of open valvuloplasty is less than 5% and the 10-year survival is 90%. Long-term freedom from endocarditis and thromboembolism is excellent and the functional results are good. Recurrent mitral stenosis/insufficiency requiring a second operative procedure may occur (8% at 5 years, 17% at 10 years). Valve replacement for mitral stenosis is associated with a slightly higher operative mortality and worse long-term result. Prosthetic valve–related complications (endocarditis, thromboembolism, tissue degeneration, and mechanical failure) can be source of long-term morbidity and mortality.

D. MITRAL INSUFFICIENCY. Mitral insufficiency may be either an acute or a chronic process. In acute mitral insufficiency the pathophysiology is due to increased left atrial pressure and low cardiac output as a result of the loss of left ventricular stroke volume through regurgitation into the left atrium. Left ventricular end-diastolic volume increases to a limited extent and, owing to the low left ventricular afterload, end-systolic volume is either low or normal. Thus, in the absence of left ventricular dysfunction the ejection fraction is usually supranormal or normal. The causes of acute mitral insufficiency include endocarditis, trauma, and acute myocardial ischemia/infarction with secondary papillary muscle dysfunction or rupture. The pathophysiology of chronic mitral insufficiency is different. The left atrium is enlarged as a result of chronic pressure and volume overload. Atrial fibrillation is common but in the absence of stasis is not usually associated with left atrial thrombus. Initially the left ventricle compensates by both hypertrophy and dilatation with preservation of systolic function. Cardiac output and left ventricular end-diastolic pressure at rest are normal. With continued volume loading the left ventricle ultimately fails, systolic function deteriorates, and end-diastolic pressure increases. Additional clinical features may include pulmonary hypertension and right ventricular dysfunction. Rheumatic fever, degenerative changes in the valve leaflets or chordae, healed endocarditis, connective tissue disorders (Marfan's syndrome, Ehlers-Danlos syndrome), IHSS, and ischemic cardiomyopathy are among the most common causes of chronic mitral insufficiency.

1. Diagnosis

a. Symptoms. The major symptoms attributable to elevated left atrial pressure include dyspnea, orthopnea, and paroxysmal nocturnal dyspnea. Fatigue and poor effort tolerance are due to inadequate cardiac output.

b. Signs. Atrial fibrillation may be present and the peripheral pulses in chronic mitral insufficiency typically exhibit a rapid upstroke and reduced volume. The apical impulse is prominent and displaced laterally. If present, a right ventricular heave is suggestive of pulmonary hypertension or right ventricular dysfunction. Signs of fluid overload or right ventricular dysfunction include an elevated jugular venous pressure, peripheral edema, hepatomegaly, or ascites. Features suggestive of endocarditis include fever, splinter/conjunctival hemorrhages, clubbing, Osler's nodes, and splenomegaly. The typical auscultatory finding is a high-pitched apical pansystolic murmur that radiates to the axilla or back. An extradiastolic filling sound (S_3) and an accentuated P_2 are also commonly heard.

c. Laboratory tests. If endocarditis is suspected, serial blood cultures from separate sites should be drawn before commencing antibiotic therapy.

d. Chest radiography. In chronic aortic insufficiency the left atrium and ventricle are invariably enlarged. Pulmonary hypertension or right ventricular dysfunction results in enlargement of the right ventricle as well. Engorgement of the superior pulmonary veins, dilation of the pulmonary arteries, and Kerley B lines are also commonly present.

e. ECG. Atrial fibrillation is common. In patients in sinus rhythm the P wave may be biphasic, indicative of left atrial enlargement. Left ventricular or biventricular hypertrophy is commonly present. In endocarditis, prolongation of the PR interval or more advanced atrioventricular block is an indication of annular involvement by the infection.

f. Echocardiography. Transthoracic or transesophageal echocardiography is diagnostic and may obviate cardiac catheterization in some patients. In addition to providing two-dimensional anatomic detail of the mitral apparatus (leaflets, annulus, chordae, and papillary muscles), Doppler flow velocity maps and contours allow assessment of the severity of the regurgitant jets and provide valuable information about ventricular function, pulmonary artery pressure, and the status of the other valves.

g. Cardiac catheterization. Injection of radiographic contrast into the body of the left ventricle is the standard technique for diagnosis and estimation of the severity of mitral insufficiency. Both the intensity of opacification and the depth of penetration into the body of the left atrium and pulmonary veins are important in quantifying mitral insufficiency as either mild ($1+$) or severe ($4+$). The left ventricle is usually imaged in one or more planes so that an assessment of both regional and overall left ventricular contraction can be made. A reduction of the global left ventricular ejection fraction to less than 40%-50% is indicative of severe left ventricular dysfunction. In chronic, well-compensated cases the left ventricular end-diastolic pressure is normal. The pulmonary artery wedge pressure trace typically show v waves, and pulmonary artery pressures are elevated. Coronary angiography is routinely performed in patients over 40 years of age and in anyone judged to be at risk for coronary artery disease.

2. Differential diagnosis. Chronic mitral insufficiency should not present much of a challenge in differential diagnosis. In acute mitral insufficiency with cardiogenic shock, the clinical findings may mimic those of acute massive pulmonary embolus with right ventricular failure or acute myocardial infarction with severe left ventricular dysfunction (>40% of the left ventricle involved) or myocardial rupture with VSD.

3. Natural history. Untreated patients ultimately develop irreversible left ventricular failure and die of low cardiac output, respiratory failure, or visceral organ hypoperfusion. Systemic thromboemboli are rare. Bacterial endocarditis is a continuing long-term risk mandating appropriate antibiotic prophylaxis at the time of invasive procedures.

4. Treatment

a. Medical. Medical treatment of acute mitral insufficiency depends upon the hemodynamic severity and underlying cause. In general, patients with a mechanical problem (endocarditis, ruptured papillary muscle or major chordae) and hemodynamically moderate to severe mitral insufficiency should be referred for mitral valve repair/replacement early in their course before they develop secondary organ failure. In the interim they may be temporarily stabilized with diuretics, vasodilators, and the intraaortic balloon pump. Patients with ischemic mitral insufficiency (posterior papillary muscle dysfunction) in the setting of acute inferior myocardial infarction may benefit from emergent thrombolytic or PTCA therapy. The mainstays of medical treatment in chronic mitral insufficiency are diuretics, digoxin, and vasodilators. Careful follow-up is essential to prevent irreversible left ventricular dysfunction.

b. Surgical. A variety of operative techniques have been used for repair of mitral valve insufficiency. Recently, the intraoperative evaluation of mitral valve function and techniques of valve repair have become much more precise, and a hemodynamically acceptable, durable repair can be performed in the majority of patients. All patients with hemodynamically significant acute mitral insufficiency should undergo operative repair/replacement unless there are compelling contraindications. In addition, patients with endocarditis and AV block (annular extension of the infection), bulky vegetation (>1 cm), fungal or *S. aureus* infection, persistent sepsis, or systemic emboli should be considered for early operation even in the absence of hemodynamically severe mitral insufficiency. In chronic mitral insufficiency, valve repair/replacement should be preformed in symptomatic patients (NYHA classes 3 and 4) as well as asymptomatic or mildly symptomatic patients (NYHA classes 1 and 2) with progressive left ventricular enlargement or decreased ejection fraction, worsening pulmonary hypertension, or the onset of atrial fibrillation.

5. Prognosis.
The operative mortality for urgent mitral valve repair/replacement in acute mitral insufficiency averages 5%-15%. It is higher in the setting of acute myocardial infarction, left ventricular dysfunction, or secondary organ failure. Among patients with chronic mitral insufficiency the average operative mortality in most institutions for mitral valve repair/

replacement is 3%-8%, the major risk factors being the patient's age, type of operation (replacement > repair), and left ventricular function. Patients who undergo valve repair have a lesser long-term risk of endocarditis and thromboembolism than those who undergo replacement with either tissue or mechanical prostheses.

E. TRICUSPID VALVE DISEASE. Diseases of the tricuspid valve are usually categorized as either functional or organic. Functional tricuspid insufficiency secondary to pulmonary hypertension can be caused by a variety of conditions that primarily affect either the lung or the left side of the heart (mitral and aortic valve disease or chronic left ventricular dysfunction). Organic disease of the tricuspid valve (stenosis or insufficiency) is usually secondary to rheumatic fever or endocarditis. Rare causes include trauma, tumors, papillary muscle rupture, carcinoid syndrome, and Marfan's syndrome. The pathophysiology is caused by elevated right atrial pressure without much effect on resting cardiac output. Cardiac output does not increase much with exercise or stress.

1. Diagnosis

a. Symptoms. The usual symptoms are fatigue, abdominal swelling (ascites), and leg edema. Fever, constitutional symptoms, pleuritic chest pain, and hemoptysis are suggestive of endocarditis.

b. Signs. Increased jugular venous pressure (v waves indicate tricuspid insufficiency), hepatomegaly (pulsation of the liver is also indicative of tricuspid insufficiency), ascites, and peripheral edema are commonly present. A right ventricular heave may be palpable. The murmurs of tricuspid valve disease are usually heard best along the left sternal border and are augmented with inspiration. An opening snap analogous to that in mitral stenosis may be audible in tricuspid stenosis, and a pansystolic murmur is indicative of tricuspid insufficiency. If pulmonary hypertension is present, P_2 may be prominent. Patients with endocarditis frequently have fever, splenomegaly, splinter hemorrhages, and pleural rubs.

c. Laboratory tests. No specific laboratory tests help in diagnosis. Patients with suspected endocarditis should have several sets of blood cultures drawn from different sites before starting antibiotic treatment.

d. Chest radiography. Enlargement of the right atrium is invariable. The right ventricle is enlarged if tricuspid insufficiency or pulmonary hypertension is present. Changes in the contour of the pulmonary arteries, pulmonary veins, left atrium, and left ventricle result from any primary left-sided valvular problem. Multiple pulmonary infiltrates/infarcts may be seen in patients with endocarditis.

e. ECG. Atrial fibrillation. Biphasic P waves in those patients with sinus rhythm. Right ventricular hypertrophy. Prolongation of the PR interval or higher degrees of AV conduction block in patients with endocarditis indicate spread of the infection to the annular tissues.

f. Echocardiography. Transthoracic or transesophageal echocardiography is extremely helpful. In addition to visualizing the tricuspid valve, right atrium, and ventricle, echocardiography permits thorough assessment of the aortic and mitral valves as well as left ventricular function.

g. Cardiac catheterization. Right atrial pressure is increased, and if tricuspid insufficiency is present v waves are seen in the right atrial pressure trace. Tricuspid stenosis is present if the mean diastolic gradient between the right atrium and ventricle is greater than 5 mm Hg. Pulmonary hypertension invariably accompanies functional disorders of the tricuspid valve. Radiographic contrast injection into the body of the right ventricle has been used to assess the severity of tricuspid insufficiency in a fashion analogous to that for mitral regurgitation.

2. Differential diagnosis. Constrictive pericarditis can mimic many of the clinical features of isolated tricuspid valve disease but should not pose much of a problem in differential diagnosis if echocardiography is available.

3. Natural history. Long-term complications include cirrhosis, renal failure, and malnutrition secondary to protein-losing enteropathy.

4. Treatment

a. Medical. For patients with functional tricuspid insufficiency, appropriate treatment of the pulmonary or left-sided cardiac problem with diuretics, digoxin, or vasodilators is all that is necessary. Patients with organic tricuspid valve insufficiency resulting from trauma, rheumatic fever, or healed endocarditis can usually be managed on a similar medical regimen and often have a satisfactory exercise tolerance as long as pulmonary vascular resistance is low.

b. Surgical. Intraoperative functional analysis and repair techniques analogous to those for the mitral valve have been developed for the tricuspid valve. At present almost all patients undergo reparative procedures unless the valve is hopelessly damaged. Patients undergoing operation for aortic or mitral valve disease who have associated functional tricuspid insufficiency (moderate to severe) should have the tricuspid valve repaired at the same time to improve perioperative cardiac function (reduce right atrial pressure and increase cardiac output). Patients with tricuspid endocarditis should undergo surgery if there is a coexisting left-sided valvular lesion, persistent sepsis despite appropriate systemic antibiotic treatment, or fungal organism. In this patient population with a high incidence of IV drug use and risk for noncompliance, tricuspid valvectomy rather than valve replacement may be a better alternative.

5. Prognosis. Tricuspid valve repair does not appear to increase the operative morbidity or mortality of other cardiac surgical procedures. If valve replacement is necessary, a tissue prostheses offers advantages in terms of freedom from valve thrombosis and thromboembolism. For patients with functional tricuspid insufficiency, long-term survival depends more upon the primary left-sided valvular problem and left ventricular function than on the type of tricuspid valve repair.

VII. CONGENITAL HEART DISEASE

ACYANOTIC DEFECTS

A. VENTRICULAR SEPTAL DEFECT. A VSD is a hole(s) in the interventricular septum. VSDs can occur either as isolated lesions or as part of another anomaly (e.g., tetralogy of Fallot, AV canal). They are the most common from of congenital cardiac anomaly, accounting for 30% to 40% of cardiac malformations at birth. They are classified by size and location. Nonrestrictive (large) VSDs are approximately the same size as the aortic orifice or larger, offering no resistance to flow. The pressures in the right and left ventricles are equal, and the magnitude of the left-to-right shunt depends upon the pulmonary vascular resistance. Smaller-sized VSDs are said to be restrictive because they offer some resistance to flow, resulting in lower pressures in the right ventricle than in the left. In small VSDs the right ventricular pressure is normal and the increase in the pulmonary blood flow (Qp/Qs) is less than 1.75. Moderate-sized VSDs raise the right ventricular pressure to half LV pressure, and the Qp/Qs is less than 3.5. VSDs may be located at the inlet, outlet, apical trabecular, or perimembranous septum when viewed from the right ventricle. In addition to the deleterious effects on the heart caused by the increased biventricular volume load, the increased pulmonary blood flow and pressure can lead to progressive obliteration of the pulmonary vascular bed. In this situation the pulmonary vascular resistance increases, the magnitude of the left-to-right shunt decreases until over time the direction of flow through the defect is reversed, and cyanosis develops (Eisenmenger's syndrome). VSDs can close spontaneously, even large ones, as a result of ingrowth of fibrous tissue or adherence of the septal leaflet of the tricuspid valve. The probability of spontaneous closure depends on the age of the child (80% at 1 month, 60% at 3 months, 50% at 6 months, and 25% at 12 months).

1. Diagnosis

a. Symptoms. Infants become symptomatic within 6 weeks to 3 months of birth as the pulmonary vascular resistance falls. They present with tachypnea, poor feeding, sweating, and failure to grow. Older children may be asymptomatic or present with effort dyspnea and failure to grow. Progressive pulmonary vascular disease causes severe exercise limitation and cyanosis.

b. Signs. In infants the typical findings are tachypnea with subcostal retractions, growth failure, increased jugular venous distention, hepatomegaly, and diminished peripheral pulses. There is usually a prominent apical impulse and right ventricular heave. The characteristic systolic murmur is best heard in the left third to fifth interspace and is often accompanied by a thrill. Older children may present only because of the systolic murmur, and they seldom have severe signs of heart failure. A prominent apical impulse and right ventricular heave may be present. S_2 is usually widely split, and the degree of splitting increases on inspiration. As pulmonary vascular resistance develops the prominence of the apical impulse, the intensity of the systolic murmur decreases until it disappears completely. The right ventricular heave becomes more pronounced and S_2 is markedly increased in intensity. Cyanosis and clubbing may then also be seen.

c. Laboratory tests. No specific diagnostic laboratory tests are available. Patients with Eisenmenger's syndrome have hypoxemia and polycythemia.

d. Chest radiography. Patients with small VSDs usually have normal chest radiographs. Those with large VSDs and shunts have large central pulmonary arteries and increased pulmonary vascular markings overall. Infants may show typical pulmonary edema. The right ventricle, left ventricle, and left atrium are usually enlarged. With the development of pulmonary vascular disease there is a reduction in peripheral pulmonary vascular markings, normalization of the left atrial and ventricular size, and further right ventricular enlargement.

e. ECG. The ECG is normal in patients with small VSDs. As the size of the shunt increases, left followed by right ventricular hypertrophy is seen. Patients with pulmonary vascular disease show regression of left ventricular hypertrophy, and right ventricular hypertrophy persists.

f. Echocardiography. Echocardiography has replaced catheterization for diagnosis of isolated VSDs in many institutions. With Doppler flow velocity techniques, the magnitude and direction of the shunt can also be measured. Echocardiography is also helpful in following patients for spontaneous VSD closure and the development of aortic valve insufficiency or infundibular stenosis.

g. Cardiac catheterization. Catheterization is used mostly to confirm the diagnosis in equivocal cases, to measure pulmonary and systemic flows and resistances in patients with suspected pulmonary vascular disease, or to evaluate other cardiac anomalies. The characteristic features of a large VSD and large shunt include a step-up in venous oxygen saturation in the right ventricle, equalization of pressures between the right and left ventricle, and a Qp/Qs greater than 3.5.

2. Differential diagnosis. VSD is usually fairly easily distinguished from atrial septal defect and patent ductus arteriosus, two other major causes of left-to-right intracardiac shunting in children. In infants with severe heart failure, the differential diagnosis includes critical aortic stenosis.

3. Natural history. Most patients have small VSDs and shunt flows that either close spontaneously or do not cause significant problems during childhood. However, everyone with persistent large VSDs and shunt flows eventually develops pulmonary vascular disease (probability 10% at 10 years, 50% at 20 years, 90% at 40 years), but it is extremly unusual within the first year of life. Bacterial endocarditis can also occur but is rare. Infants with large VSDs and shunts who develop heart failure within the first 2-3 months of life have a poor prognosis without surgical closure, with death ultimately the result of heart failure or recurrent pulmonary infections. A small number of patients develop aortic insufficiency or infundibular stenosis as a complication of their VSD.

4. Treatment

a. Medical. In symptomatic infants, heart failure is treated with diuretics and fluid and salt restriction. Older children with small to moderate-sized VSDs are usually followed serially until the defect closes spontaneously. Antibiotic prophylaxis is required for everyone prior to significant dental or other procedures. The management of patients with Eisenmenger's syndrome can be very challenging and includes optimization of hematocrit, fluid status, and right ventricular function.

b. Surgical. The two indications for surgical repair of large VSDs in infancy/early childhood are symptoms of heart failure, including retarded growth, and evidence of increasing pulmonary vascular resistance on serial follow-up even in the absence of significant symtoms. In older children, operative repair is usually recommended only after a period of observation to determine that the VSD will not close spontaneously and Qp/Qs >1.5. The development of aortic insufficiency is also an indication for prompt repair so that valve function can be preserved. Surgical closure is not recommended when the pulmonary vascular resistance is greater than 10-12 Wood units/m^2.

5. Prognosis. The operative mortality for patients with isolated VSDs is very low, even in the first 3-6 months of life. The long-term outcome in terms of growth, relief of symptoms, and recovery of normal biventricular function, and freedom from pulmonary vascular disease is particularly good for those who are operated on before 2 years of age. Patients with elevated pulmonary vascular resistance have a much higher operative mortality and a worse long-term survival (25% mortality within 5 years if pulmonary vascular resistance >10 Wood units/m^2).

B. ATRIAL SEPTAL DEFECT. ASD is a hole of variable size in the interatrial septum through which blood may shunt in either direction. An ASD is normally present in utero and postnatally may be an essential pathway if there is right-side obstruction to flow (tricuspid atresia, pulmonary stenosis with intact ventricular septum) or transposition of the great vessels. ASDs account for approximately 7% of all congenital heart disease at birth and are usually classified according to the site of the defect (fossa ovalis or secundum ASD, posterior ASD, AV septal defect or ostium primum ASD, coronary sinus ASD, sinus venosus defect or subcaval ASD, and confluent ASD). They are associated with almost every other type of cardiac anomaly. Fossa ovalis defects, the most common type overall, have a female predominance (3:1); otherwise, no gender predilection occurs among the other types. Anomalous drainage of some of the pulmonary veins (commonly the right superior pulmonary vein) into the right atrium or venae cavae can be a feature of some ASDs, particularly the sinus venosus type. Ostium primum ASDs comprise one end of a spectrum of malformations involving the embryologic endocardial cushions that ultimately form the mitral and tricuspid valves as well as a portion of the atrial and ventricular septum and thus account for the frequent occurrence of anomalies of the AV valves and proximal portion of the ventricular septum with this particular type of ASD. In spite of the different sites within the interatrial septum, the major hemodynamic effect produced by an ASD is a left-to-right shunt with volume loading of the right ventricle and increased pulmonary blood flow. The increased pulmonary blood flow rarely causes pulmonary hypertension or pulmonary vascular disease during childhood. Adults with neglected ASDs can develop right ventricular failure and supraventricular tachyarrhythmias. Careful studies have shown that although the bulk of flow across the ASD is from left to right, in some phases of the cardiac cycle the direction of flow is reversed, either as a result of the instantaneous pressure difference between the left and right atrium or as a result of streaming of inferior vena caval flow toward the atrial septum by the eustachian valve at the cavoatrial junction. The overall magnitude of the shunt depends upon the size of the communication, the pulmonary vascular resistance, and the relative diastolic compliance of the two ventricles. In early infancy the compliance of the two ventricles is similar, and the shunt may not be clinically apparent. However, as pulmonary vascular resistance declines to its normal level over the first 3 months of life accompanied by a parallel increase in right ventricular diastolic compliance, shunt flow increases. The increased flow through the right ventricular outflow tract and pulmonary artery gives rise to the systolic murmur and many of the other diagnostic clinical features.

1. Diagnosis

a. Symptoms. Most infants and young children are asymptomatic. Older children and adults can present with exertional dyspnea, fatigue, and palpitations as a result of pulmonary hypertension or right ventricular failure. There may also be a tendency to develop recurrent respiratory infections.

b. Signs. Cyanosis is usually absent and peripheral pulses are normal. A right ventricular heave, fixed splitting of S_2, midsystolic pulmonary flow murmur, and mid-diastolic tricuspid flow murmur are characteristic. Increased jugular venous pressure, hepatomegaly, ascites, and peripheral edema occur with right ventricular dysfunction. Concomitant pulmonary hypertension is suggested by a loud P_2. Prominent v waves in the jugular venous pulse and a pulsatile liver are indicative of clinically significant tricuspid insufficiency.

c. Laboratory tests. No laboratory tests are specific for ASD. Systemic arterial oxygen saturation is either normal or only slightly reduced.

d. Chest radiography. The pulmonary arteries are enlarged with prominent vascular markings consistent with increased pulmonary blood flow. The right ventricle and atrium are enlarged, suggesting volume overload.

e. ECG. Sinus rhythm, prominent p waves, and right ventricular hypertrophy are common. The majority of patients with uncomplicated ASDs have incomplete right bundle branch block and a clockwise frontal loop. Left ventricular hypertrophy suggests mitral insufficiency or systemic hypertension. Ostium primum ASDs and other AV septal defects are associated with left axis deviation and a counterclockwise frontal loop.

f. Echocardiogram. Echocardiography is diagnostic and may obviate cardiac catheterization among young patients with uncomplicated ASDs.

g. Cardiac catheterization. Cardiac catheterization may be necessary to evaluate other cardiac anomalies, to assess the pulmonary vascular resistance and status of the mitral valve, and in patients who are suspected of having anomalous pulmonary venous drainage. Patients over the age of 40 years or with risk factors should also undergo coronary angiography.

2. Natural history. Survival of patients with large ASDs is not much different from that of the normal age-matched population for the first 20 years of life. Thereafter there is an excess mortality in each decade mainly from congestive heart failure. The development of hypertension or coronary artery disease in adult patients can increase the magnitude of the shunt by reducing the compliance of the left ventricle and exacerbate symptoms. In addition, progressive mitral and tricuspid valve incompetence and recurrent supraventricular tachyarrhythmias become more significant among older patients with large ASDs. Endocarditis is extremly rare.

3. Treatment
a. Medical. Fluid overload and supraventricular arrhythmias are treated with diuretics, digoxin, and other antiarrhythmics. Antibiotic prophylaxis is not recommended for uncomplicated ASDs.

b. Surgical. ASD repairs were among the first successful open heart operations to be performed using cardiopulmonary bypass. The defects may be repaired primarily or patched with autogenous pericardium, Teflon, or Dacron. The usual indication for operative closure of an uncomplicated ASD is the presence of a Qp/Qs of 1.5 or more. Recovery of right ventricular function seems to be better with earlier operative repair, so most institutions recommend that children undergo repair before 5 years of age. Operative closure is contraindicated if the pulmonary vascular resistance is greater than 12 Wood units/m^2.

4. Prognosis. The operative mortality is extremly low and usually limited to those who have severe pulmonary hypertension, right ventricular dysfunction, or complex associated malformations. If repair is done in childhood, long-term survival and functional status are identical to those of the normal aged-matched population. Even in older patients with advanced symptoms and moderate pulmonary hypertension, ASD repair can improve survival and functional ability. Older patients who are at increased risk for both systemic and pulmonary emboli postoperatively should probably receive short-term sodium warfarin anticoagulation.

C. PULMONARY STENOSIS WITH INTACT VENTRICULAR SEPTUM.

This congenital malformation includes forms of right ventricular outflow tract obstruction in which the stenosis is usually valvar or both valvar and infundibular, but rarely may be only infundibular. It accounts for about 10% of congenital heart disease, and there is usually a female preponderance. There is a spectrum which ranges from critical pulmonary stenosis (neonatal presentation, association with poorly developed right ventricle), through severe pulmonary stenosis (later presentation, normal-size or dilated right ventricle), to mild pulmonary stenosis that remains relatively stable for life. The pulmonary valve is usually the major site of obstruction. The leaflets are thickened and fused to a variable degree, resulting in a dome-shaped structure with a narrow central orifice. Post-stenotic dilation of the main pulmonary artery is commonly present. Neonates may also have hypoplastic branch pulmonary arteries. The right ventricle is hypertrophied, and in severe cases this may result in infundibular stenosis. Abnormal myocardial sinusoids may also communicate with the coronary arteries. The tricuspid valve is usually morphologically normal but is often functionally incompetent. More than 75% of patients have an ASD or patent fossa ovalis. In utero, obstruction to right ventricular outflow and reduced pulmonary artery and ductus arteriosus blood flow are of no particular consequence and are compensated by increased blood flow across the foramen ovale into the left atrium and ventricle. At birth, the pulmonary blood flow (the sum of right ventricular output and left-to-right ductus arteriosus flow) may be inadequate to sustain life, particularly as the ductus begins to close. In those who present as infants or older children, pulmonary blood flow may not be capable of increasing as the child grows or becomes more active. There may also be continued right-to-left shunting across the foramen ovale with cyanosis. Thus, although usually presented as an acyanotic congenital heart defect, cyanosis can occur in some circumstances.

1. Diagnosis

a. Symptoms. Neonates appear critically ill, irritable, and tachypneic. Older children are often asymptomatic or only mildly symptomatic (exertional dyspnea, fatigue) and develop normally. If pulmonary stenosis is severe, chest pain, dyspnea, syncope, poor growth, and cyanosis may be present.

b. Signs. Neonates have tachypnea, tachycardia, cyanosis, and poor peripheral perfusion. There may be no murmurs if cardiac output is severly reduced. Cyanosis and clubbing are present in older children with an ASD and right-to-left shunt. The jugular venous pressure is elevated, both *a* and *v* waves may be present, and P_2 is reduced or absent. A harsh systolic murmur preceded by a click can usually be best heard in the pulmonic area. Murmurs of tricuspid insufficiency and PDA may be present. A right ventricular heave and thrill are also common. Adults may present with chronic right ventricular failure manifest as elevated jugular venous pressure, hepatomegaly, and ascites.

c. Laboratory tests. Arterial blood gases may show oxygen desaturation and acidosis in critically ill neonates. Polycythemia may be associated with oxygen desaturation in older children.

d. Chest radiography. Neonates have cardiomegaly with a relative reduction in pulmonary vascular markings. Older children have post-stenotic dilatation of the main pulmonary artery.

e. ECG. Prominent P waves. Right ventricular hypertrophy. Suspect hypoplastic right ventricle if there is left ventricular predominance.

f. Echocardiogram. Echocardiography is diagnostic for both neonates and older children. The thickened, stenotic pulmonary valve is well seen, and the size of the right ventricle, the outflow tract gradient, and the function of the tricuspid valve may all be assessed.

g. Cardiac catheterization. The characteristic findings include a systolic pressure gradient between the right ventricle and the pulmonary artery without evidence of a VSD, and peak right ventricular pressures may be suprasystemic. The severity of the right ventricular outflow tract obstruction is graded according to the peak pressure gradient: mild, <50 mm Hg; moderate, 50-80 mm Hg; and severe, >80 mm Hg. Angiography is useful to show the classic dome-shaped pulmonary valve with small central aperture, the size of the right ventricle and infundibulum, the competence of the tricuspid valve, and the size of the main pulmonary trunk and branch pulmonary arteries. It may also demonstrate right ventricular sinusoids and connections to coronary arteries. An ASD is present in >75% of patients.

2. Differential diagnosis. In neonates the differential diagnosis includes transposition of the great arteries.

3. Natural history. When symptoms appear in neonates the prognosis for survival without treatment is extremly poor. Essentially all of these patients die of acute heart failure and hypoxemia within a few days to weeks of birth. Patients who remain asymptomatic throughout the neonatal period have a wide variation in the degree of pulmonary stenosis. With time infundibular hypertrophy and further degenerative changes in the pulmonary valve can add to the severity of obstruction. Heart failure and sudden death are important causes of death in the group with moderate to severe obstruction.

4. Treatment
a. Medical. Neonates require PGE$_1$ infusion to maintain ductal patency; supplemental oxygen and other resuscitative measures while diagnostic studies are being performed and in the interim before urgent surgical repair. Children need diuretics and fluid restriction for fluid overload and in the interim prior to surgical repair.

b. Surgical. The choice of surgical procedure depends upon the age of the patient, the combination of anatomic and physiologic problems, and the surgeon's preference. The goals of the operation are to achieve satisfactory pulmonary blood flow, relieve right ventricular outflow tract obstruction, and restore right ventricular function. Neonates presenting in the first few weeks of life require urgent operation (open or closed valvotomy with or without a systemic–to–pulmonary artery shunt) and careful follow-up. It is not uncommon for these patients to require reoperation for residual outflow tract obstruction and ASD closure. Among older children operation is recommended if the patient is symptomatic or if moderate to severe pulmonary stenosis is present.

5. Prognosis. The operative mortality, long-term survival, relief of obstruction, and right ventricular function among children and adults who undergo operative repair are generally excellent. The few early and late deaths usually result from preoperative advanced right ventricular dysfunction. In neonates the operative mortality has been higher (10%-60%) and the need for reoperations more frequent (30%). Right ventricular hypoplasia and abnormal sinusoids are important determinants for both operative mortality and long-term survival.

D. PATENT DUCTUS ARTERIOSUS. The ductus arteriosus is derived from the sixth aortic arch. It most commonly originates from the main or left pulmonary artery and terminates on the descending thoracic aorta just distal to the left subclavian artery. In utero deoxygenated venous blood returning from the superior vena cava is directed across the tricuspid valve into the right ventricle and from there into the main pulmonary artery. The blood is then diverted away from the atelectatic lungs and through the ductus arteriosus into the descending aorta and on its way to the placenta to be reoxygenated. At birth the ductus measures 5-10 mm in length and is as large as the aorta in diameter. At full term ductal smooth muscle is exquisitely sensitive to tissue oxygen tension and responds rapidly to the normal postnatal increase in arterial oxygen content. Thus functional closure of the ductus is normally present by 10-15 hours of life. Failure of ductal closure occurs in 1:2500 to 5000 live births and results in shunting of blood from the aorta to the pulmonary artery, increasing both pulmonary artery flow and pressure and volume loading the left ventricle. The magnitude of the shunt depends upon the size of the ductus and the pulmonary vascular resistance. Shunting occurs throughout systole and diastole, resulting in decreased systemic diastolic blood pressure and impaired visceral perfusion. There is a significant association with prematurity and low birth weight (80% incidence in infants <1000 g). Females are affected more commonly than males.

1. Diagnosis

a. Symptoms. Onset of symptoms depends upon ductal size, pulmonary vascular resistance, and associated anomalies. Full-term infants become symptomatic as pulmonary vascular resistance drops at 6-8 weeks of age. Premature infants become symptomatic much earlier. The usual presenting symptoms of heart failure in infancy are sweating, irritability, tachypnea, and poor feeding.

b. Signs. The classic signs are bounding peripheral pulses, hyperactive precordium, low diastolic blood pressure, and a "machinery" (systolic and diastolic components) murmur heard best in the left second interspace anteriorly. The characteristic murmur may be absent in premature infants or those with low cardiac output. A mid-diastolic apical rumble attributable to increased mitral flow, gallop rhythm, and hepatomegaly may also be present. Cyanosis is an indication of right-to-left shunting.

c. Laboratory tests. There are no specific diagnostic laboratory tests.

d. Chest radiography. Cardiomegaly and pulmonary congestion are usually present.

e. ECG. Left ventricular hypertrophy is present in older children and adults.

f. Echocardiography. Transthoracic echocardiography is extremely useful in neonates. Using two-dimensional imaging and Doppler techniques, it is possible to delineate the ductus and any other cardiac/great vessel anomalies. If the ratio between left atrial diameter and aortic diameter is greater than 1.4-1.5, a significant left-to-right shunt is likely.

g. Cardiac catheterization. Catheterization is usually not required in infants. It may be used in older patients and those with atypical findings, pulmonary hypertension, or other anomalies. A step-up in venous oxygen saturation in pulmonary artery and pulmonary hypertension is characteristic. Recently, nonoperative attempts at catheter closure of PDA have been attempted.

2. Differential diagnosis.
PDA must be differentiated from aortopulmonary window and from other defects associated with left-to-right shunting and left ventricular volume overload.

3. Natural history.
Untreated patients with moderate-sized PDA may remain asymptomatic for 20-30 years. Late deaths occur secondary to heart failure, endocarditis, and,

rarely, aneurysmal dilatation and rupture. Progressive pulmonary hypertension with the development of Eisenmenger's physiology occurs in some patients with an initially large PDA and pulmonary blood flow.

4. Treatment

a. Medical. There is no uniform consensus regarding management of PDA in premature infants. The ductus may close spontaneously as the infant matures. However, a persistent ductal shunt worsens any other problem that the infant has (e.g., respiratory distress, bronchpulmonary dysplasia). Pharmacologic closure with a prostaglandin synthesis inhibitor, indomethacin, has been effective in up to 70% of infants. Side effects of indomethacin treatment include platelet dysfunction, GI bleeding, hyponatremia, and renal dysfunction.

b. Surgical. The presence of a persistent PDA in a fullterm infant is an indication for operative closure to prevent late death from heart failure or endocarditis. In premature infants, operative closure is usually deferred until after a failed attempt at pharmacologic closure. The ductus may be obliterated by either simple ligation or division and ligation. Operative complications include hemorrhage, chylothorax, recurrent laryngeal nerve injury, and infection.

5. Prognosis.
Operative mortality even in critically ill neonates is extremly low, and postoperatively they have a normal life expectancy. In older children with pulmonary hypertension and right-to-left shunting, endocarditis, or a calcified ductus the mortality is greater.

E. AORTIC STENOSIS. Congenital aortic stenosis is characterized by narrowing of the left ventricular outflow tract at the valvar, subvalvar, supravalvar, or combined levels, which results in a systolic pressure gradient between the inflow portion of the left ventricle and the aorta beyond the obstruction. Aortic stenosis affects 7% of patients with congenital heart disease. In utero, obstruction of the left ventricular outflow tract is compensated by a decrease in flow across the foramen ovale into the left atrium and increase in flow across the tricuspid valve into the right ventricle and eventually across the ductus arteriosus into the descending aorta. There may also be underdevelopment of the aortic annulus, hypoplasia of the left ventricle, coarctation of the aorta, and mitral insufficiency or stenosis. Postnatally, the increased pulmonary venous return and left atrial pressure tend to close the foramen ovale, resulting in an increased volume load on the hypertrophied, noncompliant left ventricle. In neonates, the left atrial pressures may increase further and systemic perfusion become inadequate as the ductus arteriosus begins to close. Those with less severe obstruction develop concentric left ventricular hypertrophy and may remain asymptomatic for prolonged periods of time. Valvar aortic stenosis is caused by imperfect cusp development with leaflet thickening, and the valve is bicuspid about 70% of the time. This is the most common form of congenital aortic stenosis and affects males preferentially. Discrete subvalvar aortic stenosis is the next most common form and is caused by a localized fibrous/fibromuscular ridge or fibrous tunnel beneath the usually normal aortic valve. Supravalvar aortic stenosis is the least common form and is caused by localized or diffuse narrowing of the ascending aorta. The stenosis may encroach upon the coronary arteries or arch vessels.

1. Diagnosis

a. Symptoms. Neonates/infants with severe valvar stenosis present in acute distress with pallor, perspiration, feeding difficulties, tachypnea, and cyanosis. Those with subvalvar or supravalvar stenosis rarely become symptomatic during infancy. Older children and adults with severe obstruction at any site may either be asymptomatic or have angina, syncope, or dyspnea with exertion. Angina may be more prevalent among those with supravalvar stenosis.

b. Signs. Neonates/infants with severe valvar stenosis appear acutely ill and have clinical evidence of poor perfusion such as diminished pulses, pallor, and cyanosis. If the cardiac output is low, the characteristic systolic murmur may be inaudible. In older children/adults with significant obstruction at any level, the carotid pulse has a low volume and slow upstroke. The apical impulse is prominent, and the systolic murmur is best heard at the base. The murmur radiates to the carotids and may be accompanied by a palpable thrill. An S_3 or S_4 is usually indicative of severe stenosis. An ejection click is heard only in valvar stenosis and although a diastolic murmur of aortic insufficiency is uncommon in valvar or supravalvar aortic stenosis, one may be present in more than half of the patients with subvalvar stenosis. A moderate number of patients with supravalvar stenosis have a syndrome of elfin facies, low IQ, and poor growth.

c. Laboratory tests. No laboratory tests are diagnostic.

d. Chest radiography. The left ventricle is prominent, but overall cardiac size is not increased unless overt heart failure is present. Post-stenotic dilation of the ascending aorta is characteristically seen in valvar aortic stenosis but not the other types.

e. ECG. Left ventricular hypertrophy is usually present. Rarely, the ECG is normal.

f. Echocardiography. The two-dimensional echocardiogram demonstrates the anatomy of the left ventricular outflow tract, the site of obstruction, and any other associated cardiac anomalies. In patients with subvalvar obstruction the echocardiogram can also be useful in excluding hypertrophic cardiomyopathy. The pressure gradient and valve area can be estimated using Doppler flow velocity techniques.

g. Cardiac catheterization. Aortic stenosis is diagnosed by finding a systolic pressure gradient across the appropriate site in the left ventricular outflow tract at catheterization. Simultaneous measurement of the cardiac output allows calculation of the orifice area. The degree of stenosis may be classified hemodynamically as mild (gradient <50 mm Hg, area >0.8 cm^2/m^2), moderate (gradient 50 to 75 mm Hg, area 0.5-0.8 cm^2/m^2), or severe (gradient >75 mm Hg, area <0.5 cm^2/m^2). Angiography allows demonstration of the site of obstruction, the presence of aortic insufficiency, and any other associated cardiac anomaly.

2. Differential diagnosis. The differential diagnosis in infants includes other forms of obstruction of the left ventricle such as coarctation of the aorta.

3. Natural history. In neonates/infants with severe valvar stenosis, rapidly progressive heart failure ultimately results in death within a few days to weeks of birth. Among children/adults with other forms of aortic stenosis, the onset of clinical heart failure may be delayed for a long time. However, there is usually an increase in the severity of the stenosis with time (moderate valvar stenosis progresses to severe stenosis within 10 years in approximately 60% of patients). The progression to severe stenosis among those with subvalvar stenosis may occur more rapidly. Those with severe stenosis, particularly supravalvar stenosis, are also at greatest risk of sudden death (1%-20%). In patients with subaortic stenosis post-stenotic turbulence may lead to leaflet thickening and aortic insufficiency. Spontaneous bacterial endocarditis is also occasionally (1%) a cause of late morbidity and mortality among patients with valvar and subvalvar stenosis.

4. Treatment

a. Medical. In neonates infusion of PGE$_1$ and correction of metabolic acidosis may temporarily stabilize the patient while diagnostic studies are being performed and in the interim before urgent valvotomy.

b. Surgical. Urgent valvotomy is required for all symptomatic infants/neonates with valvar stenosis. The usual indications for operation among older children/adults with valvar stenosis are the presence of symptoms or clinical evidence of severe stenosis (gradient, valve area, severe left ventricular hypertrophy, or progressive left ventricular dilatation). An initial valvotomy can nearly always be performed with at least partial relief of the obstruction. Repeat valvotomies may be required in those who restenose but are often preferable to prosthetic valve replacement in a young child. In teenagers and adults, if the valve is badly deformed aortic valve replacement with or without annular enlargement may be a more reasonable approach. Indications for operation among patients with subvalvar and supravalvar obstruction include symptoms or, given the more rapid progression and greater risk of sudden death, clinical evidence of moderate stenosis. A variety of operative procedures have been performed in these patients directed toward either resecting discrete sites of obstruction or patching diffuse sites. Select patients have even undergone placement of a valved conduit between the apex of the left ventricle and the descending aorta.

5. Prognosis. The operative mortality for valvotomy for valvar aortic stenosis depends upon the age of the patient (neonates/infants, 10%-80%; children/adults, <5%). Late survival is good, although nearly one third of patients require reoperation within 15-20 years and a significant number of these reoperations result in prosthetic valve replacement. Among patients with subvalvar and supravalvar stenosis, the operative mortality and long-term survival are somewhat better with the discrete than with the diffuse forms of stenosis.

F. COARCTATION OF THE AORTA. Coarctation of the aorta is a localized narrowing of the aorta which obstructs blood flow. Although any aortic segment can be involved, it is most common in the descending thoracic aorta at the site of insertion of the ductus arteriosus. The obstruction may be caused by tubular hypoplasia or a ridge of infolded hyperplastic intima and media. Coarctation of the aorta accounts for 5%-10% of congenital heart defects, and at autopsy the incidence is about 1 in 3000-4000. Isolated coarctation is more common in boys, but coarctation is associated with more complex congenital heart disease (bicuspid aortic valve, VSD, PDA, mitral valve anomalies), and both genders are affected equally. It is occasionally seen among members of the same family and the incidence is over 30% in patients with Turner's syndrome. The pathophysiology of coarctation results from the effects of increased afterload on the left ventricle and the adequacy of systemic aortic perfusion distal to the site of obstruction. There are no major hemodynamic consequences in utero and no stimulus for the development of collaterals until the ductus begins to close postnatally.

1. Diagnosis

a. Symptoms. Infants with preductal coarctation or interrupted aortic arch commonly present with heart failure shortly after birth, either secondary to other frequently associated cardiac anomalies or as a result of the dependence of distal aortic perfusion on continued ductal patency. Heart failure in these infants is manifested by irritability, sweating, tachypnea, and poor feeding. Among older children the symptoms are more often due to hypertension (headache, epistaxis, visual disturbances) or left ventricular dysfunction (exertional dyspnea).

b. Signs. In older children the cardinal signs are upper extremity hypertension and a differential in systolic blood pressure between the arms and the legs. The femoral pulses are either absent or diminished and the upstroke is delayed. A systolic murmur may be audible over the precordium and posteriorly between the scapulas. Collateral vessels can often be observed, palpated, or auscultated in the infrascapular region. Critically ill infants may not have an audible murmur and present instead with evidence of poor systemic perfusion (hypotension, oliguria, metabolic acidosis).

c. Laboratory tests. No laboratory tests are diagnostic. Plasma renin levels have not been consistently elevated.

d. Chest radiography. Cardiomegaly with prominence of the left ventricle is common. Pulmonary congestion indicates fluid overload or left ventricular dysfunction. In older children collateral circulation produces rib notching. The "3" sign is considered characteristic and consists of enlargement of the segment of aorta proximal to the coarctation, followed by the coarcted segment, and finally the distal segment affected by post-stenotic dilatation.

e. ECG. In infancy right, left, or biventricular hypertrophy may be seen. Among older children with hypertension left ventricular hypertrophy with strain is more common.

f. Echocardiography. Transthoracic or transesophageal echocardiography is an effective means of diagnosis and follow-up after repair. Doppler techniques enable measurement of flow velocity from which the pressure gradient across the site of obstruction and the cross-sectional area can be calculated. In addition, any associated cardiac anomalies can be readily detected.

g. Cardiac catheterization. Cardiac catheterization may be required to determine the location and hemodynamic severity, potential arch vessel involvement, and extent of collateral blood vessels. Recently there have been reports of balloon catheter dilatation both as primary treatment and for recurrences after previous repair of coarctation of the aorta.

2. Differential diagnosis. In infants coarctation must be distinguished from other lesions producing severe heart failure such as aortic stenosis. The differential diagnosis in older children includes other causes of hypertension (e.g., pheochromocytoma, renal disease).

3. Natural history. Without operative treatment virtually all symptomatic infants die of heart failure within a few days or weeks. Among those who are asymptomatic at birth and do not have operative correction, the average life expectancy is 30-40 years. The major causes of death among older patients are aortic rupture, bacterial endocarditis, cerebral hemorrhage, and heart failure.

4. Treatment

a. Medical. Critically ill infants with heart failure require aggressive medical treatment including the use of prostaglandins to maintain ductal patency prior to definitive repair. Pharmacologic management is also required if hypertension persists following a technically adequate repair in children and adults.

b. Surgical. The indications for immediate surgical repair in symptomatic infants are compelling, but no consensus exists regarding the optimal timing of surgery in asymptomatic children. Repairs in late childhood are associated with an increased incidence of persistent hypertension, whereas those performed in infancy have a higher rate of recurrent coarctation. Several surgical techniques have evolved. The major ones include resection with end-to-end anastomosis, resection and grafting (homograft or prosthetic tube graft), incision and prosthetic "onlay" patch, and subclavian flap aortoplasty. Each technique has its own unique features as well as complications. Paraplegia occurs in 0.5%-1% of patients and does not appear to be related to the choice of operative technique.

5. Prognosis. The operative mortality among critically ill infants is 5%-10% and is lower in older children and patients with isolated coarctation. Long-term survival and freedom from persistent hypertension and hypertensive vascular disease are good. Recurrence of coarctation following an initially successful repair is uncommon and may be related either to failure of a circumferential suture line to grow at the same rate as the adjacent aortic normal segments or to suture line thrombosis.

CYANOTIC DEFECTS

A. TETRALOGY OF FALLOT. Tetralogy of Fallot is part of the spectrum of congenital malformations characterized by pulmonary stenosis or atresia and VSD. The classic lesion consists of four major defects—right ventricular outflow tract obstruction as a result of muscular infundibular stenosis, a large perimembranous VSD, dextroposition of the aorta, and right ventricular hypertrophy. Physiologically, the VSD is nonrestrictive and pressures in the right and left ventricle are equal. Pulmonary blood flow depends upon the severity of the infundibular stenosis and the extent of systemic-to-pulmonary artery collaterals such as the ductus arteriosus. The predominant intracardiac shunt is from right to left, producing systemic cyanosis. A variety of additional anomalies may be present including an ASD, muscular VSDs, valvar, main, or branch pulmonary artery stenosis, coronary artery anomalies, and right-sided aortic arch.

1. Diagnosis

a. Symptoms. The symptoms depend upon the severity of the anatomic malformation. Cyanosis is the most common initial presentation. Infants with pulmonary atresia deteriorate hemodynamically as the ductus closes unless bronchial collaterals are already well developed. Rarely, cyanosis may become apparent only as the child outgrows the available pulmonary blood flow. Some children experience intense cyanotic "spells" that may lead to unconsciousness and cerebrovascular injury. Ambulatory children often exhibit a characteristic periodic "squatting" posture that increases systemic vascular resistance and reduces the right-to-left shunt.

b. Signs. Cyanosis, nail clubbing, and growth retardation are present. A precordial thrill is usually palpable. A harsh right ventricular outflow murmur is audible in the pulmonary area and along the left sternal border. The intensity of the murmur may change depending upon pulmonary blood flow. Continuous murmurs are characteristic of either naturally occurring or surgically created systemic-to-pulmonary shunts.

c. Laboratory tests. Polycythemia and systemic arterial hypoxemia are present.

d. Chest radiography. The usual appearance is diminished pulmonary vascularity and size of the main pulmonary artery. Classically the heart is boot shaped (coeur en sabot). Up to one quarter of patients have a right-sided aortic arch.

e. ECG. Right ventricular hypertrophy is characteristic.

f. Echocardiography. Transthoracic or transesophageal echocardiography provides almost all of the anatomic and physiologic information necessary to diagnose and plan treatment for tetralogy of Fallot. It also provides valuable information about associated anomalies.

g. Cardiac catheterization. Catheterization and angiography provide information about intraventricular pressures and the anatomy of the aorta, right ventricular outflow tract, and pulmonary arteries. It is also useful to define the status of surgically created systemic-to-pulmonary artery shunts as well as naturally occurring sources of pulmonary collateral blood flow.

2. Natural history. Untreated, most patients with tetralogy of Fallot die before adulthood; the average age at death is 12 years among those who survive infancy. Often death occurs during an hypoxic spell or as the result of a thrombotic event associated with severe polycythemia. In the preantibiotic era endocarditis and cerebral abscess were also frequent causes of death. Currently, almost every patient is a candidate for either palliative or definitive repair during infancy or early childhood.

3. Treatment

a. Medical. The initial medical treatment is directed toward stabilizing the infant until a systemic-to-pulmonary artery shunt or definitive repair is performed. This may include systemic administration of PGE_1 to maintain ductal patency and correction of hypoglycemia and metabolic acidosis. If a shunt is performed prior to definitive repair, children require careful follow-up in the interim. Heart failure may occur as a consequence of the additional volume loading imposed by the shunt, and it is important to maintain an adequate but not excessive hematocrit.

b. Surgical. The current trend is to perform definitive repair of tetralogy of Fallot in infancy. Pulmonary atresia, diminutive branch pulmonary arteries, a small left ventricle, or an anomalous left anterior descending coronary artery originating from the right coronary artery may preclude definitive repair at the time of initial presentation. Such patients may be palliated without the need for cardiopulmonary bypass by a surgically created systemic-to-pulmonary shunt (Blalock-Taussig shunt or a central aortopulmonary shunt using prosthetic graft material). Definitive repair of tetralogy of Fallot consists of patch closure of the VSD and resection or patching of all obstruction between the right ventricle and pulmonary arteries to restore normal pulmonary blood flow. Patients with pulmonary atresia require synthetic or homograft conduits to reestablish continuity between the right ventricle and main pulmonary artery. Major systemic-to-pulmonary collaterals should also be obliterated at the time of definitive repair. The operative mortality for the definitive repair of uncomplicated tetralogy of Fallot is between 1% and 5%.

4. Prognosis. The long-term survival and functional ability of most patients following repair are excellent. Heart block occurs in about 1%, and a residual VSD is detectable in about 4% of patients. Persistent elevation of right ventricular pressure above 60 mm Hg, a right bundle branch block, or frequent premature ventricular contractions are associated with an increased risk of sudden death during follow-up.

B. TRANSPOSITION OF THE GREAT ARTERIES. TGA is a severe cardiac malformation in which the aorta arises from the morphologic right ventricle and the pulmonary artery arises from the morphologic left ventricle. Up to one third of the patients have associated cardiac defects such as a VSD or left ventricular outflow tract obstruction. From birth systemic oxygenation and carbon dioxide elimination depend upon the extent of mixing of blood between the two parallel circulations through shunts across septal defects or a PDA.

1. Diagnosis

a. *Symptoms.* Older children with TGA and the combination of a VSD and left ventricular outflow tract obstruction may have hypoxic spells similar to those seen in tetralogy of Fallot.

b. *Signs.* The most striking sign is usually persistent cyanosis in the newborn period which does respond to a increase in inspired oxygen concentration. Ductal closure may lead to rapid clinical deterioration. Congestive heart failure manifested by tachypnea, dyspnea, tachycardia, and hepatomegaly may also be present. The heart is usually overactive and has a prominent left parasternal lift. The heart sounds are usually loud and crisp. A systolic ejection or shunt murmur may be present.

c. Laboratory tests. Polycythemia, systemic arterial hypoxemia, and in severe cases lactic acidosis are evident.

d. Chest radiography. In the AP projection the cardiac silhouette is enlarged and looks like an egg on its side. The cardiac pedicle is characteristically narrow. A pattern of increased pulmonary blood flow may also be present.

e. ECG. Normal sinus rhythm or sinus tachycardia with right-axis deviation (left axis is distinctly uncommon in uncomplicated TGA). Right ventricular hypertrophy is commonly seen. ST-T wave abnormalities may reflect myocardial ischemia, especially in the critically ill neonate.

f. Echocardiography. Transthoracic or transesophageal echocardiography is diagnostic for TGA. It also provides valuable information about the atrial septum and the adequacy of balloon atrial septostomy, right and left ventricular contractility and wall motion, the AV junction, the left ventricular outflow tract with respect to any obstructing elements, the ventricular septum for VSD, and the aortic isthmus for associated coarctation. With current imaging techniques the origins of the coronary arteries can also be seen. The echo also provides a useful means of follow-up after corrective or palliative surgical treatment.

g. Cardiac catheterization. Angiography and hemodynamic measurements may be necessary if insufficient information is available from echocardiography. More commonly, cardiac catheterization affords an opportunity to create or enlarge an ASD via balloon atrial septostomy to facilitate mixing between the two parallel circulations and stabilize the neonate until more definitive surgical repair is performed.

2. Natural history. Untreated, 90% of patients with TGA die before their first birthday and almost half of those deaths occur in the first month of life. By itself balloon atrial septostomy improves the 1-year mortality to about 40% in infants with uncomplicated TGA. Some patients with an intact ventricular septum or an associated VSD may experience progressive left ventricular outflow tract obstruction. Pulmonary vascular obstructive disease is also occasionally seen early in the course, particularly if unrestricted pulmonary blood flow (VSD without left ventricular outflow tract obstruction or PDA) is present.

3. Treatment

a. Medical. The initial medical therapy is directed at correction of metabolic acidosis, treatment of heart failure and hypoglycemia, maintenance of normothermia, and ventilatory support. Balloon atrial septostomy should be performed if systemic oxygenation is inadequate. Some infants may require PGE_1 infusions to maintain ductal patency. Failure to maintain the systemic arterial oxygen tension above 30 mm Hg increases the risk of permanent hypoxic cerebral injury.

b. Surgical. Palliative "closed heart" surgical procedures for TGA include pulmonary artery banding if excessive pulmonary flow is present and atrial septectomy (Blalock-Hanlon procedure) to improve mixing. Definitive "open heart" procedures for uncomplicated TGA include those in which blood flow is redirected at the atrial level (Mustard or Senning operation) as well as the direct rerouting of the aorta and pulmonary artery—the arterial switch. Recently, the arterial switch has gained popularity as operative mortality rates have improved. Average operative mortality for both the arterial and atrial switch operations is 5% to 10%. Additional operative procedures may be applicable to those with more complex malformations.

4. Prognosis. Long-term survival after atrial switch procedures is approximately 80% at 10-20 years. Late complications include supraventricular arrhythmias, incompetence of the tricuspid valve, and heart failure, the right ventricle not being capable of supporting the systemic circulation over the normal life span. As experience with the arterial switch operation grows, the late technical complications relating to the aortic and pulmonary anastomoses and the reimplanted coronary arteries are being reduced. Arrhythmias are uncommon, but it is still too early to determine whether the arterial switch is superior to the atrial switch in the long term.

VIII. CARDIAC TUMORS

Primary cardiac tumors are either benign or malignant neoplasms that arise from the endocardial, myocardial, or epicardial layer of the heart. Tumors arising from the pericardium are not included. Metastatic disease or contiguous spread from lung and breast cancers to the heart occurs 20 to 30 times more commonly than primary cardiac tumors. Most primary cardiac tumors (70%) are benign, and myxoma is the most frequent benign tumor. Myxomas are intracavitary tumors that occur most commonly in the left atrium from the vicinity of the fossa ovalis. Although generally regarded as benign tumors, distant metastases and local recurrences have been reported despite seemingly adequate resection margins. They occur in older adults and are two to three times more common in women than in men. They are extremely rare in children. In children, the most frequent primary cardiac tumor is rhabdomyoma, a benign tumor whose identity as a true neoplasm or myocardial hamartoma remains controversial. Half of the affected patients have tuberous sclerosis or hamartomas in other organs. Cardiac rhabdomyomas usually occur in the ventricles, and multiple lesions may be present. Lipoma, papillary fibroelastoma, fibroma, and hemangioma constitute the bulk of the remaining benign cardiac tumors. The malignant tumors (30%) comprise various sarcomas (angiosarcoma, rhabdomyosarcoma, mesothelioma, and fibrosarcoma being among the more common). Any of the cardiac chambers may be involved, and metastases to distant organs are common.

1. Diagnosis

a. Symptoms. Symptoms of exertional dyspnea, edema, and fatigue are consistent with obstruction to blood flow. Aggravation of symptoms caused by changes in body position can result from AV valve obstruction by a mobile atrial myxoma. Syncope and palpitations can be the result of tumor-induced arrhythmias. An interesting group of constitutional symptoms associated with some myxomas includes fever, arthralgia, weight loss, and Raynaud's phenomenon.

b. Signs. Elevated jugular venous pressure, pulmonary rales, peripheral edema, ascites, and hepatomegaly are all consistent with blood flow obstruction. Acute arterial insufficiency related to tumor embolization may also be the initial presentation. Various flow murmurs and tumor plops can be heard in some patients.

c. Laboratory tests. Patients with myxomas may have hyperglobulinemia, elevated sedimentation rate, polycythemia or hemolytic anemia, and thrombocytopenia. Occasionally, pathologic analysis of embolectomy specimens reveals an unsuspected tumor.

d. Chest radiography. The chest radiographic findings are nonspecific. A primary lung tumor or pulmonary metastases may be present. Other potential findings include pulmonary congestion and an enlarged cardiac silhouette. Rarely, calcifications within the tumor may be visible on the plain chest radiograph.

e. ECG. The ECG is also nonspecific. It may show atrial fibrillation, abnormal atrioventricular conduction, or ventricular dysrhythmias related to tumor infiltration.

f. Echocardiogram. Transthoracic or transesophageal two-dimensional echocardiography is diagnostic and may obviate more invasive studies.

g. Cardiac catheterization. Myxomas are prone to embolization so that catheterization is usually performed only to visualize the coronary arteries in patients over the age of 40 years or with risk factors for coronary artery disease.

h. CT/MRI scanning. These noninvasive techniques may provide complementary information to the echocardiogram about the extent of tumor involvement locally and whether multiple sites of involvement or metastatic disease are present.

2. Differential diagnosis. The differential diagnosis of atrial myxoma includes tricuspid or mitral valve stenosis, endocarditis, collagen-vascular disease, constrictive pericarditis, cardiomyopathy, or occult malignancy.

3. Natural history. The natural history of untreated atrial myxomas is not well defined. Systemic and pulmonary emboli occur in a large number of patients, potentially resulting in lethal myocardial infarction or cerebral injury. Once obstructive symptoms have developed, the average life expectancy is probably only 1-2 years. The expected survival of children with rhabdomyomas and patients with malignant cardiac tumors is worse.

4. Treatment

a. Medical. Diuretics, transvenous pacemakers, and antiarrhythmic therapy may produce temporary relief of symptoms in some patients.

b. Surgical. Urgent surgical excision is recommended for all patients with myxomas who are otherwise reasonable operative risks. Some patients with nonresectable tumors that are otherwise well localized may be candidates for cardiac transplantation.

5. Prognosis. The operative mortality for resection of an uncomplicated atrial myxoma is less than 2%, and the mortality is probably similar for patients with resectable rhabdomyomas. The long-term survival is excellent, and the risk of recurrence in most reports is about 1%. The prognosis for patients with malignant tumors is poor. More than 80% of these patients have either distant metastases or extensive nonresectable local disease at the time of presentation. Conventional chemotherapy and radiation therapy have only a limited palliative role.

IX. TRANSPLANTATION

There has been a major growth in thoracic organ transplantation as a result of improvements in immunosuppression, notably cyclosporine. Operative and long-term survival rates are now acceptable, and substantial functional improvement is the rule. The indications for heart transplantation have remained reasonably stable, although those for combined heart-lung and lung transplantation are still undergoing modification. Prior to transplantation, all patients are carefully screened to exclude infections or diseases in other organ systems (CNS, heart, lungs, liver, kidneys, GI tract) which would be exacerbated by immunosuppression. Absolute contraindications are uncontrollable infection, including HIV, and cancer. Experience has shown that ability to understand and comply with the complex medical regimen following transplant is one of the most powerful predictors of long-term success in a given patient. Thus, a thorough psychosocial evaluation and an education program are part of the initial assessment.

Donors are screened for transmissible diseases (cancer, hepatitis, HIV infection) prior to organ harvesting. Donor and recipient are usually matched only in terms of blood group (ABO compatibility) and size. Rarely, a recipient has become sensitized to HLA antigens (blood transfusions, prior transplants, or pregnancies) and has a high level of HLA antibodies. In these cases a formal cross-match between the donor and recipient must be performed to avoid possible hyperacute rejection.

Triple-drug immunosuppression (cyclosporine, corticosteroids, and azathioprine) protocols are used chronically by most institutions for all forms of thoracic organ transplantation. The dosages of the individual drugs are carefully adjusted to achieve the desired level of immunosuppression and to avoid systemic toxicity. The efficacy of immunosuppression is determined histologically (endocardial biopsy or transbronchial biopsy) or functionally (physical examination, chest radiography, ECG, echocardiogram, blood gases, or pulmonary function studies depending upon the specific transplant). Sensitive and specific immunologic monitoring techniques are still undergoing development. Allograft rejection occurs frequently but is usually readily treated with pulse corticosteroid therapy or cytolytic drugs (OKT3 and antithymocyte globulin). Long-term survival and functional rehabilitation are excellent in most reported series. During the first year after transplant the most frequent causes of death and hospital readmission are acute allograft rejection and infection. Beyond the first year post-transplant allograft coronary artery disease or small airway obstruction as well as certain forms of cancer (skin, lymphoma, perineum) becomes more prevalent.

A. HEART. Worldwide between 2500 and 3000 heart transplants are performed each year. The real need is perhaps tenfold greater, but further growth is limited by the number of available donors. The only indication is end-stage heart disease not amenable to other, more conventional treatment. Most commonly this is the result of coronary artery disease and myocardial infarction or idiopathic dilated cardiomyopathy. Some patients with congenital heart disease, valvular heart disease, and other forms of cardiomyopathy have also been transplanted. A few patients have undergone retransplantation as a result of either a failed transplant, acute rejection, or allograft coronary artery disease. The usual presentation is severe congestive heart failure, but intractable arrhythmias and myocardial ischemia are also valid indications.

Heart transplantation can be performed orthotopically, replacing most of the recipient's own heart with the donor heart or heterotopically, preserving the recipient's own heart and attaching the donor heart to the recipient's in a piggy-back fashion so that the two hearts function in parallel. The orthotopic technique is more commonly used. However, if the recipient has preexisting pulmonary hypertension (PA_{sys} >60 mm Hg) or an elevated pulmonary vascular resistance (PA_{mean} − PCWP/CO >4 Wood units), the donor right ventricle may fail acutely. Therefore it is extremely important to assess pulmonary artery pressure and pulmonary vascular resistance prior to transplantation so that the appropriate operation is performed (heterotopic technique, combined heart-lung or orthotopic technique with a conditioned right ventricle).

Potential heart donors are carefully evaluated for a history of heart disease and risk factors for heart disease (smoking, hypertension, family history, diabetes, hyperlipidemia). A thorough cardiovascular examination is performed. Additional necessary tests include an ECG and echocardiogram. Cardiac catheterization may be performed if coronary artery disease is suspected by virtue of the donor's age or risk factors. A final evaluation is performed at the time of organ harvesting. The donor heart can be preserved satisfactorily with hypothermic crystalloid cardioplegia for periods of up to 4 to 6 hours. This generally limits the available donor pool to those within 1500 miles of the transplant center.

The operative mortality for heart transplantation is between 5% and 10% and is influenced by the recipient's pretransplant pulmonary vascular resistance and indication for transplant, those with an elevated pulmonary vascular resistance, congenital heart disease, or a prior heart transplant having a much increased operative mortality. The 1- and 5-year survivals are about 80% and 60%, respectively. Interestingly, recipient and donor age, gender, diagnosis (with the exception already noted), and donor preservation time do not seem to influence either the operative mortality or long-term survival.

B. COMBINED HEART-LUNG. For several years combined heart-lung transplantation was the only form of clinical pulmonary transplantation available and was applied to a wide variety of end-stage lung as well as heart and lung diseases. The current indications for combined heart-lung transplantation are shrinking as single and bilateral lung transplantations prove to be equally effective and technically simpler treatment for various pulmonary parenchymal and pulmonary vascular diseases. Cystic fibrosis and complex congenital heart disease with pulmonary hypertension constitute the largest groups of patients for which the combined operation is being performed at the present time. Approximately 150 combined heart-lung transplants are performed world wide each year.

Donor screening for the combined heart-lung transplant includes all of the usual criteria (e.g., history, physical examination, laboratory tests, chest radiography, ECG, echocardiogram) for both the heart and lung suitability. Size matching is very important. Oversized organs can lead to cardiac tamponade or compressive atelectasis when the thorax is closed.

Combined heart-lung transplantation is a formidable operation. Removal of the recipient's organs must be performed on cardiopulmonary bypass with strict attention to hemostasis, particularly in the posterior mediastinum and chest wall. The phrenic nerves and left recurrent laryngeal nerve must be carefully protected. The donor lungs are passed through pericardial windows behind the phrenic nerves into their respective hemithoraces. A tracheal anastomosis is performed just above the main carina. The right atrial and aortic anastomoses complete the transplant procedure. Early operative results depend upon ability to control bleeding and the quality of pulmonary and cardiac preservation. Technical modifications have reduced the operative mortality to the range of 10% to 20%.

Some combined heart-lung recipients have sufficiently good heart function that their hearts can be preserved for use in another patient, the so-called domino procedure. Combined heart-lung donors must obviously have good heart and lung function and be free of infection. Donors and recipients are matched for blood group and size exactly as for isolated heart and lung transplantation. Current methods for cardiac and pulmonary preservation provide up to 4 hours of ex vivo ischemia time, so that organ recovery at a distant hospital (within 1000 to 1500 miles) is the rule.

The long-term functional results have been influenced by the development of obliterative bronchiolitis in up to one third of patients. Five-year survival rates are approximately 40% to 50%.

C. LUNG. Isolated lung transplantation has supplanted combined heart and lung transplantation as the treatment for end-stage lung disease over the past 5 years. The only indication is end-stage disease that is not amenable to more conventional treatment. However, the exact physiologic definitions of end-stage lung disease are not as precise as for heart transplantation. Three general groups of disorders have been considered—pulmonary vascular disease (primary pulmonary hypertension or simple congenital heart disease with Eisenmenger's physiology), restrictive lung disease (e.g., idiopathic pulmonary fibrosis, fibrosing alveolitis), and obstructive lung disease (e.g., emphysema, alpha-1-antitrypsin deficiency, bronchiectasis, cystic fibrosis).

Single-lung transplants can be performed on either side, the choice being influenced by asymmetry of the recipient's disease, prior pulmonary surgery in the recipient, donor lung availability, and the anticipated need for partial cardiopulmonary bypass during transplantation. Bilateral lung replacement is necessary in patients with cystic fibrosis or bronchiectasis to eliminate all sources of recurrent sepsis or cross-infection. If partial cardiopulmonary bypass is anticipated during lung transplantation (recipient right ventricular dysfunction or severely impaired gas exchange), a right thoracotomy provides better access to the heart for cannulation. Alternately, femoral cannulation for cardiopulmonary bypass may be used from either side. If the donor is larger than the recipient, the left hemithorax more readily accommodates a larger sized lung than the right.

Potential lung donors are carefully screened for preexisting lung disease on the basis of history and physical examination. The AP portable chest radiograph is examined carefully for areas of atelectasis or consolidation as well as to obtain measurements of the height and width of the lungs. Sputum microbiology is used to exclude donors with heavy airway contamination or to direct post-transplant antimicrobial treatment in the recipient. Serial arterial blood gases and ventilator mechanics provide vital information about gas exchange and lung compliance. The arterial oxygen partial pressure should be greater than 300 or 100 mm Hg when the inspired oxygen fraction is 1.0 or 0.4, respectively, and the PEEP is 5 cm H_2O. The peak airway pressure should be less than 30 cm H_2O at a tidal volume of 15 ml/kg.

The final assessment is made at the time of organ procurement. Flexible bronchoscopy is performed to exclude anatomic variations and assess the airways for signs of inflammation or foreign body aspiration. Unilateral lung disease in the donor does not preclude procurement of the opposite lung. Pulmonary preservation techniques permit up to 8 to 10 hours of cold ischemia, with satisfactory function easily allowing time for multiple transplants (bilateral single lungs in the same patient) or long-distance procurement (>1500 miles).

Currently, the overall patient survival for pulmonary transplantation is between 60% and 70% at 2 years. Obliterative bronchiolitis has been identified among some of the long-term survivors, but it is too early to determine the ultimate impact of this on long-term survival.

11

Vascular Surgery

Cornelius Olcott IV

I. EVALUATION OF THE VASCULAR SURGICAL PATIENT

A careful history and physical examination are very important in the evaluation of the vascular surgical patient. In most cases the diagnosis can be made on the basis of these 2 modalities. Occasionally, additional information may be required from noninvasive tests and/or arteriograms.

A. HISTORY. The history should be tailored to the patient's chief complaint. However, a complete vascular history should inquire into symptoms of occlusive arterial disease, venous disease, and aneurysmal disease as well as the more unusual entities such as portal hypertension and thoracic outlet syndrome, where appropriate.

Most patients have problems related to arterial occlusive disease. The examiner should inquire about symptoms involving any segment of the arterial system: cardiac (angina, MI, CHF, past history of CABG or angioplasty), cerebrovascular (stroke, TIA, amaurosis fugax, global ischemia), visceral (postprandial pain, weight loss), renal (hypertension, renal insufficiency), extremity (claudication, rest pain, ulcers). One should also inquire about the presence of risk factors, e.g., smoking, diabetes, hypertension, hyperlipidemia, family history. Special attention should be paid to the presence or absence of CAD, as this is the principal cause of death in patients with vascular disease. Also the presence of significant CAD may alter the work-up and management of vascular patients.

B. PHYSICAL EXAMINATION. Both the arterial and venous systems should be carefully examined.

1. Pulses. The following pulses should be examined: carotid, superficial temporal, subclavian, brachial radial, ulnar, aortic, femoral, popliteal, dosalis pedis, and posterior tibial. Pulses should be graded 0 (absent) to 4+ (normal).

2. Arteries. In addition to palpating the pulse, the examiner should determine the character of the artery; i.e., is it calcified, aneurysmal?

3. Bruits. Bruits reflect turbulent flow and hence stenosis. One should auscultate for bruits over the carotid, subclavian, iliac, and femoral arteries and over the aorta.

4. Thrill is a palpable bruit and a manifestation of severe stenosis.

5. Elevation pallor. Pallor on elevation of the feet denotes significant ischemia.

6. Dependent rubor is a violacious color of the feet when they are made dependent. This also denotes significant ischemia.

7. Other signs of ischemia are ulceration, mottling, gangrene, and hair loss.

C. NONINVASIVE TESTS. These technics have greatly expanded the vascular surgeon's ability to objectively evaluate the vascular patient.

1. Cerebrovascular disease. Several technics are available to evaluate the degree of stenosis and the character of the plaque. At present, the duplex scan, especially color Doppler imaging, is the most accurate.

2. Lower extremity. Doppler studies provide waveforms and sequential pressures in the lower extremities which permit the examiner to determine the extent and location of occlusive disease. The ABI (ankle/brachial index) in the ratio of ankle systolic pressure to brachial artery pressure as determined by the Doppler scan. This ratio is frequently used to express the degree of lower extremity ischemia. The duplex scan, especially with color Doppler imaging, has proven very accurate in determining the extent and severity of stenosis in lower extremity vessels and bypass grafts.

The venous system of the lower extremities can also be accurately evaluated by means of the Doppler and duplex scans. At present, this is the most commonly used technic for detecting deep venous thrombosis.

3. CT and **MRI** are increasingly being used to image the arterial system. These are particularly useful in evaluating aneurysmal disease. Magnetic resonance angiography is still experimental but promises to provide accurate imaging without angiography.

D. ARTERIOGRAPHY is still considered the gold standard for vascular imaging. It is used to determine the vascular anatomy and the pattern of occlusive lesions in patients with arterial disease.

II. PREOPERATIVE PREPARATION AND POSTOPERATIVE CARE

Formerly, vascular patients were admitted for work-up and arteriography. Also, most patients were admitted at least 24 hours prior to reconstructive surgery. In the present climate of cost containment, most arteriograms are done on an outpatient basis, and patients are frequently admitted on the day of surgery. Hence, much of the preoperative evaluation and preparation is done prior to admission.

A. ARTERIOGRAPHY

1. Preparation. (1) Informed consent. (2) Appropriate IV should be started and run at a rate to keep the patient hydrated, 75-100 ml/hr. (3) Shave the site for arterial puncture—femoral or axillary. (4) Check renal function and clotting studies. (5) Check for history of allergic reactions to contrast agents.

2. Care after the study. (1) Bed rest for 6 hours after study. (2) Check arterial puncture site for bleeding, hematoma, false aneurysm, or A-V fistula. (3) Check distal pulses to rule out arterial thrombosis following arterial puncture. (4) Follow renal function if patient is diabetic and/or has a history of renal insufficiency. (5) Observe for urinary retention.

B. ROUTINE ADMITTING ORDERS. These should be individualized to the patient. Care should be taken to avoid unnecessary repetition of laboratory tests, as this increases cost. Typical preoperative tests include CBC, urinalysis, renal function tests, electrolytes, PT, PTT, platelet count, ECG, and chest radiography. Typing and cross-matching of blood should also be performed. Check to see if the patient has autologous blood or donor-specific blood available.

C. CEREBROVASCULAR AND ARCH RECONSTRUCTIONS

1. Preoperative. Males should shave neck the morning of surgery. Prep the chest if sternotomy or thoracotomy is anticipated. Overnight hydration. Transfusion usually not required.

2. Postoperative. Monitor blood pressure closely and maintain at preoperative levels ± 20 mm Hg. This usually means a mean arterial pressure of 80-100 mm Hg. Hypertension is usually treated with IV nipride; hypotension usually responds to IV fluids. Neurologic checks at frequent intervals to evaluate any change in postoperative neurologic status. Watch neck closely for signs of hematoma, tracheal deviation, or respiratory embarrassment.

D. MAJOR ABDOMINAL CASES

1. Preoperative. Preoperative weight, prep from nipples to toes, overnight hydration, begin prophylactic antibiotics, type and cross-match for 2-3 units of packed cells or whole blood.

2. Postoperative. In addition to the usual care after major abdominal surgery, the patient is monitored closely for proper fluid balance and cardiac/hemodynamic function. Swann-Ganz catheters are frequently used to monitor filling pressures, cardiac output, and peripheral resistance. This permits accurate fluid management. Pulses, especially those distal to the reconstruction, are monitored hourly for the first 24 hours. Pulmonary function is followed closely, and extubation is carried out as soon as permitted, usually the first postoperative morning. Ambulation is begun as soon as the patient is stable, but prolonged sitting is discouraged for reconstructions below the inguinal ligament.

E. LOWER EXTREMITY RECONSTRUCTIONS

1. Preoperative. Same as for abdominal cases except cross-match for only 1 unit.

2. Postoperative. Similar to abdominal cases. Fluid requirements are much less, and less invasive monitoring is required. Distal pulses are monitored closely to detect postoperative thrombosis.

III. TRAUMA

Penetrating wounds may injure vessels by direct laceration or from the blast effect. Blunt trauma may also disrupt vessels completely or in part. In the latter case, typically the intima is torn, resulting in delayed thrombosis.

1. Diagnosis. Injury in proximity to a major artery or vein, presence of arterial or venous bleeding, expanding hematoma, hypotension or shock, diminished or absent distal pulses (the presence of a normal distal pulse does not rule out the presence of an arterial injury), bruit at site of injury. Injury to anatomically related nerves.

2. Radiographs. Plain films may help track the path of a bullet and/or reveal associated bone injuries. Arteriograms may help in determining the presence and extent of injury. Life-saving surgery should not be delayed for arteriograms; these may be obtained in the OR if necessary.

3. Complications. Hemorrhage and shock, false aneurysm, A-V fistula, distal ischemia, venous thrombosis, compartment syndrome, bullet embolization.

4. Treatment

a. Emergency measures. These should be directed toward control of bleeding and resuscitation. Bleeding is best controlled by direct pressure. Large bore IV's should be started for fluid resuscitation. Transfusions are carried out as necessary. Monitoring lines should be established. Fractures should be splinted.

b. Surgical treatment has two primary goals—control of bleeding and reestablishment of vessel continuity to prevent distal ischemia. The latter may be accomplished by direct suture repair, excision of the injured portion with direct end-to-end anastomosis, or excision of injured area and repair with interposition autogenous graft. Ligation is seldom necessary except in cases of carotid injury in conjunction with associated neurologic deficit. Arteriovenous fistulas and direct venous injuries should also be repaired if possible. Vascular suture lines should be covered with fascia or subcutaneous tissue in addition to skin. Penetrating wounds may require debridement. A fasciotomy may be required to prevent compartment syndrome.

5. Prognosis. Proper arterial reconstruction, performed before irreversible ischemia develops, has an excellent prognosis. Ligation of major vessels carries a high risk of subsequent amputation.

IV. ARTERIOVENOUS FISTULAS

Arteriovenous fistulas are abnormal communications between arteries and veins. They may be either congenital or acquired.

A. CONGENITAL ARTERIOVENOUS FISTULAS. These are typically multiple small communications that are present from birth but may not become manifest until age 10-20 years. Frequently they become more problematic during pregnancy. They most frequently occur in the upper or lower extremity, female pelvis, or head and neck.

1. Diagnosis
a. Symptoms. Pain and swelling in the area of the fistula, bleeding from fistula, cardiac failure.

b. Signs. Mass composed of enlarged, tortuous arteries and veins, increased temperature over the lesion, continuous bruit and thrill over lesion. Venous hypertension distally, possibly associated with venous insufficiency. Increased limb length if extremity is involved. Nicoladoni-Branham sign— prompt decrease in heart rate with digital closure of the fistula.

c. Tests. Chest radiography may demonstrate cardiac enlargement; extremity radiographs may show increased bone length. Arteriograms demonstrate the anatomy of the vascular lesion. CT and MRI can be useful for delineating the extent of the lesion and the involvement of adjacent tissues.

2. Differential diagnosis.
Congenital fistulas should be differentiated from acquired fistulas. An acquired or traumatic fistula typically has only a single communication. Hemangiomas are benign tumors composed of thin-walled vessels but lacking the A-V communications.

3. Complications.
These lesions may be asymptomatic. However, they may cause pain, bleeding, extremity dysfunction, or CHF, or be cosmetically displeasing.

4. Treatment
a. Small lesions can be easily excised.

b. Large congenital lesions are usually best managed by embolization. Some large lesions (e.g., in the pelvis) may be safely excised after embolization to decrease the vascularity of the lesion.

5. Prognosis.
Completely excised lesion does not recur. Embolization does not "cure" the lesion, and recurrence with time is the rule.

B. TRAUMATIC ARTERIOVENOUS FISTULAS result from penetrating injuries that produce a connection between an adjacent artery and vein. These may be iatrogenic (e.g., fistula between femoral artery and vein after transfemoral catherization). If not corrected, these lesions slowly enlarge. However, small fistulas, particularly iatrogenic fistulas, may close spontaneously.

1. Diagnosis. History of trauma or interventional procedure, pain, CHF, bruit and/or thrill, venous hypertension distally, Nicoladoni-Branham sign.

2. Complications. These lesions slowly enlarge and may produce pain, bleeding, cardiac failure, or distal ischemia.

3. Treatment. Surgical management requires closure of the fistula and reconstruction, if necessary, of the involved artery and vein.

V. ANEURYSMS

Aneurysms are fusiform or sacular dilatations of an artery which result in a dilatation of at least 1.5 times the normal diameter. Mural thrombus is deposited on the vessel wall because of eddy currents and stagnant flow. For this reason, the functional lumen of the aneurysm, as viewed by arteriography, may not be increased.

A. THORACOABDOMINAL ANEURYSMS involve the descending thoracic aorta and abdominal aorta to a varying degree. Typically the visceral and renal arteries are involved. The aneurysms may be standard aneurysms or dissecting aneurysms.

1. Diagnosis
a. Symptoms. May be asymptomatic. However, expanding or dissecting aneurysms may cause chest, back, or abdominal pain.

b. Signs. Pulsatile abdominal mass if abdominal aorta is involved. May have associated aneurysmal disease elsewhere, e.g., femoral or popliteal arteries. Hypertension.

c. Radiographs. Chest radiography demonstrates enlargement of the thoracic aorta. Arteriograms demonstrate the extent of the aneurysm, especially involvement of the visceral and renal arteries.

d. Imaging. CT and MRI are useful for delineating extent of aneurysm and determining extent of the false lumen in dissecting aneurysms.

2. Complications. Rupture, embolization, occlusion of visceral or renal arteries.

3. Treatment. Symptomatic aneurysms or those greater than twice the diameter of the normal proximal aorta should be treated with aneurysmectomy and reconstruction. A major risk of this procedure is postoperative paraplegia secondary to spinal cord ischemia. Therefore, a conservative approach is warranted in smaller, asymptomatic aneurysms. Dissecting aneurysms of the descending aorta are usually treated medically (by control of hypertension) unless complications develop.

4. Prognosis. Resection is curative, but operative risk is great secondary to spinal cord ischemia, renal failure, and cardiac complications.

B. ABDOMINAL AORTIC ANEURYSMS involve the subdiaphragmatic aorta. Usually the aneurysm is limited to the infrarenal aorta, although the suprarenal aorta may be involved as well. The process may extend distally to involve the iliac arteries, especially the common iliacs.

1. Diagnosis

a. Symptoms. Intact aneurysms are asymptomatic except for the rare inflammatory aneurysm that may produce abdominal pain. Expanding or rupturing aneurysms may produce back and/or abdominal pain. Rupture is usually associated with hypotension or severe shock. AAA may also produce symptoms secondary to thrombosis or embolization.

b. Signs. Pulsatile and expansile abdominal mass, typically just superior to and to the left of the umbilicus. Associated aneurysmal disease involving other arteries, e.g., the femoral and popliteal arteries.

c. Radiographs. Abdominal radiographs, especially cross-table lateral views, may show calcification in the vessel wall. Arteriograms are of value in demonstrating abnormalities of associated intraabdominal arteries, e.g., renal arteries. However, the presence of mural thrombus typically produces a normal-appearing lumen on arteriography and hence may not be helpful in determining diagnosis or extent of the aneurysm. Arteriograms should be obtained if one suspects associated occlusive disease, renal artery involvement, or a thoracoabdominal component.

d. Special tests. Ultrasonography, CT, and MRI may be used to document the size and extent of the aneurysm. CT may be used to detect an aneurysm in the stable patient with abdominal pain.

2. Differential diagnosis. Other abdominal masses may be pulsatile if they lie anterior to the aorta, e.g., lymphomas, pancreatic masses, mesenteric masses. These lesions are not typically expansile, however.

3. Complications. Rupture causes death from hemorrhage. Bleeding may be contained in the retroperitoneum at first, but eventually it breaks into the free abdominal cavity and causes death. A patient with a ruptured AAA presents with abdominal and/or back pain and hypotension. A patient with a pulsatile abdominal mass and abdominal or back pain should be considered to have a ruptured AAA until proven otherwise. Other complications include distal embolization, thrombosis, A-V fistula (secondary to erosion into the inferior vena cava) or gastrointestinal bleeding (secondary to erosion into the bowel).

4. Treatment

a. Asymptomatic aneurysms <5 cm may be followed, especially if the patient is a poor surgical candidate. Aneurysms >5 cm should be resected unless there is a compelling medical reason to defer. Standard surgical technique involves replacing the aneurysmal portion with a Dacron graft. This may be a tube graft if only the aorta is involved or a bifurcated graft if the iliacs are involved.

b. Symptomatic aneurysms are a surgical emergency and should be taken to the OR emergently for exploration and resection.

C. FEMORAL ANEURYSMS involve the common femoral artery and a variable portion of the superficial or profunda femoral artery.

1. Diagnosis. These aneurysms are usually asymptomatic and are detected on physical examination. Note: An associated abdominal aortic aneurysm should be sought in any patient with a femoral artery aneurysm. Ultrasonography may be used to confirm physical findings. Arteriography may be used to evaluate associated occlusive disease.

2. Differential diagnosis. Other forms of groin masses are usually easily differentiated from a pulsatile aneurysm. False aneurysms may need to be differentiated from true aneurysms. False aneurysms may be associated with disruption of an anastomosis after an aortofemoral bypass or may occur as a complication of transfemoral catheterization.

3. Complications. Thrombosis, embolization, or rupture (rare).

4. Treatment. Most femoral aneurysms should be repaired to prevent complications. These are usually repaired using an interposition Dacron graft. False aneurysms >2 cm should be surgically repaired; those <2 cm may be treated successfully by compression until obliteration of the false aneurysm occurs.

5. Prognosis. Good.

D. POPLITEAL ANEURYSM

1. Diagnosis. A pulsatile mass palpable in the popliteal fossa. Ultrasonography may be helpful in determining the size and extent of the aneurysm. Arteriography is helpful in determining the vascular anatomy and associated occlusive disease or in detecting distal embolization.

2. Differential diagnosis. Adventitial cystic disease of the popliteal artery and Baker's cyst.

3. Complications. Thrombosis and embolization are the most frequent complications. These may result in severe lower extremity ischemia. Rupture is rare.

4. Treatment. Surgical management consists of exclusion and bypass, usually with autogenous saphenous vein. Because of the disastrous consequences of thrombosis or embolization, most surgeons consider aneurysms >2 cm as candidates for surgery.

5. Prognosis. Good following reconstruction.

E. VISCERAL ARTERY ANEURYSM.
Aneurysms may arise in the celiac axis or its branches, the mesenteric arteries, or the renal arteries. Approximately 60% of splanchnic artery aneurysms involve the splenic artery, and these occur typically in pregnant females. Aneurysms involving the splanchnic vessels may be mycotic, especially in IV drug users. Renal artery aneurysms are usually atherosclerotic or associated with fibromuscular dysplasia.

1. Diagnosis. Visceral artery aneurysms may produce abdominal pain. Renal artery aneurysms may be associated with hypertension or hematuria. Mycotic aneurysm may be associated with findings of systemic infection. These aneurysms are usually not palpable. Diagnosis is made by arteriography or CT.

2. Complications. Mycotic aneurysms are a source of sepsis and usually rupture if not treated. Other visceral aneurysms may rupture, especially splenic artery aneurysms in pregnant women. Visceral aneurysms may also compress adjacent structures, e.g., common bile duct.

3. Treatment

a. Symptomatic splanchnic artery aneurysms should be resected.

b. Mycotic aneurysms should be resected and reconstructed or approached by endoaneurysmorrhaphy with an attempt made to get rid of the infected tissue.

c. Renal artery aneurysms are considered for resection if they are symptomatic or >2 cm in diameter or lack a calcified wall. Reconstruction is also indicated for aneurysms associated with renovascular hypertension or renal artery dissection.

4. Prognosis. Surgical correction of atherosclerotic aneurysms is curative. The prognosis for mycotic aneurysms is not as good, as these patients frequently succumb to the complications of septicemia.

VI. ARTERIAL OCCLUSIVE DISEASE

A. AORTOILIOFEMORAL DISEASE. Atherosclerosis may involve singly, or in combination, any of the arteries supplying the lower extremities. Typical patterns include aortoiliac, aortoiliofemoral, or superficial femoral disease alone or in combination with inflow disease. Disease involving the popliteal artery, the trifurcation vessels, or the profunda is indicative of advanced atherosclerosis. Stenosis or occlusion may occur gradually (secondary to progressive atherosclerosis) or suddenly (secondary to an embolus or acute thrombosis of a preexisting atherosclerotic lesion). Gradual progression of stenoses permits the development of collateral circulation, which, for a time, minimizes the severity of symptoms. Acute occlusion typically causes severe ischemia because collaterals have not developed.

1. Diagnosis
a. Symptoms
Claudication. Ischemic muscle pain occurring with activity. Pain begins after variable amounts of exercise. The more advanced the ischemia, the more prompt the onset of pain. It is characteristically relieved by rest. Claudication usually involves muscle groups distal to the arterial lesion; e.g., superficial femoral artery lesions produce calf claudication, and aortoiliac disease produces buttock, thigh, and calf claudication.

*Rest pain.*This is severe pain that occurs when the limb is horizontal, e.g., when in bed at night, because gravity is no longer a factor in increasing blood flow to the distal leg. It is relieved by lowering the leg. This is a symptom of advanced ischemia.

*Ischemic ulcers and gangrene.*Tissue loss secondary to very advanced ischemia.

b. Signs. Diminished or absent pulses distal to the lesion. The greater the stenosis, the more diminished the pulse. **Bruit**—an audible systolic sound that can be auscultated over an arterial stenosis. The more severe the stenosis, the louder and more high pitched the bruit. **Thrill**—a palpable bruit. It denotes severe stenosis. Pallor with elevation of the leg and dependent rubor are also associated with significant ischemia. Tissue loss and gangrene are indicative of very advanced ischemia.

c. Noninvasive tests. Doppler ultrasonography is extremely useful for objectively evaluating the physiologic effect of occlusive disease. Waveforms are determined at the level of the common femoral, superficial femoral, popliteal, dorsalis pedal, and posterior tibial arteries. Doppler pressures are also obtained at the level of the thigh, calf, and ankle. These pressures are expressed as a fraction of the brachial artery pressure, e.g., ABI. Normal is 1.0; 0.90 is compatible with claudication; <0.5 is compatible with advanced ischemia. The duplex scan may be used to visualize the lower extremity vessels or lower extremity bypass grafts.

d. Arteriography is the most reliable modality for demonstrating the extent and pattern of occlusive arterial disease. This is usually performed by the transfemoral route, although the axillary artery may also be used.

2. Differential diagnosis. Neurogenic claudication can mimic claudication of vascular origin. It occurs secondary to spinal stenosis. Typically the patient with neurogenic claudication develops symptoms when upright. Symptoms are relieved by bending over (e.g., walking uphill) or sitting. Vascular examination, unless there is associated vascular disease, is normal.

3. Complications. Disability due to diminished exercise tolerance. Limb loss may occur secondary to gangrene, but this is rare.

4. Treatment

a. Medical. Control of risk factors—hypertension, hyperlipidemia, diabetes, smoking. Trental, which increases the pliability of red cells. A walking program to develop collaterals may completely relieve mild claudication.

b. Endovascular techniques. Transluminal angioplasty and atherectomy have both proven to be of some value in selected patients, particularly patients with focal, short-segment occlusive disease. Both procedures have an approximately 30% recurrence rate at 1 year.

c. Surgical management. Occlusive disease involving the aortoiliac system is usually managed by aortofemoral bypass. However, disease limited to the aorta and proximal common iliacs may be managed by endarterectomy, especially in young patients. Infrainguinal disease is usually managed by a bypass from the femoral vessels to the best distal vessel—either popliteal or tibial/peroneal. Autogenous saphenous vein is the conduit of choice. However, prosthetic material may be used if autogenous vein (leg or arm) is not available.

5. Prognosis. Reconstructive vascular procedures for lower extremity occlusive disease produce satisfactory results >95% of patients. Long-term results are better with aortofemoral than with infrainguinal reconstructions. The long-term prognosis for any patient with atherosclerosis is guarded, however, because atherosclerosis is a progressive systemic disease that may develop elsewhere or extend distal to the point of reconstruction. The number of vessels involved and the rate of progression are variable. The younger the patient at the time of onset and the more vessels affected by atherosclerosis, the worse the prognosis.

B. VISCERAL ARTERIES. Acute occlusion may occur secondary to emboli or dissection. Most stenoses and occlusions are secondary to atherosclerosis. The median arcuate ligament may narrow the celiac axis.

1. Diagnosis
a. Symptoms. Postprandial epigastric pain typically beginning 30 minutes after eating and lasting for 1-3 hours, weight loss. Acute occlusion may cause sudden onset of severe abdominal pain out of proportion to the physical findings.

b. Signs. Abdominal bruit, findings of occlusive disease elsewhere, especially of the aortoiliac system. Acute abdomen in cases of advanced visceral ischemia.

c. Radiographs. Arteriography is definitive for demonstrating lesions of the visceral vessels. It is essential to obtain lateral views of the aorta to image the origin of the superior mesenteric and celiac arteries.

2. Differential diagnosis. Includes entities producing abdominal pain and weight loss (e.g., carcinoma of the pancreas). However, the postprandial nature of the pain is very characteristic. Visceral ischemia should be considered in patients with unexplained abdominal pain.

3. Complications. Malnutrition, weight loss, intestinal infarction, and death.

4. Treatment. Surgical treatment involves the restoration of blood flow to at least two of the three visceral vessels. This may be accomplished by endarterectomy or grafting. Compression of the celiac axis is managed by division of the arcuate ligament and mechanical dilatation of the celiac artery. Acute embolic occlusion should be managed by embolectomy and resection of nonviable bowel. A "second look" operation at 24 hours is recommended to evaluate the viability of the remaining bowel.

5. Prognosis is good following reconstruction for chronic ischemia. Prognosis is poor in cases of acute ischemia.

C. CEREBROVASCULAR. Lesions of the extracranial cerebrovascular arteries are responsible for >65% of all strokes. Symptoms arise either from emboli originating from an arterial lesion (e.g., an atherosclerotic plaque) or from severe stenosis or occlusion of a cerebrovascular artery. Diseases affecting these arteries include atherosclerosis, fibromuscular dysplasia, spontaneous or traumatic dissections, and Takayasu's arteritis.

1. Diagnosis
  a. Symptoms
  Transient ischemic attacks (TIAs). Transient, focal neurologic deficits, e.g., weakness of an arm or leg. By definition, all symptoms resolve within 24 hours. However, these events typically last only 15 minutes or less.
  Amaurosis fugax. Temporary loss of vision in one eye.
  Stroke. Permanent neurologic deficit.
  Symptoms due to decreased cerebral perfusion. Lightheadedness, fainting.
  Vertebrobasilar insufficiency. Vertigo, drop attacks, diploplia.
  b. Signs. Reduced common carotid, superficial temporal, or subclavian pulses. The internal carotid cannot be palpated. Bruits over the carotid bifurcation or in the supraclavicular fossa.

    c. Noninvasive tests. The duplex scan permits accurate evaluation of carotid stenosis and the character of the plaque. CT is useful for excluding intracranial lesions, which can mimic extracranial arterial disease.

    d. Radiographs. Arteriography provides the best assessment of location and severity of occlusive disease of the extracranial vessels.

    2. Differential diagnosis. Other causes of decreased cerebral perfusion, e.g., heart failure, aortic valve disease, arrhythmias. Emboli of cardiac origin. Intracranial vascular disease or neoplasms.

    3. Complications. Stroke, death

    4. Treatment

    a. Medical. Asymptomatic carotid stenosis of <80% is usually followed with duplex scan. Patients with minor or nonspecific symptoms in the absence of significant stenosis are usually treated with aspirin or some other antiplatelet agent.

    b. Surgical. Patients with symptomatic carotid lesions in conjunction with significant stenosis should be operated upon. The procedure of choice is endarterectomy. The management of patients with symptoms and stenosis of 30%-70% is still controversial. However, most surgeons perform an endarterectomy if the patient has recurrent or worsening symptoms. Fibromuscular dysplasia of the carotid is usually managed by dilatation. Dissections usually resolve spontaneously and do not require surgical intervention. Vertebral lesions are usually limited to the orifice of the vessel and are treated either by endarterectomy or transposition into the adjacent carotid artery.

    5. Prognosis. Surgical stroke rate should be less than 3%. Approximately 20% of patients develop a recurrent stenosis of varying severity following endarterectomy.

D. RENOVASCULAR LESIONS. Renovascular hypertension is caused by stenosis of the renal artery, which results in decreased renal blood flow that stimulates the juxtaglomerular cells of the kidney to secrete renin. The most common causes of renovascular hypertension are atherosclerosis and fibromuscular dysplasia. Atherosclerosis characteristically involves the orifice and proximal third of the renal artery. Fibromuscular disease typically involves the middle and distal third of the renal artery and occurs in middle-aged women.

    1. Diagnosis

    a. Symptoms and signs. Hypertension, upper abdominal or flank bruit.

b. Radiographs. Arteriography demonstrates the type of pathology and the extent of disease.

c. Special tests. (1) Abdominal duplex scan is still experimental. However, data suggest that in experienced hands this technique may be a good screening test for detecting renal artery stenosis. (2) Renal vein renin studies can be helpful in documenting renovascular hypertension. A ratio of involved to uninvolved kidney of 1.5 or greater is highly suggestive of renovascular hypertension. However, renovascular hypertension may exist in the absence of lateralizing renin studies. (3) Renal artery blood flow studies using nuclear scanning techniques have proven accurate in determining relative renal artery blood flow.

2. Treatment. Usual indications for intervention include uncontrollable hypertension in conjunction with an appropriate arterial lesion or progressive renal insufficiency. Atherosclerotic lesions are usually managed by endarterectomy or bypass grafting, either with saphenous vein or Dacron graft. Fibromuscular dysplastic lesions may be managed by either transluminal dilatation or interposition graft. In the latter case either hypogastric artery or saphenous vein is preferred.

3. Prognosis. Hypertension is improved in 60%-70% of patients with atherosclerosis and approximately 90% of patients with fibromuscular dysplasia.

E. ACUTE ARTERIAL OCCLUSION. Sudden occlusion of a previously patent artery is usually a dramatic event producing severe ischemia of the distal tissues. Recovery depends upon the adequacy of the collateral circulation.

1. Diagnosis

a. Symptoms and signs. The characteristic symptoms and signs are the five Ps—pallor, pain, paresthesias, paralysis, and pulselessness. Pallor and pain, in conjunction with coolness of the limb, occur early. Loss of motor and sensory nerve function occurs later and indicates the early stages of irreversible ischemia.

b. Radiographs. Arteriograms are useful for demonstrating the site of occlusion and the potential for reconstruction.

2. Differential diagnosis. It is important to determine the cause of the acute ischemia. Possibilities include:

a. Embolus. Most frequently these are cardiac in origin, e.g., in conjunction with atrial fibrillation or from a mural thrombus after MI. May also arise from a proximal atherosclerotic lesion or aneurysm.

   b. Acute thrombosis at site of preexisting stenosis. Patient usually has history of vascular symptoms, e.g., claudication, rest pain.

   c. Trauma, either penetrating or blunt.

   3. Complications. Left untreated, acute occlusion typically leads to irreversible ischemia and limb loss. Reconstruction of acutely ischemic limbs may be complicated by reperfusion syndrome with acute tissue edema and release of toxic breakdown products into the circulation. Myoglobinuria may lead to renal failure.

   4. Treatment. Immediate anticoagulation with IV heparin to prevent propagation of the thrombus. Emergency restoration of blood flow by embolectomy or by reconstruction should be considered in all patients in whom tissue is salvageable. Fibrinolytic agents may be used but frequently take too long to restore patency. In cases of irreversible ischemia, the patient should be anticoagulated and amputation performed after the limb has demarcated.

   5. Prognosis is good if blood flow is restored prior to irreversible changes. After prolonged ischemia, >8 hours, irreversible changes have frequently occurred, and attempts at revascularization carry high morbidity and mortality.

F. THROMBOANGIITIS OBLITERANS (BUERGER'S DISEASE). This obliterative disorder of the arteries usually occurs distal to the elbow or knee. It typically occurs in young male smokers. It may be associated with migratory phlebitis.

   1. Diagnosis
   a. Symptoms and signs. Foot claudication, digital ischemia frequently leading to amputation, loss of ankle and/or wrist pulses.

   b. Radiographs. Arteriograms show obliterative lesions distal to the popliteal or brachial arteries. Characteristically there are foci of occlusions alternating with normal-appearing arteries.

   2. Differential diagnosis. Atherosclerosis which usually involves the more proximal arteries, diabetic arteriopathy, vasculitis, vasospastic disorders.

   3. Complications. Progressive ischemia of digits, hands, and feet. May eventually require amputation of hands and/or feet.

4. Treatment. Stop smoking. Sympathectomy may be helpful. Amputation for necrotic tissue. Reconstructive procedures are rarely possible owing to the distal nature of the lesions.

5. Prognosis. If patient stops smoking, the disease may stabilize. Otherwise the disease is progressive, leading to amputation.

VII. VASOSPASTIC DISORDERS

Vasospastic disorders occur secondary to vasoconstriction of small arteries, resulting in sluggish flow of deoxygenated blood through the capillary bed and consequent cyanosis, coldness, and (in severe cases) pain.

1. Diagnosis

a. Raynaud's phenomenon. Sequential pallor, cyanosis, and rubor typically after exposure to cold. May occur in association with connective tissue disorder. *Raynaud's disease* is a term applied to the same findings in the absence of an identifiable cause. May lead to digital ulcers and necrosis in severe cases.

b. Acrocyanosis. A vasoconstrictive disorder occurring in young women and characterized by cyanosis of the hands and/or feet. May be seen in association with hyperhidrosis and livedo reticularis. Is a benign condition.

c. Posttraumatic sympathetic dystrophy. Seen in association with sympathetically mediated pain syndromes. Onset follows injury to the extremity and is characterized by severe pain and findings of increased sympathetic tone—cold, moist, cyanotic extremities. Primary complication is pain; tissue loss is rare.

2. Treatment. Acrocyanosis and most cases of Raynaud's phenomenon can be treated conservatively—avoid cold, protect extremities, stop smoking. Nifedipine may provide some relief secondary to its vasodilating effect. Sympathectomy may be considered for severe cases of Raynaud's phenomenon or posttraumatic sympathetic dystrophy.

VIII. VENOUS DISEASE

A. VARICOSE VEINS are dilated, tortuous veins in the lower extremity involving the greater and/or lesser saphenous system.

They may be either primary (associated with a normal deep venous system) or secondary (associated with a diseased deep venous system).

1. Diagnosis

a. Symptoms and signs. Enlarged, tortuous veins involving the greater and/or lesser saphenous system. Dull, heavy, aching discomfort that progresses during the day and is relieved by elevation of the leg. May have findings of associated chronic venous insufficiency.

b. Special tests. Venous Doppler and duplex scans can demonstrate status of the deep system and the presence of saphenofemoral incompetence.

2. Differential diagnosis. Should determine if varices are primary or secondary. Rule out associated A-V malformation.

3. Complications. Superficial thrombophlebitis, dermatitis, bleeding.

4. Treatment. Most patients respond to a conservative regimen of elevation, exercise, and elastic support stockings. Patients with severe varicosities who are symptomatic or have developed complications should be considered for varicose vein stripping. Some patients also request stripping for cosmetic reasons. Sclerosing injections of small varicosities and "spider veins" may be helpful but may be associated with significant inflammation around the injection site.

B. DEEP VEIN THROMBOPHLEBITIS. Acute inflammation and thrombosis of the deep veins of the lower extremity. See Chapter 2.

C. SUPERFICIAL THROMBOPHLEBITIS. Acute inflammation and thrombosis of the superficial venous system. Pain, tenderness, and induration are present along the course of the involved vein. See Chapter 2.

D. POSTPHLEBITIC SYNDROME is a consequence of deep venous thrombosis—persistent obstruction of the deep venous system, incomplete recanalization, valve destruction, and reflux through incompetent perforators—and results in high pressure in the superficial system. This results in chronic edema, extravasation of red cells with breakdown of the cells and inflammation and fibrosis. The overlying skin is very susceptible to ulceration and infection.

1. Diagnosis

a. Symptoms and signs. Edema of the distal leg and ankle which is progressive during the day. Stasis dermatitis, a pruritic eczematous reaction. Hyperpigmentation, brownish discoloration secondary to hemosiderin deposition from extravasated red cells. Ulceration most commonly over the medial malleolus and associated with edema and cellulitis. Pain associated with swelling and ulceration and relieved by elevation.

b. Tests. Venous Doppler and duplex scans can detect deep venous occlusions and incompetent perforators and reflux. Venography may be used to demonstrate the anatomy and the site of valvular destruction or malfunction and areas of occlusion.

2. Treatment. Conservative treatment is directed toward avoiding venous hypertension, edema, and ulceration. This consists of custom-fitted elastic stockings, intermittent leg elevation, and intermittent pneumatic compression devices for severe cases. Small stasis ulcers can be treated on an outpatient basis with compressive dressings (Unna boot) and antibiotics. More extensive ulcers may require hospitalization, bed rest with elevation, local wound care, and IV antibiotics. Skin grafts may be required. When all conservative measures fail, subfascial ligation of perforators (Linton procedure) may be considered. Venous reconstructions with valve transplantation or repair and venous bypasses have been used with some success.

IX. LYMPHEDEMA

A. PRIMARY LYMPHEDEMA. Congenital lymphedema is present at birth. Lymphedema praecox becomes evident in the teens or twenties. Lymphedema tarda develops after age 25 years.

B. SECONDARY LYMPHEDEMA: Results from lymphatic obstruction secondary to another disease process, e.g., neoplasm, infection, or surgical procedures.

1. Diagnosis

a. Symptoms and signs. Progressive swelling of one or more extremities. Usually begins in the foot and ankle but eventually involves the entire leg. Upper extremity lymphedema is usually secondary, e.g., after axillary dissection. The edema is characteristically nonpitting and does not disappear with overnight elevation. Recurrent cellulitis is common.

b. Tests. Lymphangiograms document the site of obstruction. Venous noninvasive test can be used to rule out venous disease.

2. Differential diagnosis. Other causes of lower extremity edema—venous disease, CHF, hypoproteinemia.

3. Complications. Recurrent cellulitis usually secondary to streptococci.

4. Treatment
a. Medical: The goal is to control edema and prevent infection. This includes good foot hygiene, elevation of the lower extremities at night; an intermittent compression device may be used; elastic stocking should be worn during the day. Antibiotics should be started at the first sign of infection.

b. Surgical. Various procedures have been tried. These are aimed at resecting the subcutaneous fat and/or improving lymphatic drainage. None of these is uniformly successful, and they are rarely recommended.

5. Prognosis. Most patients have steady progression of the edema and intermittent bouts of cellulitis. There is no known "cure."

X. ACCESS FOR HEMODIALYSIS

Access to the vascular system is important for the increasing number of patients on hemodialysis. Several techniques are currently employed.

A. SUBCLAVIAN OR FEMORAL VENOUS CATHETERS.
Dual-lumen catheters may be placed in either the femoral or subclavian veins under local anesthesia. These are especially useful for temporary dialysis or when the patient is too ill for insertion of a more permanent shunt. They can be used immediately.

B. ARTERIOVENOUS FISTULAS. A variety of technics has been developed to construct A-V fistulas that can be cannulated percutaneously for hemodialysis access. These are used for cases of permanent hemodialysis.

C. CHOICE OF ACCESS PROCEDURE
1. A plan should be developed for each patient which will provide the best possible access while keeping open as many options as possible for future access.

2. Autogenous fistulas are preferred but take longer to mature.

3. Fistulas should be placed distally at first. Preference is given to the nondominate upper extremity. Upper extremities are preferable to lower extremities for fistula insertion.

4. Based on the above, our general approach is:

a. Radial-cephalic fistula is our first choice, provided that there is adequate time to allow the fistula to mature before dialysis is required.

b. A bovine or PTFE fistula placed initially in the lower arm. These can be used within days, but their durability is not as good as that of autogenous fistulas. The upper arm or leg may also be used as dictated by the anatomy and adequacy of the arteries and veins.

12

Alimentary Tract

Theodore R. Schrock

I. TRAUMA: GENERAL PRINCIPLES

Penetrating wounds made by missiles and knives may injure any structure in the abdomen. Blunt trauma is likely to damage solid organs (spleen, liver, pancreas, kidneys), although a distended hollow viscus (bladder, intestine) may be ruptured by a direct blow. Deceleration forces may avulse organs (liver, bladder, intestine) from their attachments.

A. DIAGNOSIS
1. History. Get information about the injury from the patient, relatives, ambulance attendant, police, or witnesses as resuscitation is begun.

2. Findings
a. Penetrating wounds may not be obvious. Do not overlook wounds of entry or exit in the flanks or posteriorly. Penetrating wounds of the thorax below the nipples are injuries of the abdomen as well until proved otherwise.

b. Blunt trauma to the abdomen to the abdomen typically causes pain, distention, tenderness, and muscular rigidity from leakage of blood or intestinal contents. These signs may not appear for 12 hours or more, so repeated observation is necessary in some cases. Pain from visceral injury may be difficult to distinguish from muscular or skeletal pain, and there may be no objective findings despite extensive visceral damage.

Fractures of the lower ribs are common accompaniments of splenic and hepatic injuries.

Digital rectal examination may reveal blood in the stool.

3. Laboratory tests. Hematocrit, leukocyte count, and urinalysis are obtained routinely, and other tests are ordered as necessary. Serum and urine amylase values reflect pancreatic injury or perforated viscus.

4. Radiographs
a. Plain radiographs of the abdomen may reveal free intraperitoneal air, obliteration of the psoas shadow, and other

findings, most of them nonspecific. Fractures of transverse processes indicate severe trauma and should alert one to the possibilities of extensive visceral injury.

b. Chest radiography may disclose rib fractures, hemothorax, pneumothorax, or other evidence of thoracic injury.

c. Abdominal ultrasound and/or CT is used frequently to detect injuries to solid viscera and retroperitoneal structures.

d. Contrast studies of the urinary tract are necessary if hematuria is present, although CT may answer the questions as well.

e. Angiography may be helpful in cases of injury to the spleen, liver, or pancreas, but CT may make angiography unnecessary.

5. Special tests. *Peritoneal lavage* is useful to detect intraabdominal bleeding after blunt trauma if the diagnosis is unclear from physical and radiographic signs. The test should not be used in combative or uncooperative patients or in those with previous abdominal operations. **The bladder must be empty.** *Diagnostic laparoscopy* is used increasingly to evaluate abdominal trauma.

B. TREATMENT

1. Emergency treatment of injured patients and the management of shock are discussed in Chapter 1.

2. IV antibiotics are begun in patients with penetrating injuries and in patients with blunt trauma if intestinal injury is suspected.

3. Gunshot wounds of the abdomen and lower chest demand laparotomy, and stab wounds in patients with hemodynamic instability or peritonitis also require abdominal exploration. The need for operation in stable patients with stab wounds is controversial.

4. Exploratory laparotomy in blunt trauma is prompted by peritonitis, hypovolemia without an equivocal extraabdominal source, or injuries known to carry a high risk of associated abdominal injuries (e.g., fracture of lower ribs). Beware of attributing hypovolemia to an extraabdominal injury such as a scalp laceration or long bone fracture; while these wounds indeed can account for extensive blood loss, an occult abdominal source must be considered too.

5. Laparotomy

a. Control of bleeding is the first priority. Packs may stop bleeding in one area while another, more major, bleeding site is attended to.

b. Further contamination by intestinal contents should be prevented by isolating perforated intestine between clamps as soon as possible after massive bleeding is controlled.

c. Thorough exploration is then carried out, with special care to identify all intestinal perforations in patients with penetrating wounds. Victims of blunt trauma require careful inspection of the pancreas and duodenum.

d. Retroperitoneal hematomas should be explored if they are expanding or pulsating or if urinary tract injury is known or suspected.

e. Specific injuries are treated (see sections on individual organs in this chapter).

f. The peritoneal cavity is irrigated copiously with saline solution before closure.

g. The skin and subcutaneous fat are left open if fecal contamination was found; delayed primary closure can be attempted 4-5 days later.

II. ACUTE ABDOMEN

Most severe abdominal pain which lasts 6 hours or longer in a previously well patient is caused by a surgical condition. Every effort should be made to **diagnose the problem early** by taking a careful history and performing a thorough physical examination. Laboratory tests and radiographs are supplementary.

A. HISTORY

1. Age of the patient has obvious importance in determining the probable cause of an acute abdominal problem.

2. Pain is the cardinal symptom of the acute abdomen. Note the following:

a. Time and mode of onset (explosive, rapid, gradual). Note the relationship of onset to the last meal.

b. Character (dull, burning, cramping).

c. Severity (excruciating, severe, moderate, mild).

d. Constancy (steady, intermittent).

e. Location at onset.

f. Shift (subsides in one area and reappears in another) or *radiation* (remains in original site but extends to involve adjacent areas supplied by the same somatic nerves).

g. Effect of respiration, movement, position (erect, supine, lateral decubitus, hips flexed), *eating, defecation, and micturition.*

3. Vomiting. Anorexia, nausea, and vomiting are gradations of the same mechanism. These symptoms result from irritation of the peritoneum, obstruction of a muscular tube, or absorption of toxic substances. Note these characteristics:

a. Time of onset. If vomiting *preceded* abdominal pain, a surgical cause is unlikely.

b. Frequency and persistence.

c. Character. Note especially if the appearance of the vomitus changes with repeated episodes. Patients may continue to retch (dry heaves) after the stomach is emptied. Hematemesis should be noted.

4. Defecation

a. Diarrhea (frequency, consistency, character, continence, hematochezia).

b. Constipation is infrequent bowel movements and *obstipation* is absence of bowel movements. Failure to pass any stool or flatus for 24 hours is indicative of intestinal obstruction.

5. Fever. Note the time of appearance of fever, and note especially if shaking chills (rigors) occurred. Chills are a symptom of bacteremia (or viremia) and are most typical of infection in the urinary, biliary, or portal venous systems.

6. Past history

a. Previous abdominal disease and operations.

b. Systemic diseases and diseases of other organ systems.

c. Recent trauma, even if it seemed trivial at the time.

d. Menstrual history: last menstrual period, use of contraceptives.

B. PHYSICAL EXAMINATION

1. General appearance

a. Facial expression. Flushed, pale, flaring nostrils.

b. Position and activity in bed. Lying quietly, restless, writhing, hips and knees flexed.

2. Vital signs. Fever, pulse rate, respiratory rate.

3. Chest. Look for signs of pneumonitis.

4. Abdomen. The following sequence elicits maximal information with minimal discomfort to the patient.

a. Inspection. Scars, contour (scaphoid, distended), visible peristalsis.

b. Hernia orifices. Inguinal, femoral, umbilical, incisional (if any).

c. Cough tenderness. Ask the patient to cough and then point to the painful spot. Cough tenderness is a sign of peritoneal irritation; it may also be found with tenderness in the muscles of the abdominal wall. The examiner learns the location and the degree of localization of peritoneal irritation by this simple maneuver.

d. Palpitation

(1) Muscle spasm: *Gently* place the flat of the hand over the abdomen and depress it slightly. True muscle spasm persists as the patient takes a deep inspiration; if guarding is voluntary, the muscle relaxes during inspiration. Muscle spasm indicates peritoneal irritation.

(2) One-finger palpation: Begin away from the point of cough tenderness and systemically examine the abdomen by *gently* probing with one index finger. If properly performed, this step is not painful and it localizes the peritoneal irritation. *Direct tenderness* is sensed beneath the examining finger; *referred tenderness* is felt in some other area.

(3) Deep palpation should not be performed in an area that is tender to one-finger palpation. A mass is the chief abnormality detected by deep palpation.

(4) Rebound tenderness is elicited by pressing gradually on the abdominal wall and releasing the pressure suddenly. Tenderness sensed in that area on release of pressure is *rebound tenderness;* pain felt elsewhere is *referred rebound tenderness*. Testing for rebound tenderness elicits the same information that was already obtained by gentler methods (cough and one-finger palpation).

(5) Tenderness should be sought in the costovertebral angles.

e. Percussion of the mid- and lower abdomen is just another means of detecting peritoneal irritation and usually is unnecessary. Percussion over the liver may reveal absence of dullness, a sign of free intraperitoneal air. Percussion may identify free fluid in the abdomen, but this finding usually is of little diagnostic value.

f. Auscultation is useful mainly in diagnosis of intestinal obstruction in which peristaltic rushes and high-pitched tinkles are audible. In other acute abdominal conditions, peristalsis varies from absent to hyperactive. It is clearly an error to assume that active bowel sounds exclude the possibility of peritonitis.

g. Other signs

(1) *Iliopsoas sign.* There are two methods of eliciting this sign of inflammation in or adjacent to the iliopsoas muscle. (a) With the patient supine, have the patient actively flex the hip and knee against the resistance of the examiner's hand. (b) Have the patient lie on the side opposite the area of abdominal pain. With the hip and knee straight, the examiner passively extends the thigh on the affected side.

(2) *Obturator sign.* With the patient supine, flex the hip and knee and rotate the hip internally and externally. Inflammation adjacent to the obturator internus muscle is indicated by pain on this movement.

(3) *Murphy's sign.* Inspiratory arrest during a deep breath as the examiner palpates the right upper quadrant. Classically, this sign is elicited when an acutely inflamed gallbladder comes into contact with examining fingers.

h. Pelvic and rectal examination.

Tenderness of the pelvic peritoneum is elicited rectally or vaginally. Masses, rectal bleeding, and cervical discharge may be detected also.

C. LABORATORY TESTS

1. Blood

a. Hematocrit may reflect bleeding or dehydration.

b. Leukocyte count and differential are useful if they are abnormal, but normal leukocyte profiles do not exclude a surgical condition.

c. Amylase may be elevated in many conditions other than pancreatitis, including perforated viscus, intestinal obstruction, and intestinal ischemia.

d. Serum electrolytes, creatinine, bilirubin, and so on, are helpful in ill patients.

2. Urine should be examined for specific gravity, glucose, albumin, blood, leukocytes, casts, and bacteria.

3. Peritoneal fluid. Paracentesis or peritoneal lavage is rarely used today in nontrauma cases.

D. RADIOGRAPHS. If perforation or obstruction is suspected, insert a nasogastric tube **before** sending the patient for radiographs.

1. Plain radiographs of the chest and abdomen are essential in most patients with acute abdominal disease. Abdominal films should be obtained in the supine and erect (or decubitus) positions. Look for gas pattern, masses, free air, obliteration of the properitoneal fat line or the outlines of the psoas muscles, liver and kidney shadows, and air in the biliary tree.

2. Ultrasonography is especially useful in patients with pelvic, biliary, or pancreatic problems; solid and cystic masses can be identified and differentiated. Appendicitis can be diagnosed accurately by some ultrasonographers.

3. Studies of the upper or lower GI tract with water-soluble media may diagnose intestinal obstruction or perforation. Barium should be used only when perforation is clearly absent.

4. CT is better than ultrasonography in locating and diagnosing abdominal masses because the bowel lumen can be filled with contrast.

5. Angiography diagnoses sites of intestinal bleeding.

E. RADIONUCLIDE SCANS of various kinds find application in acute abdominal conditions (e.g., HIDA scan for acute cholecystitis).

F. SPECIAL TESTS. Diagnostic laparoscopy or peritoneoscopy is performed in suspected gynecologic disease or other acute abdominal conditions. It is assuming greater importance in general surgery.

G. DIAGNOSIS BY GROUPING OF SYMPTOMS AND SIGNS. Possible causes of an acute abdominal illness can be estimated from the grouping of symptoms and signs:

1. Abdominal pain alone

a. The early stages of many conditions fall into this category, and only with repeated evaluation do other symptoms and signs appear.

b. Central, severe abdominal pain with no other abnormalities is seen in early appendicitis, intestinal obstruction, gastroenteritis, and pancreatitis.

c. Biliary and renal colic have characteristic distributions in most cases.

2. Severe central pain with shock. Consider pancreatitis, intestinal ischemia, and intraabdominal bleeding (e.g., ruptured ectopic pregnancy, ruptured aneurysm).

3. Pain, vomiting, distention but no rigidity. Small bowel obstruction.

4. Pain with obstipation and distention. Colonic obstruction.

5. Severe pain with collapse and generalized rigidity. Perforated ulcer or other perforated viscus.

6. Pain, tenderness, and rigidity.

a. Right upper quadrant. Cholecystitis, perforated ulcer, inflammation of a high-lying appendix.

b. Left upper quadrant. Ruptured spleen, perforated ulcer, and various uncommon diseases.

c. Left lower quadrant. Diverticulitis, perforated colonic cancer, pelvic peritonitis.

d. Right lower quadrant. Appendicitis, perforated ulcer, gastroenteritis, Meckel's diverticulitis, cholecystitis (low-lying gallbladder), gynecologic diseases.

H. CONDITIONS THAT MIMIC THE ACUTE ABDOMEN. Extraabdominal and systemic diseases can simulate the acute abdomen. Examples include pneumonia, myocardial infarction, and porphyria.

I. TREATMENT

1. If the diagnosis is uncertain, reevaluate the patient frequently and attempt to make a diagnosis as soon as possible. The patient should be NPO; IV fluids are given, and nasogastric suction is often advisable.

2. Narcotic analgesics should be given if needed. Seldom do analgesics mask the objective findings of surgical disease.

3. Antibiotics are not administered until a decision is made about surgery.

4. The most important decision is whether the acute abdomen is "surgical"; if so, operation should be performed as soon as the patient is prepared. Most patients with localized peritoneal irritation and muscular rigidity, and essentially all patients with generalized peritonitis, septicemia, or hemodynamic instability should have exploratory laparotomy. Precise preoperative diagnosis of the condition causing the acute abdomen is a worthy objective and helps the surgeon plan the placement of the incision, but it is less critical than recognition that some form of surgical disease is in progress and must be treated by operation.

III. PERITONITIS AND ABDOMINAL ABSCESS

Peritonitis is inflammation of the peritoneum, a thin endothelial layer with a rich vascular and lymphatic supply. Abdominal abscess is one consequence of peritonitis.

A. ACUTE PERITONITIS

1. Bacterial causes. The peritoneum is normally resistant to infection by small inocula of common bacteria; continuous contamination, virulent bacteria, diminished host resistance, and the presence of ascites, blood, foreign bodies or active digestive enzymes are addictive factors that increase the likelihood of peritonitis from bacterial contamination.

a. Primary bacterial peritonitis is the result of hematogenous bacterial contamination of the peritoneal cavity. Streptococci and pneumococci are the usual organisms. The condition occurs mainly in patients with ascites.

b. Secondary bacterial peritonitis follows acute infections or perforations of the GI or GU tracts. It is much more common than the primary form.

2. Chemical causes

a. Gastric and pancreatic juice are severely irritating to the peritoneum and may cause shock within a very short time. Eventually, secondary bacterial peritonitis is superimposed on the chemical irritation.

b. Bile, in the absence of bacteria and pancreatic juice, causes little peritoneal reaction. The addition of bacteria and/or pancreatic enzymes results in severe peritonitis.

c. Blood is a mild irritant in the peritoneal cavity.

d. Urine is only mildly irritating by itself, but urine mixed with bacteria causes a severe form of peritonitis.

3. Diagnosis. The clinical picture depends upon the cause of peritonitis, the extent of inflammation, and the interval after onset. Peritonitis may be **localized, diffuse, or generalized.** The following comments apply to chemical peritonitis and secondary bacterial peritonitis.

a. Symptoms

(1) Acute abdominal pain is a characteristic symptom. Pain is sudden, severe, and generalized in patients with chemical peritonitis due to a perforated viscus (e.g., perforated ulcer). In other conditions (e.g., appendicitis), pain is caused by the underlying disease initially, and it becomes more diffuse if peritonitis spreads. In these cases, perito-

nitis extends slowly from localized to diffuse to generalized, and if the host defenses contain the infection, peritonitis does not progress to the generalized stage.

(2) Nausea and vomiting are usually present.

(3) Sudden collapse may occur at the onset of chemical peritonitis.

b. Signs

(1) Shock (neurogenic, hypovolemic, or septic) is present in many patients with generalized peritonitis.

(2) Fever is routinely noted with advanced peritonitis, although it may be deceptively mild or even absent in elderly or immune-deficient patients.

(3) Abdominal distention becomes more marked with the passage of time.

(4) Abdominal tenderness and rigidity are localized, diffuse, or generalized depending upon the extent of peritoneal irritation.

(5) Abdomen classically is said to be silent with generalized peritonitis. This is an unreliable sign.

c. Laboratory tests.
Leukocytosis, elevated hematocrit (hemoconcentration), and metabolic acidosis are found with peritonitis. Tests reflect respiratory, hepatic, and renal failure in advanced untreated peritonitis.

d. Radiographs.
Ileus is a nonspecific finding in peritonitis; both small and large bowel are dilated. Free air may be noted in cases of perforated viscus. More specific signs of the underlying cause of peritonitis may be present. CT is very helpful if time permits.

e. Special tests.
Paracentesis or peritoneal lavage is rarely used.

4. Differential diagnosis. The surgeon's task is to differentiate peritonitis from diseases that mimic it and to distinguish between surgical and nonsurgical causes of true peritonitis. Acute edematous pancreatitis, salpingitis, and gastroenteritis are among for diseases that do not require operation ordinarily. The differential diagnosis of peritonitis is especially that of the acute abdomen. (See Section II and specific disease entities in other sections.)

5. Complications. Death may result from hypovolemia in patients with chemical peritonitis and from overwhelming sepsis in patients with bacterial peritonitis. Multiple organ failure (pulmonary, cardiac, hepatic, and renal) precedes death by hours to days.

Late complications include abdominal abscess (see below) and adhesions that may cause intestinal obstruction at some future date.

6. Treatment

a. Primary peritonitis is treated with antibiotics if the diagnosis is established with certainty.

b. Treatment of *secondary peritonitis* is directed toward the underlying cause and requires operation in most cases.

(1) Treat shock (see Chapter 1) and correct fluid and electrolyte derangements (Chapter 2).

(2) Broad-spectrum antibiotics are begun empirically and modified later as culture reports become available. The choice of antibiotics depends upon the suspected origin of peritonitis (see Chapter 4).

(3) Treat associated diseases and the systemic consequences of peritonitis (e.g., respiratory or renal insufficiency).

(4) *Operation.* Correct the inciting disease. The entire peritoneal cavity should be explored, pockets of infection emptied, foreign substances (feces, bile, blood) evacuated, and the abdomen irrigated with isotonic saline. Antibiotics such as cephalosporins are unnecessary in the lavage solution, and aminoglycosides should be avoided because they may cause prolonged neuromuscular block in patients who have received relaxing agents as part of the anesthetic technic. Drainage of the general peritoneal cavity is not recommended. Drains become isolated from the area they are supposed to drain with a few hours, they interfere with peritoneal defenses, and they may erode into viscera.

(5) *Postoperative care* is essentially the care of a critically ill patient. Antibiotics should be continued and changed as necessary. The surgeon should be alert to abscess formation. The sitting (Fowler or semi-Fowler) position has little value in patients with peritonitis and, in fact, may be harmful. The normal mechanism for clearing bacteria from the abdominal cavity is by absorption through diaphragmatic lymphatics, so circulation of peritoneal fluid under the diaphragmatic lymphatics, so circulation of peritoneal fluid under the diaphragms is desirable. Further, the size of the subdiaphragmatic space is increased in the sitting position, so Fowler's actually may cause more subphrenic (and pelvic) abscesses than the flat or head-down position.

7. Prognosis depends upon age, associated diseases, the cause of peritonitis, and the promptness and effectiveness of surgical treatment.

B. CHRONIC PERITONITIS
1. Chylous ascites
a. Congenital chylous ascites is due to abnormal communication of intestinal lymphatics with the peritoneal cavity. In some patients, chyle refluxes into the lower extremities as well. Surgical ligation and division of the abnormal lymphatic communications may be effective.

b. Acquired chylous ascites may be due to obstruction of major lymphatics (e.g., the thoracic duct) by tumor, disruption by surgical dissection, or idiopathic. Most cases resolve spontaneously, although malignant obstruction persist until death from the tumor.

2. Tuberculous peritonitis may be primary or the result of spread from a focus in the lungs or genital tract.

a. Diagnosis. Weakness, night sweats, weight loss, and abdominal distention are present for weeks to months. Ascites, masses, and a "doughy" feel to the abdomen may be noted. Peritoneal fluid has a high protein (>3 g/dl) and lymphocyte content; tubercle bacilli are identified by culture. Biopsy of the peritoneum percutaneously or by laparoscopy shows typical tuberculous granulomas and yields a diagnosis long before culture results are available.

b. Treatment. Antituberculosis chemotherapy is effective (see Chapter 4).

3. Starch peritonitis. Chronic granulomatous peritonitis may result from starch powder on surgical gloves. The disease is prevented by washing gloves thoroughly before placing the hands in the peritoneal cavity or new starch-free gloves can be used.

Severe abdominal pain, fever, and signs of peritonitis develop about 2 weeks after operation. Intestinal obstruction is prominent. Reoperation should be avoided if other causes can be excluded.

C. ABDOMINAL ABSCESSES
are common sequelae of bacterial peritonitis. Persistent fever, anorexia, malaise, and leukocytosis are typical. Other symptoms and signs and the treatment depend upon the location of the abscess. Common sites are shown in Figure 12-1.

1. Subphrenic abscess. An abscess may form in any of the subphrenic spaces. There are 3 spaces on either side of the

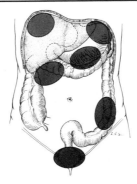

FIGURE 12-1. Common locations of peritoneal abscess formation. (From Dunphy JE, Way LW, editors: *Current surgical diagnosis and treatment,* New York, 1981, Lange.)

midline. On the right, the spaces are superior to the liver, inferior to the liver, and subhepatic. On the left, one space is anterior to the liver, one is anterior to the lesser sac, and another is the lesser sac itself.

    a. Diagnosis. The adage "pus somewhere, pus nowhere, pus under the diaphragm" was appropriate before CT became available.

    (1) *Symptoms and signs.* (a) Spiking fever that is not explained by infection elsewhere. (b) Anorexia and malaise. (c) Pain and tenderness over the lower thorax, flank, or upper abdomen in some cases. Pain can be referred to the shoulder. (d) Pleural effusion and limitation of diaphragmatic excursion.

    (2) *Radiographs.* Films of the upper abdomen and chest may show pleural effusion, stippled gas or an air-fluid level beneath the diaphragm, and an elevated and immobile diaphragm on the affected side. CT is the definitive study.

    (3) *Special tests.* Thoracentesis proves that the pleural effusion is sterile and increases the likelihood that a subphrenic abscess, rather than a primary pulmonary problem, is responsible for the effusion.

b. Treatment. Antibiotic therapy alone may resolve subphrenic cellulitis (phlegmon), but once a true abscess containing pus has formed, drainage is required. Remember also that abdominal abscesses may be multiple.

(1) *Percutaneous drainage* under CT or ultrasound guidance is preferred if a "window" exists—i.e., the abscess is adjacent to the abdominal wall so that viscera are not endangered during insertion of the needle.

(2) *Open surgical drainage* is safer for abscesses which are situated behind or among loops of bowel. Large particles of necrotic tissue and foreign bodies are removed more easily by open drainage. Solitary abscesses are drained extraperitoneally (through a subcostal incision) or extrapleurally (through the bed of the resected 12th rib posteriorly: Ochsner approach).

c. Prognosis is excellent if the abscess is well-drained. Some abscesses, particularly those in the lesser sac, are difficult to drain adequately, and repeated operations may be necessary.

2. Pelvic abscess

a. Diagnosis. Pelvic abscess is more easily diagnosed than subphrenic abscess in most cases. Symptoms are fever, pelvic discomfort, rectal pressure, diarrhea, and urinary symptoms.

A tender, boggy, or indurated mass is palpable anterior to the rectum. In women, the abscess may bulge into the vagina from the pouch of Douglas.

Ultrasonography is accurate for localization of abscesses in the pelvis. CT is needed in some patients.

b. Treatment. Antibiotics should be given to help contain the infection; pelvic cellulitis may resolve with antibiotics alone.

The classic indication of a maturing abscess is downward descent of the mass, often with gaping and incontinence of the anus. This kind of large abscess is rare today.

Pelvic abscesses are drained into the rectum or vagina. This procedure is performed under anesthesia with ultrasound guidance to be certain the cavity does not elude the probing needle. Once the cavity is entered and pus is aspirated, a large catheter is inserted and left in place for a few days.

Postoperative pelvic abscesses sometimes are drained preferentially by a transabdominal approach.

c. Prognosis. Recovery is rapid and complete in most patients.

3. Other abdominal abscesses. Abscesses may form in the lateral gutters, in the lesser sac, between loops of small bowel, or beneath an abdominal incision.

a. Diagnosis. Symptoms include fever, malaise, and pain. Repeated, careful one-finger palpation may disclose tenderness over an abscess as it develops, and a mass becomes palpable in many cases.

Plain radiographs may reveal collections of gas and fluid outside the bowel or displacement of dilated intestinal loops.

Ultrasonography, CT, and indium-111 leukocyte scan are useful tests. A recent incision limits the ability of ultrasonography to detect abscesses beneath the wound.

b. Treatment. Percutaneous drainage is used for most of these abscesses. Open operation is performed if other problems exist, i.e., a leaking anastomosis or necrotic intestine.

c. Prognosis depends upon the patient's age and general condition, the location and multiplicity of abscesses, and the adequacy of surgical drainage.

IV. UPPER GASTROINTESTINAL HEMORRHAGE

Duodenal ulcer, gastric ulcer, gastritis, esophageal varices, and Mallory-Weiss syndrome account for 95% of cases of massive bleeding from the upper GI tract.

A. MANIFESTATIONS
   1. Hematemesis is the vomiting of blood. If the blood is red, the source is proximal to the ligament of Treitz with few exceptions.

   2. Coffee-ground emesis reflects the presence of blood in the stomach for a sufficient time to allow the conversion of hemoglobin to methemoglobin by gastric acid.

   3. Melena is the passage of black stools. Blood must remain in the gut for several hours for it to change color, so most patients with melena are bleeding from the upper GI tract.

   4. Hematochezia is the passage of bright red blood per rectum. This too may originate in the upper tract. Management is discussed in Section V.

B. DIAGNOSIS AND TREATMENT. The amount of blood loss and the rate of bleeding determine the urgency of the diagnostic and therapeutic efforts. Hematemesis always implies the threat of exsanguination and requires immediate action.

Coffee-ground emesis and melena (especially if present for several days) may be evaluated more leisurely. Hematochezia is discussed in Section V. The following comments apply to severe bleeding.

1. Questions the patient about known upper GI disease or symptoms that may suggest the cause of bleeding.

2. Physical examination may reveal stigmata of cirrhosis and portal hypertension, but bleeding cannot be assumed to be variceal because about 50% of cirrhotics with acute upper GI hemorrhage are bleeding from peptic ulcer, gastritis, or other nonvariceal lesions.

3. Resuscitation with IV fluids is begun immediately, and transfusions are given as necessary. Avoid inadequate resuscitation; hypotension is a poor way to stop bleeding, and it leads to pulmonary and renal failure.

4. Pass a large Ewald (32-36 Fr) tube through the mouth into the stomach and lavage the stomach with iced saline to evacuate liquid and clotted blood. The Ewald tube can be removed and a nasogastric tube inserted after bleeding stops. Patients may bleed from a duodenal ulcer without reflux of blood into the stomach; the gastric aspirate in such patients contains no blood or bile.

5. Measure hematocrit, PT, PTT, platelets, serum creatinine, albumin, and liver function.

6. Bleeding may stop with iced saline lavage. Subsequent management is directed at the specific cause of the bleeding episode. The nasogastric tube is removed as soon as it is certain that bleeding has ceased.

7. If bleeding persists, continued nasogastric suction, careful monitoring of vital signs, and serial hematocrits are guides to the rate of bleeding and help determine the course of action.

8. If the patient is stable, fiberoptic endoscopy should be done to determine the bleeding site. Endoscopic control of bleeding from varices or peptic ulcers may be possible by sclerotherapy or one of several methods of coagulation.

9. Angiography is useful to diagnose bleeding sites if endoscopy fails (e.g., bleeding distal to the ligament of Treitz). Angiography with infusion of vasoconstricting agents is used therapeutically in selected patients who are prohibitive operative risks. Embolization of bleeding points with clot or other substances may be effective.

10. Operation to control bleeding may be needed if a patient requires more than 4 units of blood to achieve hemodynamic stability initially, or if more than 1 unit of blood is required every 8 hours thereafter and if endoscopic control is possible. These are general rules, and many exceptions must be made (e.g., jaundiced cirrhotic patients or patients with acutely bleeding varices). In potentially salvageable patients, the goal is to operate before the systemic effects (especially pulmonary and renal) of prolonged hypotension and multiple transfusions occur. Elderly patients tolerate massive hemorrhage poorly and should be operated on earlier rather than later than younger patients. Early operation also is indicated if compatible blood is not available for transfusion or if the patient refuses transfusions.

11. Management of specific causes of upper GI hemorrhage is discussed in appropriate sections in this chapter.

V. LOWER GASTROINTESTINAL HEMORRHAGE

Severe bleeding per rectum can arise from lesions at any level in the GI tract. The lower tract (distal small bowel, colon, anorectum) is the probable source of dark red to bright red blood (**hematochezia**), but it is important to keep in mind that the color of evacuated blood is a function of the length of time it resided in the bowel, and bright red blood can originate at any level. If the patient is not in shock, bright red blood is likely to be coming from the lower tract.

Colonic lesions that give rise to acute hemorrhage include vascular ectasias (angiodysplasias), diverticula, ulcerative colitis, ischemic colitis, and solitary ulcer. Neoplasms rarely cause exsanguinating hemorrhage. Severe bleeding originates with equal frequency in the right colon and the left colon.

Diagnostic and therapeutic maneuvers are performed simultaneously (Figure 12-2).

1. Resuscitation with IV fluid takes first priority.

2. A nasogastric tube should be inserted and the aspirate examined for bile and for gross occult blood. The presence of bile without blood suggests that the gastroduodenum is not the bleeding site. Endoscopy of the upper tract should be performed if the aspirate contains blood or if doubt remains about an upper tract source.

3. Anoscopy and sigmoidoscopy (rigid or flexible) are mandatory. Bleeding hemorrhoids, ulcerative colitis, or ischemia may be detected and treatment initiated.

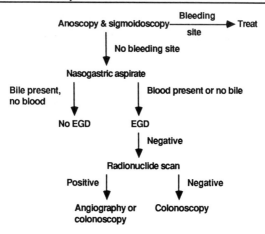

FIGURE 12-2. Plan of diagnosis and treatment of acute lower GI hemorrhage. EGD = esophagogastroduodenoscopy.

4. If bleeding stops spontaneously shortly after admission to the hospital (75% of patients), fiberoptic colonoscopy is performed after the colon is cleansed. Barium should be avoided because it interferes with angiography, which may be desirable if bleeding recurs. If the bleeding site is not found and bleeding does not recur, nothing further should be done.

5. If bleeding continues, one can perform colonoscopy or obtain a radionuclide "bleeding" scan. The choice depends on the rate of bleeding and one's experience with these diagnostic alternatives.

a. Colonoscopy in the presence of rapid bleeding requires no bowel prep because blood itself is a cathartic. This examination can be difficult.

b. Colonoscopy in patients with slower bleeding is preceded by an oral saline lavage prep using one of the products containing polyethylene glycol (e.g., Golytely or Colyte). Colonoscopy in this setting identifies a bleeding site in 30%-70% of cases.

c. Radionuclide scans using technetium ^{99m}Tc-labeled red cells are 10 times more sensitive than angiograms in detecting ongoing bleeding. Scans obtained within an hour after injection are the most useful, because active bleeding will be detected, and angiography will likely be rewarding. Delayed scans are obtained if early images are negative. If radionuclide scans are persistently normal, angiography usually is not attempted. Success with scans is not uniform and they are not used in some centers.

6. Angiography demonstrates the bleeding site in 40%-70% of patients. If the bleeding site is identified, a vasoconstrictor (epinephrine or vasopressin) is infused into the artery supplying the bleeding point. This method is successful in about 50%, and if bleeding does not recur operation may not be required. Elective operation after preparation of the colon is advisable in some instances.

7. Intraoperative colonoscopy is a useful maneuver, and intraoperative enteroscopy (examination of the small intestine) may also be helpful.

8. Operation is limited to segmental colonic resection if the bleeding site has been localized conclusively. More extensive resection is warranted in selected good-risk patients with bleeding from the right colon and multiple diverticula in the left colon. Total abdominal colectomy (subtotal colectomy) with ileorectal anastomosis is the only recourse for persistent colonic bleeding of unknown origin, but fortunately this procedure seldom is required today.

The mortality rate of lower GI bleeding is about 10%.

VI. INTESTINAL OBSTRUCTION*

Mechanical obstruction of the intestine refers to complete or partial physical blockage of the lumen. **Simple obstruction** implies one obstructing point; obstruction at two or more points is a **closed loop.** The intestine is viable in **nonstrangulating obstruction.** When the obstructing mechanism occludes the mesenteric blood supply as well as the lumen, **strangulation** may develop. It is more likely in closed loop than in simple obstruction.

About 85% of mechanical obstructions occur in the small intestine and 15% in the large intestine. The causes of obstruction in the western world are listed in Table 12-1; the relative incidence of these causes is very different in developing coun-

---

*Obstruction in infants and children is discussed in Chapter 19.

Table 12-1. Causes of mechanical intestinal
obstruction in adults

Site of obstruction	Cause	Relative incidence
Small intestine	Adhesions	60%
	External hernia	10%
	Neoplasm	20%
	Miscellaneous	10%
Large intestine	Carcinoma of colon	65%
	Diverticulitis	20%
	Volvulus	5%
	Miscellaneous	10%

tries. Miscellaneous causes of small bowel obstruction include
intussusception, internal hernia, volvulus, foreign body, gallstone, inflammatory bowel disease, and stricture from ischemia
or radiation injury. Diverticulitis seldom obstructs the colon
completely; volvulus is the second most common cause of complete colonic obstruction. Causes of large bowel obstruction include inflammatory bowel disease, benign tumors, ischemic
stricture, and fecal impaction.

A. OBSTRUCTION OF THE SMALL INTESTINE
1. Diagnosis
a. Symptoms
(1) Cramping abdominal *pain* with a crescendo-decrescendo
pattern, recurring every few minutes, is typical. Obstruction of the proximal intestine causes variable upper abdominal discomfort rather than cramps. Continuous pain
suggests strangulation.
(2) *Vomiting* occurs minutes to hours after the onset of pain,
depending on how distal the obstruction is. Vomitus becomes feculent owing to bacterial overgrowth, especially
with distal obstruction. Blood in the vomitus indicates
strangulation or an associated lesion.
(3) *Obstipation* is a feature of complete obstruction, although gas and feces in the colon can be expelled after
the obstruction begins.
b. Signs
(1) Vital signs are normal, or they reflect dehydration.
Shock or high fever suggests strangulation.
(2) Abdominal distention is minimal in proximal obstruction
and marked in prolonged distal obstruction. Mild tender-

ness is common; severe tenderness warns of strangulation. Peristaltic rushes and high-pitched tinkles are audible coincident with cramps.

(3) A tender, incarcerated external hernia (inguinal, femoral, umbilical, incisional) should be sought; femoral hernias are difficult to find in obese patients.

c. Laboratory tests. Results of blood chemistries depend upon the degree of dehydration. Leukocytosis may indicate strangulation, but the leukocyte count is occasionally normal even in patients with necrotic bowel. Urinalysis reflects dehydration.

d. Radiographic findings. Plain abdominal films in the supine and erect (or lateral decubitus) positions show dilated small bowel loops with gas-fluid levels in a ladder-like pattern. This picture is absent in proximal obstruction. The colon typically contains no gas. Gas in intestinal wall is a late sign of strangulation.

Oral contrast medium establishes the diagnosis of obstruction in equivocal cases.

2. Differential diagnosis

a. Small versus large obstruction is discussed in the following section.

b. Paralytic (adynamic) ileus follows abdominal surgery (see Chapter 2), or it is associated with peritonitis or trauma to the abdomen or back. The inciting cause, such as appendicitis or pancreatitis, should be evident. Ileus causes constant mild pain and abdominal distention. Plain films show gas mainly in the colon. Contrast radiographs help in doubtful cases.

3. Complications. Strangulation is the cause of most deaths from intestinal obstruction. The luminal contents are a lethal mixture of bacteria, bacterial products, necrotic tissue, and blood. The strangulated bowel may perforate, releasing this material into the peritoneal cavity; even if the bowel does not perforate, bacteria may transude through the ischemic bowel or enter the circulation via lymphatics and cause septic shock.

4. Treatment. With a few exceptions, complete obstruction of the small intestine is treated by operation because of the risk of strangulation. Strangulation cannot be excluded with certainty as long as obstruction persists. If obstruction is incomplete, nonoperative management may be in order.

a. Preoperative preparation

(1) *A nasogastric tube* should be inserted to relieve vomiting and to avoid further distention of the bowel by swallowed air. A long intestinal tube has no advantage if prompt operation is planned.

(2) *Fluid and electrolyte resuscitation* is crucial. Huge amounts of isotonic fluid are lost into the bowel lumen, intestinal wall, peritoneal cavity, and by vomiting. Hypovolemia is the cause of death in nonstrangulating obstruction. These losses should be replaced and the acid-base imbalances corrected before operation.

(3) *Antibiotics* are advisable. They are essential in strangulation, and strangulation is always a possibility until operation proves otherwise.

b. Operation is begun when the patient has been rehydrated and vital organs are functioning properly.

If a groin hernia is the cause of obstruction, the incision is made over that area. Otherwise, a generous abdominal incision should be made.

Operative details depend on the cause of obstruction. Adhesive bands are lysed or the obstructing lesion is removed. Strangulated bowel is resected.

5. Prognosis. Nonstrangulating obstruction has a mortality rate of about 2%; most deaths are in the elderly. Strangulation obstruction has a mortality rate of 8% if operation is performed within 36 hours after the onset of symptoms and 25% if operation is delayed beyond 36 hours.

B. OBSTRUCTION OF THE LARGE INTESTINE. In 10%-20% of patients, the ileocecal valve is incompetent, and pressure proximal to an obstructing lesion in the colon is relieved by reflux into the ileum. In other patients, however, a closed loop is formed between the obstructing point and the ileocecal valve, and perforation of the cecum may result from progressive distention with impairment of blood flow in the cecal wall.

1. Diagnosis

a. Symptoms. Cramping *pain* develops insidiously in the hypogastrium, left lower quadrant, or diffusely in the abdomen. Severe, continuous pain suggests strangulation. Loud borborygmi are common. *Obstipation* is a universal feature if obstruction is complete. *Vomiting* occurs late or not at all.

b. Signs. The abdomen is markedly distended and tympanitic; tenderness may overlie the distended colon; diffuse severe tenderness and rigidity indicate perforation. Gross or occult blood may be present in the stool. Sigmoidoscopy is mandatory; the obstructing lesion may be seen.

c. Radiographic findings. Plain films show a distended colon outlining the peritoneal cavity like a "picture frame." The small bowel is dilated also if the ileocecal valve is incompetent. Hypaque enema shows the site of obstruction. CT scans are used in certain situations.

d. Special tests. Colonoscopy or flexible sigmoidoscopy reveals the obstructing lesion. Cathartics must not be given, but gentle enema is necessary.

2. Differential diagnosis

a. Small vs large bowel obstruction. Large bowel obstruction is slower in onset, the pain is less severe, and vomiting is not always present. Radiography usually differentiates the two conditions.

b. Pseudo-obstruction. (Ogilvie's syndrome) is colonic distention in the absence of a mechanical block. It is associated with other illnesses, operations, or medications. Distention without pain is the first symptom. On plain radiographs, distention often is limited to the right and transverse colon. Contrast enema excludes a mechanical problem; the colon should not be overfilled lest perforation occur. Decompression can be accomplished by colonoscopy in most cases; cecostomy is the other option.

c. Paralytic ileus (see section on small bowel obstruction).

3. Complications.
Gangrene and perforation of the cecum are threats if the acutely dilated cecum is 12 cm or more in diameter.

4. Treatment.
Immediate resection of the obstructed segment is preferred. Decompressive cecostomy or transverse colostomy is reserved for critically ill patients who would not tolerate resection. Resection has the advantage of eliminating the offending lesion, frequently carcinoma, rather than leaving it in place for days or weeks longer.

a. Preoperative preparation requires the same measures described for small bowel obstruction; fluid and electrolyte deficits usually are less severe.

b. Operation. Obstructing cecal lesions are resected, usually with primary anastomosis. Obstructing lesions in the left colon are resected also, but most surgeons delay anastomosis to a later date. Intraoperative colonic lavage to cleanse the colon may allow immediate anastomosis.

c. Postoperative care is directed toward preparation of the patient for elective resection if the obstructing lesion is not removed initially.

5. Prognosis. Overall mortality rates of 20% are common. Cecal perforation is fatal in 40% and is the most important preventable cause of death.

C. VOLVULUS OF THE LARGE INTESTINE. Volvulus is rotation of the bowel (usually the cecum or the sigmoid colon) on its mesocolon, causing obstruction of the lumen and compromise of the circulation simultaneously. Volvulus causes 5%-10% of cases of colonic obstruction in the United States and a much higher percentage in some countries where high-residue diets are standard.

1. Cecal volvulus results from incomplete embryologic fixation of the ascending colon.

Because the cecum and the terminal ileum rotate together, the symptoms include those of small bowel obstruction. Pain in the right abdomen is severe and cramping initially, and then it becomes continuous. Vomiting and obstipation follow. The abdomen is distended.

The radiographic picture is characteristic, with a dilated cecum in the left upper quadrant. Barium enema is very helpful.

Operation is usually performed. In selected patients with severe associated diseases, colonoscopic detorsion may be attempted instead. The right colon is resected if it is strangulated; if the bowel is viable, the volvulus may be untwisted and the cecum sutured to the parietal peritoneum (cecopexy).

The operative mortality rate is 12%. Death is the consequence of delayed recognition and treatment; if the cecum is gangrenous, the death rate is 35%. Recurrence after cecopexy or resection is unusual.

2. Sigmoid volvulus results from elongation of the sigmoid in elderly, bedridden, or mentally ill patients.

Pain is cramping. Obstipation occurs immediately.

Plain films show a huge distended loop rising out of the pelvis into the right upper quadrant. Barium enema findings are pathognomonic. Unless strangulation is suspected, the first episode is treated by decompression using a flexible sigmoidoscope or placing a tube through a rigid sigmoidoscope. Resection of the sigmoid is advisable in young patients and in older patients with recurrent episodes, but preliminary deflation with a sigmoidoscope permits resection to be done electively.

The mortality rate is 25% for the first episode. Death is due to perforation (50% mortality) or associated disease in these elderly people. Only 5% die after operation if the bowel is viable.

VII. ACUTE INTESTINAL ISCHEMIA*

Acute intestinal ischemia may result from **arterial** occlusion (thrombosis or embolus), **venous** occlusion (thrombosis), or **nonocclusive** mechanisms (splanchnic hypoperfusion). **Mesenteric** ischemia involves the superior mesenteric vessels, and **colonic** ischemia results from impaired inferior mesenteric circulation.

The consequences of ischemia vary with the vessel involved, adequacy of collaterals, and other factors. The mucosa becomes ischemic first and may ulcerate, slough, and bleed. Severe ischemia leads to full-thickness infarction of the gut. The clinical course depends upon many variables and may range from mild to fulminating. Most patients are elderly.

A. DIAGNOSIS

1. Symptoms. Severe, poorly localized abdominal pain is the hallmark of intestinal ischemia. It may not respond to analgesics and is worse with movement. Vomiting, diarrhea (commonly bloody, especially if the colon is involved), or even constipation may occur.

History may reveal an underlying cause, e.g., cardiac arrhythmia, sepsis, hypercoagulable state, oral contraceptives, malignancy, portal hypertension, trauma, or intestinal angina.

2. Signs. *Pain out of proportion to objective findings* is typical of intestinal ischemia. There may be no abdominal abnormalities initially. Shock, fever, abdominal tenderness, distention, and peritonitis are late findings. Sigmoidoscopy may disclose ischemia of the rectum (uncommon) or sigmoid. An underlying cause of ischemia may be evident on physical examination (e.g., hypoperfusion in cardiogenic shock).

3. Laboratory tests. Blood is found in gastric contents or stool in 75%-95% of patients. Paracentesis fluid contains blood only in advanced cases.

Leukocytosis often is striking and hyperamylasemia is present in 50% of patients. Other tests reflect the severity of

---

*Chronic intstinal ischemia is discussed in Chapter 11.

hemoconcentration, fluid and electrolyte losses, and base deficit. Creatinine kinase (BB isoenzyme) correlates with intestinal infarction.

Hematologic studies (e.g., prothrombin time, partial thromboplastin time, antithrombin III assay, etc.) may reveal hypercoagulation in patients with no apparent cause for mesenteric venous occlusion.

4. Radiographs. Plain abdominal radiographs are nonspecific at first: diffuse distention of small bowel and/or colon, blunt plicae, thickened bowel wall, and small bowel loops that remain unchanged over several hours are suggestive. Late findings are diagnostic of intestinal necrosis: intramural gas and gas in the portal venous system.

Contrast radiographs reveal "thumbprinting" and either slow or rapid motility. These findings are most often limited to the left colon in cases of colonic ischemia. CT and MRI may be helpful. Selective mesenteric arteriography may reveal major arterial occlusion, or it may be entirely normal despite extensive infarction.

5. Special tests. Fiberoptic colonoscopy reveals colonic ischemia, but it should be reserved for subacute cases because of the risk of perforation. Indium-111 leukocyte scan is positive in many cases.

B. DIFFERENTIAL DIAGNOSIS. Acute pancreatitis is associated with a high serum amylase, but ischemic intestine may also result in hyperamylasemia. It may be impossible to differentiate the two conditions without exploring the abdomen.

Strangulation obstruction is difficult to differentiate from ischemia; both conditions require operation.

Ischemic colon may be confused with diverticulitis, ulcerative colitis, Crohn's disease, and carcinoma. Crohn's disease is the most difficult to differentiate, but ischemia usually has a more rapid onset and bleeding is more prominent than in Crohn's colitis.

C. COMPLICATIONS. Gangrene of the bowel wall leads to perforation and a high mortality rate. Massive bleeding from extensive mucosal ulceration can cause hypovolemic shock. Reperfusion injury after arterial blood flow is reestablished results from release of oxygen radicals that damage cell membranes.

D. TREATMENT. Mild ischemia may be treated expectantly with IV fluids and antibiotics. The problem is to determine which cases of ischemia are mild, and it is better to operate if there is any doubt.

Angiography with demonstrates embolic occlusion of the superior mesenteric artery can be followed by intraarterial infusion of papaverine (30-60 mg/hour). This drug seems to improve the chances of a good result if operation is then performed promptly. Embolectomy or arterial reconstruction is attempted if possible, and infarcted bowel is resected. Allopurinol prevents reperfusion injury experimentally but is unproved clinically. Venous thrombosis is managed by resection of gangrenous intestine. Ischemic colon is resected if it does not respond to antibiotics and fluids.

Nonocclusive ischemia is treated first by correcting the precipitating cause (e.g., congestive heart failure). Intraarterial papaverine has been used also, but operation is usually required to exclude other diseases and to resect infarcted bowel. The infarction may be patchy or diffuse.

Postoperative care involves close attention to maintenance of tissue perfusion by well-oxygenated blood. Anticoagulants are recommended for venous thrombosis, and antiplatelet-aggregating drugs are used by some surgeons for arterial thrombosis. A "second look" operation is performed 6-12 hours after the initial procedure if marginally viable bowel is left in.

E. PROGNOSIS. Acute intestinal ischemia is fatal in about 45% of patients overall; severe associated diseases, delay in diagnosis, and extensive infarction are factors responsible for death. Acute venous thrombosis has a mortality rate of 30%. Nonocclusive ischemia is fatal in up to 80% of patients.

VIII. ESOPHAGUS

A. PERFORATION

1. Instrumental perforation. The esophagus is most susceptible to perforation just above sites of narrowing. The normal esophagus is narrowed at the cricopharyngeal area, in its midportion where it is compressed by the aortic arch and the left mainstem bronchus, and at the diaphragmatic hiatus. Pathologic narrowing may occur at any level. Injury during endoscopy is prevented by skillful, gentle technic; the instrument should never be forced blindly.

a. Diagnosis. The manifestations depend upon the level of perforation, the extent of perforation, and the interval after perforation.

(1) *Symptoms and signs.* History of instrumentation. Pain on swallowing. Fever. Hypotension; shock may occur early after perforation of the thoracic esophagus. Pain, tenderness, and crepitus in the neck with perforation of the cervical esophagus. Pain in the chest, dyspnea, and pleural effusion with thoracic perforation; tenderness and crepitus in the neck may be minimal or absent. Pneumo-mediastinum may be reflected in the auscultatory finding of a "mediastinal crunch" (Hamman's sign).

(2) *Laboratory tests.* Leukocytosis usually develops.

(3) *Radiographs.* Depending upon the site of perforation, chest radiographs and films of the neck may show air in the soft tissues, air and fluid behind the cervical esophagus, mediastinal widening and emphysema, pneumothorax, and pleural effusion. Esophagram demonstrates the site of perforation.

b. Complications. Virulent bacteria from the oropharynx cause rapidly progressive infection in the neck, mediastinum, or pleural space. These infections are fatal if untreated.

c. Treatment. See below.

2. External trauma. The manifestations of perforation from external penetrating trauma are identical to those of instrumental perforation.

3. Spontaneous (emetogenic) perforation. Postemetic perforation of the esophagus (Boerhaave's syndrome) follows violent retching, often the consequence of an alcoholic binge. The most frequent site of perforation is the left posterior part of the distal esophagus. Men are more commonly affected than women.

a. Diagnosis. History of alcoholic binge or excessive eating. Violent retching. Sudden, severe pain in the lower chest and upper abdomen followed rapidly by shock. There may be crepitus in the neck, a rigid abdomen, and/or a mediastinal crunch. Pneumothorax, usually on the left. Esophagram demonstrates in the site of rupture.

b. Differential diagnosis. Myocardial infarction, pulmonary embolus, perforated peptic ulcer, and pancreatitis are excluded by radiographic proof of esophageal perforation.

c. Treatment. Antibiotics should be started immediately. Very small perforations, usually instrumental, with leakage confined to the mediastinum, may require no intervention. Some larger leaks may be managed by radiographically guided placement of a tube down the esophageal lumen, through the hole, and into the abscess cavity, as can be done with postoperative anastomotic leaks. Operation is required in most other patients. Suture closure of the perforation is possible if operation is performed within 24 hours of the injury. Delayed cases may require resection of the perforated esophagus, cervical esophagostomy, and later restoration of continuity by means of colonic interposition.

   d. Prognosis. About 90% of patients survive if surgical closure is carried out. Delayed treatment carries a death rate of 50%. Minor perforations do well with nonoperative therapy.

B. MALLORY-WEISS SYNDROME is a longitudinal tear at the esophagogastric junction as a result of vomiting. The laceration extends through the mucosa and submucosa. Approximately 75% are on the gastric side, and 5% are on the esophageal side of the esophagogastric junction; 20% cross the junction. About 25% have multiple tears. Nearly all patients have an associated hiatal hernia. Mallory-Weiss syndrome accounts for about 10% of cases of acute upper GI hemorrhage.

   1. Diagnosis. Vigorous vomiting of food or nonproductive retching, *followed by* hematemesis. *Endoscopy* identifies the laceration(s) and excludes other causes of bleeding.

   2. Treatment. Initial management of upper GI hemorrhage is described in Section IV above. About 90% of patients with Mallory-Weiss lesions stop bleeding with gastric lavage. IV vasopressin (0.4-0.6 units/min) may be useful. Endoscopic methods are successful in some cases. Very few patients require operation to suture the laceration.

C. FOREIGN BODIES. Children and mentally disturbed adults may ingest foreign bodies. Large chunks of meat are swallowed by edentulous patients. Depending on its size, the object may pass into the stomach or become lodged at sites of anatomic or pathologic narrowing.

   1. Diagnosis
   a. Symptoms and signs. History of ingesting a foreign body or swallowing a bolus of meat. Pain in the mediastinum or neck. Dysphagia may be mild or severe. Dyspnea in some cases.

   b. Radiographs. Opaque objects are visible on plain chest radiographs. Esophagram detects most objects.

   c. Special tests. Esophagoscopy is diagnostic and therapeutic.

   2. Complications. Infection above the impacted object, perforation, and erosion into adjacent blood vessels or the tracheobronchial tree.

3. Treatment. Esophagoscopy is performed for diagnosis and treatment.

Proteolytic enzymes (e.g., commercially available meat tenderizers) may disimpact meat, but perforations have been reported. This method of management no longer is recommended.

D. CORROSIVE ESOPHAGITIS. Ingestion of strong acid or alkali produces chemical burn of the pharynx, esophagus, and stomach.

1. Diagnosis

a. Symptoms and signs. History of ingestion of acid or alkali (determine the chemical nature of the substance). Fever and shock in severe cases. Respiratory distress if the airway is obstructed by edema or if some of the caustic material was aspirated. Severe burning pain from mouth to stomach; accentuated by swallowing. Edema and mucosal destruction of lips, tongue, pharynx, and (in some cases) larynx **(the absence of these findings does not exclude esophageal injury)**. Signs of esophageal or gastric perforation may be noted.

b. Special tests. Esophagoscopy determines the extent of injury; some patients have oropharyngeal burns only, and others have extensive damage to the esophagus and stomach. Direct laryngoscopy assesses the degree of damage to the larynx.

2. Complications. Bleeding and perforation are early complications. Late sequelae include tracheoesophageal fistula and stricture.

3. Treatment

a. Do **not** induce vomiting and **do not** perform gastric lavage.

b. Establish and maintain the airway.

c. Lavage the mouth and have the patient swallow milk, water, or **dilute** acid or alkali to neutralize the caustic substance. This procedure is probably ineffective if instituted more than a few minutes after ingestion.

d. Esophagoscopy should be performed within 12 hours of ingestion if possible, within 48 hours at the latest. Endoscopy is contraindicated in patients with severe respiratory distress or suspected perforation. The proximal point of esophageal injury should be noted and the esophagoscope advanced no farther. Depth of mucosal burn should be characterized as first, second, or third degree.

e. First-degree burns are treated with antibiotics alone.

f. Second- and third-degree burns require laparotomy to determine viability of the stomach and distal esophagus. Resection is performed for full-thickness burns, and less severe damage may be treated with corticosteroids. An esophageal stent is used in some cases.

g. Late strictures are treated by dilatations or esophagectomy.

4. Prognosis. Up to 70% of patients with oropharyngeal burns have no esophageal involvement. Superficial esophageal burns usually heal without residual stricture. Deep burns require early resection or they progress to stricture formation in nearly every case.

E. HIATAL HERNIA AND REFLUX ESOPHAGITIS. Hiatal hernia is displacement of the stomach through the esophageal hiatus into the mediastinum. There are two types of hiatal hernia, sliding and paraesophageal.

1. Sliding hiatal hernia and reflux esophagitis. About 95% of hiatal hernias are of the sliding variety in which the esophagogastric junction and the proximal stomach are displaced upward into the mediastinum. Obesity and loss of strength of the fascial attachments are contributory factors.

The clinical manifestations of sliding hiatal hernia are not caused by the hernia itself but by the **esophageal reflux** which frequently accompanies it. Sliding hiatal hernia does not strangulate. Reflux normally is prevented by mechanisms including the lower esophageal sphincter and intraabdominal segment of esophagus. In about half of patients with sliding hiatal hernia, the barrier to reflux is impaired. Reflux may occur also in the absence of any demonstrable hiatal hernia. Persistent reflux leads to **reflux esophagitis**, and continued esophagitis may result in **esophageal stricture**.

a. Diagnosis

(1) *Symptoms.* Hiatal hernia alone is asymptomatic. Esophageal reflux typically causes retrosternal burning pain (heartburn) which is exacerbated by gravity (e.g., lying supine) or by increasing pressure in the abdomen (e.g., lifting, straining). Regurgitation of sour or bitter fluid into the mouth is a common symptom. Nocturnal cough and repeated episodes of pneumonia may result from aspiration of regurgitated gastric contents. Dysphagia may be due to edema or to formation of a fibrous stricture. Bleeding is a symptom of esophagitis; it is seldom massive.

(2) *Signs.* None.

(3) *Radiographs.* Chest radiographs may show a gas-fluid shadow in the mediastinum. Esophagram may demonstrate a hiatal hernia, and cine-esophagography or fluoroscopy may document the presence of gastroesophageal reflux; strictures are evident on these studies also.

(4) *Special tests.* Esophagoscopy and biopsy reveal the presence and degree of esophagitis and the associated Barrett's epithelium (see below). Endoscopy also rules out other esophageal or gastric lesions. Esophageal motility studies measure the strength of the gastroesophageal sphincter and exclude motility disorders as a cause. Monitoring of pH in the distal esophagus is the most sensitive method of diagnosing reflux. Gastroesophageal scintigraphy is also a sensitive test for esophageal reflux. The **Bernstein test** determines whether the patient's symptoms are due to esophagitis; 0.1 N HCl instilled into the distal esophagus reproduces the patient's pain if esophagitis is responsible for it. This test is unreliable and is seldom used today.

b. Differential diagnosis. Myocardial ischemia, peptic ulcer, and cholelithiasis are just a few of the other diseases that can be confused with gastroesophageal reflux. Esophagitis is also caused by drugs and infections (e.g., monilia).

c. Complications. Esophagitis, sometimes progressing to stricture formation, is the most common complication of reflux. Pulmonary complications from repeated aspiration also occur. Esophageal carcinoma is an occasional late development. Barrett's epithelium is also a consequence of reflux.

d. Medical treatment. Asymptomatic sliding hiatal hernia requires no treatment. Antacids, H_2-receptor antagonists, and omeprazole are the mainstays of medical treatment of reflux. Bethanechol and metoclopramide seem to strengthen the sphincter.

The heal of the bed should be elevated about 15 cm to prevent nocturnal reflux. Patients should not lie down after meals and should not eat before bedtime. Strictures are treated by endoscopic dilatation.

e. Surgical treatment. Surgical repair is indicated for refractory esophagitis, severe unresponsive stricture, or recurrent pneumonia. Operation is performed through the abdomen or through the thorax depending upon the patient's obesity, previous operations, associated diseases, and the surgeon's preference.

Surgical antireflux procedures aim to reduce the hiatal hernia, restore the intraabdominal segment of esophagus, and anchor the gastroesophageal area in the abdomen. The **Nissen fundoplication** (360-degree fundic wrap around the distal esophagus) is the most popular procedure. The **Hill repair** (posterior gastropexy) and the **Belsey fundoplication** (270-degree fundic wrap) have fewer proponents. The **Angelchik prosthesis** is a plastic collar that is fastened around the distal esophagus. This foreign body may erode, migrate, or constrict the esophagus, and it cannot be recommended. Antireflux procedures can be performed laparoscopically.

An acid-reducing procedure is added to the antireflux operation if the patient has associated gastric or duodenal ulcer. Strictures may respond to an antireflux procedure and esophageal dilatation during and after operation; rarely, strictures require esophageal resection and replacement.

f. Prognosis. Most patients with gastroesophageal reflux respond to medical therapy. Surgical repairs of the three types mentioned are successful in about 90% of patients.

2. Paraesophageal hiatal hernia. In this type of hiatal hernia, the esophagogastric junction remains in the normal position, and the fundus of the stomach herniates through the hiatus to the left of the esophagus. With time, increasing amounts of stomach are included in the hernia.

Reflux is uncommon in paraesophageal hiatal hernia, and the clinical manifestations are due to obstruction of the herniated stomach. Eructation and postprandial pain in the lower chest are typical symptoms. If untreated, the herniated stomach may ulcerate, bleed, or strangulate.

The diagnosis often is unsuspected in a patient with nonspecific complaints. Chest radiography shows a gas-fluid level in the mediastinum, and esophagram establishes the diagnosis.

Unlike sliding hiatal hernia, paraesophageal hiatal hernia should be repaired surgically in nearly every instance.

3. Columnar-lined (Barrett's) esophagus is epithelial metaplasia caused by reflux esophagitis. It may be patchy or confluent, and it extends a variable distance from the gastroesophageal junction. Endoscopy and biopsy make the diagnosis. Esophageal ulcer or stricture nearly always reflects the presence of Barrett's epithelium. Treatment is the same as for simple reflux esophagitis. Adenocarcinoma of the esophagus develops in a small percentage of cases (perhaps 1%-2% instead of the 10% reported earlier), and periodic endoscopic surveillance is recommended. Prophylactic esophagectomy is the subject of debate and is not widely practiced.

F. MOTILITY DISORDERS

1. Achalasia is a motility disorder in which primary peristalsis is deficient, and the gastroesophageal sphincter fails to relax with swallowing. The circular muscle of the distal esophagus is thickened, and the esophagus dilates progressively above this point. The ganglion cells of Auerbach's plexuses in the esophagus are absent in many of these patients, but the cause is unknown.

a. Diagnosis

(1) *Symptoms and signs.* **Dysphagia** is the most common symptom. Pain is not prominent, and weight loss is not severe. Regurgitation and aspiration occur when the patient is recumbent. **Vigorous achalaisa** is a variant of this disease characterized by chest pain due to muscular esophageal spasms.

(2) *Radiographs.* Esophagrams show dilatation above a narrow distal esophagus. Barium does not empty readily into the stomach. Peristalsis is abnormal. In advanced cases, the esophagus is markedly dilated and tortuous ("sigmoid esophagus").

(3) *Special tests.* Esophagoscopy excludes organic obstruction; the instrument advances into the stomach with minimal force despite the narrowing. Motility studies reveal the following: peristalsis in the esophagus is uncoordinated, and primary peristalsis is absent; the gastroesophageal sphincter has above-normal resting pressure and does not relax completely when the patient swallows; bethanechol given subcutaneously causes strong contraction of the distal esophagus because it is autonomically denervated.

b. Differential diagnosis.

Carcinoma is excluded by esophagoscopy, biopsy, and cytology. Benign stricture from reflux esophagitis is not associated with as marked proximal dilatation, and peristalsis is normal in the body of the esophagus. Scleroderma is associated with gastroesophageal reflux in the early stages, but when esophagitis progresses to stricture, the radiographic findings resemble those of achalasia with a dilated body and narrow distal segment; scleroderma is distinguished by the persistence of peristalsis in the upper third of the esophagus and by the lack of response to bethanechol. Chagas' disease, caused by *Trypanosoma cruzi,* may destroy ganglion cells and produce a condition identical with achalasia. Diffuse spasm is discussed below. About 25% of patients with motility disorders are not readily classifiable as either achalasia or diffuse spasm and probably represent intermediate forms.

c. Complications. Progressive esophageal dilatation and repeated aspiration. Carcinoma occasionally is associated with achalasia, but the etiologic relationship has not been proved. Malnutrition is rarely marked.

d. Medical treatment. Patients with early achalasia, before the esophagus becomes tortuous, are often treated by pneumatic dilatation. A special balloon is positioned through the narrow distal segment and inflated sufficiently to partially disrupt the hypertrophied muscle.

e. Surgical treatment. Longitudinal esophageal myotomy (Heller procedure) is the surgical method of choice. It is usually performed through the left chest, but it can be accomplished through the abdomen. Thoracoscopic or laparoscopic procedures are performed in large centers. Gastroesophageal reflux is avoided by limiting the distal extent of the myotomy.

f. Prognosis. 85% of patients are relieved by one or more pneumatic dilatations; perforation occurs in about 5% of cases. Good to excellent results are obtained in 85% of surgically treated patients; incomplete myotomy and gastroesophageal reflux are the two chief sources of poor results.

2. Cricopharyngeal achalasia (upper esophageal sphincter dysfunction). In this condition, the cricopharyngeal sphincter does not relax completely, and dysphagia results. The diagnosis is made by esophagram, endoscopy, and motility studies. Treatment is by cricopharyngeal myotomy. Results of operation are excellent.

3. Diffuse esophageal spasm is associated with intermittent retrosternal pain and dysphagia. The esophagram shows segmental spasms that may take a "corkscrew" configuration. The esophagus is not dilated. Motility studies demonstrate disorganized peristalsis, usually involving only the lower half or third of the esophagus. There may be a response to bethanechol. A few patients progress to typical achalasia.

Patients may benefit from long-acting nitrates (e.g., Isordil). Pneumatic dilatation is successful in some patients. A long esophageal myotomy gives lasting relief in 90% of cases of diffuse spasm.

G. DIVERTICULA. Most esophageal diverticula are of the **pulsion** variety; they are protrusions of mucosa and submucosa through defects in the muscle layers. They are usually manifestations of abnormal motility. **Traction** diverticula are pulled out by healing of inflamed adjacent nodes.

1. Pharyngoesophageal (Zenker's) diverticulum. Pressures generated by swallowing may cause a diverticulum to form above the cricopharyngeal sphincter. The diverticulum arises posteriorly in the midline and projects laterally, usually to the left. Most patients are men over age 60 years.

Dysphagia, regurgitation of undigested food, and halitosis are typical symptoms. Esophagogram reveals the diverticulum and thus excludes other causes of cervical dysphagia.

Repeated aspiration pneumonitis is the most common complication. The diverticulum may ulcerate, perforate, or fistulize.

Excision of the diverticulum, with or without cricopharyngeal myotomy, is the treatment of choice. Results are excellent.

2. Epiphrenic diverticulum. Diverticula form in the distal esophagus in some patients with motility disorders, particularly diffuse esophageal spasm. Dysphagia, pain, and regurgitation are symptoms. The diagnosis is made by x-ray studies. The diverticulum may become inflamed, ulcerate, and bleed.

Surgical excision in combination with esophageal myotomy is successful in 80% or more of cases and is indicated for severe symptoms; minor symptoms do not warrant surgical intervention.

H. NEOPLASMS
1. Benign
a. Leiomyoma is the most common benign esophageal neoplasm. The tumor is intramural. Small leiomyomas are asymptomatic; larger ones cause dysphagia, and the mucosa may ulcerate and bleed. The radiographic appearance is distinctive: a smooth, rounded mass compressing the lumen. Symptomatic leiomyomas should be excised surgically.

b. Benign neoplasms may arise from other tissue elements: lipomas, fibromas, etc. These lesions also cause symptoms by compressing the lumen. Mucosal lesions can be excised endoscopically, but intramural tumors require a surgical approach.

c. Congenital cysts or reduplications are most common in the distal esophagus. They may require excision.

2. Malignant. Squamous cell carcinoma of the esophagus is most common in men 50-60 years of age. About 30% arise in the distal third of the esophagus, 50% in the middle third, and 20% in the upper third. They spread by lymphatics, vascular invasion, and direct extension.

a. Diagnosis

(1) *Symptoms and signs.* Progressive dysphagia is the typical symptom. Weight loss and anemia are present.

(2) *Radiographs.* Esophagram reveals an irregular mass narrowing the esophagus. Proximal dilatation is not marked. CT scan helps stage the disease.

(3) *Special tests.* Esophagoscopy with biopsy or brushings is diagnostic. Bronchoscopy is advisable for mid or upper esophageal lesions, because involvement of the tracheobronchial tree is common.

b. Differential diagnosis.

Benign strictures and neoplasms are distinguishable by radiographic and endoscopic studies, and most importantly by biopsy. Adenocarcinoma of the gastric cardia commonly involves the distal esophagus and is detected by biopsy.

c. Complications.

Obstruction of the esophagus is inevitable unless the patient dies earlier of some other complication. Extension of the lesion may lead to tracheoesophageal fistula or massive hemorrhage from major mediastinal vessels.

d. Treatment

(1) If the patient has a life expectancy of 6 months or more and is in good condition, resection is preferred for lesions in the distal or middle third (and perhaps the proximal third also). Resection provides palliation even in the presence of metastases because it maintains a swallowing mechanism. The esophagus is resected and the stomach is brought up into the chest or neck. Colon interposition is another option. Preoperative nutritional repletion may be needed.

(2) Radiation therapy may shrink bulky lesions and allow resection of otherwise inoperable tumor. Routine adjuvant radiation therapy has not proved beneficial. Combinations of radiation and chemotherapy may be advantageous, however.

(3) Many patients who have incurable tumors may be palliated by esophagectomy through the abdomen and the neck, without opening the chest. If the patient is in poor condition or clearly has an unresectable lesion, the goal of palliative treatment is maintenance of a patent esophagus. Endoscopic application of a laser (usually the Nd:YAG laser) is used to "core out" a lumen through obstructing esophageal cancer. An intraluminal plastic tube placed through the lesion by an endoscopic technic is a last resort because patients may sense the esophageal tube, and also it tends to occlude.

e. Prognosis. Only one-third to one-half of esophageal carcinomas are resectable when diagnosed. The operative mortality rate is 5%. The 5-year survival rate after curative resection is 20%. About 95% of patients, overall, die of the disease within 3 years.

IX. STOMACH AND DUODENUM

A. TRAUMA

1. Stomach. Penetrating injuries of the stomach are managed relatively easily by simple suture. Results are excellent.

2. Duodenum

a. Minor lacerations or perforations from blunt or penetrating trauma are treated by suture. Leakage from duodenal closures is fairly common.

b. Major lacerations and disruptions are sutured or resected. Duodenectomy and pancreatectomy are required for unusually extensive trauma.

B. PEPTIC ULCER. The combined effects of acid and peptic enzymes in gastric juice may produce ulceration of the gastric or duodenal mucosa.

Duodenal ulcer is most common in men 20-40 years of age. Gastric ulcer affects a group about 10 years older. The incidence of this disease declined until recently for unknown reasons; currently about 2% of adults in the United States have active peptic ulcers.

1. Cause

a. Duodenal ulcer. Patients with duodenal ulcer typically have increased gastric acid secretion, both basally and in response to stimulation. They have an increased parietal cell mass and a greater and more sustained drive to secrete acid. The fundamental cause of these abnormalities is unknown. About 95% of duodenal ulcers are located in the duodenal bulb.

b. Gastric ulcer. Patients with gastric ulcer fall into three groups. **Type I ulcers** occur in the absence of a history of duodenal ulcer and are located in the pyloric mucosa within 2 cm of the junction with the oxyntic gland area. 95% are on the lesser curvature. These patients have low or normal acid secretion. Damage to the antral mucosa by reflux of duodenal juice or other mechanisms is at least partially responsible for making the mucosa vulnerable to acid-peptic digestion. **Type II ulcers** are associated with duodenal ulcers. These patients are hypersecretors. The ulcers are prepyloric. **Type III ulcers** develop in the antrum and are caused by nonsteroidal antiinflammatory drugs.

2. Diagnosis

a. Symptoms and signs. Minor differences in the typical symptoms of gastric and duodenal ulcer are not reliable enough to allow a definite diagnosis based on history alone.

Pain in the epigastrium is relieved by food or antacids and often awakens the patient at night; paradoxically, some patients with ulcers have no pain at all. Nausea and vomiting are variable. Epigastric tenderness may be present. Symptoms tend to exacerbate and remit in cycles of a few months or a few years.

b. Laboratory tests. Anemia and occult blood in the stool may be noted. Serum calcium should be determined, because patients with hyperparathyroidism are prone to develop duodenal ulcer. Serum gastrin levels are normal in conventional peptic ulcer disease and elevated in Zollinger-Ellison syndrome. Gastric analysis is seldom helpful.

c. Radiographs. Barium study of stomach and duodenum may show a gastric or duodenal ulcer crater or deformity of the duodenal. Radiographs are about 90% reliable in diagnosing an active ulcer, and they have about the same degree of accuracy in distinguishing benign from malignant gastric ulcers.

d. Special tests. Gastroduodenoscopy is important for examination and biopsy of gastric ulcers to rule out malignancy. Duodenal ulcers do not require endoscopy unless the diagnosis is uncertain, the patient is bleeding, or the ulcer is recurrent.

3. Differential diagnosis. Nearly any other abdominal disease can mimic peptic ulcer; cholelithiasis, reflux esophagitis, pancreatitis, and functional complaints are among the conditions to be considered. It is most important to differentiate gastric cancer from benign gastric ulcer.

4. Complications

a. Hemorrhage (see Section IV of this chapter).

b. Perforation. Ulceration completely through the gastric or duodenal wall results in perforation into the peritoneal cavity if the ulcer is anterior. Posterior gastric ulcers may perforate into the lesser sac; posterior duodenal ulcers may penetrate into the pancreas but do not, as a rule, perforate freely.

Perforation causes sudden, severe abdominal pain which rapidly becomes generalized as corrosive gastric juice spreads throughout the peritoneal cavity. Eventually, bacterial peritonitis is superimposed on initial chemical peritonitis.

Examination discloses a rigid abdomen in a patient who moves cautiously and breathes shallowly. Liver dullness may be absent, and bowel sounds are quiet. The patient may be in shock.

Leukocytosis, elevated amylase, and hemoconcentration are noted. Free abdominal air is present on upright or lateral decubitus radiographs in 80%-90% of patients. Contrast radiographs of the stomach and duodenum are helpful if the diagnosis is uncertain. Barium is more accurate than water-soluble contrast, and it has proved to be safe in this situation. Small perforations may seal quickly and therefore not be apparent on the upper GI series.

c. Pyloric obstruction. The pylorus may be obstructed by edema (potentially reversible) or fibrosis (irreversible). Vomiting of food containing no bile develops progressively. Examination may reveal a succussion splash. Metabolic alkalosis and dehydration are present.

A saline load test helps determine the completeness of obstruction; 700 ml of saline are instilled through the nasogastric tube, the tube is plugged, and the residual volume is aspirated 30 minutes later; a residual of more than 350 ml is diagnostic of obstruction. Radiographs are definitive.

5. Medical treatment is preferred for uncomplicated peptic ulcer; operation is performed for complications or intractability.

a. Diet, drugs, and habits. Smoking, alcohol, and xanthines (coffee, tea, cola beverages, chocolate) should be avoided, as should all known or suspected ulcerogenic drugs (corticosteroids, reserpine, salicylates). Diet otherwise need not be restricted. "Bland" diets offer no advantage over ordinary foods.

b. Drug therapy. Five categories of drug therapy are in wide use in the United States for peptic ulcer disease.

(1) *H_2-receptor antagonists.* Cimetidine (300 mg orally, after meals and at bedtime), ranitidine (150 mg orally, twice a day), and famotidine (5-10 mg twice a day) are effective inhibitors of acid secretion. Relapse is common after cessation of therapy, but it can be prevented in many patients by a bedtime dose of ranitidine (300 mg) or cimetidine (800 mg).

(2) *Antacids.* Antacids are given as a supplement to H_2 blockers if symptoms require them. The choice of antac-

ids depends upon taste, cost, the need to avoid exacerbation of associated diseases (e.g., by giving antacids rich in sodium to cardiac patients), side-effects (e.g., diarrhea), etc. One effective type of antacids is a combination of aluminum hydroxide and magnesium hydroxide. In general, antacids should be given 1 and 3 hours after each meal and at bedtime. Liquids are preferable to tablets.

(3) *Sucralfate.* This polymer compound coats the ulcer and prevents access of acid and enzymes to the ulcer crater. Give 1 g, four times daily if the ulcer does not respond to other agents.

(4) *Bismuth compounds.* Colloidal bismuth subcitrate also coats the ulcer with a protective coagulum. Give 5 ml in 15 ml of water four times daily.

(5) *Proton pump blockers.* Omeprazole reduces acid secretion profoundly by inhibiting the proton pump in the parietal cell. Give 20 mg/day as a single dose.

6. Surgical treatment. Complications (hemorrhage, perforation, and obstruction) are indications for operation. Intractability is difficult to define and is a highly subjective indication for operation in patients with duodenal ulcer. Gastric ulcers that do not heal in 2-3 months may require surgery because of intractability and/or the possibility that the ulcer is malignant.

Several technics are currently used for surgical treatment of peptic ulcer (see below for Zollinger-Ellison syndrome).

a. Vagotomy. There are three types of vagotomy: Truncal vagotomy with a drainage procedure (pyloroplasty or gastrojejunostomy). Selective (gastric) vagotomy with a drainage procedure. Proximal gastric (parietal cell, highly selective) vagotomy, usually without a drainage procedure. Laparoscopic methods of vagotomy are undergoing tests.

b. Vagotomy and antrectomy, with gastroduodenostomy (Billroth I) or gastrojejunostomy (Billroth II). Antrectomy is a 40%-50% distal gastrectomy.

c. Subtotal gastrectomy (Billroth I or II). "Subtotal" refers to 65%-75% resection of the distal stomach. It is rarely done as the initial procedure.

d. Antrectomy alone is useful for gastric ulcer.

Note: Operative mortality is lower after vagotomy than after gastric resection (antrectomy or subtotal). Recurrent ulcer is more frequent after vagotomy than after vagotomy and antrectomy or subtotal gastrectomy. The incidence of postoperative sequelae (see below) is lowest after proximal gastric vagotomy.

Ulcers may persist or recur at the same or new sites because of (a) Inadequate operation—this may reflect a technical or anatomic problem (e.g., incomplete vagotomy), or more often, it means simply that the operation did not lower acid secretion enough to control the individual patient's ulcer diathesis. (b) Retained (excluded) antrum, a very rare problem. (c) Inadequate drainage of the stomach. (d) Loss of alkaline fluid to neutralize acid at the anastomosis. (e) Zollinger-Ellison syndrome.

The so-called **postgastrectomy syndromes** are a heterogeneous group of unpleasant consequences of gastric surgery.

(1) *Dumping syndrome.* Cardiovascular symptoms (sweating, palpitations, desire to lie down) and intestinal symptoms (nausea, cramps, diarrhea) are noted postprandially. Dumping seems to be limited to operations which destroy or bypass the pylorus.

(2) *Diarrhea.* "Postvagotomy diarrhea" is probably the result of intestinal denervation and precipitous gastric emptying.

(3) *Alkaline gastritis.* Reflux of duodenal juices into the stomach produces gastritis, pain, and bilious vomiting in some patients after gastrectomy or a drainage procedure.

(4) *Malabsorption.* Steatorrhea occurs to a mild degree after gastrectomy. Blind loop syndrome (bacterial overgrowth in the afferent limb of a Billroth II reconstruction) may lead to severe malabsorption.

(5) *Anemia.* Iron deficiency or vitamin B_{12} deficiency may produce anemia after gastric surgery.

(6) *Others* include early satiety and vomiting of food.

7. Treatment of complications

a. Hemorrhage (see also Section IV). Emergency operation is required if bleeding peptic ulcer does not respond to ice-water lavage or endoscopic methods of treatment. Bleeding duodenal ulcer is usually treated by truncal vagotomy, pyloroplasty, and suture of the bleeding vessel in the ulcer crater. Proximal gastric vagotomy is preferred if the pylorus can be left intact. Gastric ulcer is managed in the same way or by gastrectomy (gastric ulcers should be biopsied).

b. Perforation. Operation is undertaken as soon as the patient is resuscitated. (a) Acute duodenal ulcers (less than 1-month history before perforation) can be treated by simple suture. This is the safest course also in patients who have severe associated diseases or who have bacterial peritonitis at the time of operation. (b) A definitive acid-reducing procedure (e.g., proximal gastric vagotomy with suture of the perforation) is favored in the majority of patients with a longer history of ulcer. About 75% of patients with perforated chronic duodenal ulcer have further ulcer problems after simple suture alone. (c) Gastric ulcers can be locally excised (to exclude cancer) and the defect sutured, or an antrectomy can be performed.

c. Pyloric obstruction is treated initially with nasogastric suction. Endoscopic balloon dilatation is often successful. If obstruction persists, vagotomy and drainage or antrectomy are suitable procedures.

C. ZOLLINGER-ELLISON SYNDROME is peptic ulcer disease caused by excessive production of gastrin by a pancreatic islet cell carcinoma (60%), solitary pancreatic adenoma (25%), microadenomatosis or hyperplasia (10%), or a duodenal adenoma (5%). The gastrin-producing tumor is called a gastrinoma, one of the **apudomas.** About 30% of patients have associated insulinomas and/or tumors of the parathyroids, pituitary, and adrenal cortex (MEN-I syndrome).

1. Diagnosis

a. Symptoms and signs of peptic ulcer. Diarrhea from massive outpouring of gastric acid. Complications (bleeding, perforation, obstruction). Recurrent ulcer after acid-reducing surgery.

b. Laboratory tests. Serum gastrin levels are elevated. Conditions such as pernicious anemia and gastric ulcer also cause high serum gastrin levels, but they are associated with acid hyposecretion in contrast to the hypersecretion of ZE syndrome. Borderline gastrin values are clarified by response to a secretin provocative test; a rise in serum gastrin of 150 pg/ml within 15 minutes after IV infusion of secretin (2 units/kg) indicates the presence of ZE syndrome.

Gastric analysis shows basal hypersecretion (>15 mEq H^+/hour in patients with an intact stomach, and little increase in acid secretion with stimulation by pentagastrin. The ratio of basal to maximal acid output (BAO/MAO) is >0.6 in most cases. Serum Ca^{++} is elevated in patients with hyperparathyroidism (a component of MEN-I).

c. Radiographs. Upper GI series demonstrates ulcer(s) in stomach, duodenum, and/or jejunum. Gastric folds are prominent, and liquid is present in stomach even in fasting patients. The duodenal and jejunal mucosa may be edematous.

CT may show the pancreatic tumor. False-negative and false-positive findings are frequent with angiography. Gastrin levels in blood obtained by transhepatic portal venous puncture may have localizing value.

2. Treatment

a. Medical. Antacids alone are inadequate. Cimetidine (300-600 mg orally, four times/day) or ranitidine (300-450 mg, four times/day) is effective in 85% of patients over the short term. Omeprazole (80-120 mg/day) is especially effective in controlling acid hypersecretion.

b. Surgical. Total gastrectomy is unnecessary because acid secretion can be controlled with medications. Surgical excision of the tumor(s) is the only curative treatment. The pancreas and duodenum are the likely sites. The surgical cure rate should be 60%-90% in the short term, and the long-term cure rate approaches 50%.

3. Prognosis. Patients with localized but unresectable gastrinoma have excellent survival if acid secretion is controlled. Patients with metastatic disease ultimately die of this disease.

D. STRESS ULCER. Acute ulceration of the stomach and/or the duodenum develops in some severely ill patients. Ulcers occurring in burned patients are termed **Curling's ulcers**. Other patients with stress ulcers have had extensive trauma or major surgical procedures, often complicated by shock and sepsis, and the ulceration results from a combination of mucosal ischemia and acid hypersecretion. Ulcers associated with CNS lesions (Cushing's ulcers) are related to elevated gastrin levels and are not included in the stress ulcer category. Gastritis induced by alcohol **(hemorrhagic alcoholic gastritis)** or salicylates is a related condition in which the gastric mucosa is damaged by the pharmacologic agent; these lesions should not be termed stress ulcers either.

1. Diagnosis. Hemorrhage is the most common mode of presentation. Perforation is the first manifestation in some cases. Diagnostic evaluation of upper GI hemorrhage is discussed in Section IV of this chapter.

2. Prevention. Antacids by constant instillation through a nasogastric tube are effective but cumbersome, and therefore H_2 blockers are used more often. Neither type of agent seems effective in septic patients. For unclear reasons, stress ulcers are much less common in recent years.

3. Treatment

a. Medical. (1) Gastric lavage with iced saline may stop the bleeding. (2) Cimetidine is ineffective in the presence of bleeding. (3) Selective abdominal angiography with infusion of a vasoconstricting agent (vasopressin or epinephrine) into the left gastric artery is worth a trial in critically ill patients.

b. Surgical. Operation is necessary if bleeding is not controlled medically. Vagotomy, pyloroplasty, and suture of bleeding sites carry a high risk of recurrent bleeding (40%). If the patient's condition allows it, vagotomy and subtotal gastrectomy are probably more effective. Total gastrectomy is indicated in rare instances.

4. Prognosis. Stress ulcer is a grave complication, and emphasis should be on prevention.

E. GASTRIC NEOPLASMS

1. Adenocarcinoma of the stomach is declining in frequency in western countries, but it remains a common disease in Japan and some European countries.

Cancer arises in the pyloric area in about two thirds of cases. Morphologically, gastric carcinoma may be ulcerating (25%), polypoid (25%), superficial spreading (15%), linitis plastica (10%), or so advanced that it cannot be classified into one of the other four groups (25%).

a. Diagnosis

(1) *Symptoms.* Vague postprandial discomfort. Anorexia and weight loss. Vomiting. Chronic bleeding (vomiting small amounts of blood; melena).

(2) *Signs.* Epigastric mass in 25%, hepatomegaly in 10%. Evidence of metastases: Virchow node in the neck, Blumer shelf on rectal examination, enlarged ovaries (Krukenberg tumors). Gross or occult blood in the stool in 50% of patients.

(3) *Laboratory tests.* Anemia is common (40%). Elevated CEA reflects large tumor bulk.

(4) *Radiographs.* Most gastric cancers are visible on upper GI series. Benign ulcers may be difficult to distinguish from malignant ones.

(5) *Special tests.* Gastroscopy with biopsy or brushings usually proves the diagnosis.

b. Differential diagnosis. Benign ulcers must be differentiated from malignant ulcers. Other gastric malignancies (lymphoma, leiomyosarcoma) are discussed below. Rarely, cancer arising in the pancreas or colon invades the stomach and mimics a primary gastric lesion.

c. Treatment

(1) *Surgical.* Resection of the stomach, omentum, and regional lymph nodes is performed for cure if there is no distant spread or unresectable local extension. About half of operated patients have resectable lesions, and 50% of these resections are classified as curative (all gross tumor removed). Subtotal gastrectomy is sufficient for distal tumors. Total gastrectomy is required if lesser resection does not encompass the tumor. Esophagogastrectomy is performed for tumors arising in the proximal stomach. Palliative resection is preferable to gastrojejunostomy for incurable distal cancers if it is feasible.

(2) *Chemotherapy.* Combination chemotherapy is reserved for unresectable or recurrent disease.

d. Prognosis.
The overall 5-year survival rate is about 13%. Resected cancers without lymph node metastases are cured in 50% of cases; with lymph node involvement, the survival rate after curative resection falls to about 35%.

2. Polyps. About 30% of adenomatous gastric polyps are malignant and cancer is found in some other part of the stomach in 20% of patients with adenomatous polyps. Hyperplastic polyps have no malignant implications; hyperplasia is the histologic pattern in 75% of patients. Achlorhydria is found in most patients with polyps. Anemia from chronic bleeding or from vitamin B_{12} deficiency may be noted. Gastric cytology should be obtained.

One or a few pedunculated polyps can be excised through an endoscope. A polyp >2 cm in diameter is an indication for laparotomy if endoscopic excision is unsuccessful. Partial gastrectomy should be done for multiple adenomatous polyps confined to one part of the stomach, and total gastrectomy is performed in rare instances of diffuse polyposis. Resection is unnecessary in asymptomatic patients with hyperplastic polyps.

3. Leiomyoma and leiomyosarcoma

a. Leiomyoma of the stomach may bleed and should be excised.

b. Leiomyosarcoma often ulcerates centrally and bleeds. These tumors may be very large. Gastrectomy is required. 5-year survival rate is 25%.

4. Lymphomas.
Symptoms of gastric lymphoma are the same as for adenocarcinoma. Half of gastric lymphomas are palpable in the epigastrium. Upper GI series, endoscopy, biopsy, and cytology should lead to the diagnosis. Treatment is by resection followed by radiation therapy and sometimes che-

motherapy. Prognosis is relatively good; about 50% of patients survive 5 years.

F. DUODENAL LESIONS

1. Diverticula. Acquired false diverticula of the duodenum are common. They usually occur on the medial wall of the duodenum near the ampulla of Vater. Most diverticula are asymptomatic. Bleeding, perforation, obstruction of the bile duct, and acute pancreatitis are rare complications. Diverticula should be excised if they cause one of these complications, but otherwise diverticula can be ignored.

2. Neoplasms

a. Benign. Gastrinomas, Brunner's gland adenomas, leiomyomas, carcinoids, and pancreatic rests may occur in the duodenum.

b. Malignant. Adenocarcinoma of the duodenum is rare. It may arise near the bile duct and cause obstructive jaundice. Malignancies arising in other tissue elements (e.g., leiomyosarcoma) are very rare.

3. Superior mesenteric artery syndrome. Compression of the third portion of the duodenum by the superior mesenteric artery may cause obstruction in patients who have lost a great deal of weight from illness or injury. Assuming the prone position after eating may allow the artery to fall away from the duodenum, and the condition improves as weight is gained.

X. SMALL INTESTINE (JEJUNUM AND ILEUM)*

A. TRAUMA. Penetrating injuries from knives and low-velocity missiles are simply sutured. High-velocity missiles and blunt trauma cause extensive damage to the bowel wall and the mesentery; these injuries require resection with end-to-end anastomosis.

B. FISTULAS. Most external fistulas of the small bowel are complications of surgical procedures.

1. Diagnosis

a. Symptoms and signs. Postoperative fever, abdominal pain. Leakage of intestinal contents through the abdomi-

---

*Obstruction is discussed in Section VI. Regional enteritis (Crohn's disease) is discussed in Section XI. Intestinal stomas are covered in Section XI. Ischemia is covered in Section VII.

nal incision. Persistent sepsis if abscess drainage is incomplete. Excoriation of the skin by intestinal juices. Fluid and electrolyte losses, most marked with proximal fistulas. Rapid weight loss.

b. Laboratory tests. Studies reflect the presence of sepsis and the degree of dehydration and malnutrition.

c. Radiographs. Plain abdominal films may show intestinal obstruction or suggest the presence of abscess. Contrast given orally, by enema, or through the fistula (fistulogram) delineates the anatomy, including location and number of fistulas, intrinsic bowel disease, associated abscesses, and obstruction of the bowel distal to the fistula. CT scans and sonograms are helpful also, especially to search for abscesses.

2. Complications. Death in the early stages is the result of hypovolemia and sepsis. Late death is due to sepsis or underlying disease.

3. Treatment. An orderly program should follow this sequence:

a. Fluids and electrolytes. In addition to the usual measures for resuscitation of profoundly depleted patients (Chapters 1 and 2), losses from the fistula should be collected and the volume and electrolyte content measured at least daily. H_2 blockers help reduce fluid output through proximal fistulas. Somatostatin analogue also may reduce fistula drainage.

b. Control of fistula drainage is necessary to minimize excoriation of the skin. Stoma appliances are useful. An interventional radiologist can place a catheter into the fistula and position it close to the intestinal opening to collect fistula drainage.

c. Treatment of sepsis. Abscesses should be sought and drained when discovered. Here too, a fistulogram may show the abscess and a catheter can be manipulated into it.

d. Nutrition. Oral intake should be avoided initially; a nasogastric tube may be required. Parenteral nutrition is begun when the patient is stable hemodynamically. If possible, alimentary feedings should be instituted later, orally or through the fistula; however, many patients never reach the stage of enteric feedings as long as the fistula remains.

e. Operation. About 30% of fistulas close spontaneously. Causes of failure to close include distal obstruction, neoplasm or foreign body at the fistula site, intrinsic bowel disease (e.g., Crohn's, radiation), extensive disruption of the bowel wall, and a short (less than 2 cm) fistula tract. Operation is required in these cases and usually consists of resection with anastomosis.

4. Prognosis. Eighty to ninety percent of patients survive. Sepsis and untreatable underlying disease (e.g., malignancy, radiation damage) are the chief causes of death.

C. BLIND LOOP SYNDROME (contaminated small bowel syndrome) is a form of malabsorption caused by bacterial proliferation in stagnant intestinal contents in a variety of situations, including blind (poorly emptying) loops. The syndrome consists of steatorrhea, diarrhea, macrocytic (vitamin B_{12} deficiency) anemia, hypocalcemia, and malnutrition.

Standard laboratory tests show high fecal fat content and abnormal absorption of orally administered vitamin B_{12} (Schilling test) and D-xylose. More than 10^6 bacteria/ml in upper intestinal aspirates is evidence of bacterial overgrowth in the region sampled. Several types of breath tests are available to help make the diagnosis of blind loop syndrome.

Oral broad-spectrum antibiotics improve the results of laboratory tests and relieve symptoms, at least temporarily. Surgical treatment of the underlying disorder is carried out in those patients with a correctable anatomic lesion.

D. SHORT BOWEL SYNDROME. Extensive resection of the small intestine produces a group of deficiencies from loss of absorptive surface. Severity of the syndrome depends on the length of gut removed, the site of resection, the underlying disease, and other factors. Loss of ileum is poorly tolerated because transport of bile salts, vitamin B_{12}, and cholesterol is limited to this area. If jejunum is resected there is decreased stimulation of pancreatic and biliary secretion because sites of cholecystokinin and secretin release are lost; this change may contribute to malabsorption of fat.

1. Clinical course and treatment

a. Stage I. Huge fluid and electrolyte losses from diarrhea require careful replacement therapy. No food should be given orally; IV feeding is required. H_2 blockers should be given IV. Codeine helps control the diarrhea. Somatostatin injections may be beneficial. This stage lasts from 1-3 months.

b. Stage II. Parenteral nutrition continues as isotonic fluids are begun orally after stool volume diminishes to 2500 ml/day. Hypertonic oral fluids exacerbate diarrhea and dilute defined formula diets may be helpful. Foods are added to the diet by trial and error; fat is poorly absorbed after ileal resection because the pool of bile salts shrinks, and less than 30 g of fat should be allowed each day. Milk is avoided because lactose deficiency is common in short bowel syndrome.

c. Stage III. Complete dependence on oral intake is expected eventually if the intestinal remnant is sufficiently long; 6 months to 2 years may be necessary for full adaptation. After ileal resection, patients need injections of vitamin B_{12} (1000 µg IM every 2-3 months) for life. Other vitamin deficiencies should be prevented. Enteric hyperoxaluria, causing urinary tract stones, is prevented by a low-oxalate, low-fat diet plus oral calcium or citrate. H_2 blockers should be given. Blind loop syndrome requires treatment if it appears. Surgical procedures such as reversed intestinal segments are seldom helpful. Patients who are unable to maintain nutrition orally are candidates for chronic parenteral nutrition on an outpatient basis.

E. BYPASS FOR OBESITY. Morbidly obese patients (those weighing more than 45 kg over the ideal) have been treated by jejunoileal bypass. This operation has been replaced almost entirely by gastric bypass, a reversible exclusion of most of the stomach, or partitioning (gastroplasty).

F. DIVERTICULA
  1. Meckel's diverticulum is a congenital anomaly due to persistence of the omphalomesenteric duct. It is a true diverticulum and is located within 100 cm of the ileocecal valve. About half of Meckel's diverticula contain heterotopic gastric, pancreatic, or other alimentary tissue. Only 4% become symptomatic, usually in childhood, and nearly always before age 30 years.

  a. Manifestations. Lower GI bleeding results from erosion by heterotopic gastric tissue in early childhood. Meckel's diverticulitis resembles appendicitis in its pathogenesis, symptoms, and signs; perforation is common. Intestinal obstruction is caused by intussusception, entrapment of bowel beneath a mesodiverticular band, or other mechanisms.

  b. Treatment. Demonstration of the diverticulum by x-rays or ^{99m}Tc sodium pertechnetate is unreliable. Laparotomy is performed to find and remove the diverticulum. About 6% of patients with symptomatic Meckel's diverticula die of the disease due to delayed recognition and treatment.

  2. Acquired diverticula are uncommon false diverticula, often found in the jejunum. Motility disorders may contribute to development of these lesions. They cause bleeding, diverticulitis, or blind loop syndrome. Barium radiographs demonstrate the diverticula which are treated by resection of involved segment.

G. RADIATION ENTEROPATHY. Radiation therapy for abdominal or pelvic malignancy injures the proliferating intestinal epithelium transiently. If large doses of radiation are given, the intestinal blood vessels are gradually obliterated and the intestine becomes ischemic. Symptoms may begin months to years after radiation and consist of obstruction due to stricture, bleeding from ulcerated mucosa, or necrosis with perforation and formation of abscesses and fistulas. Surgical treatment is required for these complications. The operative mortality rate is high (10%-15%); the long-term outlook depends upon the presence of residual malignancy and extent of the radiation injuries.

H. TUMORS. The jejunum and ileum give rise to 1%-5% of all tumors of the alimentary tract. Only 10% become symptomatic, and most of the symptomatic ones are malignant despite the fact that benign tumors outnumber malignant lesions by 10 to 1. Bleeding and obstruction are the usual symptoms.

1. Benign tumors include leiomyomas, lipomas, neurofibromas, to name a few. **Polyps** may be adenomatous or villous, but more often they are **hamartomas.** Hamartomas are multiple in 50% of cases, and 10% of these patients have a familial disorder. **Peutz-Jeghers** syndrome (intestinal polyposis and mucocutaneous pigmentation). These polyps have little malignant potential. Symptomatic polyps are removed by operation. Polyps occur in the small intestine in **Gardner's syndrome** also.

2. Malignant tumors

a. Adenocarcinoma is rare in the small bowel; it usually occurs in the jejunum, but in Crohn's disease it may be distal. Carcinoma is seldom diagnosed preoperatively and is fatal in the majority of patients.

b. Lymphoma arises in the terminal ileum and causes obstruction, fever, and malabsorption. Segmental resection is the preferred treatment.

c. Leiomyosarcoma ulcerates centrally and bleeds.

d. Carcinoid tumor of the ileum grows slowly, but 80% of tumors greater than 2 cm in diameter have metastasized at the time of operation. **Carcinoid syndrome** (cutaneous flushing diarrhea, bronchoconstriction, and right-sided cardiac valvular disease) is due to vasoactive substances released by hepatic metastases or by primary ovarian or bronchial carcinoids; it may be the first symptom. Urinary levels of 5-hydroxyindoleacetic acid are elevated in some patients if serotonin is one of the substances released. Primary small bowel carcinoids are resected; hepatic metastases are treated medically. The 5-year survival rate is 70% for small bowel carcinoids; only 20% of those with liver metastases live 5 years.

e. Metastases to the small bowel occur in malignant melanoma, breast cancer, and others. Occasionally operation is needed to relieve symptoms of obstruction or bleeding.

XI. LARGE INTESTINE*

A. GENERAL PRINCIPLES

1. Diagnostic evaluation. In addition to a complete history and thorough physical examination, including digital rectal examination, anoscopy and proctosigmoidoscopy are required in nearly all patients. Colonoscopy is the direct study of choice in many conditions. Testing of stool for occult blood and ova, parasites, and enteric pathogens is necessary in some situations. Plain abdominal radiographs, barium enema radiographs, CT, MRI, ultrasonography, and mesenteric angiography are used selectively.

2. Preoperative preparation

a. Bowel preparation. Elective operations on the large intestine require mechanical evacuation of feces. Antibiotic suppression of fecal bacteria is also recommended. The regimen must be modified if the colon is obstructed or if the patient has inflammatory bowel disease.

(1) *Mechanical preparation.* (a) Clear liquid diet all day on the day before operation. (b) Metoclopramide 10 mg orally at 4 PM. (c) Polyethylene glycol-sodium sulfate solution (Golytely or Colyte) chilled, beginning 20 minutes after the dose of metoclopramide. The patient should drink one glass every 10 minutes if possible until 4-6 L are consumed. If the patient is unable to tolerate this solution, instill it through a nasogastric tube or use the alternative preparation. (d) The *alternative preparation* is one bottle (7 oz) of magnesium citrate at 3 PM **and** tapwater enemas until clear in the early evening.

---

*Obstruction is covered in Section VI. Ischemia is covered in Section VII. Bleeding is covered in Section V. Anorectum is covered in Section XII.

(2) *Antibiotic preparation.* (a) Neomycin 1 g and erythromycin base 1 g, both to be given at 2 PM, 6 PM, and 11 PM.

b. Patients may require IV fluids to avoid dehydration.

c. Systemic antibiotic prophylaxis is used by many surgeons instead of, or in addition to, the oral antibiotics listed here.

d. After induction of anesthesia, a Foley catheter is inserted. Some surgeons do not use a nasogastric tube at all, but others use a tube to evacuate gas that enters the stomach during induction of anesthesia.

3. Postoperative care
a. Nasogastric tube (if any) is removed on the first postoperative day.

b. Oral fluids and then food are begun when flatus is passed per rectum or intestinal stoma, usually 2-5 days after operation. Laxatives and enemas are contraindicated if a colonic anastomosis has been done.

4. Complications
a. Important complications to look for are wound infection, intraabdominal abscess, and anastomotic leakage.

b. Anastomotic leakage (dehiscence) is suggested when a previously afebrile patient suddenly develops a high fever, abdominal pain and tenderness. CT or water-soluble contrast enema radiograph is obtained to confirm the diagnosis. Systemic antibiotics are sufficient treatment for small localized leaks; operation to exteriorize the anastomosis or divert the fecal stream is necessary for large leaks associated with diffuse or generalized peritonitis.

B. TRAUMA
1. Preoperative preparation.
IV antibiotics are begun preoperatively when colonic injury is suspected.

2. Operation.
Surgical treatment depends upon the portion of bowel injured, size of colonic wound, associated damage to the mesocolon, fecal contamination, shock, and other injuries. These principles generally apply:

a. Right colon. Small perforations are sutured primarily. Large wounds require right colectomy with immediate anastomosis or with ileostomy and a delayed anastomosis.

b. Left colon. Small wounds are sutured primarily if conditions are ideal, but often they are sutured and exteriorized or just exteriorized as a colostomy. Large injuries are resected and the ends of the bowel fashioned as a colostomy and a mucous fistula; anastomosis is done later.

c. Intraperitoneal rectum. Diverting sigmoid colostomy and suture of the perforation are the treatment of choice. Intraoperative irrigation of the rectum to cleanse it of feces is controversial. The colostomy is taken down a few weeks later.

d. Extraperitoneal rectum. See Anorectum (Section XII below).

C. CARCINOMA. Adenocarcinoma of the colon or rectum is the most common visceral malignancy that affects both sexes in western countries. Other large bowel malignancies comprise no more than 5% of the total. Adenocarcinoma reaches a peak incidence between the ages of 60 and 75 years. These tumors spread by direct extension, hematogenous metastases, lymphatic metastases to regional nodes, gravitational metastases (seeding from tumor on the serosal surface), and perineural invasion. Multiple synchronous cancers occur in 5% of patients.

1. Diagnosis

a. Symptoms depend upon location and the size of tumor and the presence of complications. Cancer of the colon or rectum remains asymptomatic for a long period. Routine screening procedures are methods of detecting asymptomatic cancers. Current recommendations include digital rectal examination annually after age 40 years, guaiac slide test for fecal occult blood annually after age 50 years, and sigmoidoscopy at age 50 and 51 years, then every 3-5 years. The presence of risk factors for cancer indicate the need for earlier and more intensive screening.

(1) *Right colon.* Fatiguability and weakness due to chronic anemia, vague abdominal discomfort, and weight loss.

(2) *Left colon.* Change in bowel habits (alternating constipation and diarrhea), colicky abdominal pain, and gross blood and/or mucus in stool.

(3) *Rectum.* Blood and mucus in the stool, change in bowel habits, and tenesmus (painful urgent desire to evacuate the rectum).

b. Signs. The tumor may be palpable abdominally; this is more often true in cancer of the right colon. Occult or gross blood in the stool. Digital rectal and flexible sigmoidoscopic examination reveal only two thirds of cancers of the large bowel; biopsy should be obtained. Metastases to supraclavicular and groin nodes, umbilicus, and liver should be noted.

c. Laboratory tests. Iron deficiency anemia is common, especially with right-sided lesions. Liver function tests (e.g., elevated alkaline phosphatase) may suggest that hepatic metastases are present. CEA is elevated in large tumors but is normal in more than half of patients with tumors confined to the bowel wall. A baseline value should be obtained.

d. Colonoscopy. Fiberoptic colonoscopy is performed to confirm the diagnosis in patients with proximal lesions not reached by sigmoidoscopy and to detect synchronous polyps and cancers. If a distal lesion is so obstructive that the instrument will not pass, colonoscopy should be done a few weeks after operation to clear the colon of unsuspected neoplasms.

e. Radiographs. Air-contrast barium enema is unnecessary if the lesion is seen on colonoscopy. Chest x-ray should be obtained. Abdominal and pelvic CT and/or MRI are obtained selectively to search for metastases. Endorectal ultrasound helps stage rectal cancer.

2. Differential diagnosis. Symptoms may be mistakenly attributed to benign GI disorders, functional problems, primary hematologic diseases, or benign anorectal conditions. Diverticular disease, Crohn's colitis, amebiasis, and ischemic colitis are ruled out by colonoscopic biopsy of the cancer.

3. Complications

a. Obstruction is most common in the left colon because the lumen is smaller in that location. Treatment is discussed in Section VI.

b. Perforation can occur into the general peritoneal cavity, or it can form a localized abscess or fistula. Treatment is by resection.

c. Bleeding from cancer is rarely massive.

d. Spread to adjacent organs (bladder, small bowel, uterus, vagina, prostate, spleen, pancreas, and so on) is treated by removing the involved organ or a part of it whenever possible.

4. Treatment

a. Cancer of the **colon** is resected together with the regional lymphatic drainage of the affected part. Primary anastomosis is usually done. Distant metastases do not contraindicate resection of the primary tumor for palliation. Postoperative adjuvant chemotherapy is recommended for Stage II or III cancers.

b. Cancer of the **rectum** is resected with primary anastomosis if possible; for lesions situated very low in the rectum, abdominoperineal resection with permanent colostomy is standard. Postoperative radiation therapy is recommended for most resectable patients. Selected small cancers, especially polypoid ones, can be treated by local excision or radiation therapy. Fulguration and/or radiation is used for distal lesions in patients who represent prohibitive surgical risk or who refuse standard therapy.

5. Prognosis. The operative mortality rate is 2%-6%. Five-year survival rates after resection depend on the stage of the lesion. The TNM system has replaced the older Dukes' system (see Figure 5-2 p. 260).

Stage I (limited to bowel wall): 80%.

Stage II (through the entire wall): 60%.

Stage III (lymph nodes positive): 30%.

Stage IV (distant metastases or unresectable local spread): 5%.

Long-term follow-up is essential to detect recurrent and metachronous lesions. Sigmoidoscopy, examination of stool for occult blood, colonoscopy, serial CEA values, and sometimes barium enema are obtained. Details of the follow-up program vary widely. If the CEA level is normal after curative resection, a sustained rise subsequently is presumptive evidence of recurrence.

D. POLYPS are lesions that project into the lumen. Epithelial polyps are classified into four types: **neoplastic** (adenoma or carcinoma); **hamartoma** (juvenile polyp or Peutz-Jeghers polyp); **inflammatory** (inflammatory polyp or benign lymphoid polyp); and **hyperplastic.** There are three types of adenomas: tubular adenoma (adenomatous polyp), tubulovillous adenoma (villoglandular adenoma), and villous adenoma (villous papilloma). Lipomas, leiomyomas, and carcinoids are nonepithelial polypoid lesions. About 5% of tubular adenomas, 15% of tubulovillous adenomas, and 30% of villous adenomas become malignant. The majority of adenocarcinomas of large bowel are believed to evolve from an adenoma. Epithelial polyps should be removed in order to make a histologic diagnosis, relieve symptoms, and prevent transformation into cancer.

1. Diagnosis

a. Symptoms. Many polyps are asymptomatic. Rectal bleeding is the most common symptom; bleeding is rarely massive. Altered bowel habits, mucus in the stool, and tenesmus are noted in some patients with large polyps, especially in the rectum.

b. Signs. Colonic polyps are not evident on physical examination; polyps in the lower rectum are palpable. Villous adenoma in rectum is a soft, velvety mass. Sigmoidoscopy reveals many of these lesions; if a polyp is found in the rectum, there is a 50% chance of another polyp elsewhere in the large bowel.

Stigmata of familial polyposis syndromes may be present (see below).

c. Radiographs. Barium enema or pneumocolon shows about 80% of polyps, including most of the large ones.

d. Special tests. Colonoscopy is the most accurate method of detecting polyps, and it should be performed in every patient with a neoplastic polyp found anywhere in the colon or rectum.

2. Differential diagnosis. Artifacts on the barium enema include bits of stool and air bubbles. Colonoscopy resolves these questions.

3. Treatment. If a polyp is found during sigmoidoscopy, it should not be removed because of the explosion hazard in an incompletely prepared colon. This lesion—and any others—can be excised during the required colonoscopy.

Tiny lesions are excised or destroyed. Pedunculated polyps are excised at colonoscopy. If invasive cancer is found in a specimen, resection of that segment generally is not necessary if the margins are clear grossly and histologically, the tumor is well-differentiated, and there is no vascular or lymphatic invasion.

Large sessile lesions in the rectum are excised surgically through the anus in most cases. Radical operation is required only for invasive cancer. Large sessile lesions in the colon may be excised colonoscopically or resected surgically. Multiple colonic polyps may be an indication for resection of all or part of the colon.

4. Prognosis. Villous adenomas recur in about 15% of patients, and new polyps may develop. Patients should be followed with colonoscopy every 2-3 years.

5. Familial polyposis syndromes

a. Familial adenomatous polyposis is an autosomal dominant generalized tissue growth disorder. Multiple adenomatous polyps are scattered throughout the colon and rectum. **Gardner's syndrome** is familial adenomatous polyposis with expression of other abnormalities including desmoid tumors, osteomas of the skull or mandible, sebaceous cysts, medulloblastoma, thyroid cancer, periampullary neoplasms, and others.

Colorectal cancer develops before age 40 years in nearly all untreated patients. Colectomy and ileorectal anastomosis is the preferred treatment if the rectum has very few polyps. If the rectum is carpeted with lesions, ileoanal anastomosis is performed instead. Perhaps 12% of patients eventually develop periampullary malignancy. Desmoid tumors are difficult to treat; progesterone, tamoxifen, sulindac, and prednisone are successful in some cases.

b. Peutz-Jeghers syndrome consists of mucocutaneous pigmentation of the lips, gums, and axillae, and polyps throughout the GI tract. The polyps are hamartomas and have a low malignant potential.

E. DIVERTICULAR DISEASE. True diverticula of the colon (containing all layers of the bowel wall) are rare; false diverticula are acquired herniations of mucosa and submucosa through the muscular coats. The prevalence increases from 10% at age 40 years to 65% at age 80 years. In some people, diverticula result from high pressures in the colon, perhaps as a consequence of firm, tenacious stools in response to a fiber-deficient diet. In other people, however, weakness of the colonic wall is a more important factor than high pressure. Diverticula are present in the sigmoid colon in 95% of those affected, with or without involvement of the more proximal colon.

1. Diverticulosis refers to the presence of diverticula.

a. Diagnosis

(1) *Symptoms and signs.* Most patients with diverticulosis due to weakness of the colonic wall are asymptomatic. Some patients with the high-pressure or hypermotility type of diverticular disease develop cramping lower abdominal pain and constipation, diarrhea, or both; these symptoms are caused by contractions of the thickened muscle, and the diverticula themselves are merely coincidental. A mildly tender tubular structure (sigmoid colon) is sometimes palpable in the left lower quadrant in patients with pain. There are no systemic symptoms or signs of infection.

(2) *Radiographs.* Barium enema shows diverticula. In patients with pain, radiographs may reveal segmental spasm which gives a "sawtooth" appearance to the colon.

b. Differential diagnosis. Diverticulosis with pain may be difficult to distinguish from diverticulitis. The absence of systemic signs of infection (fever, leukocytosis), and the relatively rapid subsidence of pain, exclude diverticulitis in most cases.

c. Complications. Diverticula bleed (see Section V) or perforate (see Diverticulitis, below) in 15%-40% of patients.

d. Treatment. Asymptomatic patients require no treatment. Patients with painful diverticular disease without diverticulitis may benefit from a high-bulk diet. Unprocessed bran (10-25 g/day added to food) is the least expensive way to increase fiber in the diet, but commercial bulk agents may be more convenient.

Surgical treatment is not indicated in the absence of complications.

2. Diverticulitis is more accurately termed "peridiverticulitis"; it results from perforation of a diverticulum which causes infection in the adjacent tissue, or, occasionally, in the entire peritoneal cavity. The sigmoid colon is nearly always the site of perforation. Microperforation results in localized inflammation, and macroperforation contaminates a wider area.

a. Diagnosis

(1) *Symptoms and signs.* Mild to severe, steady, aching or cramping pain develops abruptly in the left lower quadrant. Constipation, diarrhea, abdominal distention, nausea, and vomiting depend upon the extent and severity of the inflammation. Dysuria is noted if inflammation is adjacent to the bladder. Physical examination shows fever, abdominal distention, tenderness, and sometimes a mass in the left lower quadrant. Tenderness on rectal examination and gross or occult blood in the stools are common. Sigmoidoscopy shows erythema, edema, spasm, and angulation at the rectosigmoid. Perforation into the free peritoneal cavity produces symptoms and signs of generalized peritonitis. In some patients, the acute attack is insidious and patients first seek medical care for a complication such as colovesical fistula or large bowel obstruction.

(2) *Laboratory test.* Leukocytosis.

(3) *Radiographs.* Plain abdominal films may show ileus, colonic obstruction, or abdominal mass; free air is present rarely. CT may be very helpful in showing inflamed colon and inflammation or abscess adjacent to it; CT is the preferred initial study. Water-soluble contrast enema radiographs may be obtained if CT is nondiagnostic. If the colon contains no diverticula, it is difficult to sustain a diagnosis of diverticulitis, and some other acute condition (see below) should be entertained. Barium enema

should not be obtained because of the risk of precipitating barium peritonitis.

b. Differential diagnosis. Many other acute abdominal diseases can produce the same picture; appendicitis, colonic ischemia, Crohn's disease, and perforated carcinoma are the most difficult to distinguish. Colonoscopy may differentiate these diseases in the chronic phase, but it is not likely to help in an acutely ill patient.

c. Complications

(1) *Abscess* may form in the colonic wall, in the mesocolon, or in the paracolic tissues.

(2) *Fistula* results from erosion of an abscess into a hollow viscus such as the bladder, vagina, or small bowel. Colovesical fistula causes dysuria, fecaluria, and pneumaturia (passage of gas in the urine).

(3) *Colonic obstruction* is usually partial.

(4) *Massive bleeding* rarely is a complication of diverticulitis; bleeding diverticula usually have not perforated.

d. Medical treatment. Acutely ill patients should be hospitalized. Nothing is allowed by mouth; nasogastric suction is instituted if the abdomen is distended. IV fluid and electrolyte therapy is important. Broad-spectrum antibiotics are given IV.

e. Surgical treatment. Operation is performed immediately if the patient has free perforation with generalized fecal peritonitis or if an abscess ruptures later and causes purulent peritonitis. Resection or exteriorization of the perforated segment (without anastomosis) is the usual procedure.

Patients who fail to improve on expectant management of contained perforations are candidates for more aggressive intervention. Percutaneous catheter drainage of abscesses under CT guidance is possible in many patients, and if so it is an excellent temporary solution to a serious dilemma. Good risk patients should have resection subsequently.

A deep abscess that is not accessible to catheter drainage in a patient who does not improve on IV antibiotics requires resection of the diseased segment. Primary anastomosis may not be possible, and instead a temporary end colostomy is established and the distal stump is oversewn (Hartmann). Anastomosis is carried out 3 months later. Therefore, this is a two-stage approach. The old three-stage operation involving transverse colostomy is seldom indicated today. A one-stage resection with primary anastomosis is preferred in the presence of colovesical fistula and in elective operations for resolved diverticulitis.

f. Prognosis. The mortality rate for the first attack of diverticulitis is 5%. About 25% of hospitalized patients require operation for the first attack. Elective interval resection of the sigmoid colon, after the first attack subsides, is indicated in young patients (under age 50) or if the symptoms persist or recur. Recurrent diverticulitis after colonic resection is rare; recurrence after medical therapy is about 30%.

F. INFLAMMATORY DISEASE OF THE BOWEL. Ulcerative colitis and Crohn's disease (regional enteritis, granulomatous colitis) are idiopathic inflammatory diseases that affect the small bowel, large intestine, or both. About 10% of patients have features of both diseases (indeterminate colitis). Comparison of the two diseases is shown in Table 12-2. Antibiotic-associated colitis is another entity described below, and ischemic colitis is discussed in Section VII.

1. Ulcerative colitis
a. Diagnosis
(1) *Symptoms and signs.* (a) Onset between 15 and 30 years of age usually; it can appear earlier or later. (b) Onset may be fulminating or insidious. Typical symptoms are frequent watery stools mixed with pus, blood, and mucus. Rectal urgency and tenesmus are common. Cramping abdominal pain, vomiting, fever, weight loss, and dehydration are variable. (c) Abdominal distention and tenderness in serious cases. Superficial anal fissures and gritty rectal mucosa on rectal examination; blood, pus, or mucus are seen on the examining finger. (d) Sigmoidoscopy is essential; enemas are not given beforehand. The rectum is involved in nearly all cases and in some the disease is limited to the rectum (ulcerative proctitis). The rectal mucosa is granular, dull, erythematous, and friable (bleeds when wiped with a swab). The submucosal vascular pattern is obliterated. Gross large ulcers are rare. Mucosal involvement is confluent.

(2) *Laboratory tests.* Anemia and leukocytosis are typical. Severe illness results in derangements of fluid and electrolyte balance, hypoalbuminemia, etc.

(3) *Colonoscopy.* Colonoscopy should be done cautiously or not at all in fulminating disease. It is helpful in chronic disease to investigate strictures, carry out surveillance for cancer, assess extent of involvement, or determine re-

Table 12-2. Comparison of ulcerative colitis and Crohn's disease

	Ulcerative colitis	Crohn's disease
Symptoms and signs		
Diarrhea	Severe	Less severe
Rectal bleeding	Typical	Uncommon
Anal lesions	Occasional	Frequent, complex
X-ray findings		
	Colon only	Colon and/or small bowel
	Confluent, concentric	Skip areas, eccentric
	Serrations, pseudopolyps	Longitudinal ulcers, "cobblestoning"
	Internal fistulas very rare	Internal fistulas common
Complications		
Toxic dilatation	3%-10%	2%-5%
Carcinoma	Greatly increased incidence	Increased incidence
Systemic	Common	Common
Massive hemorrhage	Uncommon	Rare

Morphology		
Gross	Confluent	Skip areas
	Rectum involved	Rectum often spared
	Thin mesentery	Thickened mesentery
	Diffuse superficial ulceration	Deep longitudinal ulcers or transverse fissures
Microscopic	Bowel wall thin	Bowel wall greatly thickened
	Pseudopolyps common	Pseudopolyps uncommon
	Inflammation limited to mucosa and submucosa	Transmural inflammation with submucosal fibrosis
	Crypt abscesses common	Crypt abscesses uncommon
	Granulomas rare	Granulomas frequent
Prognosis	Exacerbations, remissions	Indolent, progressive
	Good response to medical treatment	Poor response to medical treatment
	Seldom recurs after proctocolectomy with ileostomy	Often recurs after resection of involved bowel

sponse to treatment. Occasionally, it makes the initial diagnosis when other tests fail.

(4) *Radiographs.* Barium enema is not required in most patients. It should not be performed in acutely ill patients and should not be preceded by vigorous catharsis. In acute colitis, the mucosa is serrated. In chronic disease, haustrations are effaced and the colon is shortened and narrowed. Pseudopolyposis reflects severe ulceration. Strictures raise the suspicion of malignancy.

b. Differential diagnosis. Crohn's disease (see Table 12-2). Bacillary infections (e.g., those caused by *Salmonella, Shigella, Campylobacter, Chlamydia,* or gonococcus) and parasitic diseases (amebiasis, schistosomiasis) are excluded by bacterial culture, serologic tests, and examination of stools for ova and parasites. Ischemic colitis has a segmental distribution.

c. Complications

(1) Systemic or *extracolonic manifestations* occur as part of the disease. They include hepatobiliary lesions (steatosis, pericholangitis, gallstones, bile duct carcinoma); skin and mucous membrane lesions (erythema nodosum, pyoderma gangrenosum, aphthous stomatitis); bone and joint lesions (arthralgia, arthritis, ankylosing spondylitis); uveitis; delayed growth and maturation in children.

(2) *Acute colonic dilatation* (toxic megacolon) occurs in 3%-5% of cases. Patients are seriously ill (toxic), and plain abdominal films show dilatation of the transverse colon to greater than 6 cm in diameter.

(3) *Perforation* occurs with or without preceding acute dilatation and is often lethal. The appearance of this complication is masked by corticosteroids.

(4) *Massive hemorrhage* is rare.

(5) *Carcinoma* of the colon has a greatly increased incidence after the disease has been present for 10 years or longer.

d. Medical management

(1) *Mild attacks* often respond to outpatient management, including reduced physical activity, milk-free diet, and oral sulfonamides (sulfasalazine [Azulfidine] 2-8 g/day). If response is not prompt, topical hydrocortisone should be administered as a retention enema at bedtime (60 ml saline containing 100 mg of hydrocortisone or hydrocortisone acetate rectal foam). 5-ASA enemas are also effective.

(2) *Severe attacks* require hospitalization. Nothing is given by mouth, and nasogastric suction may be needed. Careful attention to fluid and electrolyte balance (especially hypokalemia) is essential; transfusions may be necessary. IV broad-spectrum antibiotics are given. Corticosteroids are administered IV as hydrocortisone (100-300 mg/day) or prednisolone (20-80 mg/day). Parenteral nutrition is required if the disease does not respond promptly.

Oral food and medications (corticosteroids and antibacterials) are resumed as symptoms subside.

(3) *Maintenance* on sulfasalazine (2 g/day orally) reduces relapse rates. Oral forms of 5-ASA (e.g., mesalamine) are under study. Topical hydrocortisone (by enema) or oral prednisone (20-40 mg/day) may be helpful; long-term maintenance on high-dose steroids causes complications and should be avoided. Azathioprine and 6-mercaptopurine are advocated in some situations. Cyclosporine has been used recently.

e. Surgical treatment

(1) Emergency colectomy is required for severe attacks or complications (hemorrhage, toxic dilatation) that do not respond promptly to medical management.

(2) Elective operation is indicated for chronic symptoms, frequent exacerbations, or prevention or treatment of cancer in long-standing disease. The preferred operation in most cases is total colectomy and ileoanal anastomosis with an ileal reservoir (restorative proctocolectomy, ileal pouch–anal anastomosis). Complete excision of the distal rectal mucosa is accomplished by mucosal stripping transanally or by deep dissection from the pelvic side to ensure that this goal is met. A temporary ileostomy is sometimes used to protect the anastomosis for 2-3 months. The outcome is four to six stools per day on average; sepsis is the most serious complication. **Pouchitis,** inflammation of the ileal reservoir from bacterial overgrowth, occurs to some extent in about 20% of patients but is treatable with antibiotics in the majority. Total proctocolectomy is removal of the entire colon, rectum, and anus; a permanent end ileostomy or continent ileostomy (see below) is required. Today this operation is reserved for patients who do not qualify for the ileoanal procedure because of advanced age or associated diseases.

f. Prognosis. The mortality rate is 1% during the year after onset of colitis; nearly all of these deaths occur in the course of a fulminating attack. Approximately 15% undergo colectomy at some time. Mortality rate is <1% for elective operations and 2%-3% for emergency colectomy. Impotence occurs in <5% of men after proctectomy; most of those affected are over 50 years of age.

2. Crohn's disease
a. Diagnosis
(1) *Symptoms and signs.* (a) The peak incidence is between 15 and 20 years of age. (b) Continuous or episodic diarrhea occurs in 90% of patients. (c) Blood in stools is unusual if only the small bowel is diseased; bleeding is more common with colonic involvement. (d) Postprandial cramping midabdominal pain, weight loss, fever, and anemia. (e) Large and complex anal lesions (abscess, fistula, fissure) may precede the appearance of intestinal symptoms. (f) A mass is palpable in the right lower quadrant in some patients. (g) Sigmoidoscopy shows a normal rectum in 50% of cases. Mucosal disease is patchy, with gross irregular ulcerations separated by edematous or even normal-appearing mucosa.

(2) *Radiographs.* The involvement is limited to the distal small bowel in 25%, large bowel in 30%, and both distal ileum and colon in 45%. Barium enema and small bowel contrast studies are required. Small bowel enema or enteroclysis shows mucosal detail. Thickened, strictured bowel wall with deep, undermining longitudinal ulcers, transverse fissures which look like spicules, and cobblestoning are characteristic. **Skip lesions** with normal intervening bowel, abscesses, and internal fistulas are important findings.

b. Differential diagnosis. Ulcerative colitis (see Table 12-2), *Chlamydia trachomatis* infections, tuberculous enteritis, lymphoma, diverticulitis, and intestinal ischemia need to be differentiated.

c. Complications. Extraintestinal manifestations are the same as in ulcerative colitis. Acute colonic dilatation can occur. Abscesses and internal fistulas are present routinely. Carcinoma of the colon or small bowel is associated with chronic Crohn's disease.

d. Medical treatment. Initial treatment in most cases is medical, and the regimen is similar to that for ulcerative colitis. Total parenteral nutrition is a useful adjunct. Metronidazole may be effective for anorectal Crohn's disease.

e. Surgical treatment. Operation is required for complications of the disease. Involved intestine is resected or strictured areas in the small bowel are widened (stricturoplasty), especially if there are multiple skip lesions. The rectum can be preserved in many cases.

f. Prognosis. Crohn's disease is an indolent disease which responds to medical therapy less well than does ulcerative colitis. Recurrence rate after surgical resection with anastomosis is 50%-75% at 15 years; it is lower after proctocolectomy with ileostomy.

3. Antibiotic-associated colitis is a spectrum of abnormal colonic responses to antibiotic therapy. The mildest form is diarrhea without gross mucosal abnormality; obvious inflammation of the mucosa is seen in a more severe stage of the disease, and at the most extreme, there are whitish-green or yellow plaques on the inflamed mucosa (**pseudomembranous colitis**). Antibiotic-associated colitis involves just the colon, and the small bowel is spared. Pseudomembranous colitis is caused by *Clostridium difficile,* which may be cultured from stool; a cytotoxin is detectable in feces also. Sigmoidoscopy or colonoscopy reveals a characteristic appearance.

The offending antibiotic should be discontinued. In mild cases, colitis resolves in 1-2 weeks, but severe symptoms require active treatment. Oral cholestyramine (4 g orally every 6 hours for 5 days) is useful. Metronidazole (1.5-2 g/day for 7-14 days) is effective. Vancomycin (125-500 mg orally four times daily for 7-10 days) is expensive and usually unnecessary. Antidiarrheal drugs may prolong the symptoms and should not be used. Pseudomembranous colitis, if untreated, may lead to colonic dilatation, or even colonic perforation; surgical intervention is required for these complications. Mortality rates up to 20% have been reported in complicated cases.

G. INTESTINAL STOMAS are temporary or permanent openings of the bowel onto the surface of the abdomen. Ileostomy and colostomy are the most common types.

1. Ileostomy. Permanent end ileostomy is required when proctocolectomy is performed for familial polyposis or inflammatory bowel disease. It is usually placed in the right lower quadrant and projects about 3 cm above the skin level to permit adherence of an appliance. **Loop ileostomy** is constructed for temporary fecal diversion; an opening is made in the side of an exteriorized loop. Small amounts of liquid and gas are expelled from an ileostomy intermittently, and the appliance must be worn constantly. Patients lead normal lives in every other way. Problems and complications include the following:

a. Dehydration and electrolyte depletion if the patient does not take sufficient salt and water to replace the fixed losses that are a consequence of removing the colon. Ileostomates should take fluids in large quantities and should salt their food liberally. They should not get into a position (e.g., hiking in the desert) where water is unavailable. Viral gastroenteritis, with vomiting and large losses through ileostomy, requires aggressive treatment, even hospitalization in some cases.

b. Ileostomy dysfunction is profuse watery discharge from the ileostomy due to obstruction. A minor surgical procedure to release the subcutaneous cicatrix may be necessary.

c. Stenosis due to circumferential scarring should be revised.

d. Retraction of the stoma causes leakage beneath the appliance.

e. Prolapse is usually preventable by good operative technic.

f. Periileostomy fistula results from an ill-fitting appliance or recurrent inflammatory disease.

g. Skin irritation is common and is due to leakage and soiling of the skin. An enterostomal therapist may treat this and other stoma problems.

h. Odor is minimal with modern appliances.

i. Uric acid urinary tract calculi may result from chronic dehydration.

2. Continent ileostomy (Kock pouch) is a technic in which a reservoir is constructed within the abdomen and a valve is made of intestine to prevent leakage from the reservoir. Gas and fluid are emptied by inserting a catheter into the stoma several times a day; an appliance is unnecessary. Failure of the valve mechanism requires surgical revision. Ileitis due to bacterial overgrowth (pouchitis) may require antibiotic therapy.

3. Colostomy. Temporary colostomies are made to decompress the colon and/or divert the fecal stream; permanent colostomy is required when the rectum is removed, usually for carcinoma. The permanent type is an **end colostomy** and is made by bringing the end of the colon out to the skin. A temporary colostomy may be an end colostomy or a **loop colostomy**.

A permanent sigmoid colostomy expels stool once or twice a day. An appliance is not required, but many patients wear a light plastic pouch for reassurance. Many surgeons instruct patients to irrigate end-colostomies by carefully inserting a lubricated catheter with a conical tip and instilling water, 500 ml at a time, by gravity flow from a reservoir held at shoulder height. Irrigations should not begin until at least 1 week after operation. Most patients are able to eat the same foods they enjoyed before. Colostomies do not require dilatation.

Many of the same complications occur with colostomy as with ileostomy, e.g., stenosis and prolapse. Paracolostomy hernia is common in these generally elderly patients with weak tissues.

XII. ANORECTUM*

A. EXAMINATION. The following sequence should be followed in the physical examination of patients with anorectal complaints. Occasionally, a step may be deferred (e.g., if a painful lesion is present), but all maneuvers should be completed eventually.

1. Preparation

a. Rapport is important; the examiner must describe the expected sensations before they appear.

b. The inverted (knee-chest, prone jackknife) position requires a special examining table; the left lateral decubitus (Sims') position is also satisfactory.

c. Good lighting, an assistant, and conveniently arranged instruments are essential.

2. Inspection

a. The buttocks are retracted with the fingers of both hands, and the perineum is inspected.

b. Anal orifice is gently everted by lateral retraction on each side of the anus.

3. Palpation

a. The perineal and perianal tissues are gently palpated to search for a mass, induration, or tenderness.

---

*Pilonidal sinus and hidradenitis suppurativa are discussed in Chapter 4.

b. The lubricated index finger is placed at the anal orifice and gently inserted, and digital examination of the anorectum is accomplished.

4. Anoscopy

a. A tubular metal or plastic anoscope (proctoscope) is lubricated and gently inserted, aiming toward the umbilicus. After the sphincteric ring is passed, the tip of the instrument is directed posteriorly to negotiate the anorectal angle.

b. Obturator is removed and lower rectum and anal canal are inspected.

5. Sigmoidoscopy

a. Rigid sigmoidoscopy is performed with a rigid metal or plastic instrument 25 cm long. It can be done with or without laxatives or enemas.

  (1) The instrument is lubricated and inserted, changing the direction after the sphincters are passed as with anoscopy.
  (2) The obturator is removed and the instrument is advanced, following the lumen under direct vision.
  (3) At the rectosigmoid junction, about 12-15 cm from the anal verge, the lumen bends sharply forward and to the left. Anterior pressure with the tip of the instrument usually straightens this turn, and the sigmoid colon is entered.
  (4) The bowel is examined by sweeping the tip circumferentially as the instrument is withdrawn. Care must be taken to flatten out the rectal valves, two on the left and one on the right, because lesions may be hidden above them.

b. Flexible sigmoidoscopy uses an instrument 60 cm long. The diagnostic yield is two to three times that of rigid sigmoidoscopy and complication rate is low. Flexible sigmoidoscopy is preferred for screening examinations in asymptomatic patients or in patients with suspected distal colonic lesions.

B. TRAUMA. Perforation of the intraperitoneal rectum is managed as described in the section on Large Intestine. Perforating injuries of the extraperitoneal rectum caused by sharp trauma are diagnosed by anoscopy and sigmoidoscopy. Blood is present in the lumen, and the perforation can be seen in most cases. If there is doubt, a water-soluble contrast medium can be instilled and radiographs obtained. Look for injury of associated structures, especially urinary tract.

Patients should be placed on IV broad-spectrum antibiotics. Operative treatment consists of diverting sigmoid colostomy; irrigation of the rectum to cleanse it of feces; and drainage of the area of perforation, usually by presacral sump drains. No attempt should be made to suture perforations. The colostomy is taken down after the rectal wound heals. Wounds that disrupt the sphincters extensively are managed in the same way, deferring definitive repair until conditions improve. Sphincters can be repaired primarily if injury is not severe.

C. HEMORRHOIDS, or piles, are enlarged vascular cushions in the lower rectum and anal canal. They are not simply varicose veins. **Internal hemorrhoids** arise above the pectinate line; **external hemorrhoids** arise below the pectinate line. Many patients have **mixed** (interno-external) hemorrhoids.

1. Diagnosis
a. Symptoms
(1) *Bleeding* with defecation is a cardinal symptom. Typically, bright red blood is noted on toilet tissue, stool, or in the water of the toilet bowl. Blood may drip from anus for a few moments after defecation.

(2) *Prolapse* of a mass with defecation is the second cardinal symptom. The mass slips back spontaneously after defecation at first, but later it must be reduced manually, and eventually it may become irreducible.

(3) *Mucoid discharge* is noted by some patients with prolapsing hemorrhoids.

(4) Difficulty with hygiene is common when there are large external components.

(5) Pain is not a symptom of internal hemorrhoids, except when they prolapse and thrombose. Pain is nearly always due to another associated condition.

b. Signs
(1) External hemorrhoids are visible beneath the perianal skin or anoderm.

(2) Internal hemorrhoids are found by inspection if they prolapse. The three primary locations of internal hemorrhoids are left lateral, right anterior, and right posterior.

(3) Internal hemorrhoids usually are not palpable in the anal canal. Anoscopy is required to diagnose nonprolapsing internal hemorrhoids.

2. Differential diagnosis.
Other causes of rectal bleeding (e.g., carcinoma) are ruled out by colonoscopy or flexible sigmoidoscopy. Other prolapsing lesions and other causes of anorectal symptoms should be apparent on examination.

3. Complications.
Anemia from chronic bleeding is uncommon and acute massive hemorrhage is rare. Prolapsed hem-

orrhoids may thrombose, become inflamed, and cause severe pain.

4. Treatment. Methods of treatment and the purpose of each method are listed in Table 12-3 and are discussed here.

a. Reduce downward pressure. A high-residue diet minimizes straining at stool. Patients should avoid sitting on toilet for prolonged periods. Prolapse should be reduced. Topical ointments and suppositories have little value.

b. Fixation of cushions

(1) *Injection* of sclerosing solutions (e.g., 5% phenol in oil) into the submucosal tissue at the upper pole of each hemorrhoid is effective for small bleeding internal hemorrhoids.

(2) *Ligation* with rubber bands using a special instrument causes slough of the hemorrhoid and tethers the mucosa within the anal canal to prevent prolapse. Care must be taken to place bands in an insensitive area at least 0.5 cm above the pectinate line. Rare, fatal infections have been reported.

(3) *Photocoagulation and electrocoagulation* create heat and then scarring to hold the hemorrhoids within the anal canal.

(4) *Heater probe* is a small device at the tip of a probe that heats the tissue and achieves the desired result.

c. Reduce sphincter pressure. Sphincterotomy is not used much because high sphincter pressure is not believed responsible for hemorrhoid symptoms.

d. Excision of hemorrhoids is used mainly for large

Table 12-3. Treatment of internal hemorrhoids

Purpose	Method
1. Reduce downward pressure	Diet, bulk agents. Avoid prolonged sitting on toilet
2. Fixation of hemorrhoid cushions	Sclerosing injections. Rubber band ligations. Photocoagulation (infrared, laser). Electrocoagulation (bipolar, DC). Heater probe
3. Reduce sphincter pressure	Internal sphincterotomy
4. Excision of hemorrhoids	Hemorrhoidectomy

prolapsing hemorrhoids where the skin-covered external components are a source of difficulty.

e. Acutely prolapsed, inflamed, thrombosed hemorrhoids can be treated by bed rest, ice packs, analgesics, and bulk laxatives. If prolapsed tissues are still viable, effective immediate relief is easily provided by injection of bupivacaine 0.25% containing epinephrine and hyaluronidase (150 units in each 10 ml of anesthetic). This usually permits reduction of the prolapse. Emergency hemorrhoidectomy is required in some cases.

5. Prognosis. Most methods of treatment are successful in controlling bleeding, although repeated injections or ligations may be required at intervals over the years. Hemorrhoidectomy is more permanently effective, but has disadvantages of cost and time lost from work.

D. THROMBOSED EXTERNAL HEMORRHOID. An external hemorrhoid may thrombose acutely as a result of vigorous exercise, straining to defecate, or unknown causes. A severely painful mass appears suddenly at the anus; pain is aggravated by sitting, walking, and defecation, and it begins to subside in a few days. Bleeding is noted if the thrombosed hemorrhoid ulcerates and extrudes the clot.

On examination, one or more bluish, tender, spherical masses varying from a few mm to several cm in diameter are seen at the anal verge. Anoderm covers the upper portion of the mass, thus distinguishing it from a prolapsed internal hemorrhoid which has pink rectal mucosa on the upper portion.

These lesions subside spontaneously, but severe pain is relieved and recovery hastened by excising the mass under local anesthesia. Alternatively, the mass can be incised and the clot extracted from the thrombosed veins with a hemostat. The incision should not be sutured.

E. FISSURE. Anal fissure (fissure-in-ano) is a tear in the anoderm. More than 90% occur in the posterior midline; the remainder are in the anterior midline.

1. Diagnosis. Pain with defecation is the typical symptom. In some patients there is a second type of pain that begins an hour or so after defecation. A few spots of blood may be noted on the toilet tissue.

An **acute fissure** is visible as a tear in the anoderm when the anus is gently everted. **Chronic fissure** has the white transverse fibers of the internal sphincter exposed in its base. A **sentinal tag** or pile (a swollen tag of skin at the anal verge) and a **hypertrophied papilla** at the upper end of the fissure complete the triad of chronic fissure. Fissures located off the midline suggest that inflammatory bowel disease, carcinoma, venereal disease, or immunologic deficiency may underlie the problem.

2. Treatment

a. Acute fissures usually heal in 2-3 weeks with bulk laxatives, analgesics, and sitz baths. Topical application of silver nitrate may help.

b. Chronic fissures that do not respond to simple measures may be treated surgically. Lateral subcutaneous sphincterotomy is the method of choice. It can be performed under local or general anesthesia and is successful in more than 95% of patients.

F. ABSCESS. An abscess can develop in any of the tissue spaces adjacent to the anorectum. A typical anorectal abscess begins as infection in an anal crypt (cryptoglandular) which then spreads along tissue planes. Abscesses are named according to their location in the anatomic spaces, e.g., **perianal** (beneath the anoderm or perianal skin); **ischiorectal** (in the ischiorectal fossa); **intersphincteric** (between the internal and external sphincters); and others.

1. Diagnosis. Throbbing, constant pain made worse by sitting or walking is typical of superficial abscesses. Deeper abscesses may cause pain high in the rectum or in the lower abdomen. Fever is common.

An indurated, tender mass is visible and palpable externally or by digital rectal examination. Often, fluctuance cannot be appreciated in the mass although it is filled with pus.

2. Complications. Abscesses may extend along tissue planes to adjacent areas, e.g., scrotum or lower abdominal wall.

3. Treatment. There is no medical treatment for anorectal abscess, and antibiotics have little place in treatment of drainable abscesses in otherwise healthy patients. Prompt surgical drainage must be done when the diagnosis is made. It is incorrect to assume that a mass contains no pus because it is not fluctuant; these lesions are ready to drain when first seen. Patients with immunologic deficiency or hematologic malignancy are exceptions.

Small abscesses may be drained under local anesthesia; large ones require a general anesthetic. Care must be taken to avoid cutting the sphincters; an incision parallel to the anus is safe in this regard.

4. Prognosis. About 66% of anorectal abscesses heal with formation of an anorectal fistula. Abscesses in immune-deficient patients can be lethal.

G. FISTULA. An anorectal fistula (fistula-in-ano) is a hollow tract filled with granulation tissue. It has an opening (primary or internal) inside the anal canal and one or more orifices (secondary or external) in the perianal skin. An anorectal **sinus** has only one opening and is blind at the other end.

Most fistulas begin with infection in a crypt as for anorectal abscesses, so most primary openings are at the pectinate line. Fistulas from Crohn's disease, carcinoma, and *Chlamydia* may be complex.

Secondary openings appearing anterior to a transverse line through the center of the anus arise from primary openings which are located radially in the anal canal. If the secondary orifice is posterior to this imaginary line, the primary opening is in the posterior midline. This useful guide is the Goodsall-Salmon rule. Anterior secondary openings >3 cm from the anal verge may be exceptions to the rule; they arise from the posterior midline.

Fistulas may be classified according to their relationship to the sphincters: *intersphincteric* (tract runs between internal and external), *transsphincteric* (tract passes through both internal and external), *suprasphincteric* (tract loops over the puborectalis), and *extrasphincteric* (tract arises from the rectum above the levators and bypasses the sphincters on its course to the skin of the perineum).

1. Diagnosis

a. Symptoms. There may be a history of abscess which drained spontaneously or was drained surgically. Drainage of pus, blood, mucus, and occasionally stool is the chief complaint; drainage is intermittent if the fistula seals and reopens.

b. Signs. Secondary openings are raised, reddish papules; a drop of pus can be expressed if the fistula is patent. The tract is palpated as an indurated cord extending toward the anus. Anoscopy reveals the primary opening, and a hooked probe can be inserted into it; probing the tract from the secondary orifice is helpful sometimes. The relationship of the fistula to the sphincters is important and should be assessed in the unanesthetized patient. Sigmoidoscopy is done to rule out other rectal diseases. Barium enema or colonoscopy is indicated in patients with unusual fistulas or a history suggesting inflammatory bowel disease.

2. Differential diagnosis. Hidradenitis suppurativa and pilonidal sinus (Chap. 4) are easily distinguished because there is no communication with anal canal in these conditions. Presacral teratoma may be difficult to differentiate.

3. Complications. Recurrent abscess, systemic infection, carcinoma.

4. Treatment. Surgical **fistulotomy** is the treatment of choice because established fistulas do not heal. All tracts must be identified and exposed. Great care must be taken to avoid division of the puborectalis muscle because incontinence invariably results; fortunately, suprasphincteric fistulas are rare. They require management by a specialist. Fistulotomy usually should not be performed in the presence of active Crohn's disease.

5. Prognosis. Recurrent fistula after surgical treatment is due to an overlooked primary opening, inadequate exposure of the tracts, failure to care for the wound to ensure healing from the base outward, or underlying intestinal disease.

H. DISORDERS OF THE PELVIC FLOOR are a group of conditions related to abnormal structure or function of the levators ani and the anal sphincters. Table 12-4 lists these conditions; the inclusion of some of them is debatable. Hemorrhoids are discussed above, and rectal prolapse is described below. The other conditions are not dealt with here.

I. RECTAL PROLAPSE (procidentia) is protrusion of the entire thickness of the rectum through the anus. It should be distinguished from partial or mucosal prolapse, which is protrusion of just the mucosa. Rectal prolapse is more common in women; it increases with age in women but not in men. Responsible factors include chronic straining to defecate and laxity of pelvic musculature from aging, neurologic disease, or

Table 12-4. Disorders of the pelvic floor

Solitary rectal ulcer syndrome	Descending perineum syndrome
Rectal prolapse	Anal fissure
Constipation (some types)	Chronic anal pain syndromes
Fecal incontinence	

trauma. Procidentia in children is related to growth and development.

1. Diagnosis

a. Symptoms. A mass protrudes from anus during defecation. Initially it reduces spontaneously, but eventually it protrudes with standing and is difficult to reduce. Blood and mucus from exposed mucosa are common. Partial or complete incontinence is typical in adults with chronic prolapse.

b. Signs. Examine the patient in the squatting position and in the prone-jackknife or lateral decubitus position.

Mucosal prolapse (partial prolapse) is a symmetrical protrusion 2-4 cm long with radial folds. Palpation between finger and thumb reveals two layers of mucosa. The sphincters often are lax. The anus is everted.

Procidentia (complete prolapse) is an asymmetrical projection up to 12 cm long with concentric folds. The lumen points posteriorly due to the presence of small bowel and omentum in a hernia sac on the anterior wall; this large mass of tissue anteriorly is palpable. The anal orifice may gape widely even with the prolapse reduced, and the patient may be unable to contract the sphincter muscles. There is a sulcus between the anus and the protruding rectum, and the anus is normally positioned.

2. Differential diagnosis.
Prolapsing hemorrhoids and polyps are easily differentiated.

3. Complications.
Chronic procidentia impairs the sphincters so that incontinence may be a problem even if the prolapse is repaired.

4. Treatment.
Prolapse in children is treated by correction of constipation, instruction not to strain, defecation in a recumbent position, and strapping the buttocks together between bowel movements.

Mucosal prolapse is treated by fixation of the sliding mucosa by submucosal injections of sclerosing solution (e.g., 5% phenol in oil). Excision of the prolapsing mucosa is also successful.

Procidentia in adults is treated by surgical repair. Resection of redundant sigmoid combined with posterior fixation of the rectum to the sacrum (proctopexy) is the most popular method. Transabdominal posterior proctopexy alone is used in some individuals who have no redundant sigmoid, no history of constipation, and no diverticulosis. Perineal proctosigmoidectomy (Delorme procedure) is an alternative in poor surgical candidates. Encircling the anus with a plastic suture, mesh, or band (Thiersch procedure) is reserved for aged or debilitated patients.

5. Prognosis. Prolapse in children usually is self-correcting. Partial prolapse in adults responds well to treatment. Surgical repair of complete prolapse is successful in most cases, but residual incontinence due to chronic stretching of the sphincters is difficult to treat, especially in elderly patients.

J. PRURITUS ANI. Itching of perianal skin is a symptom, not a diagnosis.

1. Causes

a. Anorectal diseases (fistulas, condylomata acuminata, neoplasms).

b. Dermatologic diseases (e.g., psoriasis, atopic eczema).

c. Contact dermatitis from ointments, deodorants, soaps, and so on.

d. Infections (fungal, bacterial).

e. Parasitic infestations (*Enterobius vermicularis,* scabies, lice).

f. Oral antibiotics, especially tetracyclines; the mechanism may be the frequent, loose, irritating stools resulting from oral antibiotics.

g. Systemic diseases (diabetes, liver disease).

h. Hygiene (Poor hygiene or vigorous rubbing and cleaning with irritant soaps.)

i. Warmth and moisture. Tight clothing, obesity, hot climate, exercise.

j. Dietary (alcoholic beverages, coffee, milk).

k. Psychogenic.

l. Idiopathic. Some patients probably have pruritus from seepage of irritant stools which have an alkaline pH and contain active digestive enzymes.

2. Diagnosis

a. Symptoms. Pruritus is worse at night regardless of cause; it may spread to involve the entire perineum and vulva or scrotum. Relationships of pruritus to foods (peppers, citrus fruits) and beverages (coffee, milk, alcohol) should be ascertained. Ask about bowel habits, hygienic practices, topical medications, oral antibiotics, types of clothing, pruritus elsewhere.

b. Signs. Perianal skin may be completely normal, or it may be erythematous, lichenified, moist, and macerated. Dermatologic disease (especially psoriasis) may be evident. Anorectal disease is sought by anoscopy.

c. Laboratory tests. Candidiasis is diagnosed by mixing scrapings with 10% KOH, warming the preparation, and examining it microscopically. Because fungi grow secondarily on moist surfaces, it is difficult to prove that fungi are the primary problem. Scabies and pediculosis are diagnosed by identifying the parasites or nits. *Enterobius* is identified by finding eggs on the perianal skin. The patient should place transparent adhesive tape against the skin on awakening in the morning and then affix the tape to a glass slide.

3. Treatment
a. Specific treatment is used for systemic, dermatologic, malignant, anorectal, fungal, or parasitic disease.

b. Nonspecific treatment
(1) Stop all current antibiotics and topical medications.
(2) Modify diet if certain foods or beverages are contributory.
(3) If stools are loose, prescribe a bulk agent (e.g., unprocessed bran) and discontinue all laxatives.
(4) Tight underclothing and heavy bedclothing should be avoided.
(5) Cleansing after defecation is best accomplished by moist cotton or cloth or commercially prepared wipes (e.g., Flings). Avoid the use of soap in the affected area.
(6) Apply a lubricating lotion such as Balneol.
(7) Nonmedicated talcum powder is used and a piece of cotton is placed against the anus to absorb moisture.
(8) Refractory patients benefit from 1% hydrocortisone cream applied sparingly four times daily.

4. Prognosis. Most patients respond to treatment, but a few seem resistant to all therapy.

K. SEXUALLY TRANSMITTED DISEASES
1. Condylomata acuminata are caused by HPV. They are found on the perianal skin of patients who have no anal sexual contact, but inoculation of the virus into the anal canal probably requires anal intercourse or instrumentation.

Condylomata are small warts initially but gradually enlarge to form confluent exophytic masses in some patients. Bleeding, pruritus, and difficulty with hygiene are the main symptoms. Anoscopy must be done to detect warts at or just above the pectinate line; these lesions are pink and velvety.

Small external warts can be painted with 25% podophyllin in tincture of benzoin, although results are often disappointing. Apply podophyllin only to the warts, and have the patient bathe within a few hours to avoid ulcerating normal skin. Condylomata are eradicated more effectively by excision or fulguration. Interferons are promising but unproved.

Recurrence, even after thorough treatment, is the rule, and patients must be followed closely for months after the last known sexual contact. There is an association between condylomata acuminata and subsequent epidermoid cancer of the anus.

2. Gonococcal proctitis. Rectal gonorrhea causes inflammation of the rectal mucosa, sparing the anoderm. Pain, diarrhea, bleeding, and purulent discharge are the symptoms. Anoscopy shows friable ulcerated mucosa, and thick pus often exudes from the crypts.

Obtain cultures to confirm the diagnosis. Cervical gonorrhea and syphilis must be investigated also.

a. Treatment
(1) Aqueous procaine penicillin G, 4.8 million units IM (2.4 million units in each buttock) 1 hour after probenecid 1 g orally.
(2) Alternative: Ampicillin 3.5 g orally and probenecid 1 g orally at the same time.
(3) **Never** treat gonorrhea with benzathine penicillin G.
(4) Penicillin-resistant gonorrhea requires treatment with drugs selected on the basis of sensitivity testing.

b. Follow-up. Get a rectal specimen for culture 7 days after completion of treatment.

3. Syphilis. Primary anorectal syphilis is an ulcer which resembles an anal fissure; the lesion heals in 3-4 weeks. Secondary lesions are multiple plaques with a wet odorous discharge. The diagnosis is made by darkfield examination and serologic tests.

Benzathine penicillin G is the drug of choice. For primary or secondary syphilis, give 1.2 million units IM in each buttock (total 2.4 million units). Erythromycin and tetracycline are alternative drugs.

4. *Chlamydia trachomatis* proctitis caused by LGV immunotypes resembles Crohn's disease clinically and endoscopically. Non-LGV immunotypes of *C. trachomatis* produce a milder inflammation that may be asymptomatic. The organisms are identified by culture. Tetracycline (2 g daily for 2-3 weeks) is effective treatment.

5. Other. *Campylobacter jejuni, Shigella, Salmonella, Yersinia,* herpes simplex, chancroid, granuloma inguinale, hepatitis, amebiasis, and HIV are among the organisms and diseases that are transmitted by anorectal sexual contact.

L. MALIGNANT TUMORS OF THE ANUS. Epidermoid carcinomas are the most common anal malignancies. Melanoma, mucinous adenocarcinoma, Bowen's disease, and Paget's disease are other malignant lesions that can arise in the anal canal or on the perianal skin. Invasive epidermoid cancer of the anus, carcinoma-in-situ, dysplasia, and condylomata acuminata are related diseases that can be caused by human papillomavirus. Male homosexuals, particularly those who are HIV-positive, have a high prevalence of one or more of these conditions.

Anal cancer is categorized as cancer of the anal margin (the anal verge and perianal skin) or cancer of the anal canal (involving the anoderm up to and including the dentate line and the transitional epithelium just proximal to that).

1. Diagnosis. Bleeding, pruritus, pain, drainage, and a mass are the usual symptoms that bring a patient to the physician complaining of hemorrhoids. The tumor is visible and/or palpable. Its size, location, and depth of invasion should be noted. Biopsy confirms the diagnosis.

Anal cancer can metastasize to lymph nodes in the groins as well as to the retrorectal nodes and by the hematogenous route to liver, lungs, and so on.

2. Treatment. Small lesions at the anal margin can be excised locally. Radiation therapy in combination with chemotherapy is the preferred treatment for larger tumors of the anal margin and all lesions in the anal canal. Inguinal metastases are treated by irradiation also. Persistence or recurrence may require abdominoperineal resection.

3. Prognosis. The 5-year survival rate is about 60% after treatment of epidermoid cancer.

XIII. APPENDIX

A. ACUTE APPENDICITIS is the most common abdominal surgical emergency in western countries. The incidence is highest in young adults, but any age may be affected. Appendicitis results from obstruction of the lumen by a fecalith, foreign body, tumor, or parasite. The mucosa secretes fluid behind the obstruction, the intraluminal pressure rises, the mucosa becomes hypoxic and ulcerates, and bacteria invade into the wall.

The appendix is viable and intact in **simple** appendicitis. **Gangrenous** appendicitis implies necrosis of the wall. **Perforated** appendicitis refers to gross disruption. Gangrene and perforation are likely to occur after 24-36 hours.

1. Diagnosis.

a. Symptoms

(1) Pain in the epigastrium, periumbilical area, generalized in the abdomen, or in the right lower quadrant is the first symptom. This pain is vague, mild to moderate in severity, and sometimes colicky. It subsides gradually after 4 hours, then **shifts** to the right lower quadrant where it is a steady, progressively severe ache made worse by movement.

(2) Anorexia, nausea, or vomiting follows start of pain by a few hours.

(3) Other symptoms include low-grade fever and constipation.

(4) Infants with appendicitis are lethargic, irritable and anorexic.

(5) In the elderly, symptoms are less marked than in younger adults.

b. Signs

(1) Localized tenderness in the right lower quadrant is the most important finding. Tenderness may be in the right flank if appendix is retrocecal. Tenderness to rectal or vaginal examination is detected in pelvic appendicitis. If appendix is bizarrely situated, tenderness is localized to other sites.

(2) Other signs include fever (<38° C), muscular rigidity, rebound tenderness, referred tenderness, and positive psoas and obturator signs. (See Acute Abdomen, Section II of this chapter.)

(3) Infants may require sedation; localized tenderness is present. In the elderly, tenderness may be deceptively mild. In pregnant women, tenderness is localized higher in the abdomen than usual.

c. Laboratory tests.
The leukocyte count averages between 10,000 and 16,000/mm^3 with a "shift to the left" (>75% neutrophils) in 75% of cases. Ninety-six percent have leukocytosis or an abnormal differential white cell count; the important corollary is that some patients with appendicitis have an entirely normal leukocyte profile. Urinalysis may show small numbers of erythrocytes or leukocytes.

d. Radiographic findings. No specific abnormalities on plain abdominal films. Ultrasonography is not as reliable as claimed initially.

e. Special tests. Laparoscopy is used increasingly to clinch the diagnosis, and today many appendectomies are performed laparoscopically too. The entire appendix must be seen in order to rule out appendicitis.

2. Differential diagnosis
a. Gastrointestinal diseases
(1) *Medical.* Gastroenteritis and mesenteric lymphadenitis usually occur in children or young adults. Nausea and vomiting precede abdominal pain; high fever, malaise, and other symptoms of viral illness are prominent. Pain and tenderness are poorly localized and vary during a period of observation.

(2) *Surgical.* Meckel's diverticulitis is rare; associated symptoms of bowel obstruction, vaguely localized pain, and tenderness near the umbilicus are hints to this diagnosis. Other surgical diseases include perforated peptic ulcer, cholecystitis, sigmoid diverticulitis, and so on.

b. Gynecologic diseases
(1) Acute salpingitis begins in the lower abdomen without the characteristic shift. High fever, diffuse bilateral lower abdominal tenderness, cervical tenderness, and vaginal discharge containing gram-negative intracellular diplococci are clues to the diagnosis.

(2) Mittelschmerz is pain caused by rupture of an ovarian follicle at the time of ovulation; sudden pain in the middle of the menstrual cycle, minimal GI symptoms, and spontaneous improvement are the rule.

(3) Ruptured ectopic pregnancy causes sudden pain, shock (if blood loss is massive), and diffuse pelvic tenderness. The enlarged tube may be palpable; culdocentesis returns bloody fluid.

(4) Twisted ovarian cyst causes sudden pain and simultaneous vomiting; the mass may not be palpable without an anesthetic.

c. Urinary tract disease
(1) Ureteral colic radiates into the groin; there is no muscular rigidity and little direct tenderness. The urine contains erythrocytes. IV urography makes the diagnosis.

(2) Acute pyelonephritis is associated with high fever, chills, and tenderness in the costovertebral angle. Pyuria, white cell casts, and gross bacteria are seen in the urine.

d. Systemic diseases include basilar pneumonia, diabetic ketoacidosis, acute porphyria, and tabetic crisis. In most cases, abdominal pain and tenderness are diffuse.

3. Complications

a. Perforation occurs in 20% of patients (80%-90% in infants and 40%-75% in patients >60 years of age). Increased pain, high fever, diffuse tenderness, and high leukocyte counts suggest that perforation has occurred.

b. Peritonitis, diffuse or generalized, is one consequence of perforation. Increasing pain, tenderness, distention, fever, and toxicity occur.

c. Appendiceal abscess is another result of perforation. A tender mass is palpable in the right lower quadrant or in the pelvis. The mass is a phlegmon initially, but it may progress to a cavity containing pus.

d. Pylephlebitis (septic thrombophlebitis of the portal vein) causes high fever, shaking, chills, and jaundice.

4. Treatment

a. Preoperative preparation

(1) If the diagnosis is uncertain, the patient should be observed and examination of the abdomen and pelvis repeated at intervals. Little is gained by prolonging observation beyond a few hours. Nothing is given by mouth; analgesics are withheld until a decision is reached if the patient is not in severe pain.

(2) Nasogastric tube is inserted if abdomen is distended or patient is toxic.

(3) IV fluid and electrolyte repletion often is not required in young adults with simple appendicitis. Infants, the elderly, and the severely ill must have deficits replaced before operation.

(4) IV antibiotics are administered for perforation or pylephlebitis.

(5) High fever, particularly in children, must be lowered before anesthesia is induced.

b. Operation

(1) Appendectomy is the only acceptable treatment for simple appendicitis or performed appendicitis with peritonitis if adequate facilities and personnel are available. If not, large doses of IV antibiotics should be given instead. If the team is skilled at laparoscopic surgery, that approach may be used for diagnosis and treatment.

(2) The appendix is removed. If the appendix has perforated freely, the abdomen is lavaged with saline or antibiotics. Drains are not used unless there is a well-defined abscess.

(3) Appendiceal abscess is treated with IV antibiotics and, in most cases, immediate operation.

c. Postoperative care

(1) *Simple appendicitis.* Ambulation is begun on the first day. Nasogastric suction is unnecessary. Antibiotics are not required. IV fluids are discontinued when oral fluids are begun (second or third day); diet is advanced rapidly. Strong cathartics and enemas are contraindicated. Patients leave hospital in 3-5 days and are back to full activity in 3 weeks.

(2) *Perforated appendicitis.* Treatment varies with severity of illness. Nasogastric suction, antibiotics for 5-7 days, and prolonged IV fluids are usually necessary. Critically ill patients require intensive care.

d. Complications.

Wound infection occurs in 10% or more of patients with perforated appendicitis if the skin incision is closed primarily. Abdominal abscesses, particularly in the pelvis or subphrenic space, result from perforation with peritonitis. Small bowel obstruction from adhesions may occur. Hepatic abscesses are consequences of pylephlebitis.

5. Prognosis. The mortality rate is 0%-0.3% in simple appendicitis and about 1% in perforated cases. Perforation causes death in up to 15% of elderly patients. Perforation (and death) result from delay by patient, physician, or surgeon. There is an inverse correlation between the rate of perforation and the rate of negative abdominal exploration. If appendicitis cannot be excluded, it is advisable to operate.

B. NEOPLASMS

1. Adenocarcinoma of the appendix is rare and seldom is diagnosed preoperatively. Right colectomy is required.

2. Carcinoid tumor is fairly common. If it does not involve the cecum or regional lymph nodes and is <2 cm in diameter, appendectomy is sufficient. Right colectomy is advisable for larger or metastatic tumors.

3. Mucocele of the appendix is a simple cyst in some cases, resulting from previous appendicitis. Other mucoceles are malignant, and if they perforate, pseudomyxoma peritonei may develop.

XIV. LIVER AND BILIARY TRACT

A. HEPATIC TRAUMA

1. Diagnosis. Blunt or penetrating trauma to the liver causes intraabdominal bleeding. Symptoms and signs depend upon the amount of blood loss; severe injuries produce hypovolemic shock. Occasionally, the liver is ruptured centrally with little or no bleeding into the abdomen; CT is useful in these cases. Fractured ribs on the right should raise the suspicion of hepatic injury.

2. Treatment. Patients with significant hepatic trauma should have laparotomy. A few carefully selected patients may be managed nonoperatively, at least initially.

a. Small lacerations or penetrating wounds may have stopped bleeding by the time operation is performed. These wounds require no treatment.

b. Actively bleeding wounds are explored and the bleeding points ligated or coagulated. Large sutures to approximate the edges of the liver are ill-advised because of the risk of creating a closed space in which bile collection, abscess, or hematoma can develop. Devitalized tissue should be debrided and external drainage provided.

c. The Pringle maneuver (occlusion of hepatic artery and portal vein in duodenohepatic ligament) is useful for temporary control in patients with massive hemorrhage. Pringle maneuver plus cannulation of the inferior vena cava through right atrial appendage is used to isolate the liver from its vascular supply temporarily to facilitate suture of lacerations of the hepatic veins.

d. Large stellate lacerations should be debrided and drained after bleeding is controlled.

e. Subcapsular hematomas should be opened and explored if there is concern about extensive disruption of hepatic parenchyma.

3. Prognosis. Overall mortality rate for hepatic injuries is 10% or more; most deaths follow blunt trauma. *Postoperative complications* include the following:

a. Recurrent bleeding requires operation.

b. Infection within the hepatic parenchyma and/or in the subphrenic or subhepatic spaces is common. External drainage is necessary.

c. Hemobilia is bleeding into the bile duct; the cause is inadequately treated hepatic parenchymal disruption. Patients have GI hemorrhage, often with biliary colic, jaundice, and fever. Treatment consists of surgically ligating or embolizing the artery that feeds the bleeding site; in some cases lobectomy is necessary.

B. HEPATIC NEOPLASMS

1. Primary malignant tumors. Primary malignant hepatic tumors are common in Africa and the Orient and uncommon in USA and Europe. Young children and older adults are affected. Cirrhosis predisposes to hepatic malignancy. Chronic hepatitis B is an important risk factor for hepatoma.

a. Types

(1) Hepatocellular carcinoma (hepatoma) comprises 80% of primary hepatic cancers. Metastases to extrahepatic lymph nodes, lung, and other sites occur early in the course. In children this type of tumor is also known as hepatoblastoma. Fibrolamellar hepatoma is an uncommon variety of hepatoma with a more favorable prognosis.

(2) Cholangiocellular carcinoma (cholangiocarcinoma) spreads throughout the liver and metastasizes early.

(3) Mixed cell type (hepatocholangioma).

b. Diagnosis

(1) *Symptoms.* Abdominal pain, anorexia, weight loss, fullness or distention, and jaundice (in some cases) are most common symptoms. Massive intraabdominal hemorrhage from rupture of the tumor may be the initial manifestation. Fever and severe pain, due to necrosis, may occur. Obstruction of hepatic veins produces Budd-Chiari syndrome.

(2) *Signs.* Hepatomegaly; bruit or friction rub over liver; ascites in 30%.

(3) *Laboratory tests.* Elevated serum alkaline phosphatase and/or serum bilirubin in 60%. Alpha-fetoprotein is elevated in the serum of 80% of patients with hepatomas. One half are positive for HBsAg.

(4) *Radiographs.* CT show the extent and location of tumor masses. MRI is used increasingly. Arteriography helps evaluate patients for surgery. Most hepatomas are supplied by hepatic artery and are demonstrated by this study.

(5) *Special tests.* Percutaneous needle biopsy is diagnostic if positive. Laparoscopy is used for staging and guided biopsy.

c. Differential diagnosis.
Primary hepatic malignancy must be differentiated from benign tumors, metastatic cancer, hepatic abscesses, and cysts.

d. Complications. Intraabdominal hemorrhage, Budd-Chiari syndrome, acute portal hypertension, and necrosis of the tumor.

e. Treatment. Resection rates vary from 15%-60%. Small lesions are excised locally, and larger ones are resected by lobectomy or trisegmentectomy if the procedure has a possibility of removing all of the gross tumor. Liver transplantation is used increasingly in some centers, sometimes preceded by chemoembolization. Chemoembolization is used alone in advanced hepatomas with no hope of surgical cure. Chemotherapeutic agents can be delivered into the hepatic artery as well.

f. Prognosis. Three-year survival after curative surgical resection is 30%; 5-year survival is 15%. Early results of transplantation are promising.

2. Metastatic malignant tumors. Cancers of the GI tract, lung, breast, ovary, uterus, and kidney commonly spread to the liver by hematogenous or lymphatic routes. More than 90% of patients with hepatic metastases have metastases elsewhere.

a. Diagnosis

(1) *Symptoms and signs.* Most patients have symptoms and signs of the primary tumor. Weakness, anorexia, and weight loss. Right upper quadrant abdominal discomfort. Ascites and/or jaundice in advanced cases. A large, irregular liver is palpable in about 60% of patients. A friction rub may be audible over the liver.

(2) *Laboratory tests.* Anemia is common. Elevated serum alkaline phosphatase and bilirubin. CEA is elevated in many patients with metastases from colon cancer.

(3) *Other tests.* CT scan is essential. Needle biopsy is diagnostic. Laparoscopy with biopsy is performed in some centers in patients with nondiagnostic studies. Angiography is helpful if operation is planned.

b. Treatment. Partial hepatectomy (varies from excision of the mass to formal lobectomy) is performed in highly selected patients with metastases confined to one lobe. This operation is most often done for metastatic cancer of the colon or rectum.

Intraarterial chemotherapy using a constant infusion pump gives a response rate of 30%-50% in patients with metastatic colon cancer.

c. Prognosis. Life expectancy depends upon the type of metastatic tumor. Cancer of the large bowel permits longer survival than other primary malignancies. Most patients are dead by 2 years after hepatic metastases are diagnosed, and many die within a few months.

3. Benign tumors

a. Adenomas. Hepatic adenomas occur mainly in young women, and oral contraceptives are believed to be an important etiologic factor. About one third of patients have multiple adenomas.

Hepatic adenomas are asymptomatic until they reach 10 cm in diameter or larger. Spontaneous rupture of these large tumors produces acute abdominal pain that mimics other acute upper abdominal diseases, or they can bleed massively into the peritoneal cavity. Asymptomatic lesions may be discovered during abdominal operations for other reasons.

CT and angiography are useful diagnostic tests unless the patient is bleeding massively.

These tumors have no malignant potential. If the lesion is small (<7 cm) and asymptomatic, oral contraceptives should be discontinued and the patient observed for regression of the tumor. Continued enlargement of the lesion requires more aggressive treatment. Large or symptomatic adenomas should be resected. Recurrence is rare.

b. Focal nodular hyperplasia is usually asymptomatic and does not become malignant. Hepatic scintiscan may not show a filling defect because the lesion contains normal numbers of Kupffer's cells. Arteriography reveals an extremely rich blood supply to the mass. Most lesions do not need to be excised.

c. Hemangiomas. Small hemangiomas are found beneath the liver capsule in many patients undergoing abdominal operation. These incidental lesions can be ignored; large lesions may rupture or cause symptoms and signs of an arteriovenous fistula and should be resected.

d. Cysts. Congenital solitary hepatic cysts are usually asymptomatic, but in some instances they cause pain or are palpable. Symptomatic cysts should be drained into the peritoneal cavity or into the intestine (Roux-en-Y). Congenital polycystic liver is associated with polycystic kidneys in one half of patients. No treatment is required in most cases, although symptoms caused by progressive enlargement may be relieved by operation. The laparoscopic approach works well for single or multiple simple cysts.

C. HEPATIC ABSCESS

1. Pyogenic (bacterial) abscess usually follows an acute abdominal infection (e.g., appendicitis, diverticulitis) in which the liver becomes infected via the portal vein. Abscesses may also develop from the biliary tract or by bacteremia from distant sites. In 10% of cases, a pyogenic abscess has no apparent underlying cause and is termed "cryptogenic."

a. Diagnosis

(1) *Symptoms and signs.* Fever, malaise, anorexia, toxicity, chills, jaundice, and right upper abdominal pain referred to the right shoulder. Large, tender liver.

(2) *Laboratory tests.* Leukocytosis, anemia, elevated alkaline phosphatase, elevated bilirubin (in some cases). Blood cultures may identify the responsible organism(s).

(3) *Radiographs.* Chest films show elevation of the right diaphragm and pleural effusion in 30% of patients. Abdominal films may show a gas-fluid level in the liver. Ultrasonography and CT reveal the size, number, and position of hepatic abscesses. Angiography is seldom required.

b. Differential diagnosis. Hepatic tumor is distinguishable from abscess because it is solid. Patients with vague complaints have various other diagnoses considered before the hepatic abscess is recognized.

Amebic abscess is very difficult to exclude, although a positive blood culture is strong presumptive evidence of pyogenic abscess (see below).

c. Complications. Persistent hepatic abscess may rupture, cause septic shock, bleed into the bile ducts, or progressively impair hepatic function.

d. Medical treatment. If amebic abscess is a possibility, antiamebic therapy should be given. IV antibiotics in large doses are required for pyogenic abscess. Percutaneous catheter placement under radiologic guidance is the preferred method of drainage for most hepatic abscesses.

e. Surgical treatment. If percutaneous methods fail, or if associated problems require operation anyway, open surgical drainage is performed.

f. Prognosis. Solitary abscess has an excellent prognosis if diagnosed and treated promptly. Multiple abscesses are a grave complication.

2. Amebic abscess appears in the absence of amebic dysentery in 80% of cases. The abscess is solitary and in the right lobe usually.

Fever, pain, and tenderness in the right upper quadrant are typical manifestations. Alkaline phosphatase is elevated; bilirubin is normal. Studies show a fluid-filled mass in the liver.

Treatment is medical. Metronidazole (Flagyl) 750 mg orally, three times daily for 10 days is preferred. It should be followed by diloxanide furoate (500 mg three times daily for 10 days) and chloroquine (500 mg daily for 2 weeks). Alternatively, dehydroemetine (1-1.5 mg/kg IM daily for 10 days) and chloroquine (500 mg orally twice daily for 2 days) plus diloxanide furoate (500 mg three times daily for 10 days). Percutaneous aspiration of large amebic abscess prevents rupture and speeds healing. Surgical drainage is rarely necessary.

3. Echinococcal cyst (hydatid disease). Echinococcosis of the liver produces a cyst which is manifested by pain, hepatomegaly, and (if the cyst has ruptured into the bile ducts) fever, jaundice, and biliary colic. Most cysts are solitary and in the right lobe. Surgical excision is the treatment of choice. Care must be taken to avoid spilling the contents into the peritoneal cavity.

D. PORTAL HYPERTENSION is present when the portal venous pressure equals or exceeds 20 cm water (15 mm Hg). Collateral channels dilate between portal and systemic venous circulations; the most important of these routes is at the gastroesophageal junction, leading to formation of **esophageal varices** which may rupture and bleed into the GI tract. Ascites, hepatic encephalopathy, and hypersplenism are other consequences of portal hypertension.

1. Causes. Increased portal blood flow (Banti's syndrome, certain types of splenomegaly) is rarely the cause of portal hypertension. Increased resistance to portal flow is much more often responsible; the site of high resistance may be at prehepatic, hepatic, or posthepatic levels.

a. Prehepatic (obstruction of the portal vein). Congenital atresia, thrombosis, or extrinsic compression.

b. Hepatic. Cirrhosis (e.g., alcoholic, biliary, hemochromatosis), congenital fibrosis, schistosomiasis, acute alcoholic hepatitis, or idiopathic.

c. Posthepatic. Budd-Chiari syndrome or constrictive pericarditis.

2. Cirrhosis and variceal hemorrhage. Cirrhosis is responsible for 85% of portal hypertension in the United States, and alcoholism is the most common cause of cirrhosis. About 40% of cirrhotic patients experience variceal hemorrhage eventually and 30% die of variceal hemorrhage or hepatic failure within a year after diagnosis is established. The first episode of variceal bleeding is fatal to 50%-80% of cirrhotic patients, and 66% of those who survive the first episode will bleed again with about the same risk of death from the recurrent episode as from the initial one. A portosystemic shunt aims to prevent variceal bleeding.

Prophylactic portosystemic shunt (shunt performed in a patient who has never bled from varices) does not improve long-term survival.

Therapeutic portosystemic shunt is performed in a patient who is bleeding (emergency shunt) or has bled from varices (elective shunt).

3. Acute variceal hemorrhage. Assessment and initial treatment of massive upper GI hemorrhage are discussed in Section VI of this chapter.

a. Diagnosis. History may disclose chronic alcoholism, acute alcoholic binge, known cirrhosis, previous episodes of bleeding, or ingestion of drugs (e.g., aspirin) that bear on the acute bleeding problem.

Physical examination may reveal stigmata of cirrhosis (spider angiomata, palmar erythema, testicular atrophy, gynecomastia, hepatomegaly) or portal hypertension (ascites, splenomegaly, venous collaterals radiating from the umbilicus). Jaundice is an important finding.

Liver function tests are usually deranged in acutely bleeding alcoholics, regardless of the source of bleeding.

One cannot assume that patients with varices are bleeding from that source, so **endoscopy** is essential to identify the bleeding site. Upper GI series should be done if the bleeding site is not found endoscopically.

b. Treatment. Specific measures for the treatment of variceal hemorrhage include injection sclerotherapy, vasopressin infusion, balloon tamponade, and emergency portosystemic shunt. In general, shunting is done only in patients who are uncontrolled by the other measures.

(1) *Vasopressin infusion.* Vasopressin constricts mesenteric arterioles and lowers portal venous pressure by about 25%. The drug is given into a peripheral vein at the rate of 0.4-0.6 units/minute for 1 hour, and the treatment can be repeated every 3 hours if needed.

(2) *Balloon tamponade.* A Sengstaken-Blakemore tube is a triple-lumen tube with a gastric balloon, an esophageal balloon, and a lumen for suction of gastric contents. Before placement, a nasogastric tube is tied to the

Sengstaken-Blakemore tube with its tip just proximal to the esophageal balloon to permit suction of esophageal secretions. The Minnesota tube is a different version; it contains 4 lumens with a tube for esophageal aspiration incorporated into it (Fig. 12-3).

(3) *Injection sclerotherapy.* Injection of sclerosing solutions into varices can be accomplished through a flexible esophagoscope. Bleeding is controlled in 80% of patients; reinjection may be necessary within a few days and again within 1-2 months. Sclerotherapy is recommended in the majority of patients who are bleeding from varices.

(4) *Transjugular intrahepatic portosystemic shunts (TIPS).* Portal decompression is achieved by percutaneously creating a channel between the hepatic vein and the portal vein by means of a catheter passed through the jugular vein. Safety and effectiveness are being evaluated. Currently it is most useful as a preliminary to liver transplantation (see Chapter 20).

(5) *Emergency portosystemic shunt.* Ligation of varices is seldom useful because bleeding recurs in most cases.

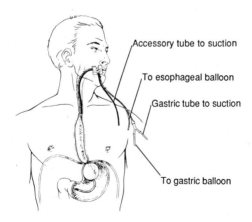

Accessory tube to suction

To esophageal balloon

Gastric tube to suction

To gastric balloon

FIGURE 12-3. Sengstaken-Blakemore tube with both gastric and esophageal balloons inflated. (From Dunphy JE, Way LE, editors: *Current surgical diagnosis and treatment,* New York, 1981, Lange)

Recent attempts to occlude varices by using the end-to-end stapling device have been unsuccessful. Therefore, emergency surgical control of variceal bleeding requires decompression of the hypertensive portal venous system.

In the presence of acute massive bleeding, the surgeon usually chooses one of the types of shunt that can be performed quickly (e.g., end-to-side portacaval shunt). Results vary widely, depending upon the patient population. Poor liver function, encephalopathy, ascites, malnutrition, and acute alcoholic liver disease indicate poor prognosis. Operative survival rates are about 50%; good-risk patients do much better than the average.

4. Elective portosystemic shunt. Patients who survive an episode of documented variceal hemorrhage should be considered for an elective portosystemic shunt. Prime candidates are patients under the age of 60 years with good liver function, although patients who lack these attributes are also shunted in some centers. Portosystemic shunt is followed by only marginally improved long-term survival, but recurrent bleeding, with its attendant demands on blood banks and other resources, is effectively prevented.

a. Preoperative evaluation and preparation. Alcoholic patients should abstain from alcohol and should consume a nutritious diet in preparation for elective operation. The goal is to allow the liver to recover from acute damage inflicted by alcohol, malnutrition, hypotension, and massive transfusion. Operative mortality correlates with preoperative liver function (Table 12-5).

Table 12-5. Relation of hepatic function and nutrition to operative mortality after portacaval shunt (Child's criteria)

Group	A	B	C
Operative mortality	**2%**	**10%**	**50%**
Serum bilirubin (mg/dl)	<2.0	2.0-3.0	>3.0
Serum albumin (g/dl)	>3.5	3.0-3.5	<3.0
Ascites	None	Easily controlled	Poorly controlled
Encephalopathy	None	Minimal	Advanced
Nutrition	Excellent	Good	Poor

Selective splenic and superior mesenteric arteriography is performed, and films are exposed until portal venous anatomy is demonstrated. This information is essential in planning operation. If the proposed shunt involves anastomosis to the left renal vein, that structure should be seen on the films.

Liver biopsy should be done to diagnose acute alcoholic hepatitis, schistosomiasis, hepatoma, and other lesions that influence the decision to perform a shunt or the type of shunt.

Preoperative measurement of portal pressure is not essential. Wedged hepatic vein pressure is the safest to obtain; alternatives are direct percutaneous splenic puncture and umbilical vein cannulation.

b. Choice of shunt. There are three types of portosystemic shunt in physiologic terms.

(1) *End-to-side portacaval shunt.* The portal vein is divided, the hepatic stump is oversewn, and the splanchnic end is anastomosed to the side of the vena cava. This has long been the standard operation against which others are measured.

(2) *Side-to-side shunts.* There are many variations on this theme: side-to-side portacaval, mesocaval, central splenorenal, and renosplenic. All share the feature of permitting blood to flow away from the liver through the portal vein (hepatofugal flow) and via the anastomosis into the systemic circulation; this may impair liver function to a greater extent than the end-to-side shunt, but the differences are small.

One type of mesocaval shunt is constructed by anastomosing a Dacron graft between the side of the vena cava and the side of the superior mesenteric vein.

Mesocaval shunts are necessary when the portal and splenic veins are too small to work with (e.g., children). Side-to-side shunts are preferred when ascites is present, because they reduce sinusoidal pressure.

(3) *Selective.* The distal splenorenal (Warren) shunt is the most common of these technics in which pressure is lowered in the esophageal varices while portal blood flow to the liver is unchanged. In the Warren shunt, the splenic vein is divided and the end nearest the portal vein is oversewn. The splenic end is anastomosed to the side of the left renal vein. This shunt is more difficult to perform than most other kinds of shunts, but the avoidance of further liver damage and the lower incidence of encephalopathy make it attractive. It should not be used in patients with marked ascites.

c. Prognosis. Operative mortality rate in elective shunts is 5%-10%. Bleeding recurs in about 8% of patients, usually because the shunt has thrombosed. Hepatic failure and encephalopathy are the most important complications.

5. Liver transplantation is effective treatment and has gained a larger role in the management of cirrhotic patients (see Chapter 20).

6. Ascites is usually controllable by use of diuretics.

The **peritoneal-jugular (LeVeen) shunt** is used for the treatment of refractory ascites. One end of the plastic tube is inserted into the peritoneal cavity, and the other end of the LeVeen shunt is placed into the jugular vein. The entire tubing is buried subcutaneously, and the flow of ascites from peritoneal cavity to jugular vein is regulated by a one-way valve. Peritoneal infection is a contraindication. Disseminated intravascular coagulation is common but mild. Thrombosis of the valve is another problem.

7. Encephalopathy. Hepatic encephalopathy is a major complication of portosystemic shunts; it also occurs in nonshunted patients, particularly during acute bleeding episodes. Factors contributing to the appearance of encephalopathy include age, poor liver function, azotemia, type of shunt, amount of protein in diet (or in blood within gut lumen), intestinal flora, and many others.

Symptoms vary from mild lethargy or personality changes to psychosis or coma. Asterixis may be present.

Encephalopathy precipitated by acute variceal hemorrhage is treated by laxatives (to remove blood from the gut) and antibiotics (e.g., neomycin) administered orally or through a gastric tube.

After portosystemic shunt, protein intake is limited to 40 g/day initially to minimize the incidence of encephalopathy. Protein restriction is eased gradually if symptoms do not develop. Chronic encephalopathy is treated by lactulose, a disaccharide that reduces production of nitrogenous compounds in the colon. Give 20-30 g orally three to four times daily.

E. EVALUATION OF OBSTRUCTIVE JAUNDICE. Jaundice may be due to prehepatic, hepatic, or posthepatic causes. Prehepatic jaundice is usually the result of hemolysis. Hepatic jaundice may arise from hepatocellular disease (viral hepatitis, alcoholic cirrhosis) or intrahepatic cholestasis (primary biliary cirrhosis, toxic effects of drugs). Posthepatic jaundice is caused by obstruction of the bile ducts; extrahepatic and obstructive jaundice are synonyms. In general, obstructive jaundice requires surgical treatment, and prehepatic and hepatic are managed medically. The goal of evaluation is to identify patients with biliary obstruction.

Specific disease entities are described individually later in this section. Some general guidelines are discussed here.

1. History

a. Age and sex. Older people are more likely to have obstructive jaundice. Primary biliary cirrhosis is almost exclusively limited to women.

b. Drugs. Alcohol, phenothiazines, and sex hormones are among the drugs that may cause jaundice. Viral hepatitis is common among people who inject illicit drugs.

c. Pain beginning in the epigastrium or right upper quadrant and radiating to the right scapula is typical of acute biliary obstruction (biliary colic). Chronic, dull, aching upper abdominal pain suggests malignancy. Diffuse pain in the right upper quadrant may result from distention of the hepatic capsule by hepatitis, acute alcoholic injury, or passive congestion from cardiac disease.

d. Fever. High fever, especially when accompanied by shaking chills (rigors), is characteristic of cholangitis from biliary obstruction.

e. Light stools and dark urine are more common in patients with extrahepatic obstruction.

f. Pruritus. Severe itching of the extremities may precede jaundice or coincide with it. Pruritus is a symptom of cholestasis of any cause.

2. Physical examination.
Hepatomegaly is not a distinguishing feature. Stigmata of cirrhosis (e.g., spider angiomata) may be found. Splenomegaly suggests the presence of portal hypertension. A nontender palpable gallbladder indicates that the cause of jaundice is malignant obstruction of the common duct (Courvoisier's law). The gallbladder is not palpable in malignant obstruction at the cystic duct level or higher.

3. Liver function tests.
Standard LFTs usually permit separation of patients into two groups: those with prehepatic or hepatocellular jaundice, and those with cholestatic jaundice. Because cholestasis may be hepatic (medical) or posthepatic (surgical), these tests merely identify patients who need further evaluation for biliary obstruction.

Cholestatic jaundice is typically associated with an elevated direct (conjugated) fraction of bilirubin, normal or mildly elevated AST, elevated alkaline phosphatase, normal albumin, and prolonged PT. Many variations occur, and there is substantial overlap of findings in cholestatic and hepatocellular jaundice.

Hepatitis antigens and/or antibodies and antimitochondrial antibodies (elevated in primary biliary cirrhosis) may be helpful.

4. Plain abdominal radiographs. About 10%-15% of gallstones are radiopaque and thus are visible on plain abdominal films. An enlarged gallbladder may be seen as soft tissue mass.

5. Ultrasonography is a safe, simple, inexpensive, and fairly reliable method of demonstrating the bile duct in obstructive jaundice. Dilated ducts and gallstones may be evident. If ducts are dilated, biliary obstruction is present. If ducts are not dilated, obstruction is not ruled out.

6. CT may demonstrate dilated bile ducts, hepatic masses, and retroperitoneal (e.g., pancreatic) masses. It is usually ordered if the ultrasound study is equivocal.

7. Percutaneous transhepatic cholangiography is a good way to demonstrate the upper level of obstruction if ducts are dilated, although even ducts of normal caliber can be entered. Coagulation defects, ascites, and cholangitis are contraindications.

8. Endoscopic retrograde cholangiopancreatography. Cannulation of the common bile duct and/or the pancreatic duct through the ampulla of Vater can be accomplished endoscopically. The lower end of obstructing lesions is demonstrated. In some cases, additional valuable information is obtained (e.g., ampullary tumor, stone eroding through the ampulla, carcinoma invading the duodenum, etc.). Cholangitis and pancreatitis are complications. It is very useful in patients with nondilated ducts or contraindications to transhepatic cholangiography. The potential for treating the cause of obstruction at the same time (e.g., sphincterotomy for retained common duct stones) makes endoscopic retrograde cholangiopancreatography even more attractive.

9. Selection of studies. Redundant studies should be avoided. The most important question to be answered is: **are the bile ducts obstructed?** The **level of obstruction** and the **cause of obstruction** are also important questions. Delineation of the ductal anatomy can help the surgeon plan the operation, and for that reason one or the other of these cholangiographic procedures is performed preoperatively.

F. CHOLELITHIASIS is the presence of gallstones in the gallbladder. Gallstones are composed predominantly of cholesterol in 75% of patients in the United States. The incidence of stones increases with age and is associated with race (highest in American Indians, lowest in blacks), sex (more common in women until menopause, thereafter about equal), multiparity, obesity, oral contraceptives, and certain intestinal diseases (inflammatory bowel disease).

The remaining 25% of gallstones are composed of calcium bilirubinate and bile acids (pigment stones). Hemolytic diseases, biliary stasis, and cirrhosis are the usual predisposing conditions.

1. Diagnosis. About 50% of pigment stones are radiopaque and can be seen on plain films. Most cholesterol stones are radiolucent. Ultrasonography is 95% accurate in detecting stones in the gallbladder.

2. Complications. Gallstones cause problems eventually in about 30% of patients. Chronic and acute cholecystitis, obstruction of the common bile duct, cholangitis, gallstone ileus, carcinoma of the gallbladder, and pancreatitis are among the complications of cholelithiasis.

3. Medical treatment. Dissolution of cholesterol gallstones by oral administration of **chenodeoxycholic acid** or **ursodeoxycholic acid** has been pushed into the background since the advent of laparoscopic cholecystectomy. The same may be said of percutaneous injection of terbutylether and biliary lithotripsy.

4. Surgical treatment. Prophylactic cholecystectomy for asymptomatic cholelithiasis is recommended in diabetics, in any patient whose gallbladder does not opacify, in patients with large gallstones or multiple tiny gallstones, or if there is a calcified gallbladder. Prophylactic cholecystectomy in the absence of these factors is controversial, but the apparent advantages of laparoscopic cholecystectomy have shifted many patients from resistance to acceptance of definitive surgical treatment.

G. CHRONIC CHOLECYSTITIS is the most common manifestation of gallstones. The term is imprecise and often applied to symptomatic gallbladders containing stones, whether or not there is inflammation or scarring.

1. Diagnosis
a. Symptoms. Pain is the characteristic symptom and is due to transient obstruction of the cystic duct by stones. Although termed biliary "colic," the pain is steady. Often it be-

gins abruptly after a meal, is centered in the epigastrium or right upper quadrant, and radiates to the right scapula. Other pain patterns occur. The pain intensifies and subsides over a few minutes to a few hours. Attacks may be frequent or separated by long asymptomatic intervals.

Nausea and vomiting in some patients.

"Fatty food intolerance" bears no specific relationship to gallstones.

b. Signs. There are usually no abdominal findings. Tenderness in the right upper quadrant is present occasionally.

c. Radiographs. Ultrasonography shows gallstones in most patients.

2. Differential diagnosis. Chronic cholecystitis should be differentiated from other upper GI diseases. An upper GI series or endoscopy may be needed. Radicular pain, angina pectoris, pancreatitis, irritable colon, and carcinoma of the gallbladder are also considered.

3. Complications. Acute cholecystitis, choledocholithiasis, and carcinoma of the gallbladder.

4. Treatment. Cholecystectomy is the treatment of choice. Increasingly, most of these operations are performed laparoscopically. Operative cholangiography is recommended by most experts for safety of the dissection and detection of common duct stones. If cholangiography demonstrates stones in the duct, experienced surgeons may explore the common duct by one of several laparoscopic techniques. Alternatively, the operation may be converted to an open procedure to accomplish duct exploration, or the stones may be left for subsequent ERCP and endoscopic extraction.

5. Prognosis. The mortality rate for elective cholecystectomy is <1%. Failure to relieve symptoms usually means that the symptoms are related to some condition other than gallstones. Postoperative jaundice may be due to retained common duct stones or operative injury to the bile ducts. Bile duct injury during laparoscopic cholecystectomy can be minimized by adequate training before undertaking unsupervised procedures.

H. ACUTE CHOLECYSTITIS. Cholelithiasis is responsible for 95% of cases. A stone impacts in the cystic duct, inflammation develops, and bacterial infection supervenes in some instances. Acalculous cholecystitis is associated with one of the following: obstruction of the cystic duct by another mechanism (e.g., tumor); occlusion of the cystic artery; primary bacterial infection; or prolonged fasting (e.g., in patients receiving parenteral nutrition).

1. Diagnosis

a. Symptoms. History of biliary colic in 75% of cases. Pain is typical of biliary colic initially, but persists. Nausea and vomiting in about 50%. Fever up to 38.5° C or rigors indicate a complication or some other diagnosis.

b. Signs. Tenderness and spasm in the right upper quadrant. Murphy's sign: arrest of a deep inspiratory effort as the examiner palpates the right upper quadrant. An enlarged, tender gallbladder is palpable (and sometimes visible) in about 35%. Mild jaundice is noted in 10%.

c. Laboratory tests. Leukocytosis in the range of 12,000-15,000/µl. Mild elevation of bilirubin (rarely >4 mg/dl with acute cholecystitis alone). Serum amylase may be elevated.

d. Radiographs. Plain abdominal films may show radiopaque gallstones or a mass. Ultrasound study usually demonstrates gallstones and should be obtained as soon as diagnosis is suspected. Oral cholecystogram is unreliable in patients with acute abdominal illnesses. HIDA scan which images the common duct but not the gallbladder is very strong evidence for cystic duct obstruction (i.e., acute cholecystitis in the appropriate clinical setting).

2. Differential diagnosis.
Other acute GI diseases; perforated peptic ulcer, acute appendicitis, acute pancreatitis. Acute distention of the liver by viral hepatitis, passive congestion, or alcoholic hepatitis. Gonococcal perihepatitis (Curtis and Fitz-Hugh syndrome) is associated with high fever and pelvic findings of salpingitis. Gonococci are seen in the cervical smear. Acute pneumonitis or myocardial infarction.

3. Complications

a. Empyema. Gallbladder is filled with pus. Patient is toxic, with a high fever and sometimes rigors. The leukocyte count is high.

b. Perforation. Gallbladder becomes gangrenous and perforates in about 10%. Interval from onset to perforation is seldom <72 hours.

(1) *Localized perforation.* Perforation is contained by surrounding omentum, liver, duodenum, colon, and a *pericholecystic abscess* is formed in about 6% of patients with acute cholecystitis. High fever, toxicity, and leukocytosis are usually present. Sometimes a mass is palpable.

(2) *Free perforation.* Perforation into the general peritoneal cavity occurs in about 1%. Spreading or generalized peritonitis and deterioration of the patient's overall condition suggest the diagnosis.

(3) *Cholecystoenteric fistula.* The gallbladder perforates and fistulizes into adjacent duodenum, colon, or stomach (3% of cases). The obstructed gallbladder is thus decompressed, and the cholecystitis may subside. Few symptoms are attributable to chronic cholecystoenteric fistulas; the main clinical problem occurs when a gallstone passes through the fistula and obstructs the intestine (gallstone ileus).

Gallstone ileus. Symptoms are those of mechanical obstruction of the small intestine (rarely the colon). More than 50% have no history suggesting recent acute cholecystitis. Diagnosis is made by plain abdominal radiographs; a radiopaque stone may be seen in mid or lower abdomen, and gas is seen in the biliary tree in about 50%. Treatment is simply to open the intestine to extract the stone; cholecystectomy is not performed at the same operation but may be required subsequently. Mortality rate is high because patients are elderly and in poor condition.

4. Treatment

a. IV fluids, nasogastric tube, and analgesics are given routinely. Antibiotics are recommended because bacteria are present in 75% of acutely inflamed gallbladders, although inflammation is usually nonbacterial initially.

b. If the diagnosis is securely established, operation should be done at an early convenient time. Although acute cholecystitis usually resolves without operation, delay of cholecystectomy to a later date prolongs the total illness without much benefit.

c. If the diagnosis is unclear or the patient is in poor general condition, expectant management can be used until a diagnosis is reached or the associated problems are corrected.

d. A true *emergency* exists, and operation must be done immediately, in patients with empyema or perforation. *Emphysematous cholecystitis* (anaerobic infection producing gas bubbles in the wall and lumen of the gallbladder) is a virulent form of cholecystitis, and it also should be treated by urgent operation.

e. Choice of operation.

(1) *Cholecystectomy* is definitive treatment and should be performed in patients who are in good condition. Some

experienced surgeons perform the procedure laparoscopically unless severe inflammation forces conversion to open operation. Operative cholangiography is recommended.

(2) *Cholecysostomy* is selected in a few elderly or poor-risk patients. Gallbladder is approached through a small subcostal incision, opened, stones extracted if possible, and a large tube is sutured into the gallbladder. Cholecystectomy is necessary later if tube cholecystography demonstrates obstruction of cystic duct or stones in the gallbladder or common duct. In other patients, the tube can be removed and cholecystectomy performed if symptoms recur. Cholecystostomy also can be done percutaneously by the interventional radiologist.

5. Prognosis is excellent in young patients with uncomplicated acute cholecystitis. Advanced age, associated diseases (especially diabetes), perforation, and other complications of gallstone diseases (e.g., choledocholithiasis and pancreatitis) are responsible for the overall mortality rate of 5%.

I. CHOLEDOCHOLITHIASIS AND CHOLANGITIS. In about 15% of patients with cholelithiasis, gallstones pass from the gallbladder through the cystic duct and into the common bile duct. Stones may form in the common bile duct itself as a consequence of stasis.

Stones may pass through the ampulla of Vater into the duodenum, or they may lodge in the ampulla, causing obstruction. About 50% of patients with choledocholithiasis have no symptoms related to the common duct. In the other 50%, choledocholithiasis causes biliary colic, cholangitis, obstructive jaundice, pancreatitis, or a combination of these problems.

1. Syndromes
a. Biliary colic. Episodes of biliary colic due to intermittent obstruction of the common duct by gallstones are similar to the attacks seen in patients with chronic cholecystitis. If the stone passes through the ampulla, or if it slips upward into the duct, thus relieving obstruction, pain subsides.

b. Cholangitis is infection in the biliary tree. There are three requirements: bacteria, obstruction, and increased pressure. Cholangitis is most commonly caused by choledocholithiasis, although other types of ductal obstruction may also be responsible. With obstruction, biliary pressure rises and cholangiovenous reflux of bacteria from the obstructed bile duct into the hepatic venous circulation results in septicemia.

Fever and chills, jaundice, and biliary colic are classic symptoms of cholangitis (Charcot's triad), although the symptom complex is incomplete in many patients. If cholangitis is very severe **(acute suppurative cholangitis),** hypotension and mental confusion may occur.

c. Obstructive jaundice is the prominent abnormality in some patients with choledocholithiasis. A history of biliary colic or cholangitis is strong evidence for this diagnosis, but the absence of such history does not exclude the possibility of obstruction by gallstones. Fluctuating jaundice, due to intermittent obstruction, is common with choledocholithiasis. Gallbladder usually is not dilated because its wall is thickened by chronic inflammation, in contrast to the marked dilatation seen in neoplastic obstruction of the common duct (Courvoisier's law).

d. Pancreatitis is discussed under Pancreas in this chapter.

2. Treatment. Patients with choledocholithiasis should have evaluation of liver function; depressed prothrombin time is treated with parenteral vitamin K preoperatively.

a. Asymptomatic choledocholithiasis is detected by palpation of a stone or cholangiographic demonstration of a stone in common duct during cholecystectomy. Treatment is cholecystectomy and choledocholithotomy. (See comments above concerning laparoscopic cholecystectomy.)

Routine use of a **choledochoscope** during open cholecystectomy and common duct exploration is recommended, and a T-tube cholangiogram is mandatory before the operation is terminated. Postoperatively, the T-tube is connected to gravity drainage and another T-tube cholangiogram is performed 7-10 days later. If the duct is normal, the tube is removed in the outpatient department about 3 weeks after operation.

b. Retained stones demonstrated on the postoperative study may be extracted by passing a ureteral stone (Dormia) basket through the T-tube tract under fluoroscopic control about 6 weeks after operation. Endoscopic sphincterotomy (division of the sphincter of Oddi) is another technic that is especially useful if the basket method fails, if the T-tube has been removed, or if the ampulla is stenotic. Dissolution of retained cholesterol stones by perfusion of the duct (through the T-tube) with monooctanoin requires lengthy hospitalization. Few patients require reoperation for retained common duct stones.

c. Biliary colic due to common duct obstruction by gallstones is treated by cholecystectomy and choledocholithotomy.

Poor-risk patients can be managed by endoscopic sphincterotomy leaving the gallbladder in situ.

d. Acute cholangitis. Usually responds to IV antibiotics. If a skilled endoscopist is available, endoscopic sphincterotomy can be attempted. If this method is unsuccessful, emergency operation is performed in patients who do not respond to antibiotics. If the acute episode subsides, plan elective operation.

e. Obstructive jaundice due to gallstones is evaluated as described earlier, and treated by cholecystectomy and choledocholithotomy or endoscopic sphincterotomy.

f. Pancreatitis associated with gallstones is cured by operation (see Pancreatitis in this chapter).

3. Prognosis. Choledocholithiasis is a life-threatening complication of gallstones. Mortality rates depend upon clinical syndrome, age, general condition, etc. Overall operative mortality rate for choledocholithotomy is about 4%.

J. CARCINOMA OF THE GALLBLADDER. Adenocarcinoma of the gallbladder is associated with gallstones in most cases. It occurs in elderly patients and causes persistent biliary colic, acute cholecystitis, or obstruction of the common duct. The gallbladder may be palpable.

Cure is seldom possible because the cancer has metastasized or extended by the time of operation. Palliation is offered by cholecystectomy or by relief of common duct obstruction. Occasionally, a small cancer is found incidentally in a gallbladder removed for symptomatic chronic cholecystitis, and long-term survival is possible in such cases.

K. MALIGNANT TUMORS OF THE BILE DUCT are rare. Most are adenocarcinomas, and they cause obstructive jaundice, usually without cholangitis. The gallbladder is palpable if obstruction is distal to the cystic duct. The diagnosis is suggested by preoperative transhepatic cholangiography or ERCP and confirmed at operation.

Tumors at the confluence of the hepatic ducts (Klatskin tumors) are often overlooked in the absence of preoperative cholangiography. Sclerosing tumors may contain a few malignant cells; biopsies occasionally are falsely negative.

Excision of the tumor (Whipple procedure for distal lesions; radical resection of ducts in the porta hepatitis for proximal lesions) is the optimal treatment, but it seldom is curative because of early metastasis or extension. If excision is not possible, palliation is provided by placement of a stent through the obstructing point by endoscopic, percutaneous, or open surgical methods. Radiation therapy is palliative in some cases.

Average survival after diagnosis is <1 year, but occasional patients survive for much longer periods.

L. STRICTURE OF THE BILE DUCT is iatrogenic in 95% of cases. Strictures caused by gallstones or nonsurgical trauma comprise the remainder. The bile ducts are especially liable to injury when cholecystectomy, either open or laparoscopic, is performed by an incompletely trained surgeon who does not appreciate the variability of ductal and vascular anatomy.

Injuries take the form of division, ligation, or excision of part or all of a segment of the duct. Postoperative fever, jaundice, and prolonged drainage of bile are indications of injury to the duct. If definitive repair is not performed at the moment of injury, stricture formation is nearly inevitable.

Cholangitis weeks to months after cholecystectomy is the typical manifestation. Transhepatic or endoscopic cholangiogram demonstrates the stricture.

Untreated stricture leads to secondary biliary cirrhosis and portal hypertension. Repeated cholangitis may result in abscess and death from sepsis.

Treatment is by surgical repair. These procedures are technically difficult and should be attempted only by experienced surgeons. One common method of repair is anastomosis of the end of the divided duct above the stricture to the side of a Roux-en-Y jejunal loop. Operation is successful in 75% of patients. Morbidity and mortality rates are high in patients with long-standing strictures.

Poor-risk patients or extremely complex strictures can be treated by endoscopic or percutaneous dilatation with a Gruntzig balloon.

M. OTHER DISEASES OF THE BILE DUCTS

1. Sclerosing cholangitis. Inflammation and fibrosis of bile ducts occur as a primary phenomenon in rare instances; there is a strong association with ulcerative colitis. Most patients have diffuse involvement of the major ducts within and outside the liver, although occasionally the process is localized. The wall is thickened and the lumen is narrowed greatly.

Cholestatic jaundice is the clinical presentation. ERCP shows multiple constrictions and areas of mild dilatation.

Operation is performed in some cases. Corticosteroids may be helpful. The disease is chronic, and biliary cirrhosis usually develops over the long term. Liver transplantation may be needed eventually.

2. Congenital anomalies

a. Choledochal cyst is a congenital development abnormality which may not cause symptoms of jaundice and cholangitis until adulthood. Excision or decompression of the cyst is the treatment of choice.

b. Caroli's disease is congenital dilatation of the intrahepatic ducts. Jaundice or portal hypertension may be the first manifestation. Surgical treatment is difficult; antibiotics are used to control cholangitis.

3. Oriental cholangiohepatitis. This chronic disease probably results from portal bacteremia. Multiple sequential strictures of the intrahepatic ducts, hepatic abscesses, and obstruction by sludge and stones are the consequences. Patients have pain, fever, jaundice, and right upper quadrant tenderness. Treatment is by cholecystectomy, extraction of stones, and diversion of bile by choledochoduodenostomy or chledochojejunostomy. Results are poor if the intrahepatic ducts are strictured and filled with stones that cannot be removed. Death occurs from persistent sepsis.

XV. PANCREAS

A. TRAUMA. Damage to the pancreas from blunt or penetrating trauma varies in severity from mild contusion to extensive disruption of the parenchyma and necrosis of the duodenum. Clinical findings may be mild and delayed; abdominal or back pain, abdominal tenderness, and elevated serum amylase are clues to the presence of pancreatic injury.

Surgical management of one common type of blunt injury, fracture of the body of the gland where it crosses the spine, consists of distal pancratectomy. Minor contusions are treated by external drainage. Extensive disruption of the pancreatic head, with preservation of blood supply to the duodenum, is sometimes treated by subtotal pancreatectomy. An alternative is a combination of antrectomy, gastrojejunostomy, tube duodenostomy, and external drainage. If the duodenum is ischemic, a Whipple procedure may be necessary.

External pancreatic fistula, infection, and traumatic pancreatitis are sources of morbidity and mortality in these difficult cases.

B. ACUTE PANCREATITIS is inflammation caused by escape of active pancreatic enzymes into the interstitial tissues of the gland. Acute **edematous pancreatitis** is characterized by marked edema of the gland and surrounding structures. **Hemorrhagic pancreatitis** is a more severe manifestation of the same process in which there is necrosis of pancreatic tissue and bleeding into the pancreas and the retroperitoneal space.

1. Causes

a. Alcohol is responsible for about 40% of cases in the United States, and in certain hospitals, the majority of cases are due to alcohol. An interval of 6 years or more from the beginning of excessive drinking to the first attack of pancreatitis is typical. Microscopic changes of chronic pancreatitis already have developed by the time of the initial attack of acute pancreatitis.

b. Gallstones are the cause of acute pancreatitis in about 40% of cases. The attack is precipitated by passage of a stone through the ampulla.

c. Hyperlipidemia, either primary or secondary to alcoholism, is a cause of pancreatitis. Lactescent serum is diagnostic.

d. Hypercalcemia due to hyperparathyroidism or other diseases may lead to pancreatitis.

e. Postoperative pancreatitis may result from direct trauma to the gland, but some cases develop after remote (e.g., pelvic) surgery.

f. Familial pancreatitis is a rare cause, beginning in childhood.

g. Pancreas divisum is an anomaly in which the dorsal and ventral pancreatic ducts do not fuse. Pancreatic secretions enter the duodenum through the duct of Santorini. This condition has been etiologically linked to pancreatitis, but the relationship is controversial.

h. Miscellaneous. Corticosteroids, azathioprine, contraceptives, protein deficiency, and others. 10%-15% of cases are idiopathic.

2. Diagnosis

a. Symptoms. Postprandial, severe, unrelenting epigastric pain radiating through to the back. Nausea, vomiting, and persistent retching. Hematemesis of a mild degree is present occasionally.

b. Signs. Shock in severe cases. Mild fever. Epigastric tenderness; sometimes generalized abdominal tenderness. Epigastric mass (edematous pancreas in the early stages). Ecchymosis in the flank (Grey-Turner's sign) or umbilicus (Cullen's signs) in hemorrhagic pancreatitis. Pleural effusion.

c. Laboratory tests
(1) Leukocytosis.
(2) Hematocrit may be high as a result of dehydration or low because of bleeding.
(3) Bilirubin and alkaline phosphatase may be mildly elevated.
(4) Serum calcium is low in severe cases.
(5) Serum may be lactescent to gross inspection.
(6) *Serum amylase* is >200 IU/dl in most cases. The rise is detected 6 hours after onset, and levels return to normal in about 48 hours. Lactescent serum interferes with amylase determination, and values may be normal in these patients. Amylase may be elevated in many other acute abdominal conditions.
(7) *Urine amylase* is a more accurate test than serum amylase. Timed collection of urine permits determination of urinary excretion of amylase; >5000 IU/24 hours is abnormal. The ratio of amylase clearance to creatinine clearance is no longer regarded as a specific diagnostic test.

d. Radiographs.
Plain abdominal films may show a dilated loop of small or large bowel (sentinal loop); distention of the right colon with no gas beyond that point (colon cut-off sign); radiopaque gallstones; pancreatic calcification in some patients with disease of long standing. Chest film may show a pleural effusion, especially on the left. CT scan may be a useful baseline study. Ultrasonography may reveal gallstones. ERCP is helpful a few weeks after the acute attack subsides if the cause is still uncertain.

3. Differential diagnosis. Acute pancreatitis must be distinguished from perforated ulcer, mesenteric vascular occlusion, strangulated small bowel obstruction, and acute cholecystitis. Some of these conditions are fatal if operation is not performed, and if there is any doubt about the diagnosis of pancreatitis, laparotomy must be done.

Chronic hyperamylasemia in the absence of pancreatitis is rare. Macroamylasemia is one variety in which amylase is bound to large molecules in serum and cannot be excreted. High serum amylase levels in a patient with low urinary amylase is suggestive; macroamylase can be measured by some laboratories.

4. Complications. Pseudocyst and abscess are discussed below. GI bleeding may result from gastritis, peptic ulcer, or Mallory-Weiss tear. Respiratory complications are frequent in severe attacks. **Ranson's criteria** are a measure of severity of pancreatitis. *Criteria present initially:* age > 55 years, WBC > 16,000, blood glucose >200 mg/dl, serum LDH >350 IU/L, AST >250 IU/dl. *Criteria developing during first 48 hours:* Hct fall >10%, BUN rise >8 mg/dl, serum calcium <8 mg/dl, arterial Po$_2$ <60 mm Hg, base deficit <4 mEq/L, fluid sequestration >600 ml. *Mortality rates* are as follows: 0-2 criteria, 2% mortality; 3-4, 15%, 5-6, 40%; 7-8, 100%.

5. Medical treatment

a. Establish and maintain an airway. Endotracheal intubation and ventilatory support may be required.

b. Replace fluid and electrolyte losses, with alertness to the appearance of hypocalcemia. Serum calcium levels <7.5 mg/dl indicate a poor prognosis and must be treated aggressively.

c. Insert a nasogastric tube to relieve the pancreas of further stimulation by gastric acid entering the duodenum.

d. Analgesics. Pentazocine is preferred because morphine and meperidine cause contraction of the sphincter of Oddi.

e. Antibiotics should not be given prophylactically.

f. Peritoneal lavage removes active enzymes and necrotic debris and may avoid some of the systemic toxicity from absorption of these substances. If lavage is planned, it should be instituted promptly. Instill 1 L of lactated Ringer's rapidly through a peritoneal dialysis catheter, and allow the fluid to return by gravity. Repeat every hour. Response should be noted within 8 hours if this treatment is to be effective. Survival rates are not greatly influenced by this maneuver.

g. Other measures. IV glucose and IV trasylol (an inhibitor of proteolytic enzymes) are not effective. TPN is needed if illness is prolonged.

6. Surgical treatment

a. Most operations in this condition are performed to exclude some other acute abdominal disease. If acute edematous pancreatitis is found, the pancreas should not be traumatized, and drains are unnecessary. If gallstones are found, cholecystectomy is performed.

b. Surgery for treatment of gallstone pancreatitis by cholecystectomy and common duct exploration is deferred until the acute attack resolves but should be performed during same hospitalization.

c. Patients with hemorrhagic pancreatitis that is not responding to medical treatment should undergo abdominal exploration to debride necrotic pancreas and provide external drainage.

7. Prognosis. Mortality rate of acute pancreatitis is about 10% overall and 35% in cases of hemorrhagic pancreatitis. Some develop chronic pancreatitis, and others have repeated attacks of acute pancreatitis without chronic changes (acute relapsing). Surgery is curative of biliary pancreatitis.

C. PANCREATIC PSEUDOCYST. About 2% of patients with acute pancreatitis develop a collection of enzyme-rich fluid in or near the pancreas. The pseudocyst is bounded by a capsule of inflamed peritoneum and adjacent structures (e.g., stomach, mesocolon, colon, liver, and diaphragm). Pseudocysts may also form, without antecedent acute pancreatitis, as a result of ductal obstruction (e.g., in alcoholics) or trauma. Pseudocysts are usually single; multiple cysts occur in 15% of cases.

1. Diagnosis

a. Symptoms and signs. Persistent or recurrent pain and fever after an attack of acute pancreatitis; appearance of epigastric pain with no history of pancreatitis in some cases. A tender epigastric mass represents swollen pancreas in the early stages of pancreatitis, but a persistent mass is likely to be a pseudocyst. Weight loss and vomiting, especially if the mass compresses the gut. Jaundice in some cases.

b. Laboratory tests. Serum amylase is elevated in 50% of patients. Leukocytosis and increased serum bilirubin are other findings.

c. Radiographs. Upper GI series shows a pancreatic mass that may displace stomach forward or widen the duodenal loop. Findings are the same whether the mass is edematous pancreas, pseudocyst, or abscess. Ultrasonography differentiates between solid and cystic masses; CT scan has the same capability.

d. Special tests. ERCP may demonstrate communication between the duct and a cyst; antibiotics should be given because of the risk of introducing infection into the cyst.

2. Differential diagnosis. Edematous pancreas (pancreatic phlegmon) is not a fluid-filled mass. Abscess must be distinguished from pseudocyst (see below). Cystic neoplasm should be suspected in patients with no history of pancreatitis; arteriography may be diagnostic, but often the presence of neoplasm is not established until the cyst wall is biopsied at operation.

3. Complications

a. Rupture of a pseudocyst into the peritoneal cavity causes generalized chemical peritonitis. It complicates 5% of cases and is fatal in many. Operation consists of draining the pseudocyst.

b. Infection of a pseudocyst results in fever and toxicity. External surgical drainage is required.

c. Hemorrhage from erosion of the cyst into adjacent major vessels is a very serious complication. Emergency operation is required, but control of the bleeding site in the midst of severe inflammation is difficult.

4. Treatment.
Uncomplicated pseudocysts developing after acute pancreatitis should be observed for about 4-6 weeks to allow resolution or thickening of the wall of the cyst. About 40% of pseudocysts resolve within 6 weeks; if the cyst persists beyond that time, operation is performed.

Small cysts can be excised, but larger ones must be drained externally or internally. External drainage is less satisfactory because 30% of such patients have prolonged drainage from a pancreatic fistula. Somatostatin analogue may speed closure of the fistula. Internal drainage may take the form of anastomosis to the stomach (cystogastrostomy) or anastomosis to a Roux-en-Y loop of jejunum.

5. Prognosis.
Internally drained pseudocysts resolve and the cavities become obliterated over several weeks. Pseudocysts recur in 10% of surgically treated cases. Death is a consequence of the complications described above.

D. PANCREATIC ABSCESS
is a collection of necrotic pancreas and pus as a result of severe pancreatitis.

1. Diagnosis.
Toxicity is the hallmark of pancreatic abscess. High fever, persistent severe pain and tenderness, and leukocytosis develop about 10 days to 2 weeks after the acute attack. A mass may be palpable. Multiple small bubbles in the region of the pancreas on plain radiography is very suggestive of abscess. Upper GI series, ultrasonography, or CT shows a mass. Percutaneous needle aspiration is helpful.

2. Treatment
is surgical drainage and debridement of necrotic pancreas. Antibiotics are given. Multiple external sump drains are placed. Repeated operations may be necessary.

Untreated pancreatic abscess is uniformly fatal. Delayed treatment and the difficulty of controlling infection contribute to the mortality rate of 30%.

E. PANCREATIC ASCITES. Chronic leakage of pancreatic fluid from a pseudocyst or pancreatic duct is responsible for this condition. The enzymes are inactive, and peritonitis does not occur. Most adults with pancreatic ascites are alcoholics, and it may be mistaken for cirrhotic ascites, but paracentesis reveals fluid with high amylase levels and protein >3 g/dl. ERCP should be done to demonstrate the site of ductal disruption. Treatment is surgical after correction of malnutrition. Internal drainage is preferred.

F. CHRONIC PANCREATITIS. Alcohol is the most common cause. Biliary tract disease rarely progresses to this stage despite acute attacks.

1. Diagnosis

a. Symptoms and signs. Persistent pain in the epigastrium and back; intensity of pain varies during the day and from one day to another. Addiction to narcotics is common. Diabetes mellitus. Steatorrhea and malnutrition.

b. Laboratory tests. Serum amylase is not high if pancreas is extensively destroyed. Bilirubin may be elevated from obstruction of the common duct by fibrosis in the head of the pancreas. Diabetes mellitus is demonstrable chemically in many cases. Steatorrhea can be proved by measuring fecal fat content over a 3-day period with the patient consuming 100 g/fat/day. Secretin stimulation of the pancreas may disclose abnormal secretion.

c. Radiographs. Plain abdominal films show pancreatic calcification in 50% of patients with chronic alcoholic pancreatitis. CT or ultrasonography is done to evaluate the pancreas and the biliary tree.

d. Special tests. ERCP reveals strictures, dilatation, calculi, etc. in the pancreatic duct. It should be performed preoperatively.

2. Differential diagnosis. Other diseases of the upper GI tract should be excluded. The possibility of factitious pain for the purpose of obtaining narcotics is a frequent concern. Objective evidence of pancreatic abnormality should be sought.

3. Complications. Diabetes, malnutrition, and narcotic addiction are common. Adenocarcinoma of the pancreas develops in up to 10% of patients with chronic alcoholic pancreatitis.

4. Medical treatment. Abstention from alcohol is essential. Diabetes requires insulin replacement. Steatorrhea responds to oral pancreatic enzymes (e.g., Viokase or Cotazym) given 1 hour before and with each meal for a total daily dose of 4-12 g. H_2 blockers minimize inactivation of ingested enzymes. Celiac plexus block with alcohol injections may relieve pain.

5. Surgical treatment. Persistent pain despite abstention from alcohol is an indication for operation. Surgical treatment takes many forms, but the procedures fall into two categories:

a. Drainage. Obstruction of the duct is relieved by providing some type of internal drainage. Obstruction at the ampulla with uniform distal dilatation sometimes is treated by sphincteroplasty. Distal pancreatectomy and anastomosis of the pancreatic stump to a Roux-en-Y loop of jejunum (DuVal procedure) is rarely done now.

Multiple constrictions and dilatations of the duct are often managed by the Puestow procedure. The duct is incised longitudinally through the anterior surface of the gland from the head to the tail, and a Roux-en-Y loop of jejunum is anastomosed to the full length of the opened duct.

b. Resection. Removal of the pancreas is necessary if the duct is not dilated. Pancreatectomy is limited to the distal gland in selected cases, and diffuse disease requires that most of the pancreas be removed (subtotal or near-total pancreatectomy). Whipple procedure is performed if the head of the gland is not severely involved.

6. Prognosis. About 75% of patients are relieved of pain by properly performed surgery. Continued consumption of alcohol makes recurrent problems likely. Diabetes and steatorrhea must be treated if they were present preoperatively or if they develop after operation (especially after pancreatectomy).

G. ADENOCARCINOMA OF THE PANCREAS. Cancer of the pancreas usually develops between age 40 and 60. The disease is rarely curable because it has extended or metastasized by the time it is detected. Two thirds of cancers arise in the head of the gland.

1. Diagnosis
a. Symptoms and signs. Pain in the epigastrium and back is deep-seated, dull, and often exacerbated by recumbency. Anorexia and weight loss are characteristic. Obstructive jaundice is caused by cancer arising in the head of the gland. Evaluation of jaundiced patients is discussed on page 592. The gallbladder often is palpable in accordance with Courvoisier's law. Cholangitis is uncommon. Migratory thrombophlebitis occasionally. Epigastric mass and hepato-

megaly (from ductal obstruction or metastases). Signs of distal spread (e.g., Virchow's node, umbilical metastases, rectal shelf).

    b. Laboratory tests. LFTs reflect metastases or ductal obstruction. Occult blood is found in the stool in many cases of pancreatic cancer. Cytologic examination of duodenal aspirates may reveal malignant cells. CEA may be elevated.

    c. Radiographs. CT shows most pancreatic tumors, and percutaneous biopsies under CT guidance are accurate in patients with advanced lesions.

    d. Special tests. ERCP shows pancreatic ductal obstruction in more than 90% of cases of pancreatic cancer, and it is very helpful in patients with bile duct obstruction.

    2. Differential diagnosis. Malignant obstructive jaundice may also be due to cancer arising in the common duct, ampulla of Vater, or duodenum. Benign biliary diseases and fibrosis from chronic pancreatitis can obstruct the duct. Pancreatic masses may be benign lesions (pseudocysts, pancreatitis) or other types of pancreatic neoplasm (cystadenoma, cystadenocarcinoma).

    3. Treatment. Diagnosis of cancer is confirmed by biopsy at operation if preoperative percutaneous cytologic specimens were not obtained or were inconclusive. A zone of pancreatitis surrounds most cancers, and the biopsy may be falsely negative. Some surgeons proceed with resection even if the biopsy is negative, if the lesion is small and resectable for cure.

    About 15% of cancers of head of the pancreas can be resected; the remainder have extended locally or metastasized so resection offers no possibility of cure. Resection of cancer arising in the body or tail is rarely possible.

    Resection of cancer in the head requires removal of the head of the pancreas (the portion to the right of the superior mesenteric vessels), the duodenum, the distal stomach (with vagotomy to avoid peptic ulcer), the distal common bile duct, and the gallbladder (Whipple procedure).

    Unresectable tumors of the head are palliated by biliary diversion (e.g., cholecystojejunostomy) and, if the duodenum is obstructed, gastrojejunostomy. Radiation therapy plus chemotherapy may be tried. Intraoperative radiation is used experimentally.

    Most patients die within a year after the diagnosis is made. Management of diabetes and exocrine insufficiency is required after pancreatectomy.

H. ENDOCRINE TUMORS OF THE PANCREAS. Gastrinoma produces Zollinger-Ellison syndrome. Two other islet cell tumors are discussed here.

1. Insulinoma. Neoplasms (or hyperplasia) of the beta cells produce hyperinsulinism. 80% of insulinomas are solitary benign lesions, 10% are malignant, and 10% are multiple benign adenomas or diffuse hyperplasia.

Whipple's triad consists of hypoglycemic symptoms with fasting, blood glucose <50 mg/dl during symptoms, and relief of symptoms by IV glucose. Other causes of hypoglycemia produce Whipple's triad, but high serum insulin levels in the presence of hypoglcyemia are diagnostic if the ratio of plasma insulin to blood glucose is >0.3. Proinsulin levels should be determined also. Arteriography localizes about half of insulinomas. CT has no value. Measurement of insulin levels in portal and splenic venous blood obtained by percutaneous transhepatic sampling may pinpoint tumor site.

Medical measures include diazoxide and streptozocin. *Surgical treatment* is recommended, however, in the absence of contraindications. Solitary tumors are excised. Multiple tumors or diffuse hyperplasia may improve after subtotal pancreatectomy.

2. Pancreatic cholera is also known as the WDHA syndrome (watery diarrhea, hypokalemia, and achlorhydria). It is caused by excessive production of VIP (vasoactive intestinal polypeptide) by a pancreatic nonbeta islet cell tumor. Other causes of diarrhea must be excluded. Surgical excision succeeds in 75% of patients.

3. Glucagonoma produces a syndrome of anemia, necrotizing dermatitis, weight loss, stomatitis, and diabetes. Serum glucagon levels are high. The majority of tumors are malignant. Resection is performed if possible.

4. Somatostatinoma produces diarrhea and diabetes.

XVI. SPLEEN

A. TRAUMA. The spleen is frequently injured by blunt trauma, penetrating wounds, and, occasionally, surgical manipulation. It may rupture spontaneously in certain diseases (e.g., leukemia, malaria, and mononucleosis).

Rupture of the splenic capsule produces intraabdominal bleeding. In some cases, a blow may contuse the spleen, a subcapsular hematoma forms, and **delayed rupture** occurs days to weeks later. Many cases of so-called delayed rupture, however, are simply delayed leakage from temporarily contained hematomas outside the spleen.

Left upper abdominal pain and tenderness should raise the suspicion of splenic rupture. Fractures of the lower ribs on the left are an important sign of trauma to the splenic region. Some patients are in shock; others have no hemodynamic instability. Pain in the left shoulder (Kehr's sign) is accentuated by the Trendelenberg position or by palpation of the left upper quadrant.

Peritoneal lavage is useful to detect blood in the peritoneal cavity. CT and ultrasonography are very reliable. Splenic scintiscan and, occasionally, arteriography are also available.

Nonoperative treatment is possible in selected patients with presumably minor splenic injuries seen on CT scan. Operation is preferred in about 75% of patients with splenic rupture. Repair of the spleen (splenorrhaphy) or partial splenectomy is preferred if these technics are feasible. The goal is preservation of viable splenic tissue without jeopardizing patient's immediate chances of recovery. Total splenectomy is necessary in cases of massive destruction.

The mortality rate of splenic rupture in the absence of other injuries is about 10%.

B. HYPERSPLENISM is abnormal splenic sequestration and destruction of red cells, leukocytes, and platelets.

1. Causes
   a. Splenic enlargement. A large spleen is capable of greater destruction of blood cells than a normal size spleen.
   (1) *Primary hypersplenism* is enlargement of the spleen for no apparent reason. It is rare.
   (2) *Secondary hypersplenism* is enlargement of the spleen as a feature of some known disease. Portal hypertension is the most common, and neoplastic involvement of the spleen (e.g., by lymphoma) is also frequent. Less common in the United States are tuberculosis, malaria, mononucleosis, and sarcoidosis. Rheumatoid arthritis may be associated with hypersplenism (Felty's syndrome).
   b. Defects of red cells. Defective red blood cells are trapped and destroyed in the spleen, leading to splenic enlargement and still more destruction of red cells and other blood cells. Spherocytosis, thalassemia, and G6PD deficiency are among these conditions.
   c. Immunologic disorders in which splenic destruction of blood cells leads to hypersplenism include autoimmune hemolytic anemia and thrombocytopenic purpura.

2. Diagnosis and treatment. Anemia, leukopenia, and thrombocytopenia are characteristic. Splenic enlargement can be demonstrated on scintiscan, ultrasonography, or CT scan. Splenic function can be evaluated by tests for destruction of labeled cells in the spleen. Treatment depends upon the underlying disease. Splenectomy is required in some hypersplenic states and recommended occasionally in others (see Table 12-6). A few of these conditions are discussed in the following section.

C. SPLENECTOMY FOR HEMATOLOGIC DISORDERS

1. Hereditary spherocytosis is the most common type of congenital hemolytic anemia. It is transmitted as an autosomal dominant trait.

Table 12-6. Indications for splenectomy

Splenectomy always indicated	Splenectomy usually indicated
Primary splenic tumor (rare)	Primary hypersplenism
Splenic abscess (rare)	Chronic ITP
Hereditary spherocytosis (congenital hemolytic anemia)	Splenic vein thrombosis causing esophageal varices
Splenectomy sometimes indicated	**Splenectomy rarely indicated**
Splenic injury (common)	Chronic lymphatic leukemia
Autoimmune hemolytic disease	Lymphosarcoma
Elliptocytosis with hemolysis	Hodgkin's disease (except staging)
Nonspherocytic congenital hemolytic anemias (e.g., pyruvate kinase deficiency)	Macroglobulinemia
	Thalassemia major
Hemoglobin H disease	Splenic artery aneurysm
Hodgkin's disease (for staging)	Sickle cell anemia
Thrombotic thrombocytopenic purpura	Splenomegaly due to portal hypertension
Myelofibrosis	

Splenectomy not indicated

Asymptomatic hypersplenism	Hereditary hemolytic anemia of moderate degree
Splenomegaly with infection	Acute leukemia
Splenomegaly associated with elevated IgM	Agranulocytosis

a. Diagnosis. Anemia, jaundice, fatigue, and spleno-megaly are usually apparent in childhood or early adulthood. Asymptomatic cases are detected when a patient's relatives are surveyed.

Mild to moderate anemia (Hgb 9-12 g/dl) and reticulocy-tosis are present. Spherocytes are seen on smear of the periph-eral blood. Bilirubin (indirect fraction) may be elevated. Spe-cial tests reveal abnormal red cell fragility. The Coombs test is negative.

b. Differential diagnosis. Spherocytes are found in the blood in other conditions, including autoimmune hemolytic anemias.

c. Complications. Gallstones in 85% of adults with spherocytosis.

d. Treatment. Splenectomy is required and should be deferred in children until age 5 years or older. Cholecystec-tomy is indicated for cholelithiasis.

e. Prognosis. Splenectomy is curative if diagnosis is correct. Persistent hemolysis is due to an overlooked accessory spleen.

2. Acquired hemolytic anemia. This may be acquired by exposure to drugs, chemical, and other agents. Nonsurgical treatment (removal of the causative agent, corticosteroids) is usually sufficient. **Autoimmune hemolytic anemia** is due to formation of antibodies against one's own red cells. This con-dition, if caused by warm antibodies, may require splenec-tomy.

Abrupt onset of anemia, fever, and jaundice in women over age 50 years is the usual presentation. The spleen is en-larged in 50% and gallstones are present in 25%. Hemolytic anemia is normochromic and normocytic. Reticulocytosis and a positive Coombs test are present.

Corticosteroid therapy leads to permanent remission in 25% of cases; splenectomy is performed in the remainder. Splenectomy is successful in 50% of patients overall, and in 80% of patients with preoperative proof (using ^{51}Cr tagged red cells) that the spleen is the site of sequestration.

3. Idiopathic (immunologic) thrombocytopenic pur-pura may be primary or secondary (e.g., to drugs, infection, lymphoproliferative disorders). Splenic destruction of platelets causes ecchymoses, petechiae, and bleeding from gingiva, gut, vagina, or urinary tract. Chronic idiopathic thrombocytopenic purpura occurs mainly in women; an acute variety appears in children.

Thrombocytopenia ($<100,000/\mu l$) is demonstrable on peripheral smear. Abundant megakaryocytes are found in the marrow. A large number of other disorders must be excluded by special studies. Some cases resolve spontaneously, and others improve with corticosteroid treatment, immunosuppressive drugs, or gamma globulin.

Splenectomy is done if steroids cannot be given, if they are ineffective, or if relapse occurs. Long-term remission is produced by splenectomy in 70% of patients, and another 15% have some favorable response. Laparoscopic splenectomy is gaining acceptance in this and other conditions.

4. Myelofibrosis is a myeloproliferative disorder related to polycythemia vera and myelogenous leukemia. Anemia, bleeding, and infection are common. Spleen is greatly enlarged and may cause local symptoms. Symptomatic cases are improved by splenectomy, but the operative mortality rate is 12%.

D. SPLENIC ABSCESS. Abscess may develop in the spleen from hematogenous seeding, by direct extension from adjacent infection, or secondary infection of a traumatic hematoma. Abscesses elsewhere are common in these cases. Splenic abscess should be suspected in a patient with unexplained sepsis, abdominal pain, and splenomegaly. Splenic scan or arteriogram reveals a filling defect. Splenectomy is the treatment in most cases; simple abscess drainage is relied upon if splenectomy would be hazardous.

E. COMPLICATIONS OF SPLENECTOMY

1. Thrombocytosis. Platelet count routinely rises after splenectomy and sometimes they exceed 1 million/μl. The peak response is about 7-10 days after operation. There is little apparent risk of thromboembolic complications, and anticoagulation is not warranted, but antiplatelet aggregating agents (e.g., aspirin) are advisable if thrombocytosis reaches very high levels.

2. Immune deficiency. Splenectomy places the patient at an increased risk of infection by encapsulated bacteria. The risk is greatest in children, but fulminant pneumococcemia has been reported after splenectomy in adults. Patients should be immunized against pneumococcus after splenectomy using a polyvalent vaccine (Pneumovax). Revaccination in 5 years is recommended.

XVII. EXTERNAL ABDOMINAL HERNIAS

Internal abdominal hernias include diaphragmatic hernia (see Chapter 19), acquired hernias caused by adhesions, and congenital hernias into the foramen of Winslow, paraduodenal spaces, etc. Intestinal obstruction is the usual manifestation, and treatment is by surgical repair.

An **external abdominal hernia** is an abnormal protrusion of intraabdominal tissues through a congenital or acquired defect in the abdominal wall. Various types are discussed individually in this section.

A. DEFINITIONS

1. Reducible. The contents of the hernia sac return to the abdomen spontaneously or with manual pressure.

2. Incarcerated (irreducible). The contents of the sac cannot be returned to the abdomen with manual pressure.

3. Strangulated. Blood supply to contents of the sac is compromised.

4. Richter's hernia. Part of the circumstance of a loop of bowel becomes incarcerated in the hernia sac.

B. INGUINAL HERNIAS. Indirect inguinal hernia is a protrusion of peritoneum, with or without abdominal viscera, through the internal inguinal ring. The defect is congenital and due to persistence of the processus vaginalis peritonei. The hernia may be apparent in infancy, or it may not become evident until later; most are diagnosed before age 50 years. Cryptorchidism and hydrocele are commonly associated with indirect hernias in male infants. Indirect inguinal hernia is more common in males than in females, but it is nevertheless the most common type of hernia of the groin in females.

Direct inguinal hernia is a protrusion through **Hesselbach's triangle,** which is bounded by the inguinal ligament inferiorly, the inferior epigastric vessels laterally and superiorly, and the border of the rectus muscle medially. Direct hernia is an acquired diffuse weakness of the transversalis fascia in the floor of the inguinal canal; it is often bilateral, and it is related to older age, obesity, persistent cough, and other conditions that chronically raise intraabdominal pressure. Direct hernia is rare in women, young men, and children of either sex. In some patients, both an indirect and direct inguinal hernia are present on the same side (pantaloon or saddlebag hernia).

1. Diagnosis

a. Symptoms. Asymptomatic hernias are discovered on routine examination. A bulge or lump in the groin, accentuated by coughing, defecation, lifting, or other physical activity; the mass extends into the scrotum in some cases. Discomfort in the groin, especially as the hernia enlarges.

b. Signs

(1) A mass in the groin, reducible or incarcerated, sometimes extending into the scrotum. In infants and women, the presence of a mass is the only finding. Small asymptomatic hernias may not be visible.

(2) In older boys and in men, the following maneuver should be performed. The scrotum is invaginated with the index finger, and the finger is placed against or through the external inguinal ring. Instruct the patient to bear down (strain) as though to defecate; this provides a sustained increase in intraabdominal pressure. The hernia sac is a balloon-like structure which impresses upon the pulp of the finger directly or from the lateral aspect. **An enlarged external ring is not a hernia,** although it is likely that a hernia is the cause of the enlargement, and a hernia must be carefully sought if the ring is large enough to admit the index finger. Inguinal hernia is most easily demonstrable with the patient standing, but examine the patient both standing and supine.

(3) *Indirect versus direct.* Indirect hernia is an elliptical mass descending obliquely in the inguinal canal. It may enter the scrotum. The mass strikes the lateral aspect of the examining finger. Pressure over the internal ring with one hand prevents the hernia from entering the inguinal canal. A direct hernia is a spherical mass which rarely descends into the scrotum. The mass impresses on the examining finger from directly in front. Manual pressure over the internal ring does not reduce the hernia.

c. Contributory factors. The history and physical examination should include a search for causes of increased intraabdominal pressure that may have contributed to development of the hernia. Bladder outlet obstruction, chronic cough, and ascites are among these underlying problems. Digital rectal examination, including palpation of the prostate, should be done.

2. Differential diagnosis. Femoral hernia (see below). "Lipoma of the cord" (properitoneal fat entering the spermatic cord) resembles a hernia and may not be recognized until operation. Hydrocele and varicocele (see Chapter 14). Lymphadenopathy.

3. Complications

a. Incarceration does not imply intestinal obstruction or strangulation.

b. Obstruction of bowel in the sac has the clinical features of any other form of intestinal obstruction. Strangulation is a risk with obstructed bowel, but it is not necessarily present.

c. Strangulation causes symptoms and signs of intestinal obstruction if the strangulated viscus is bowel. Omentum may also strangulate. There may be erythema, edema, and tenderness over the hernia; often abdominal findings mask the inguinal manifestations, especially in obese patients.

4. Treatment. All indirect inguinal hernias, regardless of age, and large or symptomatic direct hernias should be repaired unless there are strong contraindications. Coexistent respiratory and obstructive urologic disease should be improved or corrected first. Acutely incarcerated hernias should be reduced or operated on immediately. Obstruction or strangulation requires emergency operation. Common methods of surgical repair are as follows:

a. High ligation of the sac is the procedure of choice for indirect inguinal hernias in infants and children.

b. Bassini repair. The indirect sac is opened, explored, and ligated; the inguinal floor is strengthened by suture of transversalis fascia to the inguinal ligament behind the cord. Direct sacs are usually imbricated and not opened. This method is popular for indirect hernias in adults.

c. McVay or Lotheissen repair. Transversalis fascia is sutured to Cooper's ligament behind the cord after ligation of any indirect sac. This operation is often used for direct and femoral hernias.

d. Shouldice repair. Transversalis fascia is divided longitudinally and the two flaps are imbricated to the inguinal ligament. Suture of the internal oblique muscle and the conjoined tendon to the external oblique aponeurosis reinforces the repair. This technic is applicable to indirect or direct hernias.

e. Preperitoneal repairs. The preperitoneal space can be dissected through a lower abdominal incision, and the indirect or direct hernia can be repaired. Prosthetic mesh (e.g., Marlex) is usually placed as part of the repair of large direct defects; this step also is added by some surgeons to repairs done through the anterior approach. Recurrent hernias seem particularly suitable for this method.

f. Laparoscopic herniorrhaphy. Early experience with preperitoneal or transperitoneal hernia repairs by the laparoscopic approach is encouraging, but many questions remain about the durability of these procedures and the cost-benefit comparisons with more traditional repairs.

5. Prognosis. Healing is promoted by avoidance of heavy lifting or straining. Manual laborers should not return to work for 4-6 weeks; people in sedentary occupations may return to work in a few days.

Indirect inguinal hernias recur in 2%-3% of patients. Direct hernias recur in up to 10% of cases. Repair of a recurrent hernia is followed by another recurrence in 10%-20% of patients.

B. SLIDING INGUINAL HERNIA is one in which a viscus forms part of the wall of the hernia sac. The viscus may be cecum, sigmoid colon, bladder, or ovary. Sliding hernias may be indistinguishable from other types preoperatively, but large size and chronic incarceration should raise the suspicion of sliding hernia.

Because the viscus invariably comprises the posterior wall, all indirect inguinal hernia sacs should be opened anteriorly to avoid accidental entry into bowel or bladder. Standard texts should be consulted for special technics of repair of sliding hernias.

C. FEMORAL HERNIA. In this type, the sac enters the femoral canal on the medial side of the femoral vein deep to the inguinal ligament. The sac then may curve anteriorly and superiorly around the inguinal ligament to present in the inguinal area. Femoral hernia is more common in women.

The mass is visible or palpable in the upper medial thigh, or it may appear to reside above the inguinal ligament where it is difficult to distinguish from inguinal hernia. Femoral hernia must also be distinguished from lymphadenopathy and saphenous varix. Because the neck is narrow, femoral hernia is prone to incarceration and strangulation. The hernia is often overlooked in obese patients with intestinal obstruction.

Treatment is by surgical repair through a standard inguinal incision. If it is difficult to reduce the hernia though the small neck, special maneuvers are required. Strangulated bowel is an indication to open the abdomen through a separate incision. Recurrences develop in about 10% of patients.

D. UMBILICAL HERNIA in children is discussed in Chapter 19. After spontaneous closure of the umbilical ring in infancy, some adults gradually develop widening of the ring and formation of an umbilical hernia. Increased intraabdominal pressure is responsible (obesity, pregnancy, ascites, etc.)

The hernia is diagnosed by inspection and palpation. Omentum is the usual content of the sac, although bowel is present in large ones. Strangulation is common because of the unyielding fascia and small size of the defect.

Surgical repair should be done to prevent strangulation. Small hernias can be sutured transversely under local anesthesia. The skin should be tacked to the fascia to preserve the umbilicus. Large umbilical hernias require general anesthesia and more elaborate repair.

E. EPIGASTRIC HERNIA is protrusion through the linea alba in the upper abdomen. A mass (usually properitoneal fat, sometimes omentum and bowel) is palpable in the midline or just to the left. Many are asymptomatic, but epigastric hernia can be the source of unexplained pain and GI symptoms. Repair under local anesthesia is simple and effective for small hernias; larger ones are best repaired under general anesthesia.

F. INCISIONAL (VENTRAL) HERNIA. Dehiscence of fascia in an abdominal incision results in a hernia. Infection, technical errors, and associated diseases (obesity, malnutrition) account for most incisional hernias. Dehiscence may be a dramatic event in the early postoperative period (see Wound Complications in Chapter 2), or it may develop slowly over a period of weeks.

Incisional hernia is an uncomfortable and unsightly protrusion which is prone to incarceration and strangulation, especially if the defect is small. Repair is recommended for most of them. Care must be taken to excise attenuated fascia and to approximate healthy structures with nonabsorbable sutures; tension on the suture line should be avoided.

Large ventral hernias pose technical problems. Contents of the hernia cannot be returned to the peritoneal cavity in extreme cases; preoperative injections of air (pneumoperitoneum) may expand the peritoneal cavity and aid in surgical reduction. The same factors which contributed to dehiscence initially may still be present (e.g., obesity, chronic respiratory disease), and, in some cases, it is wise to avoid repair unless or until the associated problems can be corrected. Marlex mesh may be needed to bridge the fascial defect if wide mobilization and relaxing incisions do not bring the margins together without tension. Recurrence rate is high after repair of large defects.

G. OTHER HERNIAS

1. Spigelian hernia is a hernia through the linea semilunaris (where the layers of investing fascia of the oblique muscles fuse to form the rectus sheath). The most common site is in the lower abdomen at the junction of the linea semilunaris and the semicircular line of Douglas; at this point, all of the fascia of the oblique muscles passes anterior to the rectus muscle, and the posterior rectus sheath is deficient. Spigelian hernia causes discomfort and is prone to strangulation. The sac often protrudes laterally between deep layers and is difficult to palpate. For this reason, the diagnosis is frequently missed. Spigelian hernia should be repaired.

2. Lumbar hernia is a hernia through one of the lumbar triangles in the posterior abdominal wall.

3. Littre's hernia. This oddity is an external abdominal hernia (at any site) containing only a Meckel's diverticulum.

13

Gynecology

Edward C. Hill

I. EXAMINATION OF THE GYNECOLOGIC PATIENT

A. HISTORY. A complete history should be taken on all gynecologic patients with particular emphasis on menstrual history, sexual activity, past pregnancy, previous gynecologic disorders, vaginal bleeding or discharge, and pelvic pain.

B. PHYSICAL EXAMINATION should also be complete, including the breasts. In addition to a speculum and bimanual examination, the pelvic examination includes a careful combined rectovaginal palpation to detect small lesions occupying the cul-de-sac and the rectovaginal septum.

C. GYNECOLOGIC LABORATORY TESTS

1. Wet smear. A suspension of vaginal discharge in a drop of isotonic saline solution placed on a slide and coverslipped will confirm the diagnosis of *Trichomona vaginalis* vaginitis or *Gardnerella (Haemophilus)* infections. A suspension in 10% KOH solution should be done for suspected monilial vulvovaginitis.

2. Exfoliative cytology. Sampling of the squamocolumnar junction of the cervix for cytologic examination is a vital part of the routine pelvic examination to screen for early neoplastic lesions (dysplasia and carcinoma-in-situ). The exocervix is scraped with an appropriately designed spatula, and an endocervical sample is obtained with a cotton-tipped applicator or specially designed endocervical brush. The material is spread uniformly on a slide and fixed immediately.

3. Tissue biopsy. Samples of tissue may be obtained from the vulva with a dermatologist's skin punch, under local anesthesia. A punch biopsy forceps may be used to obtain tissue from the vagina or exocervix; local anesthesia usually is not necessary in these locations. The endocervix and endometrial cavity can be sampled with small curettes specifically designed for this purpose.

4. Tests of endocrine function. Hormonal studies include vaginal cell maturation index on cytologic specimens obtained from the lateral vaginal wall at the level of the cervix, fern test of cervical mucus, biologic tests for pregnancy, and a variety of special hormone assays.

D. SPECIAL TESTS

1. Schiller test. When neoplastic disease is suspected, the cervical and vaginal mucosa is painted with a strong iodine solution such as Lugol's. Nonstaining areas represent nonglycogenated cells which should be biopsied.

2. Colposcopy. The colposcope is a low-power microscope with a long focal distance used to identify areas of intraepithelial neoplasia. This examination requires special training.

3. Culdocentesis. Needle aspiration of the peritoneal cul-de-sac through the posterior vaginal fornix is a simple but informative procedure in a variety of clinical circumstances—e.g., suspected intraperitoneal bleeding or pelvic infection.

4. Laparoscopy. Examination of the internal genitalia and surrounding organs with a fiberoptic instrument after the introduction of CO_2 or NO_2 gas is a useful diagnostic procedure.

5. Hysteroscopy. Inspection of the endometrial cavity with a specially designed fiberoptic instrument has recently been added to diagnostic methods.

6. Pelvic sonography. Use of high-frequency sound waves to outline pelvic structures has proved extremely useful as a gynecologic diagnostic aid.

E. RADIOGRAPHIC STUDIES

1. Hysterosalpingography. A contrast medium is introduced through the cervical canal to outline radiographically the endometrial cavity and fallopian tubes. It is the test most frequently used to determine patency of the fallopian tubes in patients who are infertile.

2. Computerized tomography. This highly specialized radiographic technic affords cross-sectional examination of the abdomen and pelvis.

3. Magnetic resonance imaging allows a high-resolution detail of the pelvic organs and avoids radiation exposure.

4. Screening mammography following the guidelines of the American Cancer Society.

II. LEUKORRHEA

Leukorrhea is excessive nonbloody vaginal discharge. It may be mucoid or purulent, thick or thin, malodorous or inoffensive, nonirritating or accompanied by itching or burning. The causes are numerous:

1. Excess mucus due to hyperestrinism. Mid-cycle production; pregnancy; exogenous hormone; foreign bodies in the vagina.

2. Infection. *T. vaginalis;* moniliasis; *Gardnerella (Haemophilus)* vaginitis; *Herpes hominis* type 2 infection (see Section IV.D); human papilloma virus (HPV) producing flat condyloma on mucous membrane surfaces; gonorrhea; *Chlamydia trachomatis* cervicitis; mixed infections (atrophic vaginitis); bacterial vaginosis.

3. Cervical inflammation (see Section V). Cervicitis due to old obstetric lacerations; ectopy (columnar epithelium on exocervix).

A. FOREIGN BODIES. Forgotten tampons are a frequent cause of foul, purulent discharge in adults. Crayons, safety pins, paper clips, and so on, may be deposited in the vagina by children. Speculum examination reveals the source. Anesthetic may be required in children. Treatment is removal of foreign body.

B. *TRICHOMONAS VAGINALIS VAGINITIS.* *T. vaginalis* causes a thick, yellow-to-green frothy discharge with vulvar itching or burning. The vaginal mucosa may show typical punctate, erythematous "strawberry" marks. Diagnosis is confirmed by a microscopic wet smear examination.

Metronidazole (Flagyl) is the treatment of choice. The organism is transmitted by sexual congress, so both partners should be treated simultaneously with 250 mg orally three times daily for 7 days, or 2 g in 1 day in a single dose; it is contraindicated during pregnancy and lactation.

C. MONILIASIS. Vaginal yeast infections usually are caused by *Candida albicans.* Diabetics and women who eat many sweets are particularly susceptible. Other predisposing factors include pregnancy, oral contraceptives, and administration of antibiotics for some unrelated condition. Vulvar itching and a nonodorous discharge like cottage cheese are common symptoms. The vulvar mucosa is fiery red, and a thick white exudate is present in the vagina.

The exudate or scrapings from the vulva are suspended in 10% KOH to reveal the spores and/or mycelia of the organism. Nickerson's medium is best for culturing *Candida;* typical brown colonies develop.

Either clotrimazole 1% vaginal cream (Mycelex-G or Gyne-Lotrimin) or miconazole nitrate 2% cream (Monistat) applied intravaginally at bedtime each night for 1 week. Treatment should be continued for 2 weeks in refractory cases. The cream should be applied to the vulva three to four times daily for the control of pruritus. Vaginal tablets of clotrimazole may be substituted for the cream.

D. GARDNERELLA (HAEMOPHILUS) VAGINITIS, also known as "bacterial vaginosis," is a specific bacterial infection producing a thin, grey discharge with a "fishy" odor, often without local irritation. The diagnosis is made by finding the so-called "clue-cell" (a squamous epithelial cell speckled by numerous dark (gram negative) bacilli on a wet smear [saline] preparation). Clumps of *G. vaginalis* organisms may also be seen floating free.

Metronidazole (Flagyl) in a dose of 250 mg, three times daily, after meals, for 7 days to the patient and her sexual partner. Ampicillin or tetracycline in doses of 250 mg, four times daily for 2 weeks may also be used, but precautions should be taken to prevent overgrowth of monilia in the lower reproductive tract (clotrimazole vaginal tablets each night).

E. GONORRHEA. *Neisseria gonorrhoeae* infection of the cervix produces a creamy yellow discharge. A history of exposure to gonorrhea frequently is absent. A Gram's stain of the exudate may show the typical coffee bean–shaped, gram-negative, intracellular diplococci. Culture is essential for a definitive diagnosis because of similar nonpathogenic diplococci found in the lower reproductive tract. Thayer-Martin and blood agar are the best culture media.

Cervical gonorrhea may lead to ascending infection, producing acute and chronic salpingitis and pelvic peritonitis (see page 645). A serologic test for syphilis should be obtained whenever a diagnosis of gonorrhea is made.

Treatment of gonorrheal cervicitis is best carried out by giving probenecid (1 g orally) 30 minutes before the IM injection of aqueous procaine penicillin G (4.8 million units in two or more divided doses at different sites). If the patient is allergic to penicillin, oral tetracycline HCl (1.5 g initially followed by 500 mg four times daily for 4 days) should be administered. Follow-up cultures should be obtained 7-14 days after completion of treatment.

F. CHLAMYDIA CERVICITIS. The columnar cells of the cervix serve as a reservoir for *C. trachomatis,* the microorganism responsible for **trachoma inclusion conjunctivitis,** the urethral syndrome, mucopurulent cervicitis, salpingitis, and the Fitz-Hugh-Curtis syndrome. The agent is transmitted by sexual intercourse and causes a cervicitis which may be asymptomatic or produce a mucopurulent discharge. As with gonorrhea, ascending infection of the fallopian tubes occurs frequently. If suspected, the diagnosis is made by culturing the organism. Treatment is by administration of tetracycline, 250 mg 4 times daily for 2 weeks.

G. ATROPHIC VAGINITIS is encountered in postmenopausal women, whether the menopause is natural or secondary to surgical or radiation castration. The discharge often is thick and yellow and accompanied by vulvar burning and dyspareunia. Examination reveals a diffusely erythematous, smooth, atrophic mucosa. Pap smear for estrogen effect (best taken from the lateral vaginal wall at the level of the cervix) shows a predominance of immature squamous epithelial cells and few superficial cells.

Treat with estrogen vaginal cream (Premarin) or dienestrol vaginal cream, ½ applicatorful each night at bedtime for 2 weeks, then twice weekly.

III. ABNORMALITIES OF MENSTRUATION

A. DYSFUNCTIONAL UTERINE BLEEDING is irregular, frequent, or prolonged bleeding due to chronic failure to ovulate (progesterone deficiency), resulting eventually in endometrial hyperplasia. It occurs most often in adolescents and premenopausal women. It is also encountered in association with polycystic ovaries (Stein-Leventhal syndrome) and with uncommon granulosa-theca cell tumors of the ovary.

1. Diagnosis. Organic causes of bleeding must be excluded. A sample of the endometrium obtained either by dilatation and curettage or endometrial biopsy reveals proliferative endometrium in the second half of the menstrual cycle or cystic and/or adenomatous hyperplasia of the endometrium.

2. Complications. Anemia secondary to acute or chronic blood loss. Hypovolemic shock in patients with acute severe bleeding episodes. Hyperplasia with atypia (in a small number of patients) is a premalignant condition leading to the development of endometrial carcinoma.

3. Treatment

a. Mild to moderate bleeding can be controlled with a combination estrogen-progestin (mestranol and norethynodrel). Two tablets/day for 4 days of 1 mg of norethynodrel and 150 μg of mestranol, then one tablet daily for 3 weeks. Subsequent cycles are then given using combinations containing 50 μg or less of the estrogen.

b. Severe bleeding. Transfuse if hypovolemic shock is present. Conjugated estrogens (20 mg IV) to control acute bleeding, then oral estrogen-progestin combination by mouth daily for 3 weeks. Dilatation and curettage.

B. DYSMENORRHEA (PRIMARY) is incapacitating painful menstruation in the absence of organic disease. The condition always is preceded by ovulation and may be related to increased amplitude of uterine contractions associated with prostaglandin effect on the myometrium. There may be some degree of myometrial ischemia.

1. Diagnosis. *Symptoms:* Intermittent cramping lower abdominal pain radiating to the back and thighs beginning with or just prior to the onset of menstruation. *Signs:* Absence of organic disease, e.g., pelvic endometriosis or chronic salpingo-oophoritis.

2. Treatment. Simple analgesics (aspirin or acetaminophen, with or without codeine) every 3-4 hours. Prostaglandin inhibitors such as indomethacin (25 mg, three times daily), ibuprofen (400 mg, three times daily), naproxen sodium (250 mg, twice daily), or mefenamic acid (250 mg, four times daily). Suppression of ovulation: estrogen-progestin contraceptive routine.

C. AMENORRHEA. The failure to menstruate may be either primary or secondary. **Primary amenorrhea** is the failure of menstruation in a postpubertal female. Causes include congenital abnormalities (imperforate hymen and congenital absence of the vagina and/or uterus) and inherited endocrine disorders such as gonadal dysgenesis (Turner's syndrome) and androgen insensitivity syndrome. **Secondary amenorrhea** is the cessation of menses once menstrual function has become established. Pregnancy is by far the most common cause. Other causes are polycystic ovary (Stein-Leventhal) syndrome, premature menopause, cervical stricture, intrauterine synechiae (Asherman's syndrome), and pituitary adenomas.

Amenorrhea is merely a symptom and not a disease. The diagnosis often can be made on the basis of a careful history and physical examination. In some instances, a host of laboratory tests and special procedures are required to arrive at the correct diagnosis.

IV. DISORDERS OF EXTERNAL FEMALE GENITALIA

A. IMPERFORATE HYMEN is a developmental failure of the vagina to canalize at the hymeneal ring.

   1. Diagnosis. *Symptoms:* usually not recognized until the menarche; amenorrhea with cyclic lower abdominal cramping pain. *Signs:* hymeneal bulge may be evident on physical examination; a tender lower abdominal and pelvic cystic mass (hematometra and hematocolpos). Pelvic sonography is confirmative.

   2. Treatment. Surgical incision of the imperforate hymen under local anesthesia is definitive.

B. BARTHOLIN GLAND ABSCESS AND CYST. Acute bartholinitis results from pyogenic infection by *Neisseria,* staphylococci, streptococci, or coliform organisms. Inflammatory occlusion of the duct leads to an abscess. Closure of the duct in the absence of infection produces mucus retention and cyst formation.

   1. Diagnosis
   a. Abscess. Pain and swelling in the area of the posterior portion of the labia; dyspareunia; examination reveals a tender, fluctuant mass with surrounding cellulitis.

   b. Cyst. A mass noted by the patient; a soft nontender, fluctuant mass on examination.

   2. Treatment
   a. Abscess. Incision and drainage, culture and sensitivity should be obtained and appropriate antibiotic therapy begun.

   b. Cyst. No treatment if small and asymptomatic; large symptomatic cysts require marsupialization (see Figure 13-1); it is rarely necessary to excise the gland and duct.

C. HERPES GENITALIS. Venereal infection by herpesvirus hominis, type 2, is an increasingly common vulvar disease. During pregnancy it may be responsible for stillbirth and neonatal death. It has been associated with cervical intraepithelial neoplasia and may be a carcinogen.

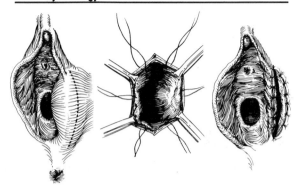

FIGURE 13-1. Marsupialization of Bartholin's cyst.

1. Diagnosis

a. Painful, erythematous papules, vesicles, and/or super-ficial ulcers of the vagina, vulva, and cervix; malaise, fever, anorexia, dysuria, urinary retention, and inguinofemoral ade-nopathy in severe cases, particularly first infections.

b. Laboratory tests. Cytologic smears of the lesions of-ten are diagnostic; the organism can be cultured, but this is rarely necessary; serum antibodies are indicative of previous infection.

2. Treatment. Acyclovir is beneficial in primary infec-tions when administered orally, parenterally, or topically. Top-ical therapy of recurrent infections has not been helpful, but there is some promise for oral acyclovir. Topical 2.5% lido-caine (Xylocaine) affords temporary relief of pain.

D. CONDYLOMATA ACUMINATA (VENEREAL WARTS)

are warty excrescenses caused by human papilloma virus (HPV) involving the vulvar and perianal skin and mucous membranes of the vulva, vagina, and cervix. In the vagina and on the cervix they are often flat and difficult to recognize grossly. The application of 3% acetic acid and colposcopy are helpful. The growths may coalesce to produce large conglomerations, particularly during pregnancy. Condylomata are often associated with leukorrhea-producing conditions. The diagnosis is made by inspection, but in doubtful cases biopsy should be done.

1. Treatment. Podophyllum resin (10%-25% solution in tincture of benzoin) is applied topically to the warts, protecting the surrounding skin and mucous membrane with petrolatum; patient should be instructed to wash the area with soap and water 6 hours after application. Patient application of 0.5 podofilox, a purified and less toxic preparation, is also effective. Electrodessication or laser therapy in extensive lesions. Liquid nitrogen can also be used. Interferon therapy in persistent disease. Treat cause of leukorrhea.

E. SOLID BENIGN TUMORS OF THE VULVA. Papillomas, fibromas, lipomas, hidradenomas, angiomas, and leiomyomas may be found on the vulva. Small asymptomatic tumors may require no treatment. Any tumor should be biopsied and/or excised if there is suspicion of malignancy.

F. MALIGNANT CONDITIONS OF THE VULVA

1. Squamous cell carcinoma is the most common malignancy. In its early stages, it appears as dysplasia or carcinoma-in-situ, often in the presence of long-standing vulvar irritation with pruritus (chronic vulvar dystrophy) or HPV infection.

a. Diagnosis. (1) Any chronic, irritating lesion of the vulva may represent a malignancy; **biopsy is essential** if malignancy is to be recognized early. (2) Dysplasia and carcinoma-in-situ often appear as red, white, or brown patches **(leukoplakia);** a benign lesion, lichen sclerosis et atrophicus, is a more common cause of white patches; biopsy is necessary to differentiate these lesions. (3) Squamous cell carcinoma occurs most often after the menopause; the lesions are papillary, cauliflower-like, nodular, or ulcerative; metastases are found in the inguinofemoral lymph nodes in 45% of patients; biopsy is diagnostic.

b. Stage grouping of vulvar carcinoma
DEFINITIONS OF CLINICAL STAGES IN CARCINOMA OF THE VULVA (FIGO 1988)

Stage 0
    Tis   Carcinoma in situ; intraepithelial carcinoma.

Stage I
T1, N0, M0 Tumor confined to the vulva;
T1, N1, M0 ≤2 cm in greatest dimension.
Nodes are not palpable, or are
palpable in either groin, not enlarged, mobile (not clinically
suspicious of neoplasm).

Stage II
T2, N0, M0 Tumor confined to the vulva
and/or perineum; >2 cm in
greatest dimension. No nodal
metastasis.

Stage III
T3, N0, M0 Tumor of any size with
T3, N1, M0 (1) Adjacent spread to the
T1, N1, M0 lower urethra and/or
T2, N1, M0 the vagina, or the anus
and/or
(2) Unilateral regional
lymph node metasta-
sis.

Stage IVA
T1, N2, M0 Tumor invades any of the fol-
T2, N2, M0 lowing:
T3, N2, M0 Upper urethra, bladder mu-
T4, N2, M0 cosa, rectal mucosa, pel-
vic bone, and/or bilat-
eral regional node me-
tastases.

Stage IVB
Any T or N Any distant metastasis in-
M1 cluding pelvic lymph nodes.

c. Treatment. (1) Local incision, laser therapy, or skin-
ning vulvectomy prevents progression of dysplasia or
carcinoma-in-situ to invasive carcinoma; (2) Carcinoma requires radical vulvectomy with bilateral inguinofemoral (and
possibly iliac-obturator) lymph node dissection.

d. Prognosis. The 5-year survival rate for squamous cell
carcinoma of the vulva varies from 95% in lesions <2 cm in
diameter without lymph node metastases to about 60% in more

extensive lesions localized to the vulva and the superficial inguinal lymph nodes. When the process has extended to the deep pelvic (iliac and obturator) lymph nodes, the chances of cure are poor.

2. Paget's disease of the vulva is an in-situ malignancy. Chronic, red, weeping, scaling, eczematoid lesions should be biopsied to make the diagnosis. Wide excision of the entire lesion, often requiring radical vulvectomy, is adequate treatment.

3. Other malignancies, including melanoma, basal cell carcinoma, Bartholin's gland cancer, and sarcoma, are rare in the vulva. The vulva may be the site of secondary cancer from the endometrium, cervix, vagina, or distant sites (e.g., lymphoma and leukemia).

V. DISORDERS OF THE CERVIX

A. CERVICITIS

1. Acute gonorrheal cervicitis is infection of the columnar epithelium of the endocervix by *N. gonorrhoeae.* The primary symptom is a purulent, thick creamy, yellow discharge, although many infections are asymptomatic. Cervicitis is often associated with infection of the periurethral (Skene's) glands. (See Section II for treatment.)

2. Chronic nonspecific cervicitis (see chlamydia cervicitis, page 627). In the majority of adolescents the columnar epithelium of the endocervix is found on the portio vaginalis of the cervix surrounding the external os. This epithelium is gradually undergoing transformation to a metaplastic type of squamous epithelium, but it is only a single cell layer in thickness, so infection of the underlying cervical stroma by organisms which normally inhabit the vagina is common. The transformation process leads to a plugging of the numerous crypts and tunnels of endocervical mucosa by squamous epithelium, giving rise to **nabothian cysts.**

a. Diagnosis. Symptoms: many patients are asymptomatic; a mucoid type of discharge is frequently the only symptom. Signs: a red, granular, friable area surrounding the external cervical os; excessive mucus production. Colposcopy is confirmative.

b. Laboratory tests: Cytologic examination reveals columnar and metaplastic squamous epithelial cells scattered among the normal squamous epithelial cells; biopsy demonstrates endocervical type of mucosa and rules out neoplasia.

c. Treatment. No treatment is required in asymptomatic patients. The endocervical mucosa will eventually be replaced physiologically by a stratified squamous epithelium. If leukorrhea is a complaint, cryosurgery, electrocoagulation, or laser vaporization of the columnar epithelium is beneficial.

B. CERVICAL POLYPS. These benign neoplasms usually arise from the endocervix and present as fleshy, polypoid structures at or near the external cervical os.

1. Diagnosis

a. Symptoms. May be asymptomatic and discovered during a routine pelvic examination; intermenstrual or postcoital bleeding.

b. Signs. A red, polypoid structure in the cervical canal at or near the external cervical os.

c. Differential diagnosis. Distinguish from polypoid cancers and sarcomas arising from the cervix or endometrial cavity.

2. Treatment. Most polyps are pedunculated and have a small base; they can be removed by grasping the pedicle with a clamp and rotating the polyp until it separates. All polyps should be submitted for pathologic examination because of the small risk of malignancy (<1%). All cervical polyps are infected. Acute salpingitis rarely follows polypectomy. Antibiotic therapy should be given if it occurs.

C. DYSPLASIA AND CARCINOMA-IN-SITU OF THE CERVIX. Dysplasia is a disorder in the maturation of the squamous epithelium of the cervix which in some patients becomes progressively more severe and results in malignancy. It is graded cytologically and histologically as mild, moderate, or severe. The endstage of the dysplastic process is carcinoma-in-situ which will eventually lead to invasive squamous cell cancer of the cervix if it is not treated (see Figure 13-2).

1. Diagnosis. Usually there are no symptoms or signs of dysplasia or carcinoma-in-situ. The cervix appears normal to gross inspection. The mucosa involved in the intraepithelial neoplastic process is nonstaining to strong iodine (Lugol's) solution (Schiller test).

Colposcopic findings are often abnormal: white epithelium, coarse punctation, mosaicism, and atypical blood vessels.

Cervical punch biopsy of nonstaining areas on the Schiller test is moderately accurate. Colposcopically-directed biopsies

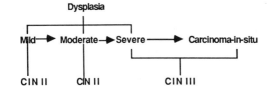

FIGURE 13-2. The spectrum of intraepithelial neoplasia of the cervix (CIN = cervical intraepithelial neoplasia).

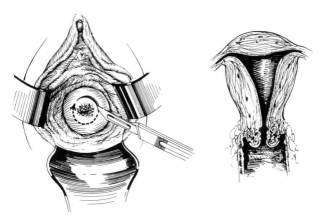

FIGURE 13-3. Conization of the cervix.

are more accurate. Cold-knife cone biopsy (Figure 13-3) with dilatation and curettage may be necessary if the process extends into the endocervical canal.

   2. Treatment. Mild dysplasia is managed by careful observation with repeated clinical and cytologic examinations every 6 months in the expectation of spontaneous regression.

   Persistent mild, moderate, and **severe dysplasia** and **carcinoma-in-situ** should be treated by eradication of the abnormal epithelium. This requires accurate identification of the involved area. Colposcopy is helpful in this regard. Small areas may be completely removed with the punch biopsy forceps. More extensive lesions require electrocoagulation, cryosurgery, laser therapy, loop electrosurgical excision, or cold-knife cone biopsy.

3. Warning. Dysplasia and carcinoma-in-situ may be found on the periphery of an invasive carcinoma. The accepted treatment of intraepithelial neoplasia is totally inadequate for invasive cancer of the cervix.

D. CANCER OF THE CERVIX is the second most common malignancy of the female reproductive tract (after endometrial carcinoma). It is rare before 20 years of age and reaches a peak between the ages of 45 and 55 years. Squamous cell cancer comprises 80% of cervical cancers. The remainder are adenocarcinomas, mixed types (adenosquamous) sarcomas, and metastatic neoplasms. Squamous cell cancer is related to sexual activity; early sexual exposure and promiscuity are prominent factors in the epidemiology. An association has been established between cancer of the cervix and infection with herpesvirus hominis, type 2, and with HPV producing flat condylomata. The neoplasm extends directly to adjacent structures and metastasizes via lymphatics to the pelvic lymph nodes thence to the para-aortic lymph nodes.

1. Diagnosis

a. Symptoms. Abnormal vaginal bleeding or discharge, particularly intermenstrual or postcoital bleeding, is often the only symptom. Pain, anorexia, and weight loss are manifestations of far-advanced disease.

b. Signs. An exophytic, ulcerative, papillary or indurative lesion on the cervix; induration of the adjacent vagina and parametria if the cancer spreads beyond the cervix.

c. Laboratory tests. Cytologic examination (6% of Pap smears are falsely negative in patients with invasive cancer), histopathologic examination of a punch biopsy is usually diagnostic.

d. Radiographs. Intravenous urography may show ureteral obstruction with hydronephrosis or a nonfunctioning kidney in advanced disease. Chest radiography may show metastases. CT with contrast may be substituted for IVP and may be more informative.

e. Special tests. Cystoscopy to evaluate the degree of bladder involvement. Proctosigmoidoscopy to determine if there is invasion of the bowel wall. MRI may help determine extent of disease.

2. Stage grouping of cervical cancer is judged clinically and is defined according to the following international classification.

Stage 0	Carcinoma-in-situ.
Stage I	Carcinoma confined to the cervix (extension to the corpus should be disregarded).
Ia1	Minimal microscopically evident stromal invasion.
Ia2	Lesions detected microscopically that can be measured. The upper limit of measurement should not show a depth of invasion of >5 mm taken from the base of the epithelium, either surface or glandular, from which it originates, and the horizontal spread must **not** exceed 7 mm.
Ib	Lesions >Ia
Stage II	Carcinoma extends beyond the cervix but not onto the pelvic wall.
IIa	No parametrial involvement. The cancer involves the vagina, but not the lower one third.
IIb	Parametrial involvement.
Stage III	Carcinoma extends onto the pelvic wall. No cancer-free space between tumor and pelvic wall. Or, the tumor involves the lower one third of the vagina. Or, hydronephrosis or nonfunctioning kidney.
IIIa	No extension onto the pelvic wall. Vaginal involvement of the lower third.
IIb	Extension onto the pelvic wall and/or hydronephrosis or nonfunctioning kidney.
Stage IV	Carcinoma extends beyond the true pelvis or clinically involves the mucosa of the bladder or rectum.
IVa	Spread of growth to adjacent organs (bladder or rectum with positive biopsy).
IVb	Spread of growth to distant organs.

3. Treatment

a. Stage I. Radiation therapy or radical hysterectomy with bilateral pelvic lymph node dissection can be used in stage I disease. The surgical approach is preferable in the young patient because of the possibility of ovarian preservation and freedom from the interference with sexual function which frequently follows radiation therapy. Radical hysterectomy and lymph node removal are also the treatment of choice in patients who are poor candidates for radiotherapy (e.g., those with ulcerative colitis, chronic pelvic infections, pelvic endometriosis with bowel adhesions, diverticulitis, or pregnancy).

Preoperative preparation: A complete work-up for metastatic disease is carried out (chest radiography, IV urography, cystoscopy, and sigmoidoscopy); the patient must be in optimal general condition with normal circulating blood volume and laboratory values.

Postoperative care: Particular attention must be paid to monitoring vital signs, urinary output, and retroperitoneal suction-drainage output. The bladder should be decompressed by indwelling catheter (urethral or suprapubic) until bladder function returns.

Complications of radical hysterectomy include fistulas (ureterovaginal, vesicovaginal, rectovaginal), urinary tract infection, lymphocysts in the retroperitoneal space, and postoperative hemorrhage. Operative mortality is <1%.

b. Stages II, III, IV. Radiation therapy is the treatment of choice for cervical cancer beyond stage I as well as many cases of stage I disease. Both external therapy and intracavitary radiation are required in order to deliver a cancericidal dose to the primary tumor, the parametria, and the pelvic lymph nodes. Additional radiation therapy to the para-aortic nodes is given in more advanced disease.

Complications of radiation therapy are castration, radiation bowel injury (see Chapter 12), radiation cystitis, vaginal stenosis, and radiation necrosis of soft tissues.

4. Recurrent cervical cancer.
Most recurrences are peripheral (in the regional pelvic lymph nodes or at distant sites) and are not amenable to therapy. Central recurrences can be effectively treated by pelvic exenteration. **Total pelvic exenteration** involves the surgical removal of the bladder and urethra, rectum and anus, vagina and part of the vulva, along with a radical hysterectomy and pelvic lymph node dissection. The patient is left with two abdominal stomas, one for the elimination of urine and the other for the fecal stream (colostomy).

This operation has an operative mortality of 2%-5%, and the morbidity is high with complications of intestinal obstruction, hemorrhage, sepsis, fistulas, pyelonephritis, thromboembolism, and electrolyte disturbances. Chemotherapy, in general, has not been effective in recurrent cervical cancer.

5. Prognosis. With optimal therapy, 5-year survival rates are as follows: stage I, 85%-90%; stage II, 50%; stage III, 30%; stage IV, 10%.

E. CLEAR-CELL CARCINOMA OF THE CERVIX OR VAGINA.

The in utero exposure to DES or related nonsteroidal estrogens has been cited as producing, in the majority of such young women, benign vaginal and cervical anomalies such as cervical hoods or collars, ridges and furrows, cockscomb appearance of the anterior cervical lip, vaginal septa, and vaginal adenosis (columnar epithelium containing mucin or metaplastic squamous epithelium). These abnormalities usually require no treatment.

A small number of these patients (estimated at <1/1000 exposed individuals) have developed clear-cell adenocarcinomas of the vagina or cervix. All exposed female offspring should be carefully examined for evidence of malignancy at intervals of not less than 6 months. The examination should include cytologic sampling of the vagina and cervix, careful palpation for evidence of submucosal nodules or induration, iodine staining, and colposcopy if available. Suspicious areas should be biopsied. Clear-cell cancers should be treated by radical surgery or irradiation.

F. SARCOMA OF THE CERVIX.

These malignancies are rare connective tissue tumors arising from mullerian duct elements which differentiate into mesodermal structures. Sarcoma botryoides, mixed mesodermal tumors, leiomyosarcoma, lymphosarcoma, and angiosarcoma are varieties. They may be encountered at any age but most often occur in postmenopausal women.

1. Diagnosis. *Symptoms:* abnormal vaginal bleeding or discharge. *Signs:* a polypoid, fleshy tumor protruding from the cervix. *Laboratory tests:* biopsy of the lesion confirms the diagnosis.

2. Treatment. These tumors respond poorly to radiation therapy. Surgical excision is preferred and may vary from simple hysterectomy to total pelvic exenteration, depending upon the extent of disease.

3. Prognosis. Leiomyosarcoma arising in a cervical myoma carries the best prognosis, with 5-year survival rates in excess of 50%. Survival figures in the other sarcomas are considerably lower.

VI. DISORDERS OF THE CORPUS UTERI

A. LEIOMYOMA (FIBROID, FIBROMYOMA). These benign smooth muscle tumors arise from the myometrial cells. They are found in about one fifth of women over the age of 35 years. Leiomyomas are more frequent in blacks than whites by a ratio of 3:1. They are usually multiple and are classified by their location in the uterine wall: submucous, intramural, or subserous. The submucous and subserous varieties may become pedunculated. Degenerative changes (hyalin, cystic, carneous, myxomatous, calcific, septic, and atrophic) may occur within the tumor. Because estrogens stimulate growth, and progestins predispose to carneous degeneration, oral contraceptive agents should be used with caution in patients with leiomyomas. Malignant degeneration (leiomyosarcoma) is rare, occurring in 0.1%-0.5% of cases. The tumors undergo atrophy with the menopause.

1. Diagnosis

a. Symptoms. Often asymptomatic. Abnormal bleeding (hypermenorrhea or intermenstrual bleeding). Symptoms due to pressure on neighboring structures, e.g., urinary frequency and urgency, constipation, and pain on defecation. Severe pain is unusual and often is associated with carneous degeneration (during pregnancy), infection, or torsion of a pedunculated tumor. Large tumors may produce a sense of pressure or pelvic heaviness. Infertility (submucous myomas interfere with implantation).

b. Signs. Enlarged, irregular contour of the uterus on bimanual examination. Pedunculated subserous myomas are palpable as adnexal masses. Pedunculated submucous myomas may be extended through the cervix and come to lie in the upper part of the vagina.

c. Laboratory tests. Chronic excessive blood loss may lead to anemia. Carneous degeneration and infection cause leukocytosis and elevation of the sedimentation rate.

d. Radiographic findings. Plain abdominal films show a soft tissue tumor displacing bladder and/or rectum. Characteristic calcifications appear in the pelvis in some cases. IV urography may demonstrate hydronephrosis and hydroureter due to compression by a large myomatous uterus.

e. Special tests. Sonography defines a solid tumor enlarging the corpus. Sounding of the uterus confirms enlargement with elongation of the endometrial cavity. Hysterography demonstrates enlargement and/or distortion of the endometrial cavity.

2. Differential diagnosis. A myoma which is single and soft (due to cystic degeneration) may produce a symmetrical uterine enlargement simulating intrauterine pregnancy. MRI is helpful in distinguishing leimyomata uteri from adenomyosis. Laparoscopic examination may be necessary to distinguish a pedunculated subserous myoma from a solid ovarian tumor.

3. Treatment. Small asymptomatic leiomyomas require no treatment other than periodic examinations to estimate the growth rate. Myomectomy should be considered in the young, infertile woman who wishes to preserve reproductive function. Total hysterectomy is curative. Indications for hysterectomy are evidence of rapid growth; hypermenorrhea producing anemia; pressure symptoms.

B. SARCOMA OF THE UTERUS (LEIOMYOSARCOMA, MIXED MESODERMAL TUMOR, STROMAL-CELL SARCOMA). These rare connective tissue tumors arise from mesodermal differentiation of mullerian duct origin. Sarcoma botryoides occurs in infancy; the other sarcomas occur at any age, but are more frequent in postmenopausal women. A number of varieties of sarcoma are encountered in the uterus: leiomyosarcoma, mixed mesodermal tumors, stromal-cell sarcoma (including endolymphatic stromal myosis), carcinosarcoma, reticulum sarcoma, and angiosarcoma.

1. Diagnosis

a. Symptoms. Abnormal bleeding or vaginal discharge; abdominal distention; urinary frequency and urgency; pelvic pressure.

b. Signs. A fleshy, polypoid tumor protruding from the cervical canal; a rapidly enlarging myomatous uterus.

c. Laboratory tests. Anemia and elevated sedimentation rate. Cytologic examination may show sarcoma cells. Histopathologic examination of a biopsy or curettings is usually diagnostic.

d. Radiographic findings. Chest radiography may demonstrate pulmonary metastases.

2. Differential diagnosis. Rapidly growing leiomyomas and endometrial carcinoma simulate uterine sarcoma.

3. Treatment

a. Surgical. Leiomyosarcoma: total hysterectomy and bilateral salpingo-oophorectomy. Mixed mesodermal tumors: preoperative irradiation followed by total abdominal hysterectomy and bilateral salpingo-oophorectomy. Stromal cell sarcomas: preoperative irradiation followed by total abdominal hysterectomy and bilateral salpingo-oophorectomy.

b. Radiation therapy may be of some palliative value in advanced disease.

c. Chemotherapy has palliative benefit only. Progestin therapy may be beneficial in low-grade stromal sarcoma (endolymphatic stromal myosis).

4. Prognosis. Leiomyosarcomas arising in preexisting leiomyomas have a relatively good prognosis, particularly if they are "low grade." Mixed mesodermal tumors and stromal cell sarcomas carry a poor prognosis with <20% 5-year survival.

C. ENDOMETRIAL CARCINOMA is an epithelial malignancy arising from the columnar cells of the endometrium; it represents the most common cancer of the female reproductive tract. It occurs primarily in postmenopausal women; in premenopausal women, it usually is associated with chronic anovulation (Stein-Leventhal syndrome). Adenomatous hyperplasia of the endometrium appears to be a precursor in some women. Chronic endogenous or exogenous estrogen stimulation of the endometrium in the absence of progesterone has been postulated as a possible cause. Obesity, hypertension, and diabetes are frequent related conditions.

Histologically the tumor varies from slight atypia (carcinoma-in-situ) to large masses of poorly differentiated malignant endometrium deeply invading the myometrial wall, cervix, and adnexa. Metastases occur via the lymphatics to the regional pelvic and para-aortic lymph nodes, by peritoneal implantation, and by hematogenous spread to the lungs, liver, bone, and brain.

1. Diagnosis

a. Symptoms. Postmenopausal bleeding; serous or sanguinous vaginal discharge; hypermenorrhea (prolonged bleeding) in the premenopausal patient.

b. Signs. Uterus may be normal size or enlarged. Symmetrical enlargement suggests myometrial involvement. Bloody discharge from cervical canal.

c. Laboratory tests. Cytologic examination is positive in only 40%-80%.

d. Radiographic findings. Hysterosalpingography can be suspicious for endometrial carcinoma, but this test is unnecessary in most cases.

e. Special tests. Cytologic sampling of the endometrial cavity. Endometrial biopsy. Fractional D and C is the most definitive diagnostic procedure. MRI is helpful in revealing the depth of myometrial invasion.

2. Differential diagnosis. Bleeding due to hormonal therapy. Cervical polyps. Cervical cancer. Atrophic vaginitis with bleeding. Uterine sarcoma.

3. Surgical staging (classification adopted by FIGO, 1988)*

Staging for Carcinoma of the Corpus Uteri

Stage IA G123	Tumor limited to endometrium
IB G123	Invasion to less than one half of the myometrium
IC G123	Invasion to more than one half of the myometrium
Stage IIA G123	Endocervical glandular involvement only
IIB G123	Cervical stromal invasion
Stage IIIA G123	Tumor invades serosa and/or adnexa, and/or positive peritoneal cytology
IIIB G123	Vaginal metastasis
IIIC G123	Metastases to pelvic and/or para-aortic lymph nodes
Stage IVA G123	Tumor invasion of bladder and/or bowel mucosa
IV B	Distant metastases including intra-abdominal and/or inguinal lymph nodes

*International Federation of Gynecology and Obstetrics. Annual report on the results of treatment in gynecological cancer. Int J Gynecol Obstet 28:189, 1989.

Histopathology—degree of differentiation:

Cases of carcinoma of the corpus should be classified (or graded) according to the degree of histologic differentiation as follows:

G1 5% or less of a nonsquamous or nonmorular solid growth pattern

G2 6-50% of a nonsquamous or nonmorular solid growth pattern

G3 More than 50% of a nonsquamous or nonmorular solid growth pattern

Notable that nuclear atypia, inappropriate for architectural grade, raises the grade of a grade 1 or 2 tumor by 1.

In serous adenocarcinomas, clear-cell adenocarcinomas, and squamous cell carcinomas, nuclear grading takes precedence.

Adenocarcinomas with squamous differentiation are graded according to the nuclear grade of the glandular component.

4. Treatment. Total abdominal hysterectomy and bilateral salpingo-oophorectomy. The uterus should be opened in the operating room and examined with the pathologist. If the depth of myometrial invasion is >50% or if the tumor is poorly differentiated (G₃), selective pelvic and para-aortic node dissection should be done. Obtain estrogen/progesterone receptor assay. Postoperative radiation therapy is given (1) if the tumor invades >50% into the myometrium; (2) if there is vascular space involvement; or (3) if target lymph nodes contain metastatic tumor. Radical hysterectomy with bilateral pelvic node dissection may be chosen in selected good surgical risk patients with stage II disease. High-dose progestin therapy provides effective palliation in some patients with widespread metastases. This may be given orally in the form of megestrol (Megace). Combination chemotherapy (platinum, doxorubicin, 5-FU) is given to those with absent hormone receptors.

5. Prognosis. Small, well-differentiated tumors confined to the endometrium have 5-year survival rates in the 95% range. Anaplastic lesions with extrauterine spread have <10% 5-year survival.

VII. DISORDERS OF THE FALLOPIAN TUBES

A. ACUTE SALPINGITIS. Acute infection of the oviducts (and adjacent ovaries and pelvic peritoneum) most often is due to *N. gonorrhoeae* ascending via the endometrial cavity. Initially, the endosalpinx is involved with a purulent exudate which escapes from the fimbriated extremity and bathes the ovaries and pelvic peritoneum in pus. Infection by secondary organisms (*Escherichia coli, B. fragilis, Peptostreptococcus, Chlamydia*) may complicate the clinical picture.

1. Diagnosis

a. Symptoms. Insidious onset of bilateral lower abdominal and pelvic pain, often following a menstrual period; fever with or without chills; nausea with or without vomiting; fatigue and general malaise.

b. Signs. Temperature elevation up to 40° C; bilateral lower abdominal tenderness, rigidity and rebound tenderness; abdominal distention with hypoactive peristalsis; purulent cervical discharge; pain on motion of the cervix; bilateral adnexal tenderness on bimanual examination.

c. Laboratory tests. Leukocytosis with a shift to the left; elevated sedimentation rate; Gram's stain of a cervical smear may show gram-negative intracellular diplococci, but culture identification of *N. gonorrhoeae* is necessary.

d. Radiographic findings. Plain films of the abdomen are nonspecific; ileus usually is present. Pelvic sonography may be helpful in defining inflammatory adnexal masses.

e. Special tests. Culdocentesis produces cloudy fluid with numerous polymorphonuclear leukocytes on microscopic examination. This material should be cultured. Laparoscopy may be necessary.

2. Differential diagnosis: Acute appendicitis; ectopic pregnancy; septic abortion; endometriosis; acute gastroenteritis; regional ileitis; diverticulitis.

3. Treatment. Uncomplicated mild infections may be treated on an outpatient basis with bedrest at home and a single injection of aqueous penicillin G (4.8 million units) 1 hour after oral administration of 1 g probenecid. Alternatively, oral tetracycline HCl (500 mg four times daily for 10 days) may be used.

Patients with severe infections should be hospitalized at bedrest in semi-Fowler's position. IV fluids are necessary to correct dehydration. Doxycycline 100 mg IV twice daily plus cefoxitin 2 g IV four times daily until 48 hours afebrile, then doxycycline 100 mg orally twice daily for a total of 10-14 days.

Superimposed anaerobic infection or pelvic abscess formation should be suspected in patients who fail to respond. Anaerobic culture and sensitivity studies may reveal *B. fragilis,* in which case clindamycin, chloramphenicol, or carbenicillin should be added to the treatment regimen. Pelvic (tubo-ovarian) abscess can be palpated as a mass in the adnexa or cul-de-sac. Failure of the mass to regress under intensive antibiotic therapy requires laparotomy. A total hysterectomy and bilateral salpingo-oophorectomy usually are necessary.

B. CHRONIC SALPINGITIS. Low-grade infection of the fallopian tubes results from recurrent acute infections producing altered pathophysiologic states such as pyosalpinges, hydrosalpinges, extensive pelvic adhesions, and fibrosis.

1. Diagnosis

a. Symptoms. A history of previous pelvic infections; chronic pelvic pain; dysmenorrhea of an acquired type; dyspareunia; infertility.

b. Signs. Fever is absent or minimal; tenderness on motion of the cervix; adnexal masses or thickening.

c. Laboratory tests. Leukocyte count and sedimentation rate are normal unless there is an acute reinfection.

d. Special tests. Laparoscopic examination may be necessary.

2. Differential diagnosis. Chronic pelvic pain of obscure etiology. Ectopic pregnancy, ovarian neoplasm. Pelvic endometriosis and inflammatory bowel disease should be considered.

3. Treatment. Mild to moderate cases may be treated symptomatically with bedrest, heat to the abdomen, and mild analgesics. The relief of infertility due to bilateral tubal occlusion requires tuboplastic surgery.

Severe cases resulting in incapacitating pain require laparotomy. Total hysterectomy with bilateral salpingo-oophorectomy usually is necessary. Estrogen replacement therapy (conjugated estrogens 0.625 mg daily for 25 days each month) should be given postoperatively to prevent menopausal atrophy of the vulva and vagina and loss of mineral from the bones.

VIII. OVARIAN TUMORS

The ovary gives rise to a greater variety of tumors than any other organ in the body. These tumors may develop at any time in life, although they are more frequent in peri- and postmenopausal women. They may be cystic or solid, benign or malignant (or of borderline malignancy), and hormonally active or inactive. One of the best classifications of these tumors is based on their cell or tissue origin in the ovary:

Coelomic (surface) epithelium. Serous cystadenoma-cystadeno-carcinoma; endometrioid cystadenoma (endometrial cyst)-endometrioid carcinoma; mucinous cystadenoma-cystadenocarcinoma. Intermediate between the frankly benign cystadenomas and the cystadenocarcinomas are the "tumors of low malignant potential." Brenner tumors also arise from coelomic epithelium.

Specialized stroma. Granulosa-theca cell tumor; Sertoli-Leydig cell tumor; thecoma (luteoma).

Nonspecialized stroma. Fibroma; fibromyoma; fibroadenoma; cystadenofibroma; sarcoma.

Germ cell. Dysgerminoma. Teratoma: benign cystic (dermoid); malignant (embryonal carcinoma, endodermal sinus tumor, choriocarcinoma, various mature and immature teratomas). Gonadoblastoma.

Parovarian tumors. Parovarian cyst; mesonephroma; hilar cell tumor; adrenal rest tumor.

Functional cysts of the ovary (follicular and corpus luteum cysts) are the most frequent cause of ovarian enlargement in women during the reproductive years. They rarely are larger than 5 cm in diameter and usually regress within 1 menstrual cycle. They are not true neoplasms.

Ovarian cysts >5 cm in diameter or smaller cysts which enlarge or fail to regress after 2 months' observation should be considered neoplastic in women during the reproductive years. Any degree of ovarian enlargement in the prepubertal or postmenopausal patient should be considered neoplastic. Cancer of the ovary, although it is third in the order of frequency of female genital malignancies, is the leading cause of death.

1. Diagnosis
a. Symptoms. The ovary is a "silent organ"; small tumors are usually asymptomatic and are discovered during routine physical examination. Larger tumors may produce abdominal distention or a sense of weight or pressure in the pelvis.

Symptoms of ovarian cancer often do not appear until there are widespread peritoneal metastases which cause malignant ascites with abdominal distention and interference with bowel function. Menstrual disturbances secondary to ovarian tumors are infrequent (17%). Torsion of an ovarian tumor may cause sudden, severe abdominal and pelvic pain.

   b. Signs. Cystic or solid adnexal mass on pelvic examination. Bilaterality, nodularity, and fixation are signs suspicious of malignancy. Ascites accompanying a pelvic mass suggests malignancy with peritoneal spread (exception: Meig's syndrome is ascites and right hydrothorax secondary to benign ovarian tumors such as fibroma or thecoma). Huge ovarian tumors, particularly those of the mucinous variety, may distend the entire abdomen and simulate ascites.

   c. Laboratory tests. There are no specific abnormalities.

   d. Radiographic findings. Chest radiographs may show metastases or hydrothorax. A plain film of the abdomen may demonstrate a benign cyst teratoma (dermoid) with tooth structure or relative radiolucency of the contents (sebum) (it also helps to demonstrate ascites). IV urography defines the course of the ureters and detects bladder compression. Barium enema shows the relationship of the large intestine to the lesion and excludes primary disease of the colon (e.g., diverticulitis and primary bowel cancer). Upper GI and small bowel series help in certain cases by demonstrating small bowel involvement by the tumor; it also excludes gastric carcinoma with metastases to the pelvis (Krukenberg tumor). CT scan is useful in selected cases.

   e. Special tests. Sonography may define the nature of an adnexal mass, whether solid or cystic, and its relationship to the uterine corpus. Laparoscopy. Paracentesis or thoracentesis with examination of cell button for malignant cells may be diagnostic. Ca 125 may be elevated.

   2. Differential diagnosis includes leiomyomata uteri; chronic salpingo-oophoritis; diverticulitis; colon cancer; pelvic kidney; and metastatic cancer to ovaries from breast, endometrium, GI tract, pancreas, thyroid, kidney, adrenal.

   3. Treatment. Surgical removal is the primary treatment of all ovarian neoplasms. Preservation of ovarian tissue is desirable in young women with benign or "borderline" tumors. Malignant tumors require total hysterectomy, bilateral salpingo-oophorectomy and removal of as much extraovarian neoplastic tissue as possible. Adjunctive therapy includes chemotherapy and radiation to the pelvis or entire abdomen.

4. Stage grouping of patients with ovarian cancer is based upon the findings at the time of operation:

Stage I	Growth limited to the ovaries.
Ia	Limited to one ovary; no ascites; no tumor on external surface; capsule intact.
Ib	Limited to both ovaries; no ascites; no tumor on external surface; capsule intact.
Ic*	Tumor either stage Ia or Ib with tumor on surface of one or both ovaries; or with capsule ruptured; or with ascites or peritoneal washings containing malignant cells.
Stage II	Growth involving one or both ovaries with pelvic extension.
IIa	Extension and/or metastases to uterus and/or tubes.
IIb	Extension to other pelvic tissues.
IIc*	Tumor either stage IIa or IIb with tumor on surface of one or both ovaries; or capsule(s) ruptured; or with ascites or peritoneal washings containing malignant cells.
Stage III	Tumor involving one or both ovaries with peritoneal implants outside the pelvis and/or positive retroperitoneal or inguinal lymph nodes. Superficial liver metastases equals stage III. Tumor is limited to the true pelvis but histologically proven malignant extension to small bowel or omentum.
IIIa	Tumor grossly limited to the true pelvis with negative nodes but with histologically confirmed microscopic seeding of abdominal peritoneal surfaces.
IIIb	Tumor of one or both ovaries with histologically confirmed implants of abdominal peritoneal surfaces not exceeding 2 cm in diameter. Nodes are negative.
IIIc	Abdominal implants >2 cm in diameter and/or positive retroperitoneal or inguinal nodes.

---

*Note whether rupture is spontaneous or iatrogenic and if source of malignant cells is from ascites or washings.

Stage IV Growth involving one or both ovaries, with distant metastases. (Malignant pleural effusion or parenchymal liver metastases.)

5. Prognosis. Benign tumors are cured by surgical removal. The overall survival for ovarian cancer, however, is only 20%-30% because most are diagnosed in the late stages. Survival rates in the range of 80% can be expected if ovarian cancer is detected when it is confined to one ovary (stage I).

IX. ENDOMETRIOSIS

Endometriosis is the occurrence of functional endometrial tissue outside the uterus, usually involving the pelvic peritoneum (cul-de-sac, ovaries, serosa of the uterus, bladder, or colon), although it may be found at distant sites (umbilicus, cesarean section scars, perineum, inguinal canal).

There are three theories of pathogenesis, all of which may be operative: retrograde flow of endometrial fragments through the fallopian tubes at the time of menstruation (Sampson's theory); differentiation of the peritoneum into endometrium (coelomic metaplasia); and vascular dissemination (endometrial tissue has been found in lymph nodes as well as in the lung, suggesting spread via lymphatics and venous channels).

It is diagnosed most often in women during the fourth decade, although it is seen as early as the second decade. It occurs more often in the higher socioeconomic levels (college graduates), and the ratio of whites to blacks is 2:1.

Ectopic endometrium is responsive to cyclic hormonal stimulation by the ovaries with periodic micromenstruation causing inflammation and dense adhesions. Grossly, lesions are small, dark blue or purplish areas on the peritoneal surfaces resembling "powder burns" or "blueberry spots." Large endometriotic cysts of the ovary, filled with chocolate-brown old blood, are often called "chocolate cysts." Microscopically, endometrial tissue (glands, stroma) can often be identified. Malignant change in peritoneal endometriosis is uncommon.

1. Diagnosis
a. Symptoms. May be asymptomatic and found incidentally at laparotomy for some other condition. Acquired dysmenorrhea is the most frequent symptom—typically, severe, disabling pain of a grinding character starts several days prior to the onset of menses and reaches a peak during menstrua-

tion; as the process progresses, the pain may be present throughout the menstrual cycle. Rectal or bladder tenesmus (rarely, there is rectal bleeding). Deep dyspareunia. Infertility is a frequently associated problem.

b. Signs. Shotty, tender nodules in the cul-de-sac are best appreciated by combined rectovaginal examination just prior to menstruation. Large adherent, cystic adnexal masses (unilateral or bilateral) may be palpable bimanually.

c. Laboratory findings are not distinctive.

d. Radiographic findings. IVP may reveal ureteral displacement or constriction with hydroureter and hydronephrosis in severe cases; barium enema may reveal constricting or submucosal lesion of the colon.

e. Special tests. Sigmoidoscopy or colonoscopy may show extrinsic compression; cystoscopy; laparoscopy often helps to establish the diagnosis.

2. Differential diagnosis includes salpingitis, ovarian cancer, colon cancer, diverticulitis, and inflammatory bowel disease.

3. Complications. Infertility. Rupture of endometrioma produces a chemical peritonitis (15% of female patients who enter hospital with acute abdominal pain have endometriosis). Obstruction of the small or large intestine. Ureteral obstruction.

4. Treatment

a. Medical. Mild endometriosis may require only analgesics during periods of dysmenorrhea. Pregnancy is beneficial because it interrupts the cyclic hormonal stimulus and episodic micromenstruation.

Hormonal treatment (pseudopregnancy) produces several months of amenorrhea: (a) Norethynodrel with mestranol (Enovid): 2.5 mg daily for 1 week, 5 mg daily for 1 week, 10 mg daily for 2 weeks, then 20 mg daily for 6-9 months. (b) Danazol: 400 mg twice daily for 3-9 months (this agent inhibits pituitary gonadotropins and has possible side-effects of masculinization and fluid retention). (c) GnRH analogs produce a temporary "artificial menopause" interfering with the cyclic hormonal stimulation of endometriosis.

b. Surgical. Conservative—excision or cauterization of implants, suspension of retroverted uterus in the young patient who desires preservation of child-bearing potential. This can often be accomplished by laparoscopy.

Modified radical—hysterectomy with ovarian preservation.

Radical—hysterectomy with bilateral salpingo-oophorectomy. This operation is required in very extensive endometriosis or in symptomatic patients over 40 years of age.

5. Prognosis. Hormonal therapy does not cure endometriosis but most patients are "improved" and some may be able to conceive. However, a significantly higher proportion of infertile patients conceive after conservative surgery, so this approach is preferable. 50% of patients undergoing conservative surgery require subsequent therapy for symptoms due to progression of the disease. Surgical castration is curative but is a drastic step in the younger woman with endometriosis. Only 6% of patients have further difficulties after hysterectomy alone, so preservation of the ovaries is desirable in patients <40 years of age unless the ovaries are involved in large endometriotic cysts.

X. PELVIC FLOOR RELAXATION

Weakening of the connective and muscular tissues supporting the pelvic viscera results in various combinations and degrees of prolapse of the uterus, vagina, bladder, urethra, rectum, and peritoneum of the cul-de-sac (uterine descensus, cystocele, urethrocele, rectocele, and enterocele).

Etiologic factors are childbirth injuries (submucosal stretching and tearing) to the supporting structures during childbirth in multiparas; the forces of gravity imposed by the upright position; increased intraabdominal pressure with various physical activities such as climbing, lifting, coughing, straining, sneezing; obesity; loss of hormonal influence on the tissues postmenopausally; congenital weaknesses (the condition is occasionally encountered in nulligravidas, and spina bifida occulta is often an associated anomaly in these patients).

1. Diagnosis

a. Symptoms. Sense of pelvic pressure or "falling out." Mass protruding from the vaginal introitus. Various urinary complaints in patients with cystourethrocele (incomplete emptying; loss of urine with coughing, straining, sneezing [stress incontinence]; inability to void without digital pressure against the vagina). Problems associated with defecation in those with rectocele (constipation, incomplete evacuation without digital compression against the vagina). Low backache.

b. Signs. A soft, compressible mass which bulges through the vaginal introitus with straining may represent the anterior vaginal wall (cystourethrocele) or posterior vaginal wall (rectocele and/or enterocele).

A firm mass presenting at or protruding through the vaginal introitus usually represents the cervix (and corpus) uteri. A first-degree prolapse is one in which the cervix descends to the lower third of the vagina. In second- and third-degree prolapse, the cervix protrudes through the vaginal introitus, and a fourth-degree prolapse involves a protrusion of the entire uterus.

There may be ulceration of the vaginal and/or cervical mucosa due to pressure and vascular stasis. Stress incontinence of urine can be demonstrated by having the patient cough during examination.

A rectocele is diagnosed by finding a large anterior sacculation of the rectum on combined rectovaginal examination. The external anal sphincter muscle may be disrupted.

Enterocele is a downward herniation of the cul-de-sac peritoneum into the rectovaginal septum and is best demonstrated as a bulge in the septum which does not admit the rectal finger. The detection of a small, high enterocele may require examining the patient rectovaginally in the standing position. A large enterocele may present as a soft, compressible mass bulging through the vaginal introitus. Small bowel may occupy the mass.

c. Laboratory tests. Urinalysis may reveal evidence of cystitis due to infection of residual urine in large cystoceles.

d. Radiographic findings. Cystography may be helpful in demonstrating cystocele, urethrocele, and loss of the vesicourethral angle. Small bowel series may demonstrate intestine in an enterocele when diagnosis is in doubt.

e. Special tests. Cystoscopy. Cystometrogram helps distinguish atonic and hypertonic (neurogenic) bladder problems. Cine studies with intravesical and intraurethral pressure studies at rest, while straining, and during micturition may be required in some individuals with complex voiding problems (combined urge and stress incontinence). Biopsy of ulcerating lesions in prolapsed tissues should be done to rule out neoplastic disease.

2. Complications. Chronic urinary tract infection in large cystoceles with large volumes of residual urine. Acute urinary retention. Fecal impaction. Rupture of enterocele with evisceration. Trophic ulceration of cervical and/or vaginal mucosa.

3. Treatment

a. Medical. Kegel exercises to strengthen the levator ani and perineal muscles. Correct obesity and chronic cough. Treat urinary tract infections. Topical estrogens (conjugated estrogen or dienestrol cream applied to the vagina each night at bedtime) if the patient is postmenopausal and the mucosa is estrogen deficient. Pessaries, in patients who are poor surgical risks.

b. Surgical. Operative intervention is best deferred in the young individual until there is no longer a desire for childbearing.

Vaginal hysterectomy with anterior colporrhaphy and posterior colpoperineoplasty is the operation most commonly performed because the condition is usually a combination of uterine prolapse, cystourethrocele, and rectocele. Any portion of this operation can be omitted if the condition does not warrant it.

Vaginal obliterative procedures, such as the LeFort colpocleisis, should be avoided. Retropubic urethral suspension (Marshall-Marchetti-Krantz, Burch, or Pereyra operations) are indicated in patients with severe stress incontinence; they may be combined with vaginal repair when necessary.

4. Prognosis.
A properly selected and executed surgical procedure provides good support with relief of symptoms and maintenance of sexual function. A frequent cause of recurrence is the failure to recognize and repair an enterocele at the time of the operative procedure.

XI. DISORDERS OF PREGNANCY

A. ECTOPIC PREGNANCY is the implantation of a fertilized ovum outside the endometrial cavity. The majority (90%) occur in the fallopian tube; the remainder are in the uterine cornu, cervix, ovary, or peritoneal cavity (abdominal pregnancy). The incidence is about one in 150 pregnancies. Factors which favor extrauterine implantation are previous salpingitis or tuboplastic surgery, in utero DES exposure, congenital abnormalities, and endometriosis.

When an ovum implants in the fallopian tube, the invading trophoblast weakens the thin wall of the tube and rupture occurs, or the pregnancy separates intraluminally, leading to tubal abortion into the peritoneal cavity. This usually takes place before the 12th week of gestation. Cornual pregnancies may develop for 4 or 5 months, and rupture of such a pregnancy is often catastrophic because of the massive hemorrhage.

The rare abdominal pregnancy results from primary implantation of the egg or from peritoneal reimplantation of a conceptus following tubal abortion. Abdominal pregnancies may progress to term although the vast majority of such fetuses succumb and undergo calcification with the formation of a lithopedion, or they become necrotic and infected.

Decidual and myometrial changes occur in the uterus even though the pregnancy is extrauterine.

1. Diagnosis

a. Symptoms. Amenorrhea—one or two missed periods or a scanty last menstrual period. Irregular vaginal bleeding. Abdominal pain—usually unilateral (pain may be absent or mild and cramping in unruptured tubal pregnancy, sudden and severe pain occurs with rupture); extravasation of blood within the peritoneal cavity causes upper abdominal or shoulder pain (referred from diaphragmatic irritation).

b. Signs. Presumptive signs of pregnancy:

Chadwick's sign: bluish discoloration of the vaginal mucosa.

Hegar's sign: softening of the uterine isthmus; slight enlargement and softness of the uterine corpus.

Pain on palpation of the adnexal area or on motion of the cervix; cul-de-sac or adnexal mass (usually soft and ill-defined); afebrile or low-grade fever (usually <38° C); signs of hypovolemia in the presence of intraperitoneal hemorrhage; Cullen's sign—bluish discoloration around the umbilicus—is sometimes present in ruptured ectopic pregnancies.

c. Laboratory tests. Radioimmunoassay for β-subunit of HCG may be helpful in establishing the diagnosis of early pregnancy. In ruptured cases mild leukocytosis and acute anemia from blood loss.

d. Special tests. Transvaginal sonography combined with β-subunit HCG assay is particularly effective in detecting unruptured tubal pregnancy. Laparoscopy may be required for confirmation. Nonclotting blood is obtained by culdocentesis in the presence of rupture. Laparotomy is indicated as a diagnostic step when ectopic pregnancy is suspected but cannot be proved.

2. Differential diagnosis.
Ruptured corpus luteum cyst with intraperitoneal bleeding. Abortion of uterine pregnancy. Salpingitis. Appendicitis. Twisted ovarian cyst.

3. Complications.
Exsanguination and death may occur if ruptured ectopic pregnancy is not recognized and treated.

4. Treatment. Unruptured: Methotrexate (50 mg/m^2 IM) is effective in the management of early ($\leq$3.5 cm in greatest diameter) unruptured tubal pregnancy. When surgery is required, salpingectomy may be necessary, but the tube can be salvaged by salpingotomy in some cases.

Ruptured ectopic pregnancy: Transfuse as necessary; immediate laparotomy to control the bleeding; rupture of an interstitial (uterine portion of fallopian tube) pregnancy may call for massive blood replacement and hysterectomy if the defect in the ruptured uterus cannot be rapidly and safely repaired.

B. ABORTION is the termination of pregnancy before viability of the fetus (about 24 weeks' gestation). Between 10% and 15% of all intrauterine pregnancies abort spontaneously, usually before the 16th week of pregnancy. The majority of these are related to anomalous development of the fertilized egg. Often only the trophoblastic elements develop and the embryo is absent (blighted ovum). Late (second trimester) abortion, on the other hand, is frequently related to uterine factors, e.g., incompetent internal cervical os, congenital anomalies, or uterine tumors (myomas).

1. Diagnosis. Threatened abortion—slight bleeding or cramping. **Inevitable abortion**—bleeding, cramping, and cervical effacement and dilatation. **Incomplete abortion**—expulsion of a portion of the products of conception, usually accompanied by heavy bleeding. **Complete abortion**—expulsion of the entire conceptus with cessation of cramping and marked diminution in bleeding.

2. Differential diagnosis includes ectopic pregnancy; hydatidiform mole; leiomyomata uteri; and membranous dysmenorrhea.

3. Complications. Anemia, hypovolemic shock (if bleeding is severe), and sepsis (if secondary infection occurs).

4. Treatment. Threatened abortion should be treated conservatively with bed rest and analgesics. Fifty percent progress to inevitable, incomplete, or complete abortion.

Inevitable and incomplete abortions are potentially serious. Blood should be typed and cross-matched if the bleeding is severe. The uterus should be evacuated by suction or by dilatation and curettage. Oxytocin should be administered (10-20 units in an IV infusion of 5% dextrose in 0%-0.9% saline).

C. HYDATIDIFORM MOLE is a degenerative process in the developing trophoblast characterized by trophoblastic proliferation and hydropic enlargement of the chorionic villi producing many grape-like vesicles. The embryo is usually absent. Bilateral theca-lutein cysts of the ovaries are a frequent accompaniment due to the stimulus of excessive chorionic gonadotropin.

1. Diagnosis

a. Symptoms. Presumptive symptoms of pregnancy (missed menses, nausea, urinary frequency, breast tenderness). Vaginal bleeding (usually begins by 6-8 weeks). Grape-like tissue may be expelled.

b. Signs. Uterus is larger than expected in 50% of patients. Bilateral cystic enlargement of ovaries in 50% of patients. Clusters of grape-like tissue may be found in vagina. Toxemia of pregnancy (hypertension, edema, proteinuria) may occur in the second trimester.

c. Laboratory tests. Pregnancy test is positive. HCG titer in the urine is markedly elevated, it may be as high as 1-2 million IU/24 hours. Anemia if bleeding is prolonged.

d. Special tests. Ultrasonography is the most easily performed and reliable diagnostic test, it is virtually diagnostic.

2. Differential diagnosis. Intrauterine pregnancy with twins, polyhydramnios, or leiomyomata uteri. Ovarian tumors complicating intrauterine pregnancy.

3. Complications. Hemorrhage; infection; or malignant change, 20% progress to chorioadenoma destruens (invasive mole) or choriocarcinoma.

4. Treatment. Suction evacuation of the uterus with simultaneous IV infusion of oxytocin (40-50 units/L of 5% dextrose). Dilatation and curettage 1 week postevacuation. Follow-up: contraception for at least 1 year; HCG titers weekly until negative for 3 weeks, then monthly for 6 months, and bimonthly for another 6 months; periodic chest radiography.

D. CHORIOADENOMA DESTRUENS (INVASIVE MOLE) AND CHORIOCARCINOMA. Chorioadenoma destruens exists when chorionic tissue capable of forming villi remains in the uterine wall or elsewhere following evacuation of a hydatidiform mole. If only proliferating trophoblastic cells without villi are found after a mole or a "normal" pregnancy, the process is classified as a choriocarcinoma.

1. Diagnosis

a. Symptoms. Recent term pregnancy, abortion or mole; persistent bleeding; failure to resume normal menstrual pattern.

  b. Signs. Persistent bilateral ovarian cystic enlargement.

  c. Laboratory tests. Persistence of HCG titers or reappearance of abnormal titers after a period of normalcy.

  d. Radiographic findings. Pulmonary metastases.

  e. Special tests to search for metastases; liver-spleen scan; CT scan; brain scan, EEG, cerebral arteriogram.

  2. Complications. Massive bleeding from invasion of the uterine wall or from metastatic deposits. Widespread metastases.

  3. Treatment. *Chemotherapy* is the treatment of choice. Single-agent therapy is used except in the "high-risk group" (see below) and is continued until the HCG titer has been normal for 12 consecutive weeks. Either of these regimens is recommended:

  (1) Methotrexate: 0.4 mg/kg/day IM for 5 days; repeated at intervals of 2-4 weeks, depending upon the recovery from toxic side-effects (bone marrow depression).
  (2) Actinomycin D: 12 μg/kg/day by IV infusion daily for 5 days; repeated at intervals of 2-4 weeks as above.

  In the high-risk group (trophoblastic neoplasia following term pregnancy; tumor resistance to previous chemotherapy; treatment delayed for more than 4 months; urinary HCG >100,000 IU/24 hours or serum β-HCG >40,000 mIU/ml; metastasis to brain or liver), combination therapy with methotrexate, actinomycin-D, and chlorambucil should be used.

  4. Prognosis. Before chemotherapy, choriocarcinoma was a uniformly fatal disease. Now survival rates of >50% can be expected.

14

Urology

Emil A. Tanagho

I. GENERAL PRINCIPLES OF DIAGNOSIS

Essential steps for the evaluation of a urologic patient include:
- Complete history with emphasis on urologic symptoms.
- Complete physical examination with emphasis on the abdomen, external genitalia, and rectum.
- Examination of the urine and prostatic or urethral secretions.
- Kidney function tests, especially the PSP (phenolsulfonphthalein) test.
- Radiographic studies, including excretory urography and CT scan.
- Special tests: cystography, urethrography, retrograde pyelography, sonography, nuclear scanning, or endoscopic examinations

A. COMMON SYMPTOMS OF GENITOURINARY DISORDERS

1. Pain. One must differentiate between kidney pain (dull, aching pain in the costovertebral angle) and ureteral pain (acute, colicky, radicular pain referred from the costovertebral angle to the pubic region or the scrotum). Suprapubic pain in spasms is typical of excessive bladder distention; this pain can be extremely severe. Prostatic pain is sensed as heaviness in the perineum or discomfort deep in the rectum. Testicular pain is felt in the scrotum (unilaterally or bilaterally).

2. Hematuria. This symptom can be initial (blood at the start of voiding), terminal (blood at the end of voiding), or total (blood throughout voiding).

3. Voiding symptoms are frequency, difficulty in initiation of urination, hesitancy, terminal dribbling, burning, urgency, urge incontinence, and interrupted weak stream.

4. Other symptoms. Urinary incontinence, retention of urine, pyuria, hematuria, chyluria, oliguria, or anuria. Genital symptoms in the male include partial or unsustained erection, penile curvature, premature ejaculation, or hemospermia. In the female, genital symptoms are primarily vaginal pain, ure-thral pain, and dyspareunia.

B. UROLOGIC LABORATORY EXAMINATION

1. Examination of the urine is essential. In the male, examine a clean midstream specimen; in the female, obtain a specimen by catheterization.

Test the urine for pH, albumin, sugar, RBCs, and ketones.

Microscopic examination. Place a drop of the centri-fuged urine sediment under a cover slip on a glass slide and examine microscopically. Normal urine contains no RBCs, no pus cells, no bacteria, and no crystals.

A drop of the sediment is spread on a slide, dried lightly under medium heat, flooded with triple-strength methylene blue for about 20 seconds, washed, dried again, and examined under the microscope. Look particularly for **bacteria** or **pus cells** (white blood cells). The presence of either requires fur-ther evaluation. Bacteria on the stained smear indicates that there are at least 10,000 organisms per ml of urine; this is pa-thognomonic of clinical infection. (If infection is suspected, obtain a urine culture.) The stained specimen should also be scrutinized for epithelial cells and possibly **malignant cells.**

Urine can be tested for its **calcium content** by the Sulkowitch test. Two milliliters of Sulkowitch reagent are added to 5 ml of urine, and the amount of calcium is estimated by the speed of precipitation and the intensity of the cloud. It is graded from 0 to 4.

C. RADIOGRAPHIC EXAMINATION

1. Plain film of the abdomen, also called KUB (kidney, ureter, and bladder), is an essential preliminary step to rule out calcifications within the system and to delineate the kidneys (position, shape, size, outline, and axis).

2. Excretory urography is fundamental; it is a test of kidney function as well as a means of delineating the anatomy of the urinary system. It is indicated whenever uropathology is suspected, especially obstruction, tumors, infection, congeni-tal anomalies, neuropathy, or trauma. **Tomograms** may be re-quired to see details. The only contraindication to excretory urography is allergy to the contrast medium. If the study must be done in allergic patients, hydration, antihistaminics, and ste-roids may be helpful.

3. Sonography for detection of masses (and to determine whether they are cystic or solid), residual urine, hydronephrotic kidney, and stones.

4. CT scan for renal, pararenal, retroperitoneal and pelvic masses, and lymphadenopathy.

5. MRI for same indications as CT, plus vascular lesions.

6. Renal angiography less commonly used for the diagnosis of kidney masses and to outline renal vasculature in hypertensive patients and those with suspected renal tumor.

7. Instrumental radiographic studies

a. Urethrograms are done by injecting contrast medium through the external meatus to opacify the entire urethra.

b. Cystograms are obtained by filling the bladder with contrast medium under gravity flow until full capacity is reached. Bladder contour, vesicoureteral reflux, diverticula, and trabeculation can be assessed. A voiding film outlines the bladder outlet and the urethral canal, and a postvoiding film demonstrates residual urine.

c. Retrograde pyelograms are done by passing a ureteral catheter through a cystoscope and injecting contrast; the outline of the pelvicalyceal system and the ureteral lumen are clearly seen. This is necessary in patients with impaired renal function, poor concentration of contrast, and incomplete filling of collecting structures. It is also used to collect urine for cytologic examination.

D. ENDOSCOPY. Endoscopic evaluation includes cystoscopy, urethroscopy, ureterorenoscopy, and any associated procedures such as biopsy or retrograde injection of contrast medium.

Urinary instrumentation is sometimes a therapeutic maneuver, e.g., to manipulate and extract ureteral stones, to crush and evacuate vesical calculi, to fulgurate sites of bleeding, to resect tumors, to dilate urethral strictures, or to treat urethral stricture by urethrotomy or endoscopic incision.

II. TRAUMA

A. THE KIDNEY is protected by the rib cage and the strong posterior abdominal muscles. It can be injured by blunt or penetrating trauma. Renal injuries range in severity; contusion, parenchymal tear (partial or complete), or even rupture of the renal pedicle may occur.

1. Diagnosis

a. Symptoms and signs. Hematuria; pain in the flank; shock, especially with multiple injuries; nausea and vomiting;

abdominal distention (ileus); ecchymosis and a mass in the flank by percussion.

b. Laboratory tests. Blood in the urine; falling hematocrit on serial tests if bleeding is active.

c. Radiographic findings. Plain film reveals a large area of grayness in the region of the injured organ with absence of the psoas line because of hematoma, extravasation of urine, or both. Excretory urogram might show impaired function or evidence of extravasation. It is important to note that the contralateral kidney is normal. Retrograde urograms are rarely indicated. CT scan is useful for detection of retroperitoneal hematoma and kidney configuration. If available, it is the preferred imaging study for detecting and staging the extent of lesion. Renal angiograms sometimes help make the diagnosis and plan the surgical reconstruction in special instances.

d. Special tests. Radioisotope scan of the kidneys may be valuable in doubtful cases of renal injury.

2. Differential diagnosis. Vertebral or rib fractures and retroperitoneal hematoma cause similar symptoms. Hematuria may be due to injury of some other part of the genitourinary tract.

3. Complications. *Early:* Infection, secondary hemorrhage, and progressive renal damage. *Late:* Fibrotic stenosis of the renal artery, hypertension, and hydronephrosis due to ureteral stricture.

4. Treatment. Treat blunt trauma **expectantly** with blood transfusion and complete bedrest (until hematuria subsides) unless there is an indication for operation (persistent bleeding or infection). Surgical procedures include suture of a laceration, amputation of the upper or lower pole, heminephrectomy, and total nephrectomy. Renal conservation should be attempted whenever possible.

B. URETER. The ureter is rarely injured by external trauma; most ureteral injuries occur during pelvic or abdominal surgery. A ureter (sometimes both ureters) is inadvertently cut, leading to extravasation of urine; or ligated, causing obstruction.

1. Diagnosis

a. Symptoms and signs. Anuria or severe oliguria following pelvic surgery means bilateral ureteral obstruction until proven otherwise; flank pain; persistent ileus; drainage of urine from the abdominal wound or the vagina.

b. Laboratory and radiographic findings. Abnormal renal function tests if the injury is bilateral. Excretory urography shows partial or complete obstruction or extravasation. Retrograde urography defines the site and nature of the injury.

2. Differential diagnosis. Prerenal causes of oliguria and anuria. Vesicovaginal and urethrovaginal fistulas are distinguished from ureterovaginal leakage by instillation of methylene blue into the bladder. Retrograde urography proves the injury is ureteral.

3. Complications. Ureteral fistula, retroperitoneal infection, pyelonephritis, and ureteral obstruction from stenosis. Peritonitis develops if urine leaks into the peritoneal cavity.

4. Treatment. The best "treatment" is **prevention.** Catheterization of the ureters before extensive pelvic surgery may help identification during operation.

If ureteral injury is recognized immediately, the edges should be trimmed and anastomosed over a stent with internal (double "J") or external ("T" tube) drainage. Reimplantation into the bladder is preferable if the injury occurs close to that structure.

Methods of late repair depend on the level of the injury and status of the ureter distal to the damaged area. If recognition and repair are not immediate, do not attempt early postoperative repair. Allow 2-3 months for tissue healing.

5. Prognosis. The results of immediate repair are good. Late repairs are also successful if properly done.

C. BLADDER. Blunt trauma to the full bladder is the most common cause of bladder rupture; it is frequently associated with pelvic fractures. The bladder rupture can be intraperitoneal or extraperitoneal.

1. Diagnosis

a. Symptoms and signs. Suprapubic pain; hematuria; inability to void; suprapubic tenderness and muscle rigidity; intraperitoneal rupture (rebound tenderness and ileus); extraperitoneal rupture (mass or dullness in the suprapubic region).

b. Laboratory tests. Blood in the urine; falling hematocrit if bleeding is active.

c. Radiographic findings. Cystography demonstrates extravasation of urine. The bladder may be displaced or compressed.

2. Differential diagnosis. Excretory urography and cystography differentiate extraperitoneal bladder rupture from urethral or renal injuries.

3. Treatment. The peritoneal cavity is explored in all cases, the injury is repaired, and a suprapubic cystostomy tube is inserted. The site of extraperitoneal rupture is drained externally. The prognosis is good.

D. URETHRA

1. Membranous urethra is fixed to the genitourinary diaphragm and is most commonly injured in association with pelvic fractures.

Urinary retention, bleeding from the urethra, and pain and fullness in the lower abdomen are the usual symptoms. Rectal examination reveals a boggy mass anteriorly; sometimes the back of the pubic bone and displacement of the prostate upward are palpable. The diagnosis is established by urethrography.

If the tear is partial, a catheter might pass into the bladder; it should be left in place for 10-14 days. If the tear is complete, no instrumentation should be done, and suprapubic cystostomy is required. Some surgeons attempt immediate repair and others defer repair until later. There is a high incidence of stricture after these injuries. Impotence is also a possible complication with severe injury due to neural damage.

2. Bulbous urethra. A straddle injury compresses the bulbous urethra between a firm object and the pubic arch, causing a partial or complete tear. Instrumentation is also a cause of trauma to this segment.

Urethral bleeding and hematuria are common. Extravasation of urine with voiding might fill the perineum, ascend to the scrotum, spread to the penis, and extend to the lower abdominal wall and upper thigh (areas limited by the attachment of Colles' fascia). Urethrography is diagnostic and should be done before instrumentation.

If the tear is partial, a catheter might be passed to the bladder; it remains in place as a stent. Catheterization usually is impossible in patients with complete rupture; suprapubic cystostomy, drainage of extravasated urine, and antibiotic coverage are required.

These injuries invariably result in strictures which must be repaired later.

3. Pendulous urethra. The pendulous urethra is most often injured by instrumentation and occasionally by trauma to the erect penis. Bleeding per urethra without urination is the usual symptom. Mild injuries heal promptly without treatment; more severe injuries heal if the urethra is stented with a catheter. Associated tears of the cavernosus tissue must be repaired to avoid formation of extensive hematoma around the penis, scrotum, and perineum. Strictures are a consequence of severe injuries.

E. PENIS. Trauma to the erect penis ruptures the cavernosus tissue, which should be repaired surgically. A rubber band or other constricting device can cause necrosis; these objects must be removed. Avulsion of the penile skin occurs rarely in industrial accidents; skin grafting may be required.

F. SCROTUM. Injury to freely mobile testes is uncommon. Severe pain, vomiting, and even shock occur when testes are contused, lacerated, or completely ruptured. Scrotal exploration may be necessary; lacerations should be sutured. Healing following severe injury is usually accompanied by testicular atrophy.

III. OBSTRUCTIVE UROPATHY

1. Classification. Urinary obstruction is classified according to:

a. Level. Upper tract (supravesical). Lower tract (vesical, infravesical).

b. Completeness. Partial; complete.

c. Acuteness. Acute; gradual, progressive.

d. Congenital or *acquired*.

2. Etiology

a. Congenital. Meatal stenosis, posterior urethral valves, congenital lower ureteral obstruction, ureteropelvic junction obstruction.

b. Acquired. Urethral or ureteral stricture, bladder outlet (usually prostatic disease), stones, neurogenic dysfunction, and extrinsic obstruction by tumors, inflammation, or fibrosis. Obstruction may also be iatrogenic.

3. Diagnosis

a. Symptoms and signs. Upper tract obstruction: abdominal pain (renal or ureteral type); GI symptoms; tenderness and fullness in the costovertebral angle; flank mass if hydronephrosis is marked; fever and chills if infection is present. *Lower tract obstruction:* difficulty initiating voiding (hesitancy); weak, interrupted stream; urinary frequency; distended bladder; rectal examination may show prostatic enlargement.

b. Laboratory tests. Pyuria, hematuria, crystalluria. Impaired renal function (elevated serum creatinine and BUN) in chronic severe obstruction. PSP is normal in unilateral obstruction, possibly abnormal if obstruction is bilateral or if the volume of residual urine is large.

c. Radiographic findings. Abdominal ultrasonography may show hydronephrotic changes or renal or ureteral calculi. Plain abdominal films may show enlargement of the kidney shadows or opaque calculi. *Excretory urography:* (1) Establishes the diagnosis of obstruction unless renal function is markedly impaired. (2) May show the cause of obstruction (e.g., stone, tumor). (3) May show the level of obstruction. (4) Demonstrates the extent of hydroureteronephrosis above the obstruction. (5) May show trabeculation of the bladder and residual urine (in the postvoiding film) in cases of bladder outlet obstruction. (6) High-dose infusion pyelography, delayed films, and tomograms may be needed to opacify the collecting structures if renal function is impaired. *CT scan and sonography* may show ureteropelvic dilatation. *Retrograde ureterography* defines the exact site of ureteral obstruction. *Retrograde cystography, urethrography,* and voiding *cystourethrography* may show the cause of bladder outlet obstruction; trabeculation and diverticula of the bladder are also seen.

d. Special tests. (1) Urethral calibration, retrograde urethrography. (2) Endoscopy: may identify urethral causes of obstruction; reveals changes in the bladder resulting from outlet obstruction; evaluates competency of the ureteral orifices; permits ureteral catheterization.

4. Differential diagnosis. Must rule out other causes of kidney enlargement (cysts, tumors) or other abdominal masses.

5. Complications. Complete loss of renal function if persistent bilateral obstruction is not relieved. Infection. Stones.

6. Treatment

a. Relief of obstruction occurs spontaneously in some cases (e.g., passage of a ureteral stone), but instrumental or surgical procedures are required in most patients.

b. **The presence of acute infection or marked impairment of renal function demands immediate, aggressive measures to decompress the urinary tract above the obstructing point.** Nephrostomy, ureterostomy, suprapubic cystostomy, and placement of urethral or ureteral catheters are methods of decompression.

7. Prognosis depends on duration and severity of obstruction. Results are excellent if acute obstruction is relieved promptly and infection is eradicated.

IV. VESICOURETERAL REFLUX

The lower end of the ureter is protected by a valve mechanism which permits free flow of urine from the upper tract into the bladder but prevents regurgitation in the other direction. The well-developed longitudinal muscle of the submucosal ureter continues uninterrupted into the base of the bladder at the trigone. When the trigone is stretched, it tightens the closure of the lower end of the ureter, and when the trigone contracts, the contraction extends into the submucosal ureter and seals it. Thus, ureteral tonus closes the ureteral orifice when the bladder is empty. As the bladder distends, the trigone is stretched, and the ureteral closure is tightened still further. With voiding (the time of maximal intravesical pressure), the trigone and submucosal ureter actively contract, and the ureter remains occluded by this mechanism.

Primary reflux, by far the most common type, is a developmental weakness of the ureterotrigonal musculature. It probably occurs with equal frequency in children of both sexes, but because girls have a shorter urethra, the clinical manifestations of reflux (infection of the upper tract) appear earlier in them. **Secondary reflux** is acquired from infravesical obstruction, neurogenic dysfunction, inflammatory diseases, or iatrogenic causes. A third category of reflux is due to congenital ureteral anomalies (e.g., ectopic orifices).

1. Complications. (1) Damage to the renal parenchyma from the high pressures of bladder contraction during voiding. (2) Infection in residual urine. (3) Infection is carried from the lower urinary tract to the upper tract. Reflux is found in about 50% of children with acute pyelonephritis and in 70% of patients with radiographic evidence of chronic pyelonephritis. (4) Dilatation and tortuosity of the ureters resulting from the greatly increased work load; the ureters must transport the refluxing urine as well as the newly excreted urine. (5) Stone formation.

2. Diagnosis
a. Symptoms, signs, and laboratory tests are characteristic of acute pyelonephritis (Section V.B), in children and in some adults. Other adults have the history and findings of

chronic pyelonephritis (Section V.C). PSP test is abnormal depending on the volume of residual urine and extent of renal damage.

b. Radiographic findings. Excretory urography may show dilated ureters or the scarring of pyelonephritis. Voiding cystography shows reflux conclusively.

c. Special tests. Endoscopy evaluates the trigone and the position, fixation, configuration, and orientation of the ureteral orifices. The length of the submucosal ureter can be estimated.

3. Differential diagnosis. Pyelonephritis from other causes. Ureteral dilatation due to other organic or functional causes.

4. Treatment. Conservative management (treat infection, dilate distal urethral stenosis) permits about one third of patients to undergo spontaneous reversal of the reflux. Another one third are treated conservatively for prolonged periods; many of these patients eventually require operation.

Immediate surgical repair is indicated in the one third with advanced disease. The weak distal ureter is excised, and the ureter is reimplanted into the bladder through a long submucosal tunnel by one of several technics.

5. Prognosis is good if reflux is detected early and poor if extensive renal damage has occurred. Surgical repairs succeed in preventing reflux, infection, and progression of renal injury in 90%-96% of patients.

V. INFECTIONS

Urinary tract infections are categorized as specific or nonspecific. **Specific infections** are caused by bacteria, each of which is associated with a specific pathologic tissue reaction. Examples are tuberculosis, syphilis, and parasitic infections. **Nonspecific infections** have similar manifestations regardless of the causative bacteria. They are much more frequent than the specific types. Gram-negative rods *(Escherichia coli, Proteus mirabilis, Proteus prodigalis,* and *Pseudomonas aeruginosa)* are frequently responsible; gram-positive cocci *(Streptococcus faecalis* and *Staphylococcus aureus)* occasionally cause urinary infections.

Because the urinary tract has defenses against infection (the complete washout mechanism and the bacteriostatic properties of the urothelium), infection usually has an underlying cause such as stasis, residual urine, foreign bodies, trauma, or a continuous source of infection.

The *ascending route of infection* is the most common. It occurs more often in females because of the short urethra and the potential source of infection in the vagina. Ascending urinary tract infection is frequent in girls under age 10 years and in young women as they begin sexual activity. *Hematogenous or descending infection* is less common; it is associated with underlying urologic diseases such as stones, tumors, or vesicoureteral reflux. Lymphatic spread of infection to the urinary tract from the GI tract or genital system takes place occasionally. Extension of infection from a nearby organ (e.g., in salpingitis, appendiceal abscess, vesicoenteric fistula) may occur also.

A. TUBERCULOSIS is a specific infection that reaches the genitourinary tract by hematogenous spread. The kidney is affected most often; tubercles in the parenchyma caseate and eventually communicate with the pelvicalyceal system. The lower tract (ureter, bladder, prostate, epididymis) is affected secondarily by descending infection; the fibrosis typical of healing tuberculosis may obstruct the ureter or urethra or cause contracture of the bladder. Vesicoureteral reflux results if bladder involvement is severe. Bilateral epididymitis may cause infertility, and the testis may be destroyed by direct extension.

1. Diagnosis

a. Symptoms and signs. The renal lesion is usually silent. Symptoms of cystitis are the common complaint (frequency, urgency, and sometimes hematuria). Thickened, nontender epididymis or an indurated, nodular prostate reflects TB of those structures; draining scrotal sinuses are seen sometimes.

b. Laboratory tests. "Sterile" pyuria (no organisms on stained smear or routine culture) means tuberculosis until proved otherwise. Acid-fast stains of the urine and cultures of tubercle bacilli are positive.

c. Radiographic findings. Chest film may show tuberculosis. Plain abdominal film may show punctate calcifications in the renal parenchyma. Excretory urography reveals ulcerated calyces, obliterated calyces, or fibrotic contracture of the ureters or bladder; vesicoureteral reflux may be present.

d. Special tests. Cystoscopy reveals tubercles if the bladder is involved; biopsy should be obtained.

2. Treatment

a. Medical. Genitourinary tuberculosis must be treated as a systemic disease (see Chapter 4); treatment is usually successful.

b. Surgical. Must be preceded by at least 3 months of medical treatment. Nephrectomy, repair of stricture, reimplantation of refluxing ureters, epididymectomy, or augmentation cystoplasty for contracted bladder may be necessary.

c. Urine must be examined and cultured at intervals for years; relapse may occur.

3. Prognosis is excellent with modern antituberculosis therapy.

B. ACUTE PYELONEPHRITIS is a combined infection of the renal pelvis and the renal parenchyma; the former seldom occurs alone. Bacteria reach the kidney by the ascending route most commonly; vesicoureteral reflux plays a major role. Hematogenous infection occurs in the presence of stones or other obstructions. Pyelonephritis, especially on the right side, may also be associated with atony and stasis in pregnancy.

1. Diagnosis

a. Symptoms and signs. High fever (39-40° C) and chills. Flank pain and lower abdominal pain (localized flank pain is uncommon in children with acute pyelonephritis). Nausea and vomiting. Tenderness in the costovertebral angle (may have abdominal distention and tenderness).

b. Laboratory tests. Leukocytosis with shift to the left. The urine is cloudy (white cells, white cell casts, and bacteria are seen). Urine culture identifies the organism and its sensitivity to antibiotics.

c. Radiographic findings. Excretory urography is normal or there is delay in secretion and haziness of the outline of the calyceal system. Obstruction or vesicoureteral reflux may be demonstrated. Voiding cystography shows reflux in many cases; it should be obtained after infection subsides.

2. Differential diagnosis. Appendicitis, cholecystitis, pancreatitis, diverticulitis, and lobar pneumonia.

3. Complications. The infection may become chronic.

4. Treatment. Antibacterial therapy is begun with sulfonamides or broad-spectrum antibiotics. The sensitivity of the organism should be determined and the treatment altered if necessary. If the infection does not respond within 48 hours, obstruction must be ruled out by excretory urography.

Underlying disease (especially vesicoureteral reflux) must be sought in boys and in girls after any febrile episode of infection.

Follow-up: After clinical response, the urine should be examined at intervals for 2 months to be certain the infection has been eradicated.

5. Prognosis is good if infection is controlled promptly and predisposing factors are identified and treated.

C. CHRONIC PYELONEPHRITIS. Vesicoureteral reflux is the most common cause of this disease.

1. Diagnosis

a. Symptoms and signs. May be asymptomatic except during acute exacerbations. Hypertension. Renal failure may be the presenting problem.

b. Laboratory tests. Absent, mild, or moderate pyuria. Bacteriuria is always present. Impaired renal function in advanced bilateral disease.

c. Radiographic findings. (1) Excretory urograms are normal in the early stages. Progressive parenchymal scarring leads to shrinkage of the kidney, delayed excretion, and poor concentration of the contrast medium. Narrowing of the infundibula and clubbing of the calyces also are typical. (2) Voiding cystography may reveal reflux and hydroureteronephrosis.

d. Special tests. Endoscopy and retrograde studies may demonstrate the underlying cause of chronic pyelonephritis.

2. Differential diagnosis. Chronic cystitis, tuberculous pyelonephritis, glomerulonephritis, and renal atrophy from vascular insufficiency.

3. Complications. Hypertension, stone formation, renal failure.

4. Medical treatment. Intensive antimicrobial therapy guided by culture and sensitivity tests. After infection is controlled, suppressive therapy is given for months using small daily divided doses of nitrofurantoin, sulfonamides, or acidified methenamine. Infection sometimes continues to recur (in these patients, suppressive therapy is continued for years).

D. CYSTITIS. Acute cystitis is a common ascending infection in females—it may appear 36-48 hours after sexual intercourse. In men, cystitis is never primary; it occurs only as a complication of bladder outlet obstruction, prostatitis, or pyelonephritis. Because there is intermittent complete emptying of the bladder contents, acute cystitis is self-limited in the absence of stasis, a constant source of infection, or both.

1. Diagnosis

a. Symptoms and signs. Frequency, urgency, urge incontinence, urethral burning on urination, pyuria, and terminal hematuria. Cystitis is not associated with fever. Underlying disease (e.g., prostatic enlargement) may be found.

b. Laboratory tests. Pyuria, bacteriuria, and hematuria.

2. Complications. Ascending infection to the kidney may develop if the ureterovesical junction is marginally balanced; reflux occurs in the presence of infection and ceases when the infection clears in these patients.

3. Treatment with antimicrobial agents should eradicate the infection promptly and the urine should be sterile in 14 days. If infection persists, complete urologic evaluation is essential.

E. URETHRITIS. Acute nonspecific urethritis is an ascending infection in women; in men, it usually is associated with prostatitis. Trichomonads, gonococci, viruses, and chemical irritants also cause acute urethritis.

1. Diagnosis

a. Symptoms and signs. Urethral discharge. Burning on urination. Evidence of prostatitis.

b. Laboratory tests. Urethral discharge is examined in saline (wet smear) to look for trichomonads. Methylene blue and Gram stains of the discharge reveal clumps of white cells, nonspecific bacteria, or gonococci. Some patients have no bacteria (viral, chemical, or *Mycoplasma pneumoniae* infection).

2. Treatment. Nonspecific urethritis is treated with antibiotics, e.g., tetracycline or erythromycin for 1 week. If discharge contains pus but no bacteria, assume *M. pneumoniae* is responsible and treat as nonspecific urethritis.

Gonococcal urethritis responds to penicillin (1.2 million units IM in each buttock 1 hour after probenecid 1 g orally) or tetracycline. Many patients have associated nonspecific urethritis that must be treated also. Treat trichomonal urethritis with metronidazole (250 mg orally for 10 days). Gonococcal and trichomonal urethritis require treatment of the sexual partner and discontinuance of intercourse (or the use of a condom) until the infection clears.

F. PROSTATITIS is most common in young adults. It usually is a hematogenous infection, but it may follow inadequately treated urethritis.

1. Diagnosis
a. Symptoms and signs. (1) *Acute prostatitis:* severe vesical irritability, urethral discharge, perineal heaviness and pain, fever, and sometimes urinary retention. Enlarged, edematous, tender prostate. Prostatic massage is contraindicated. (2) *Chronic prostatitis:* usually asymptomatic with occasional flare-up of symptoms. Prostate normal or indurated and irregular.

b. Laboratory tests. Leukocytosis in acute phase. White cells and bacteria in first-glass specimen of urine. Prostatic massage (in chronic phase only) yields secretions containing clumps of pus cells but usually no bacteria.

2. Complications
a. Acute prostatitis. Prostatic abscess, which may rupture into the urethra or perineum. Chronic prostatitis.

b. Chronic prostatitis. Acute epididymitis. Secondary posterior urethritis and cystitis.

3. Treatment.
Antimicrobial therapy for acute prostatitis. Response is usually prompt. Abscess may require surgical drainage. Residual chronic prostatitis must be treated.

Antibiotics are less effective in chronic prostatitis, but they should be used. Prostatic massage (two to three times at intervals of 10-14 days) and hot sitz baths are helpful. Regular sexual activity is encouraged to promote drainage. Chronic prostatitis in itself causes little harm, but its complications may be serious.

G. EPIDIDYMITIS.
Acute nonspecific epididymitis is usually secondary to prostatitis or urethritis. Occasionally it is caused by reflux of sterile urine into the ejaculatory ducts; recurrent epididymitis may be due to this mechanism.

1. Diagnosis
a. Symptoms and signs. History of instrumentation, catheterization, urethritis, or prostatitis. Acute severe pain and swelling in the scrotum extending into the inguinal canal in some cases. Fever. The epididymis is enlarged and tender; except in the early stages, it cannot be felt separate from the testis; the scrotal skin is reddened and adherent to the inflammatory mass.

2. Differential diagnosis.
Tuberculous epididymitis is usually not painful or tender. Torsion of the spermatic cord: pain is not relieved by lifting and supporting the testis; the pain of acute epididymitis is improved by this maneuver. Testicular tumor. Mumps orchitis.

3. Treatment. Infiltration of the spermatic cord with 15-20 ml of 1% procaine hydrochloride relieves the pain and speeds resolution. Antibiotics (e.g., tetracycline). Scrotal support, bedrest, cold compresses, and analgesics.

4. Prognosis. Acute epididymitis resolves slowly over 2-3 weeks, often with some residual induration and swelling. Sterility may result from bilateral severe cases that block the epididymal ductal system.

H. ORCHITIS is usually a complication of mumps parotitis. Very rarely, orchitis is a consequence of severe epididymitis.

Painful swelling of the testicle (usually unilateral), fever, and associated parotitis are the usual findings. Laboratory tests are normal except for leukocytosis. Acute epididymitis and torsion of the spermatic cord must be differentiated. Infiltration of the spermatic cord with 1% procaine, bedrest, analgesics, and scrotal support are helpful. Testicular atrophy and, if bilateral, infertility are the main complications. Androgenic function is maintained.

VI. URINARY STONES

Urinary calculi often are idiopathic. Other stones are secondary to stasis and infection, and some calculi occur in association with metabolic diseases (e.g., cystinuria, gout, and hyperparathyroidism). Stones are more frequent in men; they are rare in children and in Blacks.

A. RENAL AND URETERAL CALCULI
1. Diagnosis
a. Symptoms and signs. Nonobstructive stones are asymptomatic in most cases. Flank discomfort and hematuria occur occasionally. Obstructive stones cause severe flank pain and agonizing colic that radiates along the course of the ureter to the scrotum or medial thigh. Gross hematuria is not uncommon. Tenderness in the flank and signs of ileus are noted.

b. Laboratory tests
(1) *Urinalysis:* proteinuria if hematuria is present; pH >7.6 indicates the presence of urea-splitting organisms (low pH [6-6.5] is associated with uric acid calculi or renal tubular acidosis); erythrocytes, white cells, and bacteria are seen in the sediment; crystals (oxalate, phosphate, uric acid, cystine) should be sought in the sediment; Sulkowitch test may reveal hypercalciuria; qualitative test for

cystine should be done in cases of recurrence or family history.

(2) *Quantitative analysis* of calcium, oxalates, uric acid, and cystine should be done in a 24-hour specimen of urine. Urinary calcium (on a low-calcium diet—no dairy products) should not exceed 175 mg/24 hours. Higher values suggest hyperparathyroidism or idiopathic hypercalciuria.

(3) Renal function tests are normal unless there is bilateral obstruction, infection, or chronic underlying urologic disease.

(4) *Essential blood chemistries* include calcium, phosphate, uric acid, and proteins. Parathormone assays are indicated if hyperparathyroidism is suspected (see Chapter 6).

(5) Every recovered stone should be analyzed for *chemical composition*.

c. Radiographic findings. Plain abdominal films may show the stone (90% are radiopaque). Excretory urography localizes stones in the urinary tract, shows the level and degree of obstruction, and demonstrates renal damage.

d. Special tests. Cystoscopy and retrograde urography are seldom necessary for diagnostic purposes.

2. Complications. Infection, obstruction, and progressive renal damage.

3. Treatment

a. Conservative. Renal stones that are asymptomatic, unassociated with reinfection, and nonobstructive require no treatment. Ureteral stones are small and smooth (most pass spontaneously).

b. Instrumental or surgical. Renal stones that obstruct or cause recurrent infection are removed either surgically (pyelotomy, nephrotomy, or even nephrectomy may be necessary) or by extracorporeal shock wave lithotripsy; ureteral stones that remain impacted in the lower ureter should be removed by cystoscopic manipulation or operation (ureterolithotomy) if hydronephrosis progresses or infection persists.

c. Most renal stones lend themselves to *percutaneous removal*. After establishing a nephrostomy tract to the kidney, and helped by either ultrasonic or electrohydraulic lithotripsy, stones can be broken into small pieces and extracted without having to do open surgical procedures.

d. Extracorporeal shock wave lithotripsy is now the standard treatment for most renal and upper ureteral stones. Shock waves generated by spark plug, electromagnet, or ultrasound are focused on the stone and lead to its shattering into small fragments or sand that readily passes. Extracorporeal shock wave lithotripsy is effective in treating 85%-90% of renal stones. For large staghorn stones, it should be combined with percutaneous debulking.

e. Ureteral stones can also be removed under direct vision using the *rigid ureteroscope,* which can reach from the bladder all the way to the kidney. Small stones are removed with a basket. Large stones are broken into small pieces and removed.

4. Prophylaxis against recurrence is very important.

a. General measures. Large fluid intake to prevent precipitation of solutes (especially avoid nocturnal dehydration); treatment of infection; correction of obstruction and stasis.

b. Specific measures
(1) *Calcium stones:* parathyroidectomy for hyperparathyroidism; eliminate milk and cheese from the diet; potassium acid phosphate (3-6 g daily) reduces urinary excretion of calcium; a diuretic (e.g., hydrochlorothiazide 50 mg twice daily) reduces calcium content in the urine; ascorbic acid (1 g 4 times a day) or cranberry juice (200 ml, four times a day) acidifies the urine and makes calcium more soluble.
(2) *Oxalate stones:* low-oxalate and low-calcium diet; phosphates (potassium acid phosphate 3-6 g daily); pyridoxine (100 mg, three times/day).
(3) *Metabolic stones:* cystine and uric acid precipitate in acid urine (urine pH should be raised to >7.5 by giving 50% citrate solution, 4-8 ml, 4 times a day and prescribing an alkaline-ash diet); limit purines in the diet of uric acid stone formers (also give allopurinol [Zyloprim] 300 mg once or twice daily); in cystinurics, low methionine diet and penicillamine (4 g daily).

5. Prognosis. The high recurrence rate is minimized by correcting obstruction, treating infection, and using prophylactic measures. Progressive renal damage is the worst danger. Prolonged follow-up is necessary.

B. VESICAL CALCULI. Primary vesical stones are very rare in the United States but are not uncommon in developing countries. Vitamin B_6 deficiency may have an etiologic role. Secondary vesical stones are usually a consequence of infection by urea-splitting organisms in patients with neurogenic bladder or outlet obstruction. Stones entering the bladder from the ureter pass through the urethra unless the bladder outlet is obstructed. Foreign bodies in the bladder, whether self-introduced or a result of instrumentation, may serve as a nidus for stone formation. Ninety-five percent of vesical calculi occur in men.

1. Diagnosis

a. Symptoms and signs. Urinary frequency and occasional interruption of the urinary stream with pain radiating to the tip of the penis.

b. Laboratory tests reveal pyuria, bacteriuria, and hematuria.

c. Radiographic findings. Opaque stones are visible on a plain film; radiolucent stones are filling defects in the bladder on excretory urography or cystography.

d. Special tests. Cystoscopy reveals the number, size, and shape of stones; it is essential before a decision is made about the method of treatment.

2. Treatment. Small stones are removed cystoscopically after they are crushed with a lithotrite or disintegrated by means of an electrohydraulic lithotrite. Large, hard stones are removed by suprapubic cystostomy. Some stones (especially those that form in the presence of infection) can be dissolved by chemicals such as Renicidin or Solution G.

3. Prognosis. Recurrence is uncommon if the predisposing factors are corrected.

VII. TUMORS

Neoplasms of the prostate, bladder, and kidneys are among the most common tumors in humans. Testicular tumors are uncommon but highly malignant. Other genitourinary organs rarely give rise to neoplasia.

A. KIDNEY.* Benign renal tumors are rare. **Adenocarcinoma** (hypernephroma, Grawitz's tumor), arising from tubular cells, is the most common tumor of the kidney. It is more frequent in males. Adenocarcinoma invades the blood vessels early and spreads to liver, lungs, and long bones. It also invades and dis-

---

*See Chapter 19 for Wilms' tumor.

torts the renal pelvis and calyces, and it can metastasize to regional lymph nodes.

1. Diagnosis

a. Symptoms and signs. Painless gross total hematuria. Firm, irregular, nodular mass in the flank. Recent appearance of a varicocele in the left side of the scrotum if the left renal vein is involved. Symptoms and signs of metastases (weight loss, anemia, bone pain, fever of unknown origin).

b. Laboratory tests. Gross or microscopic hematuria. Renal function not impaired. Hypercalcemia in some cases.

c. Radiographic findings. Plain film may show an enlarged, irregular kidney. Excretory urograms show calyceal distortion and a space-occupying mass. US, CT, and MRI are helpful in diagnosing and staging. Renal angiography distinguishes tumor from cyst.

d. Special tests. Immediate cystoscopy if the patient has gross hematuria when first seen (blood from one ureter localizes the problem to one side). Retrograde study may rule out epithelial tumors. CT and MRI scanning are of great help in diagnosing and staging renal tumors.

2. Differential diagnosis. Renal cysts, metastases to the kidneys, hydronephrosis.

3. Treatment. Radical nephrectomy with regional lymphadenectomy. The primary tumor is radioresistant, but radiation therapy may palliate local recurrence or bony metastases.

4. Prognosis. The 5-year survival rate is 35%. Positive lymph nodes or involvement of the renal vein or vena cava worsens the prognosis. Tumor may recur as long as 10-15 years after removal of the primary.

B. RENAL PELVIS AND URETER.
These epithelial tumors comprise about 10% of kidney tumors. The most common variety is the transitional cell carcinoma, histologically similar to bladder tumors. Squamous cell carcinoma occurs in 15% of cases, commonly in association with chronic obstruction and irritation. Tumor metastasizes via lymphatics to regional lymph nodes. Secondary tumors may develop in the urinary tract distal to the primary.

1. Diagnosis

a. Symptoms and signs. Painless, gross total hematuria. Colicky pain if the tumor obstructs or if clot passes down the ureter.

b. Laboratory tests. Hematuria. Malignant cells on stained smear of the sediment.

c. Radiographic findings. Irregular filling defect in the renal pelvis or calyx on excretory urography. Retrograde urograms confirm the diagnosis.

d. Special tests. Cystoscopy shows unilateral hematuria (secondary tumors may be seen in the bladder). Cytologic study of unilateral urine or after ureteral brushing specimens yields a high rate of positives.

2. Treatment. Nephroureterectomy with excision of a cuff of bladder mucosa around the ureteral orifice.

3. Prognosis. Good if the tumor does not extend through the pelvic or ureteral muscle, poor in anaplastic tumors.

C. BLADDER. The bladder is the second most frequent site of genitourinary tumors (after the prostate). Bladder tumors are more common in males and usually occur after age 50 years. Known carcinogenic associations include industrial aromatic amines (many years of exposure) and smoking.

Most bladder tumors are transitional cell carcinomas. Epidermoid cancer (5%) and adenocarcinoma comprise the remainder. Transitional cell carcinomas are categorized histologically by their degree of differentiation (grade I to IV, IV being anaplastic) and the depth of penetration (stage O to D). The staging system is as follows:

Stage O: Papillary tumor not invading the lamina propria

Stage A: Invasion of the lamina propria but not the muscle.

Stage B: Superficial (B_1) or deep (B_2) invasion of the bladder muscle.

Stage C: Tumor extending outside the bladder wall to perivesical fat or overlying peritoneum.

Stage D: Distant metastases.

1. Diagnosis

a. Symptoms and signs. Hematuria is the most common symptom. Symptoms of secondary infection. Suprapubic pain if tumor extends beyond the bladder wall. Abdominal examination is negative unless the bladder outlet is obstructed (palpable bladder), the ureteral orifice is occluded (palpable kidney), or large bladder mass.

b. Laboratory tests. Hematuria and sometimes infected urine. Malignant cells on methylene blue or Papanicolaou stain of the sediment.

c. Radiographic findings. Excretory urograms may show ureteral obstruction. In the cystogram phase, large tumors create a filling defect in the bladder.

d. Special tests. Cystoscopy with biopsy makes the diagnosis.

2. Treatment

a. Surgical. Transurethral resection for low-grade superficial tumors. Partial bladder resection for localized lesions situated away from ureteral orifices and the base. Radical cystectomy, urethrectomy, and bilateral pelvic lymphadenectomy for high-grade invasive tumors; urinary diversion (e.g., ileal conduit, ureterosigmoidoscopy) is required.

b. Radiation therapy is effective for high-grade tumors with the objective of cure or as an adjunct to radical cystectomy.

c. Topical chemotherapy (e.g., 60 mg of thiotepa in 60 ml of water instilled into the bladder once a week for 6 weeks) may control differentiated superficial tumors. Mitomycin-C (Mutamycin), doxorubicin (Adriamycin), and BCG are also used in a similar regimen with favorable results and are considered the most effective.

3. Prognosis. Well-differentiated tumors frequently recur; cystoscopy at intervals is essential. Repeated transurethral resection often is successful. Anaplastic, deeply invasive cancers have a poor prognosis.

D. ADENOMATOUS HYPERPLASIA OF THE PROSTATE

is a benign lesion that arises in the periurethral glands, not the prostate gland proper. It grows within the prostate, however, compressing and displacing it laterally to form the "surgical capsule." It affects men over the age of 50 years.

1. Diagnosis

a. Symptoms and signs. "Prostatism": hesitancy, frequency, nocturia, weak stream, terminal dribbling. Acute urinary retention. Hematuria from rupture of dilated veins at the bladder neck; palpable bladder sometimes; prostate normal sometimes (usually enlarged, soft to firm).

b. Laboratory tests. Urine infection, hematuria, abnormal PSP test due to residual urine.

c. Radiographic findings. Excretory urography may show elevation of the bladder base, trabeculation, evidence of residual urine, and mild bilateral hydroureteronephrosis.

d. Special tests. Urodynamic studies or flow rate measurements reflect the degree of bladder outlet obstruction. Catheterization measures the volume of residual urine. Endoscopy shows enlargement of the prostate (lateral lobes, middle lobe, or trilobar) and the effects of obstruction on the bladder.

2. Differential diagnosis. Prostatic cancer, neurogenic bladder, acute prostatitis, and urethral stricture.

3. Complications. Acute retention, chronic retention, infection, calculi, diverticula, back pressure on the kidney, and progressive renal failure.

4. Treatment. Conservative treatment for the phase of irritative voiding symptoms: prostatic massage, sexual activity, and treatment of infection. The patient should void as soon as the urge is noted, and he should not drink large volumes of fluid in a short time. Acute retention is treated by catheterization. If the catheter is left indwelling for several days, acute congestion may reverse and normal voiding becomes possible.

The phase of obstructive voiding symptoms, with progressively increasing residual urine and back pressure on the kidney, requires prostatectomy. Prostatectomy (actually, excision of the adenomatous periurethral growth) may be done by the transurethral, suprapubic, retropubic, or perineal approach. Transurethral resection is preferred for glands under 50-60 g in size.

5. Prognosis is good if adenoma is removed. Operative mortality is low.

E. CARCINOMA OF THE PROSTATE is rare before age 60 years, but by the 8th decade it affects 25% of men. It is frequently associated with benign hyperplasia; in such cases, it arises in the "surgical capsule" (the true prostatic tissue surrounding the hyperplastic periurethral glands). The posterior lobe is the most common site of origin. It metastasizes via lymphatics and through the blood stream to vertebrae and pelvic bones. The following staging system is used:

Stage A: Incidental focal malignant tumor noted in tissue removed by transurethral resection for benign hyperplasia. Rectal examination is normal.

Stage B: Localized induration of prostate confined within capsule. Normal serum acid phosphatase.

Stage C: Extracapsular extension of tumor. Invasion of seminal vesicles. Elevation of serum acid phosphatase.

Stage D: Distant metastases.

1. Diagnosis

a. Symptoms. May be asymptomatic, found on routine rectal examination. "Prostatism" (as in benign hyperplasia) in 95%. Bone pain, pathologic fracture, radicular pain from vertebral involvement.

b. Signs by rectal examination. Early—firm nodule on lateral edge of prostate. Late—prostate is stony hard, fixed with extension of tumor to the seminal vesicles.

c. Laboratory tests. No abnormalities in early stages. Elevated prostate-specific antigen (PSA). Anemia from metastases to bone marrow or uremia. Infected urine. PSP shows residual urine. Deteriorating renal function with chronic obstruction. Serum acid phosphatase often is elevated with local extension or metastases; alkaline phosphatase is elevated with osseous metastases.

d. Radiographic findings. Sclerotic (osteoblastic) bony metastases; excretory urography may show vesical neck or ureteral obstruction. CT or MRI is helpful in staging prostatic cancer and detecting pelvic lymphadenopathy.

e. Special tests. Transrectal ultrasonography. Hypoechoic areas can be confirmed by ultrasound guided biopsy. Catheterization measures residual urine. Cystoscopy shows an irregular prostate and evidence of bladder outlet obstruction. Needle biopsy (transperineal or transrectal) proves the presence of malignancy; transurethral resection of obstructing tissue may also reveal carcinoma. MRI and transrectal ultrasonography are helpful in staging.

2. Differential diagnosis. Biopsy differentiates carcinoma from benign hyperplasia, chronic prostatitis, tuberculous prostatitis, and prostatic calculi.

3. Treatment

a. Surgical. Radical prostatectomy for early lesions. Transurethral resection palliates obstruction.

b. Endocrine. These tumors are hormone-dependent, and these measures are palliative: orchiectomy; estrogen (diethylstilbestrol 1-2 mg/day); androgen ablation therapy with flutamide or leuprolide; corticosteroids or hypophysectomy when the tumor becomes androgen-independent.

c. Radiation therapy (external, or interstitial with iodine-125 or gold seeds) may be curative or palliative. Osseous metastases also respond to radiation therapy.

4. Prognosis. The 10-year survival rate is 65% for early lesions treated by radical prostatectomy. Palliative measures relieve symptoms and prolong life for 10 years or more in a few patients, but most die within 5 years.

F. TESTIS. Testicular tumors comprise 4% of tumors of the genitourinary tract. They occur most frequently between ages 20 and 35 years. The incidence is higher in undescended testes. These malignancies metastasize via lymphatics to periaortic nodes and through the blood stream to the liver and lungs.

Seminoma is the most common malignant testicular tumor, followed by embryonal carcinoma, teratoma, and choriocarcinoma. Many tumors have mixed patterns. Secretion of chorionic gonadotropins is associated with hyperplasia of the Leydig cells.

Benign (Sertoli cell and interstitial cell) testicular tumors are rare. They elaborate androgens and estrogens, causing precocious sexual maturation in boys and gynecomastia in men. The following staging system is used:

Stage 1	Tumor confined to testis. No clinical or radiologic evidence of spread.
1A	Iliac and periaortic nodes uninvolved (determined by retroperitoneal lymphadenectomy).
1B	Iliac or periaortic nodes involved.
Stage 2	Clinical or radiographic evidence of metastases to nodes below the diaphragm. No metastases above the diaphragm.
Stage 3	Metastases above the diaphragm or to the viscera.

1. Diagnosis

a. Symptoms and signs. Painless enlargement of the testicle. Gynecomastia if the tumor secretes gonadotropins or estrogen. Symptoms and signs of metastases. Testis enlarged, heavy, firm, irregular, with loss of sensation. May be associated hydrocele (10%) or hematocele.

b. Laboratory tests. Elevated urinary gonadotropins mean that a chorioepithelioma is present (the degree of elevation and the response to orchiectomy are important prognostic signs). Elevated urinary 17-ketosteroids with interstitial cell tumors.

c. Radiographic findings. Chest radiographs may show metastases. Excretory urograms may show ureteral displacement of obstruction from periaortic lymph node involvement. CT scanning is helpful in staging.

2. Differential diagnosis. Hydrocele (transilluminates), hematocele, spermatocele, epididymitis, gumma.

3. Treatment

a. Surgical. Immediate operation through the inguinal canal to clamp and divide the spermatic cord and perform a radical orchiectomy. Bilateral radical retroperitoneal lymphadenectomy for all tumors except seminoma; this is done even if nodes are known to be involved preoperatively.

b. Radiation therapy. Treatment of choice for seminoma. An adjunct to lymphadenectomy in other tumors (may be used alone in stage 1 tumors).

c. Chemotherapy is an effective adjunct both preoperatively in the presence of large abdominal lymphadenopathy or postoperatively if hyperplastic nodes prove to be involved.

4. Prognosis. Seminoma has the best prognosis. Other stage 1 lesions, except choriocarcinoma, have an 85%-90% 5-year survival rate. Choriocarcinoma is usually fatal.

G. PENIS. Tumors of the penis are epidermoid lesions similar to epidermoid tumors elsewhere. Most arise on the glans under redundant preputial skin. Chronic inflammation and irritation in uncircumsized men are causally related. Metastases go to inguinal lymph nodes initially, then into the iliac nodes.

A firm, ulcerated, painless lesion of the glans is the usual clinical presentation. Secondary infection produces pain and a foul discharge. Biopsy of the penile lesion differentiates carcinoma from chancre, chancroid, and condyloma acuminatum. Inguinal lymph nodes may enlarge from infection or metastases.

Partial amputation of the penis or radiation therapy gives good results in small lesions. Groin dissection (inguinal lymphadenectomy) is performed only if the nodes are enlarged.

VIII. NEUROGENIC BLADDER

Intact innervation is necessary for the bladder to function normally. The detrusor muscle is innervated by parasympathetic pelvic nerves S2-S4. The sensory supply for pain, touch, and temperature in the bladder is carried by sympathetic fibers arising in the lower thoracic and upper lumbar segments. The motor and sensory supply of the trigone comes from the same sympathetic nerves. The striated external sphincter and urogenital diaphragm receive somatic motor and sensory fibers via the pudendal nerves from S2-S4.

Normally, when the bladder fills to its maximum capacity (about 400-500 ml), a sensation of fullness and a desire to urinate are experienced. The pelvic floor and voluntary external sphincter relax, the detrusor contracts, and the bladder empties completely. The bladder generates a voiding pressure of about 20 cm of water, and the urine flow rate is 20-25 ml/second. After voiding, the bladder relaxes and the sphincter contracts to ensure continence.

Cystometry yields information about bladder capacity, completeness of emptying, and the bladder's ability to accommodate increasing volumes without increasing its pressure, thus indicating whether sensation is intact and whether the bladder can initiate and sustain a contraction. A catheter is passed into the bladder, and the volume of residual urine is measured. The catheter is attached to a water manometer and the intraluminal pressure is measured after instillation of increments of fluid. A **cystometrogram** is a graph with pressure (in cm) plotted on the ordinate and volume (in ml) on the abscissa.

Neurogenic bladder is divided into two groups, depending on the level of the lesion in relation to the micturition center (S2-S4).

A. UPPER MOTOR NEURON LESION (SPASTIC NEUROGENIC BLADDER).

Lesions above S2-S4 are usually due to trauma. The micturition center loses its communication with the midbrain and cerebral cortex, but the reflex arc between the bladder and the spinal cord remains intact. The bladder wall becomes spastic, the ability to accommodate is lost, and frequent uninhibited detrusor contraction occurs in response to bladder distention or extraneous stimuli because simultaneous contraction of the pelvic floor and voluntary sphincter prevents adequate emptying. Contraction of the detrusor is elicited by trigger mechanisms, e.g., stimulation of the abdominal skin, genitalia, or thighs.

The bladder is hypertrophied and trabeculated. Eventually, vesicoureteral reflux occurs with progressive deterioration of the upper tract. Cystometry reveals a hyperactive detrusor, high intravesical pressure, diminished vesical capacity, and some residual urine.

If bladder capacity is adequate, the patient can be trained to empty the bladder by the trigger mechanism and thus minimize uncontrolled contractions and incontinence. The resistance of the bladder outlet can be reduced (by transurethral resection of the prostate or by sphincterectomy) to help the bladder empty completely. Selected cases can benefit from sacral root stimulation to evacuate the bladder and maintain continence (bladder pacemaker). If bladder capacity is small, an indwelling catheter may be needed. Urinary diversion is indicated in cases of progressive renal damage.

B. LOWER MOTOR NEURON LESION (FLACCID NEUROGENIC BLADDER). Lesions involving the spinal cord micturition center, the cauda equina, the sacral roots, or the peripheral nerves lead to an atonic or flaccid bladder. Trauma is the common cause. Meningomyelocele and disc disease also can be responsible.

The bladder is areflexic because its connections to the micturition center are lost; any detrusor activity is on a myogenic basis with weak and unsustained contractions. Cystometry reveals a low pressure curve, increased capacity, no sensation of fullness, absent detrusor contraction, and a large volume of residual urine. UTIs, stone formation, reflux, and impaired renal function are the main complications. Incontinence of the overflow type is a problem.

The patient is instructed to empty the bladder regularly by manual suprapubic compression (Credé maneuver) to avoid overflow incontinence. Surgical reduction of outlet resistance sometimes helps completeness of emptying. Intermittent self-catheterization may be of great value in controlling infection and protecting the upper tract, especially if instituted early.

IX. OTHER DISORDERS OF THE KIDNEY*

A. POLYCYSTIC KIDNEY. This familial disorder is usually bilateral and may also involve liver and pancreas. Multiple cysts scattered throughout the kidneys compress the parenchyma and cause atrophy and renal failure. Death occurs during infancy in severe cases, but most patients become symptomatic in the 30-40 age group.

---

*See Chapter 11 for renal hypertension.

1. Diagnosis

a. Symptoms and signs. Hypertension, renal insufficiency, renal pain; one or both kidneys may be palpable.

b. Laboratory tests. Hematuria, proteinuria, pyuria, bacteriuria. Anemia due to uremia. Impaired renal function.

c. Radiographic findings. Enlarged kidneys with calyceal distortion. Sonography reveals the cystic lesion.

2. Differential diagnosis. Bilateral hydronephrosis, renal tumors, simple cysts, and tuberous sclerosis.

3. Complications. Pyelonephritis, hypertension, renal failure.

4. Treatment is medical (treat infection and renal failure—see Chapter 2). Surgical intervention is done in rare instances when a cyst compresses the ureter. Renal transplantation should be considered in end-stage patients.

5. Prognosis. Death in 5-10 years after the diagnosis is made unless transplantation is successful.

B. SIMPLE SOLITARY CYST. Simple renal cysts are much more common than polycystic kidneys. The cyst is unilateral, simple, and usually is discovered incidentally on urologic evaluation. Flank pain occurs occasionally. Spontaneous rupture, infection, hemorrhage into the cyst are possible complications.

The most important **differential diagnosis** is between cyst and tumor. Sonography, CT scan, and angiography usually distinguish the two. Fluid can be aspirated through a percutaneous needle; it should be studied cytologically because 5% of cysts have associated malignancy in the wall. Surgical exploration is indicated in doubtful cases; simple unroofing is curative for benign cysts.

C. RENAL FUSION. Horseshoe kidney is the most common type of renal fusion. It usually is asymptomatic, but it can result in hydronephrosis (from urethral compression), stone formation, or infection. No treatment is indicated unless complications occur.

15

Plastic and Reconstructive Surgery

To-Nao Wang
Stephen J. Mathes

I. GENERAL PRINCIPLES

Plastic and reconstructive surgery is a specialty devoted to the functional and aesthetic restoration of physical deformities. This includes, but is not limited to, the correction of dysfunction and disfigurement from maxillofacial, hand and lower extremity trauma, burn injury (thermal, electric, and caustic), amputation of body parts (digits, scalp, ear, and penis), major cancer resection (head and neck, breast, genitalia, and extremities), pressure sores, failures of wound healing (osteoradionecrosis, osteomyelitis, and postsurgical wound dehiscence), and congenital anomalies such as cleft lip and palate, craniofacial, hand, and truncal defects.

Aesthetic plastic surgery complements reconstructive surgery and addresses the correction of body contour distortion or asymmetry, and the stigmata and deformities that result from the aging process. Aesthetic procedures include rhytidectomy, blepharoplasty, rhinoplasty, otoplasty, augmentation or reduction mammoplasty, abdominoplasty, and suction-assisted lipectomy.

An understanding of the basic sciences of anatomy, physiology of wound healing, and pathophysiology of tissue injury is fundamental to the successful application of plastic and reconstructive surgery. Major advances such as microsurgery, craniofacial surgery, and knowledge of applied functional anatomy have led to an improved ability to solve wound problems in every anatomic region of the body.

A. APPROACH TO PLASTIC TISSUE REPAIR. The planning for surgical repair begins with an accurate assessment of the tissue defect and includes the identification of factors that may be deterrents to wound healing (Table 15-1). A clear def-

Table 15-1. Deterrents of wound healing

1. Vascular insufficiency	Arterial, venous, postirradiation ischemia
2. Malnutrition	Albumin <3, starvation >7 days, >10% loss body mass
3. Infection	>10^5 bacterial count
4. Immune deficiency	Congenital, acquired, iatrogenic
5. Antimetabolites	Chemotherapy, steroids, tobacco
6. Systemic disease	Cardiopulmonary and renal insufficiency, diabetes mellitus, morbid obesity

inition of the desired reconstructive outcome is based on an analysis of the functional and cosmetic requirements of the defect (Table 15-2). The reconstructive ladder concept is to select the least complex surgical procedure(s) that will best satisfy the reconstructive demand (Table 15-3). A successful outcome depends on correct preoperative assessment, reversal of unfavorable local and systemic factors, and execution of the surgical reconstruction to restore both form and function.

B. GENERAL PLASTIC REPAIR OF ACUTE WOUNDS

1. The mechanisms of soft tissue injury include laceration, avulsion, crush, and amputation. Selecting the proper repair depends on the viability and availability of tissues adjacent to the zone of injury.

2. Tetanus immunization status is ascertained and treatment is initiated with toxoid, hyperimmune globulin, or active immunization as appropriate.

3. Preparation for repair begins with **local anesthesia** (Table 15-4) by field infiltration or peripheral nerve block, reserving general anesthesia and regional nerve block for repair of complex wounds in the operating room as defined by the necessary duration (>2 hours) and complexity of repair.

4. The wound is cleaned by saline irrigation followed by visual inspection and digital palpation to remove retained foreign body (e.g., glass, gravel).

5. Debridement is limited to conservative sharp excision of devascularized tissues. Incisions are made at right angles to the skin to minimize the area of dermal scar formation.

6. Further tissue crush and devascularization is avoided by gentle handling of tissues with fine forceps, accurate cautery

Table 15-2. Defect analysis

Mechanism of injury	Acquired: extent of tissue loss or injury; duration. Congenital: extent of anatomic abnormality or tissue deficit	Debridement of all devitalized, chronically colonized or infected tissues (see function and contour)
Size	Availability of local tissues for repair	Wound closure by direct suture, local tissue realignment, or transplantation of distant tissues.
Composition	Anatomic structures injured, exposed, or at risk (i.e., bone, joint, cartilage, vessel, nerve, viscera)	Expeditious wound coverage by vascularized tissue to preserve deep structures
Function	Durability, sensibility, motor innervation, structural stability	Restore function by repair or substitution (i.e., ORIF, nerve graft, tendon or bone graft)
Contour	Symmetry, local tissue match	Normalize contour by augmentation or reduction (i.e., implant, autogenous flap or composite graft; excision or suction-assisted lipectomy)

of bleeding points, and minimal undermining of adjacent tissues.

7. Repair is performed by accurate and tension-free coaptation of the epidermis and dermis without strangulation of the interval tissues that can result in necrosis or permanent "cross hatching" scars.

a. Absorbable sutures (plain or chromic catgut, polyglycolate, PDS) are used for approximation of mucosa, muscle, subcutaneous tissue, and dermis.

Table 15-3. Reconstructive ladder

Simple

	1. Primary closure	
	2. Skin graft	Partial or full thickness
	3. Local, regional tissue transfer	Advancement, rotation, transposition
	4. Distant tissue transplantation	Microvascular transplantation

Complex

Table 15-4. Local anesthetic agents

Agent	Maximum dose	Indication
1%, 2% Xylocaine	6 mg/kg	Field infiltration, digital nerve block, peripheral nerve block
1%, 2% Xylocaine with 1/100,000-1/400,000 epinephrine	10 mg/kg	Scalp and face; not for use in digits or end-organ without collateral circulation
0.25%-0.5% Marcaine	Minimum effective dose. Limit: 50-150 mg/dose	Peripheral nerve block, regional nerve block

b. Skin may be closed with permanent sutures in interrupted, mattress, or intracuticular fashion (Figure 15-1) and reinforced with skin tapes as desired to support exact skin edge apposition.

c. Facial sutures are removed in 4-7 days to avoid epithelialization of suture tracks that result in permanent punctate scars adjacent to the incision.

d. Sutures at other anatomic sites that require additional support may be left in place for 10-14 days or reinforced with skin tapes after earlier removal.

8. If the patient presents later than 12 hours after injury, direct suture closure of most wounds is contraindicated owing to high risk of subsequent wound infection. Facial and scalp wounds may be closed within 24 hours if there is no gross con-

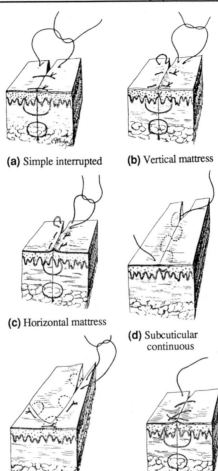

(a) Simple interrupted

(b) Vertical mattress

(c) Horizontal mattress

(d) Subcuticular continuous

(e) Half-buried horizontal mattress

(f) Continuous over and over

FIGURE 15-1. For legend see opposite page.

tamination, tissue crush, or erythema; superior tissue vascularity in this region imparts an improved capacity to resist infection.

9. Direct suture closure is contraindicated in most instances of **human bite injuries,** for which hospitalization, open wound care, parenteral antibiotics, and possible delayed closure at 3-7 days are appropriate modalities of management.

a. Immediate closure of facial bite wounds may be considered to prevent the devastating outcome of severe, visible scarring.

b. A loose closure is performed after copious irrigation, with institution of broad-spectrum antibiotic therapy and with the understanding that open wound management may become necessary if early wound infection occurs.

10. Most **animal bites** may be loosely approximated with conjoint antibiotic prophylaxis against *Pasteurella multocida.* Comprehensive care includes proper reporting to Public Health authorities and treatment for rabies depending on clinical findings.

C. METHODS OF WOUND CLOSURE

1. Direct suture of lacerations is appropriate when adjacent or deep structural injury (e.g., nerve, artery, tendon, joint) can be ruled out.

When possible, a suture line should be oriented parallel to or within natural skin creases (i.e., perpendicular to the axis of underlying muscle) to avoid tension and later scar contracture across existing vectors of stress. The most aesthetic scar alignment for facial repair is along the lines of expression or contour lines which are normally accentuated by facial animation and aging (Figure 15-2).

2. If tissue deficiency precludes a tension-free closure, addition of supplemental tissues or realignment of local tissue by elevation of local flaps may be necessary to achieve wound coverage. The technics to mobilize tissue for defect repair are categorized by the **method of transfer.**

FIGURE 15-1. Methods of suture. **A,** Simple interrupted; **B,** vertical mattress; **C,** horizontal mattress; **D,** subcuticular continuous; **E,** half-buried horizontal mattress; **F,** continuous over and over. (From Grabb, Smith, editors: *Plastic surgery,* 3rd ed, Boston, 1979, Little, Brown & Co.)

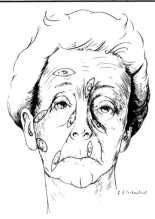

FIGURE 15-2. Sites of elliptical incisions corresponding to wrinkle lines in the face.

a. Advancement relies on adjacent tissue laxity to "reach" across the defect in a linear fashion for wound closure. Undermining of the tissue segment to be advanced (Figure 15-3**A**) or a V-Y closure may be required to achieve tension-free closure (Figure 15-3**B**).

b. Transposition and rotation closure of an adjacent defect is achieved by pivoting a segment of tissue across an arc of rotation based on a fixed point, usually located either at the flap base or at the point of entrance of the vascular pedicle into the flap. Transposition refers to the transfer of a rectangular flap of skin, muscle, or fascia. The site of origin of the flap (donor site) is either closed directly or requires skin graft coverage (Figure 15-4**A-D**). The rhomboid flap is a commonly used transposition flap for closure of small defects, particularly in the face where direct closure may distort adjacent normal structures (Figure 15-4**C-G**). Rotation implies the movement of a circular or semicircular flap of skin, fascia, or muscle (Figure 15-4**H** and **I**).

c. Transplantation refers to the complete removal of tissue from its anatomic attachment for placement at another site.

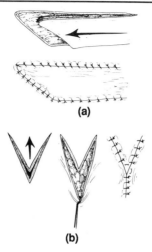

(a)

(b)

FIGURE 15-3. A, Advancement pedicle flap. **B,** V-Y advancement flap.

Nonvascularized transplants (skin, dermis, fat, bone, cartilage, tendon, nerve, or composite grafts) rely on vascular ingrowth from the recipient bed for survival. *Vascularized transplants* retain their blood supply by microvascular anastomosis of afferent and efferent vessels to recipient vessels within proximity of the defect and can enhance perfusion to the recipient bed. When there is inadequate local tissue for coverage, severe scar formation, chronic infection, or ischemia of the wound, vascularized or "free" tissue transplantation remains a superior solution to enhance wound healing and expedite wound closure. Specialized applications include the interposition of vascularized bone or jejunum to replace an incontinuity defect in the extremity or esophagus respectively.

3. Nonvascularized tissue transfer

a. Split-thickness skin grafts measure 0.012-0.024 inches (0.3-0.6 mm) in thickness and may be harvested by a Weck blade or precalibrated dermatome (Figure 15-5). Al-

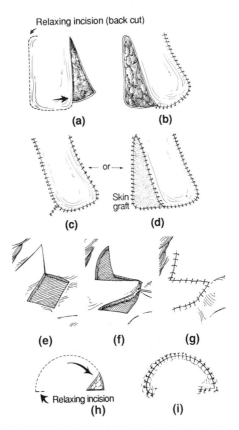

FIGURE 15-4. A-D, Transposition flap. **E,** The planned rhomboid excision is completed and the LLL flap incised. **F,** The flap is transposed into the rhomboid defect. Again, the undermining beyond the base of the flap has been performed. **G,** The defect is closed without tension and undue distortion of natural anatomic landmarks. **H-I,** Rotation flap.

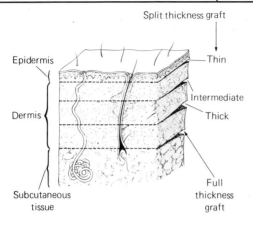

FIGURE 15-5. Depths of split-thickness grafts.

though the donor site heals spontaneously from residual dermal elements and epidermal lined skin appendages (i.e., hair follicles, sweat, and sebaceous glands), visible and permanent scar at the donor site is unavoidable. Split-thickness grafts have a tendency for hyperpigmentation and late graft contracture, making their use suboptimal for facial color match and for resurfacing areas where elastic distention is a functional requirement (e.g., over joint surfaces). Irreversible "take" or graft vascularization requires 7-14 days. The most common causes for failure of graft vascularization are motion between the graft and recipient bed, inadequate bacteriologic control of the recipient wound, and arterial or venous insufficiency of the graft bed.

b. Full-thickness skin grafts include both epidermal and dermal elements. Donor sites are closed primarily by suture. Criteria for successful vascularization of the graft at the recipient site are the same as for split-thickness grafts, but owing to an increased metabolic demand of the greater volume of tissue transplanted, clinical signs of vascularization may require longer to be apparent. The advantages of a full-thickness graft are enhanced durability, decreased graft contracture, improved sensory reinnervation, and improved color match for facial wounds, particularly if the skin is harvested from the pre- or postauricular or supraclavicular region.

c. A composite graft contains more than one tissue element (e.g., skin with fat or cartilage) and like skin grafts depends entirely on the vascularity of the recipient bed for its survival. Tissue volume exceeding 1 cm^2 may not be reliably transplanted without ischemic loss of the composite graft. Its use is indicated by specific defects of contour in specialized structures such as the nose, ear, or nipple.

4. Vascularized tissue transfer and flaps. A flap is classified by its anatomic blood supply and its soft tissue composition (Figure 15-6).

a. Random pattern skin flaps depend on dermal vasculature for viability and may be successfully elevated in all anatomic regions. The random flap may be reliably advanced, rotated, or transposed into the defect as long as the flap length does not exceed 1.5-2 times the dimension of the flap base. An example is the Z-plasty where 2 opposing random flaps are interposed for the purpose of lengthening scar contracture (Figure 15-7).

b. An axial skin flap is designed over a specific vessel that extends along the axis of the flap and sustains perfusion along the entire flap length. An axial pattern flap is more reliable than the random pattern flap, and its size is limited by the vascular territory of the underlying vessel. An example is the forehead flap where a skin flap is designed over the supratroch-

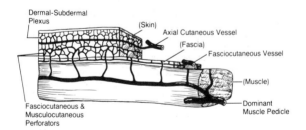

FIGURE 15-6. Skin blood supply. The anatomic basis for successful design of random pattern, axial, fasciocutaneous, muscle, and musculocutaneous flaps.

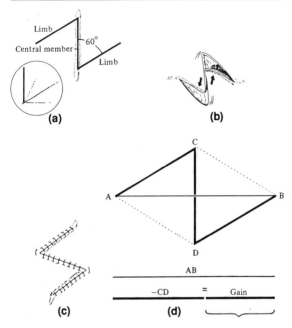

FIGURE 15-7. A-C, The classic 60-degree angle Z-plasty. Inset shows method of finding the 60° angle by first drawing a 90-degree angle, then dividing it in thirds by sighting. The limbs of the Z must be equal in length to the central member. **D,** Calculating theoretical gain in length of Z-plasty. The theoretical gain in length is the difference in length between the long diagonal and the short diagonal. In actual practice the gain in length has varied from 45% less to 25% more than calculated geometrically, due to biomechanical properties of the skin.

lear or supraorbital vessel and rotated to cover nasal defects (Figure 15-8).

c. Muscle flaps have defined patterns of blood supply by specific vascular pedicles. Muscles with major or dominant vascular pedicles may be reliably transposed or rotated locally

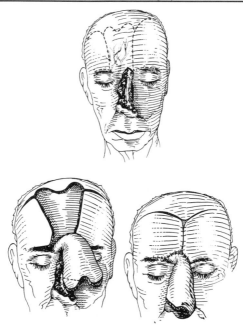

FIGURE 15-8. Forehead skin flap rotated for subtotal nasal defect coverage. Flap design based on axial pattern blood supply to the skin.

into tissue defects after release of the muscle's origin and/or insertion. Muscles may also be transplanted to cover distant defects by microvascular anastomosis of its dominant or major vascular pedicle to recipient vessels within the defect. Muscles with a single, major, or dominant vascular pedicle are more useful as a flap because the muscle is unaltered following release of its origin and/or insertions for transfer or transplantation into a defect. Frequently used muscle flaps include latissimus dorsi, pectoralis major, rectus abdominis, gracilis, and tensor fascia lata.

A *musculocutaneous flap* includes a segment of skin that

is perfused by musculocutaneous perforating vessels from the underlying muscle and may be reliably transferred as a skin and muscle unit.

d. Fasciocutaneous flaps are based on intermuscular and septal vascular pedicles that extend into deep fascia and subsequently provide cutaneous circulation. Flaps designed on fascial circulation have less bulk than musculocutaneous flaps and are not limited to a 2:1 length:width ratio of the random pattern flaps. This flap may be transposed to an adjacent defect or transplanted by microvascular defects to distant sites and is frequently used when a thin flap with skin provides more aesthetic contour when applied to surface defects. The addition of fascia is also useful when restoration of structural integrity (e.g., abdominal wall) or a biologic seal (CSF leak) is required. Unlike the musculocutaneous flap, the donor site frequently requires skin graft coverage. Reliable flaps in this category include the temporoparietal fascia, posterior gluteal thigh, radial forearm, and lateral arm flap.

e. Expanded tissue flaps are the result of serial inflation of a tissue expansion prosthesis that is implanted for the purpose of increasing the surface area of a unit of skin, fascia, or muscle intended for transfer. An interval of 6-10 weeks is needed for outpatient serial inflation (every 3-7 days) of the prosthesis with saline to achieve desired expansion of tissues. Upon removal of the prosthesis, the expanded tissues are mobilized and advanced for coverage of either an adjacent defect or retention of a permanent implant such as in postmastectomy breast reconstruction. Tissue expansion is particularly useful for restoring defects requiring specialized tissues such as hair-bearing scalp, forehead, or cheek skin, for which the quality of tissue match is aesthetically suboptimal when distant tissues are used for replacement.

II. MAXILLOFACIAL INJURY

A. SOFT TISSUE INJURY

1. Rule out underlying facial bone fracture and disruption of the lacrimal apparatus, branches of the facial nerve (VII), parotid gland and duct.

2. Irrigate to remove thrombus and debris; debride to excise devascularized tissues, remove foreign body, and convert skin edges to a perpendicular configuration.

3. Suture in layers as needed to close mucosa (oral, conjunctiva), facial muscles, and skin.

4. Adequate soft tissue coverage must be provided to preserve the viability of exposed bone and cartilage (ear, nose, calvarium).

5. Wound check in 48 hours; suture removal in 4-7 days.

6. Facial nerve, lacrimal duct, and parotid duct disruption requires anatomic repair, usually in the operating room with the assistance of loupes or microscope magnification.

7. Complications include wound infection, hypertrophic scar formation, and facial contour distortion that may require antibiotics, scar revision, or secondary reconstruction, respectively.

B. FACIAL BONE FRACTURE
1. General evaluation

a. Ascertain and secure airway; unstable facial skeleton, hemorrhage, and altered consciousness are fatal risks for aspiration and asphyxiation.

b. Rule out cervical spine injury by history (e.g., acceleration-deceleration injury), examination, and cervical spine radiography (C1-C7).

c. Palpation to evaluate the integrity of the facial skeleton (orbit, zygoma, midface, nose, and mandible).

d. Inspect the tympanic membrane, and oral and nasal cavities and palpate the temporomandibular joint for signs of hemorrhage, structural disruption, and impediment to mobility, respectively.

e. Evaluate dental occlusion by objective examination and elicit the patient's subjective assessment of altered occlusion.

f. Radiologic survey to include Water's view, basal view of the skull, and oblique views of the mandible. CT is now frequently indicated both for evaluation of possible associated intracranial injury and for analysis of complex facial fractures.

g. Defer definitive reduction or internal fixation for 5-7 days if severe edema prevents accurate assessment of facial symmetry or if multiple system trauma requires urgent stabilization of the patient's general status.

2. Nasal fracture

a. Reduce acutely under local (lidocaine to skin and 4% cocaine intranasal packs) or general anesthesia as needed.

b. Reduce by bimanual manipulation with periosteal elevator used intranasally as fulcrum.

c. Speculum intranasal inspection with repair of mucosal lacerations and drainage of septal hematoma as needed.

d. Splint reduced fracture with intranasal petrolatum gauze and molded external split (plaster or plastic) for 5-7 days.

e. Reduction after 3-4 weeks may require formal osteotomy to realign fracture segments, especially in children and young adults.

f. Complications include relapse of fracture, septal perforation, or septal deviation with nasal airway obstruction.

3. Zygoma fracture

a. Clinical signs include periorbital edema and ecchymosis, subconjunctival hemorrhage, infraorbital rim step off, malar and cheek flattening, diplopia, entrapment (inferior rectus muscle or orbital contents) preventing normal upward gaze, and ipsilateral upper lip numbness (infraorbital branch of trigeminal nerve).

b. Radiographic signs include opacified maxillary sinus and fracture at the frontal, maxillary, and temporal suture lines of the zygoma (tripod fracture pattern).

c. Accurate assessment of *visual acuity* and extraocular motion is essential to rule out globe disruption and entrapment. Ophthalmologic consultation is indicated, especially when examination is suboptimal or findings are equivocal.

d. Open reduction with three-point bony fixation with either intraosseous wires or plates and screws is indicated for displaced and unstable fractures and for positive signs of entrapment, persistent diplopia, facial asymmetry, and persistent infraorbital nerve anesthesia.

e. CT scan is indicated for assessment of orbital floor disruption and displacement of orbital contents (blowout fracture) into the maxillary sinus.

f. Complications include enophthalmos, persistent diplopia, and facial asymmetry that may require correction by secondary osteotomy and bone grafting.

4. Maxillary fractures

a. The extent of midfacial disruption is proportional to the magnitude and vector of the injuring force. Injury ranges from isolated alveolar segment fracture to craniofacial dysjunction by the Le Forte classification (Figure 15-9).

b. Urgent airway control is indicated for severe fractures with persistent hemorrhage, particularly in patients with altered consciousness due to associated neurologic injury. Neurosur-

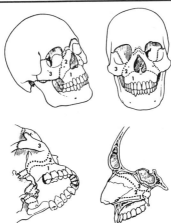

FIGURE 15-9. Fractures of the maxillas. **1:** Le Fort I (transverse or Guérin) fracture. **2:** Le Fort II (pyramidal) fracture. **3:** Le Fort III fracture (craniofacial dysjunction).

gical consultation is indicated for CSF leak and history of loss of consciousness.

c. Disimpaction and open reduction with fixation are indicated to control bleeding, CSF leak, and stabilization of fracture fragments, especially when comminution, instability, and elongation of the midface is noted. The use of mini plates and screws for bony fixation and immediate bone grafting for bone defects has significantly improved results in complex maxillary fracture management.

d. Intermaxillary fixation (arch bars) alone or with intraoral acrylic splints may be sufficient therapy for segmental, stable alveolar fractures.

e. The prevalent complications are midfacial distortion by elongation, retrusion, or malocclusion that may require secondary correction.

5. Mandible fracture
a. Clinical signs include localized tenderness on palpation, altered occlusion, and obvious disruption by external palpation or intraoral inspection.

b. Panorex radiograph to isolate mandible for assessment of teeth, mandibular body, angle, ramus and condyle, temporomandibular joints, and alterations of symmetry.

c. Subcondylar, nondisplaced, stable, isolated, or closed fractures may be treated by intermaxillary fixation with elastic traction bands and custom acrylic splints if normal occlusion can be adequately maintained for 4-6 weeks.

d. Unstable fractures with comminution and displacement or absence of teeth require open reduction and internal fixation with miniplates or wire.

e. Edentulous mandibles may require additional customized splints for anatomic reduction and union.

f. Complications include infection, nonunion, and persistent distortion of occlusion.

III. EXTREMITY DISEASE AND INJURY

A. PATHOGENESIS OF TISSUE DEFICIT

1. Traumatic crush, avulsion, or amputation may affect multiple structures at any anatomic level.

2. Arterial insufficiency by atherosclerosis or diabetes affects leg, ankle, and feet.

3. Venous insufficiency affects leg and ankle.

4. Osteomyelitis affects any level and is commonly posttraumatic in origin.

5. Osteoradionecrosis affects the zone of radiation injury.

6. Exposed bone, joint, vascular prosthesis, or orthopedic appliance may be the result of cancer resection, failure of postoperative wound healing, or infection.

B. INDICATIONS FOR RECONSTRUCTIVE COVERAGE
include preservation of exposed fracture and adjacent vital structures, limb salvage, and as definitive treatment for wounds that fail to heal spontaneously.

C. MANAGEMENT begins with aggressive surgical debridement of devitalized or infected soft tissue and bone.

1. Successful coverage depends on adequate bacteriologic control of the wound.

2. Operability depends on the adequacy of proximal arterial inflow and distal venous outflow by clinical examination and arteriography.

a. Initial priority in trauma is to restore vascularity to the distal limb by repair or interpositional replacement of disrupted major inflow vessels.

b. For severe atherosclerosis, peripheral vascular reconstruction to restore proximal inflow (aortofemoral, femoral popliteal, or femoral-distal bypass) may be necessary prior to soft tissue coverage of the distal extremity.

3. Urgent priority is indicated for coverage and preservation of exposed vessels, vascular prosthesis, bone, joint, orthopedic appliances, and tendon. Associated fractures should be stabilized with restoration of limb length by either internal or external fixation prior to definitive soft tissue coverage.

4. Choice of coverage depends on location, size, and exposed contents of the defect. Culture-specific parenteral antibiotics are indicated for all infected open wounds undergoing reconstructive coverage.

a. Skin grafting is appropriate for noninfected, well-perfused defects capable of generating granulation tissue (capillary ingrowth).

b. Local flaps (muscle, fascia, skin) are indicated by the availability of adjacent noninjured tissues.

c. Muscle or musculocutaneous flaps provide improved local wound perfusion and are preferred for coverage of infected, irradiated or ischemic wounds.

d. Free microvascular transplantation (usually muscle) is frequently the only reconstructive option for defects distal to the midtibia level. The success of elective microvascular tissue transplantation is 96%. Transplanted muscle may be anastomosed in series to distal bypass grafts to salvage the foot in diabetes and severe vascular disease. Transplanted muscle may be skin grafted directly to provide vascularized composite coverage. Restoration of sensation may be achieved by neurorrhaphy of a sensory nerve in the flap to a recipient nerve within the defect.

5. Timing of reconstructive coverage is optimal either within 1 week of acute injury or 3-4 months after onset of injury or disease.

6. Complications include infection, partial or total loss of tissues used for coverage, and limb loss.

D. SUCCESSFUL REPLANTATION OF AMPUTATED PARTS is limited by warm ischemia time of 6-8 hours and cold ischemia time up to 24 hours.

1. Multiple levels of injury in the amputated part are usually a contraindication to successful replantation.

2. Amputated parts should be transported in saline-moistened gauze placed in a watertight container. Container is transported on ice to prolong preservation.

3. Elective transplantation of toes to replace lost thumb or digits is delayed until the acute wound is healed with adequate soft tissue coverage.

IV. PRESSURE SORES

A. PATHOPHYSIOLOGY

1. The injury force is persistent pressure applied over bony prominences, resulting in the progressive ischemic necrosis of internal soft tissues (skin, fat, muscle) over the ischium, sacrum, trochanter, heels, or elbows (Table 15-5).

2. The results of pressure injury are ulceration, tissue loss, and infection.

3. Patients at risk for pressure injury have either abnormal afferent innervation to the affected part such that the pain of tissue ischemia is not perceived, or abnormal efferent motor innervation such that there is inability to alleviate pressure. Central lesions may affect both sensory and motor tracts.

a. Central deficits include quadriplegia, paraplegia, coma, and stroke.

b. Diseases with *incomplete central deficit* include multiple sclerosis, Parkinson's disease, and psychiatric pathology.

c. Peripheral sensory deficits are common in diabetes, leprosy, and chronic alcoholism.

d. Iatrogenic causes for pressure injury include injudicious cast application, failure to turn a bedridden inpatient,

Table 15-5. Clinical stages of pressure injury to skin and soft tissue over bony prominences

Observed	Duration of ischemia	Duration to resolution
I. Erythema	30 minutes	1 hour
II. Ischemia	2-6 hours	36-48 hours
III. Necrosis	>6 hours	Irreversible
IV. Ulceration	—	Irreversible

and prolonged anesthesia time for operations, especially when complicated by low-flow states (e.g., cardiopulmonary bypass, shock, high-dose vasopressors).

  e. Generalized inanition, weight loss, and flexion contractures across large joints represent additional risk factors for the development of pressure sores.

B. INDICATION FOR OPERATION is failure of spontaneous healing after the pressure has been alleviated.

  1. Partial-thickness injury heals spontaneously from residual, viable dermal elements.

  2. Full-thickness infarction requires operation to provide tissue coverage.

  3. Exposed bursa and bone require surgical resection and coverage.

  4. Invasive necrotizing infection or abscess formation requires urgent debridement and drainage.

  5. Open draining pressure sores without invasive infection to adjacent tissues is seldom the cause of systemic sepsis. Another cause commonly referrable to the pulmonary or urinary system should be considered.

C. MANAGEMENT begins with aggressive debridement of all devitalized, infected, and exposed soft tissues, bursa, and bone.

  1. All other sources of systemic infection must be controlled prior to definitive surgical coverage of the wound.

  2. Adequate nutrition is essential preoperative preparation for successful postoperative wound healing. Supplemental feeding, tube feeding, and parenteral nutrition need to be instituted as appropriate. Optimal preparation is reflected by a positive nitrogen balance before surgery.

  3. Proximal diverting colostomy is sometimes indicated to expedite postoperative wound healing in patients with severe, multiple pressure sores involving the perirectal and perineal regions.

  4. Definitive closure of open, debrided wounds can be deferred if the general patient status requires stabilization due to intercurrent systemic illness or malnutrition. Bacteriologic wound control is maintained by local wound care with Silvadene or wet-to-dry packing.

  5. Parenteral antibiotics to cover both gram-positive/negative and anaerobic flora are indicated at the time of surgical wound coverage.

6. The choice for reconstructive coverage depends on the dimensions of the debrided wound, adjacent viable tissues available for coverage, and existing incisions from previous operations performed for coverage of pressure sores.

a. Skin grafts usually lack durability and bulk necessary for the coverage of bony prominences.

b. Shallow peripelvic sores without exposed bone can be successfully covered by local skin or skin fascia rotation flaps from buttock, thigh, or back.

c. Deep ischial, sacral, and trochanteric pressure sores are frequently covered by rotation or transposition of the gluteus maximus, gracilis, tensor fascia lata, vasus lateralis, and biceps femoris muscle flaps.

d. Heel ulcers may be successfully closed by skin graft, local plantar rotation flap, intrinsic foot muscle flap, or free microvascular tissue transplantation, depending on the preexisting vascular sufficiency of the foot.

e. Reconstructive coverage achieves wound closure but does not address the basic pathology of pressure sore formation (i.e., lack of sensation).

7. The best **treatment** for pressure sores is **prevention.**

a. Avoidance of persistent pressure over bony prominences is achieved by turning or weight redistribution every 1-2 hours. Weight dispersion adjuncts such as customized wheel chair cushions and flotation beds are helpful. Patient education and spinal cord patient rehabilitation are essential mainstays of self-care.

b. Meticulous hygiene of perineum and routine skin care.

c. Avoidance of surface trauma.

V. PLASTIC SURGERY OF THE BREAST

A. POSTMASTECTOMY BREAST RECONSTRUCTION

1. Tissue deficit is determined by the antecedent operation or treatment modality.

a. Pectoralis major muscle (anterior axillary fold) is present after modified radical mastectomy and total mastectomy but is absent after radical mastectomy.

b. Nipple-areola complex is usually absent after mastectomy and preservation is usually contraindicated in the presence of cancer.

c. After primary treatment by partial breast resection and radiation therapy, the affected breast is asymmetric in volume and contour compared with the uninvolved breast. The breast and chest wall tissues are at risk for the effects of vascular insufficiency as a result of radiation injury, particularly when secondary operations need to be performed for recurrent cancer or for reconstruction to achieve improved contour.

2. Preoperative assessment includes evaluation of the adequacy and quality of the chest wall skin, the nature of the contour deficiency, the contour of the remaining breast, and the cancer risk to the remaining breast (preoperative mammography).

3. The **goal** of postmastectomy reconstruction is to simulate the best possible breast symmetry by restoration of the absent breast.

a. Reduction, mastopexy, and augmentation modification of the unaffected breast may be helpful in achieving optimal breast mound symmetry.

b. Patient input in preoperative planning is essential to her satisfaction with the postoperative outcome regarding size, contour, and symmetry.

c. Breast reconstruction is elective and must be individualized according to the patient's lifestyle and tolerance for operative morbidity.

4. Timing of breast reconstruction may be immediate (at the time of mastectomy) or delayed.

a. Delayed reconstruction allows for completion of histologic staging and decisions regarding adjuvant chemotherapy.

b. Wound healing is compromised by the antimetabolic effects of systemic chemotherapy or surface radiation therapy.

c. Mastectomy in a previously irradiated zone is an indication for immediate coverage by vascularized tissue (i.e., latissimus or rectus abduminus muscle flaps) at the time of salvage mastectomy.

5. Alternatives in reconstruction depend on the nature of the defect and patient choice.

a. Subpectoral breast implant placement is the simplest procedure with the shortest operating time. Potential complications include infection, implant exposure, and implant distortion by capsular contracture. Application is limited by deficiency or poor quality of chest wall skin, absence of the pectoralis muscle, and macromastia or extreme ptosis of the unaffected breast.

b. Tissue expansion by a two-stage operation permits the development of a greater skin surface area to accommodate the final placement of a subpectoral breast implant. Radiation is a relative contraindication for tissue expansion. Infection of the tissue expansion prosthesis requires removal of the prosthesis for resolution of the infection, and reconstruction is deferred for a minimum of 3 months.

c. Autogenous tissue breast reconstruction is achieved by either the rectus abdominus or latissimus dorsi musculocutaneous flaps. Both modalities add vascularized tissue to the chest wall and are indicated in irradiated or radical mastectomy defects.

An implant is used to augment the volume of the reconstructed breast when the latissimus is used.

Absence of excess abdominal skin, preexisting abdominal scars, and extreme obesity are contraindications to the use of the rectus abdominus flap. Potential complications include partial or total flap loss and ventral hernia formation when the rectus abdominus is used.

6. Nipple-areola reconstruction is usually deferred until satisfactory restoration of the breast mound is achieved.

B. REDUCTION MAMMOPLASTY

1. Symmetric and asymmetric macromastia occur commonly as a result of pubertal or postpartum hypertrophy.

2. Clinical morbidity includes the symptom complex of cervical musculoskeletal strain, accentuated kyphosis, inframammary intertrigo, and ulnar neuropathy.

3. Preoperative counseling includes possible postoperative loss of nipple sensation, inability to breast feed, and permanent breast scar hypertrophy.

4. Reduction prior to full pubertal breast development is relatively contraindicated owing to the risk of recurrent macromastia.

5. Aesthetic goals of operation include symmetry, cephalic transposition of the nipple-areola complex to restore its natural position, restoration of natural breast contour in relation to the inframammary fold, and preservation of nipple viability and sensation.

6. Potential complications include postoperative hemorrhage and ischemic necrosis of the nipple-areola complex.

C. AUGMENTATION MAMMOPLASTY is an aesthetic procedure to augment breast contour by placement of bilateral implants in the subcutaneous or subpectoral space. It is also the procedure of choice for correction of congenital unilateral hypomastia or correction of Poland's syndrome with the simultaneous transposition of the latissimus muscle to replace the congenitally absent pectoralis muscle. The prevalent complication is implant hardening and breast contour distortion as a result of capsular contracture.

D. GYNECOMASTIA is idiopathic in the majority of cases, but testicular and pituitary abnormalities must be ruled out prior to breast reduction. Subtotal mastectomy and lipectomy of surrounding tissues reduce the breast to simulate the normal male contour. The risk of recurrence is high for operations performed before the completion of pubertal growth. Failure to diagnose an underlying hormonal problem and drug-induced gynecomastia where cessation of medication is contraindicated are additional causes for recurrence.

VI. CUTANEOUS MALIGNANCIES

Cutaneous malignancies encountered most frequently are BCC, SCC, and melanoma.

A. PREDISPOSING RISK FACTORS in the formation of cutaneous malignancy include environmental factors, altered immune competence, and heredity.

1. Ultraviolet radiation, x-irradiation, psoralens, arsenicals, and immune deficiency (congenital, acquired, iatrogenic) are predisposing factors for the development of BCC and SCC.

2. Heredity has an unidentified, but predisposing risk for the occurrence of multiple BCC (basal cell nevus syndrome) and melanoma (BK mole syndrome)

3. Prophylaxis against UV or sun damage to skin (sunscreen) is effective in reducing the frequency of BCC.

B. BASAL CELL CARCINOMA

1. Slow growing, locally invasive tumor with rare metastasis.

2. Morphologically nodular, superficial spreading, pigmented, or morphea form. (a) Typically nodular appearance with pearly borders and central umbilication or ulceration. (b)

Indistinct demarcation of tumor margin in morphea form variety. (c) 80%-90% located in sun-exposed head and neck region.

3. Biopsy or excision is indicated by a history of growth, recurrent hyperkeratotic scale, or ulceration.

4. Excision with clear surgical margins is 98% curative. (a) Recurrence rate is higher for other modalities of treatment such as cryosurgery or curettage and is higher for morphea-form lesions regardless of the method of treatment. (b) Only two-thirds of cases with microscopically positive surgical margins result in local recurrence. (c) Excision of the recurrent lesion is curative with clearance of surgical margins. (d) Surgical excision is absolutely indicated for recurrent lesions within a previously irradiated field.

5. The excision defect is repaired by primary suture, skin grafts, or local flaps as needed.

C. SQUAMOUS CELL CARCINOMA

1. Rapidly growing lesions with propensity for perineural and perivascular extension, and hematologic or lymphatic metastasis.

2. True neoplasm with precursor lesions identified as dysplasia (erythroplakia, leukoplakia), actinic keratosis, and carcinoma in situ (Bowen's disease). Chronic inflammation and open wounds predispose to SCC formation (radiation dermatitis, draining osteomyelitis, chronic pressure sore, and nonhealing burn wounds).

3. Morphologically nodular and firm with tendency for early fixation, ulceration, and central tumor necrosis (75% head and neck location; 25% extremity and trunk location).

4. Examination for regional lymphadenopathy and chest radiographs are minimum required surveys when lesion is histologically identified as SCC.

5. Surgical margin of 5-10 mm clearance is preferred. Local recurrence is 100% if margins are positive for tumor. Local clearance does not rule out existing presence or future risk of distant metastases. Lymphadenopathy must be addressed by fine-needle aspiration for diagnosis or regional lymphadenectomy.

6. The excision defect is repaired by primary closure, skin graft, local flap transposition, or distant flap transplantation as defined by the size, depth, and location of the defect.

D. MELANOMA

1. Biopsy is indicated for lesions with a history of color change, progressive growth, pruritus, pain, or bleeding. Half of all melanomas arise within pre-existing pigmented lesions.

a. Pigmented lesions with variegated color, irregular borders, or irregular surface elevation are suspect.

b. Clinical morphology is classified as superficial spreading, nodular, lentigo maligna melanoma, or acrolentigenous.

c. Family history of melanoma and presence of multiple dysplastic nevi are increased risk factors.

d. Congenital nevocellular nevus predisposes to malignant degeneration in 10%-20% of cases.

2. Histologic staging of melanoma by Clark's or Breslow classification is prognostic of survival (Tables 15-6 and 15-7).

a. Biopsy or excision of suspicious lesion must be submitted as full-thickness specimens to determine the level of invasion.

Table 15-6. Staging of malignant melanoma (after Clark)

Level I = In situ melanoma above the basement membrane.
Level II = Invasion into the papillary dermis.
Level III = Filling the papillary layer and extending to the junction of the papillary and reticular layers but not entering the reticular layer.
Level IV = Into the reticular layer of the dermis.
Level V = Subcutaneous tissue involvement.

Table 15-7. Level of invasion, tumor thickness, and incidence of recurrence of metastasis (after Breslow)

Clark's levels	Percentage with recurrence or metastasis at 5 years	Thickness (mm)	Percentage with recurrence or metastasis at 5 years
I	0%	<0.76	0%
II	4%	0.76-1.5	33%
III	33%	1.51-2.25	32%
IV	61%	2.26-3	69%
V	78%	>3	84%

b. Regional lymphadenectomy is indicated for palpable lymphadenopathy and for thick lesions (>1.5 mm or Clark's level III).

c. Lesions located on the posterior neck, back, arms, and scalp, ulcerated lesions, and acrolentigenous melanoma carry a worse prognosis for survival.

3. The **goal of surgical excision** is to achieve local tumor control. Depending on depth and size of lesion, 0.5-3 cm margins are adequate.

Surgical resection of solitary metastasis is appropriate palliation. Adjuvant therapy for recurrent or metastatic disease includes radiation therapy, chemotherapy, and hyperthermic limb perfusion.

4. Immediate closure of the melanoma resection defect is indicated, particularly after secondary resection of recurrent or metastatic tumor in an irradiated field. Closure is accomplished by skin grafting, local flaps, or distant transplantation depending on the size, depth, and composition of the defect.

VII. CLEFT LIP AND PALATE

A. DEMOGRAPHICS and incidence vary with racial heterogeneity, gender, and heredity (Table 15-8).

B. CLASSIFICATION of lip and palate defects parallel embryonic formation of the palate (Table 15-9).

1. The primary palate includes the nostril sill, lip, and palate anterior to the incisive foramen.

2. The secondary palate includes the hard and soft palate posterior to the incisive foramen.

3. Additional designation of cleft pattern includes right or left, unilateral or bilateral, and complete or incomplete clefting of the primary and/or secondary palate.

C. PATHOPHYSIOLOGY

1. Evident congenital disruption of lip and/or palate.

2. Concomitant and characteristic deformity of the ipsilateral nose with alar flattening, deficient nasal sill, and deviation of the septum and nasal tip.

3. Abnormal formation, deficiency, and hypoplasia of palatal muscles. Functional inability to achieve separation of the nasal pharynx and oral pharynx. Persistent nasal air escape (ve-

Table 15-8. Demographics of cleft lip (CL) and palate (CP)

	Asian: 2/1000	Caucasian: 1/1000	Black: 0.4/1000 live births
Racial heterogeneity (CL and CP)			
Gender propensity	CL + CP CP	Male > female Female > male	
Inheritance	Variable genetic expression. Independent non-additive risks for clefting of the primary versus secondary palate.		

Table 15-9. Definition of primary and secondary palate

	Primary palate	**Secondary palate**
Gestational age of formation	4-7 weeks	8-12 weeks
Mechanism of formation	Mesodermal migration and reinforcement of branchial membranes	Fusion of palatal shelves
Parts	Lip, nostril sill, alveolus, palate anterior to the incisive foramen	Hard and soft palate posterior to the incisive foramen

lopharyngeal incompetence) is the basis for the typical speech pathology.

4. Abnormal function and hypoplasia of eustachian tubes with inadequate ventilation of the middle ear predisposing to middle ear infections resulting in conductive hearing deficits.

5. Abnormal teeth in the cleft line and malocclusion.

D. FEEDING PROBLEMS. Most feeding problems in infancy can be overcome by using an elongated nipple that obturates the palatal cleft, and by feeding the infant in an upright position to prevent aspiration.

E. CLEFT LIP REPAIR. The goal of repair is to create a normal appearance and to restore the upper lip to its usual position for growth and function.

1. Optimal timing is limited only by the safety of administering a general anesthesia for lip repair (i.e., infant age 10 weeks; weight 10 lbs; Hgb 10).

2. Functional repair restores the continuity of the orbicularis oris muscle such that the upper lip moves dynamically as a single continuous unit.

3. Meticulous external skin repair restores lip length while preserving all landmarks of the philtrum, vermillion, cupid's bow, and vermillion tubercle.

4. The ipsilateral nostril is repositioned to achieve symmetry with the nonaffected nostril, with or without rotation of the alar cartilage and cartilage grafts.

F. CLEFT PALATE REPAIR. The goal is to restore continuity of the palate and provide a corrected anatomic environment to promote the development of normal speech.

1. The alternative to surgical repair is to obturate the cleft with a customized prosthesis.

2. The optimal timing for surgical repair is before the development of connected speech between 6 months and 1 year of age.

3. The repair is performed in 3 layers: (a) Separate oral and nasal mucosal repairs to restore the continuity of palatal mucosa lining. (b) Palatal muscle repair with centralization and posterior advancement of muscles to simulate the normal aponeurotic muscle sling for palate mobility in swallowing and speech.

4. Concomitant examination of the middle ear under anesthesia by otolaryngology with placement of pressure-equalizing tubes as needed.

5. Speech therapy to be instituted as soon as the child has begun connected speech formation.

G. SOCIAL SERVICE and orthodontic consultation are essential resources for the child with cleft deformity from birth to adolescence.

H. SECONDARY SURGERY

1. Secondary surgery **for improved speech** is indicated when velopharyngeal insufficiency persists despite speech therapy. Construction of a static pharyngeal flap or a dynamic palatopharyngeal sphincter reduces nasal air escape and improves intelligible speech. Indications for procedures that enlarge the nasal-pharyngeal aperture such as tonsillectomy or adenoidectomy should be carefully reviewed to avoid the potential risk for increasing nasal air emission and relapse back to "cleft speech."

2. Secondary surgery to **correct any residual deformity** of the nose or midface should be deferred until full facial growth has been achieved by age 16-18 years (e.g., definitive rhinoplasty or midfacial advancement).

VIII. AESTHETIC SURGERY

Aesthetic surgery responds to an elective patient request for improvement of facial and body contour.

A. RHYTIDECTOMY AND BLEPHAROPLASTY correct the facial stigmata of the aging process as characterized by generalized cutaneous laxity (ptosis of the supratarsal skin, redundancy of the lower eyelid skin, accentuation and ptosis of the nasolabial fold, jowl formation along the mandibular border, and laxity of neck skin resulting in effacement of the normal cervical mental angle).

1. Rhytidectomy resuspends the facial and neck skin after resection of redundant skin and excess subcutaneous fat through periauricular and scalp incisions. Potential complications include hematoma and facial nerve injury.

2. Blepharoplasty resects redundant eyelid skin, removes retroseptal fat, and deepens the supratarsal fold to restore both upper and lower eyelids to a more youthful contour. Potential complications include hematoma, ectropion, and, rarely, blindness.

3. Brow lift resuspends the forehead and reduces both horizontal and vertical frown lines through a transcoronal incision behind the frontal hairline. Potential complications include hematoma and focal alopecia at the incision line.

B. AESTHETIC RHINOPLASTY corrects both congenital and traumatic contour deformities including prominent nasal dorsum convexity, the bulbous nasal tip, and the widened bony nasal pyramid. Submucous resection may be performed simultaneously to correct septal deviation commonly seen in post-traumatic or congenital cleft lip nose deformities.

C. ABDOMINOPLASTY reduces the trunk contour by resection of the abdominal panniculus, lipectomy of the abdominal skin flap, and resuspension of the reduced skin from the costal margins to the groin and pubes. Abdominoplasty, brachioplasty, and thigh lift are useful adjuncts when the need for total body skin reduction is encountered after massive weight loss as a result of gastric bypass procedures.

D. SUCTION-ASSISTED LIPECTOMY reduces subcutaneous fat by insertion of the suction cannula through 0.5 cm stab incisions that eliminate the need for the standard surgical lipectomy scar. Suction-assisted lipectomy is best applied to localized areas of firm adiposity without excessive skin laxity.

1. Common sites requested for contour reduction include the lower abdomen, waistline, flanks, hips, buttocks, and thighs.

2. Suction-assisted lipectomy is a useful adjunct for lipectomy performed for gynecomastia, abdominoplasty, and rhytidectomy/neck lift.

3. Potential complications include hemorrhage, surface irregularities, hyperpigmentation, and hypesthesia.

16

Hand Surgery

Suzanne M. Kerley, M.D.
Eugene S. Kilgore, M.D.
William L. Newmeyer III, M.D.

Any severe hand disorder should be referred to a general, plastic, or orthopedic surgeon who specializes in the hand. A Hand Surgeon is trained to manage all of the tissues and structures (skin, muscle and tendons, nerves, vessels, bones, and joints) and give them the expert care necessary to preserve or restore the function of all systems of this complex mechanism. Most hand problems are caused by trauma, but tumors, neurologic disorders, congenital anomalies, and rheumatic joint and tendon afflictions also need specialized treatment. The functional outcome depends on the quality of immediate and subsequent surgical treatment and rehabilitation.

I. TRAUMA—PRINCIPLES OF CARE

Management of the injured hand requires constant attention to the components of hand function (sensibility, mobility, placement, and power) and knowledge of how such function may be compromised or threatened by trauma or its treatment. A thorough understanding of the functional anatomy of the upper extremity is crucial to a successful outcome.

A. EVALUATION OF THE INJURED HAND. Careful records of history and examination—including a diagram detailing the problem—are invaluable aids in the initial and subsequent treatment as well as in preparing reports on temporary and permanent disability. It is essential to record in precise language everything that one knows about, plans, and actually does for the injured hand. Accurate reports can be prepared only if these details are recorded immediately at the time of evaluation and treatment.

1. History. Repeat the history-taking procedure to make certain that the data from the patient, family, employer, and other are accurate and complete. The following information is required:

a. Age, occupation, hand dominance, and preexisting hand problems.

b. Chief complaint, its duration, its previous occurrence, and whether it is getting worse, getting better, or remaining static.

c. The how, where, when, and why of the injury. A detailed history must be taken of the mechanism of injury, factors of contamination, the interval between injury and treatment, and treatment rendered to date.

d. The status of tetanus prophylaxis and allergies.

e. Review of patient's past and current state of health and treatment given.

2. Physical examination. The examination of the total patient may be cursory or complete depending on whether the history raises relevant questions or whether the patient is to be admitted to the hospital for care. In examining the hand, one must recognize significant coexisting general or local physical problems and adverse psychological conditions to plan the best treatment for the hand. The certainty of diagnosis of a hand abnormality often requires a comparison of the examination of *both* hands.

The examination of the hand should determine the following:

a. Pain or anesthesia. Note presence, type, severity of pain. Throbbing pain implies venous congestion and must be relieved by mechanical means rather than drugs. The patient must be made as comfortable as possible during the examination, often by recumbency. Anesthetic areas should be mapped, correlated with the presence or absence of sweat, and confirmed by retesting later.

b. Viability of tissues. Compare capillary filling, color, and temperature with normal skin and the opposite hand; note the quality of the pulse.

c. Deformity. Note any distortion of form by soft tissue swelling (edema, hemorrhage, infection), tumor, or bone displacement.

d. Motility. Note the status of active and passive mobility. Division of motor nerves or tendons creates characteristic deficits in active motion. Selective testing of muscle units should be done.

e. Wounding. Is the wound tidy or untidy, new or old, bleeding or dry, clean or infected, punctured or incised, deep or superficial, with or without foreign body? Probing should not be done if help is inadequate, lighting is poor, tourniquet ischemia is not instituted, or proper instruments, anesthesia, and facilities are not available. Bleeding can usually be controlled by direct pressure on the bleeding point and the release of tight garments and jewelry. If not, the bleeding point may be isolated under tourniquet (blood pressure cuff) control and carefully ligated or tagged for repair without injury to an adjacent nerve. Loupe magnification is often indispensable for this purpose.

f. Radiographs. (posterior-anterior, lateral, oblique, and special views) should be taken to determine any abnormality of bone or joint, or the presence of a radiopaque foreign body. Comparative views of both hands are often necessary to confirm a diagnosis, especially for bone detail in children.

3. Referral and deferral of treatment. The freshly injured hand should be made as comfortable as possible, usually by splinting and elevation. Constrictive dressings must be avoided. A well padded, volar splint with the wrist slightly extended with a large soft roll of gauze in the palm between thumb and fingers often gives the greatest comfort. Pain should be controlled by analgesics if necessary. Surgical toilet (irrigation and skin preparation) may be rendered and wounds closed loosely and covered with sterile dressings. If there will be more than 2 or 3 hours of delay before definitive care of an open injury, tetanus prophylaxis together with prophylactic IM or IV broad-spectrum antibiotics should be administered. Injections and IVs should not be given in the injured extremity. Nothing should be given by mouth.

An amputated part should be washed and placed in a sterile waterproof bag or other container. The container should be placed on ice (note: NOT Dry Ice) and transferred with the patient. A detailed record of the initial diagnosis and treatment should accompany the patient.

B. MANAGEMENT OF THE INJURED HAND

1. Surgical facilities. An operating room hand table, good light, magnifying loupes, specialized fine instruments, a pretested pneumatic tourniquet, and surgical assistance are essential for hand surgery. Inexperience, haste, and fatigue are serious handicaps.

2. Preparation for surgery. The patient should be supine and comfortable, with a well-padded pneumatic tourniquet on the arm. Most surgeons sit but must be readily able to shift positions as circumstances require. Microsurgery is best performed sitting, as the surgeons can then stabilize their forearms on the hand table for the most control. General, regional, or local anesthesia must be administered to keep the patient comfortable.

After skin prep and sterile draping, the freshly injured or infected extremity may then be passively elevated and the tourniquet inflated (to 250 mm Hg for adults or to 150 to 200 mm Hg for infants and children). Uncontrolled bleeding may necessitate tourniquet control before the anesthesia and skin preparation. In elective surgical cases that are not infected, the extremity is usually exsanguinated by manual compression or an elastic roll (Esmarch bandage) before inflation of the tourniquet. The patient generally tolerates the tourniquet ischemia on the unanesthetized upper arm for 20-30 minutes. When the arm is anesthetized, the tissue tolerance for ischemia is 2 to 2½ hours. The tourniquet manometer must be tested for accuracy before use because paralyses have occurred as a result of excessive tourniquet pressure. The tourniquet may be released and reinflated after the reactive hyperemia subsides (at least 20 to 30 minutes) in procedures demanding prolonged tourniquet time.

3. Anesthesia. General anesthesia (or axillary block or IV 0.5% lidocaine block) is preferred for procedures which last over 20-30 minutes. Premedication with versed and fentanyl (when not contraindicated by allergy) is ideal for its tranquilizing and analgesic effect.

Lidocaine (1%-2%) **without** epinephrine injected slowly through a fine needle (e.g., No. 26-30 gauge for the digit) is used for local blocks (into the wound) or nerve blocks (axillary, radial, ulnar, median, or digital nerve). Avoid excessive amounts that will congest the nerve, the hand, or the digit. The skin and fat should still be soft and pliable after the injection. The most one should inject at the base of an adult digit is 2.5 ml. Large-caliber needles may cut nerve tissue and should not be used.

4. Surgical techniques for fresh injuries.* Anything that touches the wound must be aseptic and both chemically and mechanically atraumatic. Starch powder should be wiped off of sterile gloves. Sponging should be by dabbing, not wiping. Instruments must be in the best condition and should consist of a selection of fine skin hooks, retractors, forceps, clamps, scissors, needle holders, atraumatic sutures, and Kirschner wires and drill. Nonreactive material should be stipu-

---

*Management of injured nerves, tendons, and so on are discussed individually later in this chapter.

lated for sutures and ligatures. Catgut should be avoided except for the closure of skin wounds in infants (e.g., 6-0 catgut). Monofilament nylon is preferred. The tissues must be kept moist, preferably with lactated Ringer's solution. Hemostasis must be complete.

a. The six fundamental precepts of dissection in the hand are as follows: (1) Dissect with at least 2 × magnification, tourniquet ischemia, and a bipolar or electrocautery available. (2) Dissect from normal tissue into abnormal. (3) Keep the tissues dissected under tension. (4) Keep the margins of the wound suspended by hooks or stay sutures. (5) Once through the dermis with a scalpel, use short-bladed, sharp, fine scissors for dissection and identify and coagulate or ligate all vessels that need to be divided. (6) Spread the tissue gently before cutting, and then cut with precision only the tensed white fascial or fibrous tissue. This prevents the inadvertent severing of nerves or vessels, which are identifiable by their soft and lax consistency, and reduces trauma to fat, which is the vital cushion of the hand.

b. Irrigation. Gross dirt on the skin should be washed off with soap and water. Skin stains do not necessarily have to be washed off. If the skin is coated with oil, ether or benzene may be necessary to remove it, but such solutions must be kept out of the wound. Tar may be removed with adhesive remover that has hydrocarbon, or using mayonnaise. Dried blood is most easily removed with hydrogen peroxide. An open wound may be irrigated with lactated Ringer's solution or antibiotic solution.

c. Debridement is the removal of blood clots, nonviable tissue, and foreign bodies which will constitute dead space. Thus, living tissue can be coapted and grafted tissue can be nourished by capillary invasion. It is occasionally necessary to debride without tourniquet ischemia so that the level of viability can be determined by the scalpel. The hand specialist knows when and how to save debrided tissue as free grafts for primary or secondary use in reconstructive surgery. The objective of debridement in the primary care of injuries is to preserve function by preserving circulation and curtailing edema and infection. Closing a wound with irregular but viable margins or with primary or delayed split-thickness grafting is far preferable to trimming the edges and forcing the closure with tight sutures. Stained but viable tissue and minute fragments of foreign material should not necessarily be removed unless the foreign material is known to be caustic.

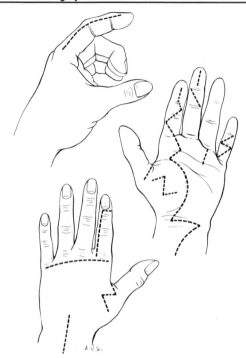

FIGURE 16-1. Proper placement of skin incisions. (From Way LE, (ed): *Current surgical diagnosis and treatment.* Lange.)

d. Exposure (Figure 16-1). Evaluation and repair demand identification of the anatomic relationships. Incisions often must be made to extend the wound beyond injured and blood-colored tissue. This should be done without injury to the blood supply, nerves, and tendons and should not predispose to secondary disabling contractures (e.g., scars crossing at right angles to flexion skin creases).

e. What to repair. After debridement and exposure, the surgeon's experience and facilities determine how much to repair deep to the skin. Skilled primary reparative or reconstructive hand surgery goes far to spare function, time, and expense. Unskilled efforts may do just the opposite. Generally speaking, skeletal distortion should be corrected, and if the tissues are not congested and the circulation is good, structures that are easily identifiable and clearly matched should be approximated. Unstable bone alignment requires some form of internal fixation. Sutures of nylon vary in caliber from 8-0 to 11-0 for digital nerves and from 3-0 to 5-0 for tendons. (Catgut is reactive and therefore should not be used except to close the skin of infants.)

Given satisfactory skeletal stability, the circulation has first priority, skin and fat second, tendons (e.g., long flexor tendons) third, and nerves the last priority in primary repair. One must avoid overloading the already injured tissues with the trauma of surgery itself.

Primary repair is that which is done within the first 24-72 hours. If circumstances of wounding suggest heavy contamination (e.g., tooth, farmyard, or sewer inflicted wound), it is probably best to irrigate and debride the wound and repair nothing primarily. When contamination is minimal but the circulation is impaired (e.g., much swelling)—or if >8 hours have passed without any surgical toilet or splinting—then it is best to prepare, dress, splint, and elevate the part and administer prophylactic broad-spectrum antibiotics. If within the first 2 weeks there is no evidence of inflammation and the tissues are soft and pliable, delayed primary repair may be considered.

Secondary repair is that which follows the first 2 weeks after injury and is usually undertaken after resolution of the swelling and induration that followed the injury.

5. Wound closure and drainage. A loosely fitting drain prevents accumulation of serum and blood and forestalls the development of "dead space" and infection or cicatrix. Therefore, drainage should be selectively used in contaminated wounds and severe compound crushing wounds. Drains should be inserted in such a way as to favor gravity drainage from the elevated extremity.

Wounds should never be closed with tension. If tension is unavoidable, it is best to leave the wound open or graft it. When tension has already built up and if uncontrolled throbbing pain has developed, it should be treated by adequate fasciotomies of **all** tight compartments, including decompression of the carpal tunnel.

Most wounds of the hand can be closed with one layer of interrupted or running everting skin sutures. Interrupted sutures are preferred if motion is to start early.

6. Prophylaxis against infection. involves prophylaxis against tetanus (see Chapter 4) and against streptococcal and staphylococcal infections. If the wound is contaminated (not necessarily clinically infected), it should be irrigated with copious amounts of lactated Ringer's or bacitracin solution at surgery and systemic antibiotics should be given for 48-72 hours afterward. The systemic drugs of choice for gram-positive organisms are penicillin, cephalosporins, or vancomycin in the penicillin-allergic patient; for gram-negative organisms, tobramycin, gentamicin, or a third-generation cephalosporin. Antibiotics must not be regarded as a substitute for the more important fundamental principles of surgical technique and protection of circulation (especially venous return).

7. Dressings and splints. The dressing should serve to keep the soft tissues at rest and prevent the development of "dead space" by gentle compression that does not obstruct venous return. A single layer of nonadherent gauze smoothed out flush with the wound facilitates dressing changes. On top of this should be placed dry gauze tailored to lie flat without folds or ridges. Dry gauze should also be placed loosely between fingers to prevent skin maceration. Up to this point nothing is wrapped circumferentially around the digit, hand, or forearm. Over this can then be placed a carefully tailored sheet of sponge rubber (e.g., Reston) to prevent congestion by the dressing. This in turn is held in place with circumferentially wrapped, loose-meshed gauze (e.g., Kling, Kerlix, Tubegauz) or cast padding. Care should be taken not to wrap the part too snugly.

Immobilization is mandatory initially in most cases of hand trauma, bearing in mind that prolonged immobilization involves a risk of stiffness. The position in immobilization must never be at the extreme of joint extension or flexion but must generally serve its need, that is, to relieve tension on a tendon or nerve suture repair. Whenever possible, immobilization should be in the position of function. This favors circulation and promotes comfort as well as early reestablishment of unimpaired function. Loosely wrapped dry cast padding covered with a volar plaster splint (10-14 thicknesses, 4 inches wide) from the midpalm across the wrist to the midforearm and held in place with one 3 or 4 inch wide roll of circumferentially wrapped bias stockinette or elastic roll makes a light and effective splint. Congestion is avoided by keeping the elbow flexed during the wrapping and the rigid component of splintage well distal to the antecubital flexion crease.

After extensive hand trauma, infection, or surgery, a well-padded forearm cast is preferred. One may put only part of the hand in such a cast—e.g., the thumb alone, or a combination of any two or three adjacent fingers. Generally speaking, such splinting is preferred for even severe fingertip injuries (e.g., amputation or crush). The wrist must be immobilized to adequately splint any part of the hand. Flat splints (e.g., tongue blade) and single digit splinting for an extensive injury impose a risk of distortion and stiffness and often fail to relieve pain. Infants and irresponsible adults usually need a long arm cast rather than a forearm cast. The elbow is immobilized at 90 degrees.

The duration of splinting varies with the problem and the age of the patient. Repair of nerves and tendons and fractures of phalanges and metacarpals usually require immobilization for 3 to 4 weeks, whereas ganglionectomy and fingertip grafting require only 6 to 8 days of casting.

8. Postinjury and postoperative care

a. Control of circulation. In serious cases where microcirculation is threatened by tissue trauma and congestion, sludging and microthrombosis may be curtailed by administering low molecular weight dextran (dextran 40) at 25 cc/hr IV. Smoking should be avoided. It is essential that the hand be constantly elevated in comfort above the heart. There must be no compression or constriction by clothing, jewelry, dressings, casts, or even skin or fascia. Throbbing and brawny induration must be mechanically (not medicinally) relieved—if necessary, by fasciotomy. Chronic (e.g., fixed) edema may be overcome by wearing an elastic glove (e.g., surgeon's glove), exercises, and elevation.

b. Movement. The patient must understand that motion inside a splint is undesirable even though possible and that vigorous movement of any part of the upper extremity may disrupt the tissues being splinted. On the other hand, gentle movement of all unsplinted joints helps the circulation of the whole upper extremity. When immobilization is discontinued, exercise should be started on an organized routine under the direction of a qualified hand therapist. Communication between surgeon and therapist is critical to establish an appropriate protocol for rehabilitation.

c. Chronic stiffness. Pain is often the chief deterrent to overcoming stiffness caused by tight scar tissue and contracted ligaments. Passive stretching is possible by the use of dynamic splints carefully adjusted and tailored to the needs of the specific problems, but these must be worn intermittently rather than continuously and should not be permitted to cause pressure sores, nerve injury, or edema. In selected cases, arthrolysis, tenolysis, or modification of skin scars may be required.

d. Care of the paralyzed hand. During the recovery stage following anesthesia or nerve injury, the patient must take care not to injure anesthetic skin by burns or cuts, or pain-free joints by sprains and subluxations. Splints should be used to keep paralyzed muscles from being overstretched and uninvolved muscles from overcontracting without antagonism. An example is the cock-up splint for the wrist and metacarpophalangeal joints in radial nerve palsy.

II. CONTUSION AND COMPRESSION INJURIES

A crushing or compressive force to the forearm, hand, or digit causing skeletal or soft-tissue injury can result in severe stiffness and even impairment of nerve function. Impaired circulation in such cases results from bleeding and serous effusion, then swelling, and finally venous obstruction and microvascular thrombosis caused by tissue tension. This **compartment syndrome** can lead to irreversible ischemic fibrosis, as in Volkmann's ischemic paralysis and contracture. This process can occur in any fascial compartment of the upper extremity—even that of any of the intrinsic muscles or digital fat pads. It can usually be prevented by attending promptly to throbbing pain and relieving it mechanically. Brawny (rocky hard) congestion must be prevented even if it means slitting the skin and fascia extensively. It is both useless and harmful to try to squeeze infiltrated blood out of tissues, although clearly defined clots can occasionally be extracted.

III. LACERATIONS AND SKIN AVULSIONS

Most wounds should be inspected and closed under tourniquet control. Magnifying loupes should be available. Blood clots should be gently removed, and easily accessible foreign bodies should be searched for by inspection or probing. It is often impractical and unnecessary to remove all foreign bodies; secondary removal is often preferable after the surrounding blood has been absorbed. Vessels that need ligation must be identified and isolated, and ligatures must be placed accurately to avoid damage to an adjacent nerve. A drain should be inserted if there is likelihood of infection or continued oozing. If a full-thickness of skin has been lost, the wound may be primarily closed with a skin graft. If oozing is too great, grafting should be delayed for 1 or 2 days. Split-thickness grafts are the most certain to take, but a full-thickness graft may be prepared by defatting an avulsed piece of skin or by taking some from the hairless portion of the groin. Very long distally based flaps and flaps that have been significantly traumatized are preferably defatted and applied as free full-thickness grafts or replaced by a split-thickness graft. Immobilization is crucial to the healing of lacerations and grafts.

IV. TENDON INJURIES

Any laceration must be assumed to have divided a tendon until proved otherwise by inspection of the wound under tourniquet ischemia with prior or simultaneous systematic testing of all tendons as they are actively tensed. An abnormal digital stance created by a tendon injury can often be demonstrated by extreme passive flexion or extension of the wrist. Penetrating glass and metal wounds can damage tendons far in excess of what is apparent and at sites far removed from the skin wound.

Tendon constriction is a common cause of pain at the site of the offending tendon sheath (pulley). The pain may coincide with a jog in the excursion of the tendon (usually a flexor tendon, e.g., trigger finger); or it may be merely associated with stretch and tension of the synovial bursa when the tendon is tensed (DeQuervain's stenosing tenosynovitis of the abductor pollicis longus). Tendon rupture occurring from a sudden stretching force and tendon adherence due to adhesions (tenodesis) are common after all forms of trauma or infection.

A. TREATMENT. Because of the complexity of restoring tendon and joint function after injury or other impairment, most problems of the flexor or extensor musculotendinous systems should be referred to the hand specialist for definitive treatment.

Stenosing tenosynovitis or trigger finger is usually treated first by injecting a small amount of lidocaine mixed with triamcinolone into the tendon sheath at the trigger point. If that fails, the tendon must be liberated surgically (tenovaginotomy). Ruptures that materially affect digital function often present complex reconstruction problems. Tenolysis can be effective in restoring tendon glide if early active postoperative movement is instituted.

The restoration of function after division of tendons requires surgical judgment and skill and the subsequent perseverance of the patient in the rehabilitation effort. Tendon repair must not be at the expense of mobility of uninjured tendons and joints. The surgeon may appropriately elect no treatment, tenorrhaphy, tendon transfer, tenodesis, or arthrodesis. Tenorrhaphy may be done primarily or secondarily by direct suture, by tendon graft, or by tendon transfer, followed by immobilization for 3 to 4 weeks. Cases referred to the specialist should receive primary wound toilet, closure, splinting, and prophylactic antibiotics. Joints must be freely mobile and skin- and fat-cover healthy and pliable for tenorrhaphy or tendon transfer to be considered.

The handling of tendons and their fibro-osseous sheaths should be atraumatic. Sponges, forceps, clamps, and needles all invite adhesions where they contact these structures. The long flexor tendons require pulleys for mechanical efficiency and to prevent bowstringing; however, in order to make certain that this pulley system does not choke and prevent excursion of a tenorrhaphy callus, rather than being repaired, enough fibro-osseous sheath must sometimes be slit or removed to correspond to the expected amplitude of glide of the callus; or the tendon(s) should be transposed superficial to the retinaculum (e.g., extensor(s) at the wrist).

The technic of suturing a tendon must be meticulous. The amount of suturing required depends on the amount of separation of the proximal stump from its distal attachment and the force necessary to hold the suture line. Retraction of the proximal stump may be prevented while placing the tendon suture by skewering the stump with a straight needle. Atraumatic nonreactive 3-0 to 4-0 sutures (e.g., monofilament nylon) should be used and can be threaded (see Figure 16-2) in a mattress, figure-of-eight, or once or twice criss-crossing fashion through the tendon stumps. The rim of a tendon juncture may be reinforced and evened up by a 6-0 or 7-0 running over-and-over suture. Nylon sutures are usually buried except when anchoring a tendon into bone, in which case the suture ends may pass through the bone and overlying epithelial layer (e.g., fingernail) to be tied over a bolster and then withdrawn in 4 to 6 weeks (Figure 16-3). When the size of two tendons to be joined is disproportionate, the smaller one may be woven once or twice through the larger one. The normal stance of the digit in repose must be preserved in executing any tendon surgery and must not be compromised by having the repaired tendon too loose (long) or too tight (short). This can be judged by passive extension and flexion of the wrist.

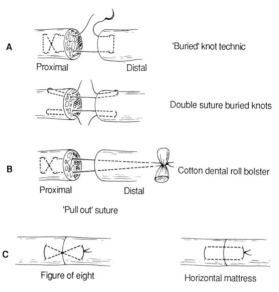

A, 'Buried' knot technic

Proximal   Distal

Double suture buried knots

B, 'Pull out' suture

Proximal   Distal

Cotton dental roll bolster

C, Figure of eight   Horizontal mattress

FIGURE 16-2. Methods of tenorrhaphy. **A,** For large caliber tendons. **B,** As the knot is tied down on the bolster at the tip of the finger, the proximal stump advances to meet the distal one. **C,** These suture techniques are best for thin tendons with limited separation of stumps (e.g., distal extensors).

Immobilization should be in a position that takes tension off the tendon repair without putting any joints in extreme flexion or extension. The wrist is most often the principal joint to be positioned.

1. Extensor tendon injury. If injury to an extensor tendon is recognized immediately and proper treatment is given, the prognosis for recovered function is usually more favorable than is the case with flexor tendons. This is because there is no sheath to contend with except at the wrist (extensor retinaculum); and, over the digit, there is less glide (e.g., 1 to 15 mm). The danger with the extensor hood over the digit lies in

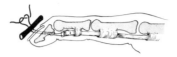

FIGURE 16-3. Flexor tenorrhaphy by reattachment, advancement, or graft.

the fact that it is very complex and at first may fully compensate for a major interruption only to decompensate insidiously later (e.g., stretch out) owing to inadequate treatment.

Exposure (often by proximal and distal extension of the wound) is important for the proper assay and repair of the injury. Because retraction of the proximal stump may be physically negligible but functionally significant, reapproximation of ends and immobilization are usually essential.

Buried 4-0 to 6-0 monofilament nylon sutures are placed as figure-of-eight, horizontal mattress, or (on the dorsum of the hand and forearm) criss-cross weaving sutures. Immobilization should be maintained for 4 to 6 weeks.

a. Mallet (baseball) finger. (Figure 16-4) is a flexion stance of the distal joint resulting from separation of the attachment of the extensor to the distal phalanx. Bone or tendon may be separated, and active extension may be partially or completely lost. A splint across the distal joint for 6 to 8 weeks may be all that is needed in fresh cases; this may be in the form of a dorsal or volar padded splint or a plastic thimble-type Stack splint. Hyperextension and excessive skin pressure must be avoided. Intractable cases may cause a secondary change in the proximal interphalangeal joint, which goes into hyperextension (recurvatum), resulting in **swan neck deformity.**

b. Buttonhole (boutonniere) deformity. (Figure 16-5) is the converse of the swan neck habitus. It results from blunt or sharp injury to the dorsum of the proximal interphalangeal joint (or metacarpophalangeal joint of the thumb). By attenuation of the extensor hood and volar migration of the lateral band mechanism the injured joint fails to extend while the distal joint overextends. Anticipation of the deformity and immobilization of the injured joint in full extension by a padded dorsal or volar splint or by Kirschner wires for 4 to 6 weeks is the recommended treatment.

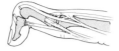

FIGURE 16-4. Mallet finger with swan neck deformity.

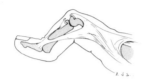

FIGURE 16-5. Buttonhole deformity.

2. Flexor tendon injury. Anatomic zones of injury that have important implications for prognosis and management are shown in Figure 16-6. The principal difference between the zones is not only the existence or nonexistence of a fibrous flexor sheath and its nature but also the number of tendons within it. Thus, in zone 2 of the finger ("no man's land") there is a snug sheath around two tendons, one of which (the superficialis) forms a tunnel around the other (the profundus). Because of the unselective involvement of all structures in reparative scar, tendon injuries in this zone often defy subsequent excursion by virtue of intractable tenodesis. Consequently, considerable experience and judgment are required for successful management of such tendon injuries.

Instead of stump-to-stump approximation, tendon advancement (Figure 16-3) with sacrifice of the distal stump is occasionally favored for division of the flexor within 1 cm of the distal phalanx (zone 1). It may be combined with tendon lengthening in the case of the flexor pollicis longus. Other alternatives are tenodesis of the distal stump, arthrodesis of the distal joint, or no treatment.

Primary tendon repair (within 72 hours) or delayed primary repair (within 2 weeks) is favored for midpalm (zone 3), wrist (zone 4), and forearm (zone 5) injuries. It is also favored

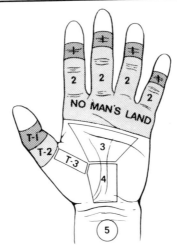

FIGURE 16-6. Flexor and tendon zones.

in tidy injuries in the digits (zones 1 and 2). When the wound in this area is untidy or when several weeks or months have elapsed since the injury, a tendon graft is generally preferred in zone 2, and tenodesis or arthrodesis may be the preferred treatment for zone 1. The amount of retraction of a proximal stump, coupled with its fixation in scar and loss of elasticity of its muscle 2 to 4 weeks after injury, may preclude bringing proximal and distal stumps back together again. A tendon graft or transfer may then be required.

When multiple tendons are divided in one zone, it may be preferable to repair only the more important ones. This is especially true in injuries in zone 2, where the profundus is usually the preferred one to be repaired.

Access to the tendons is gained via lateral (midaxial) digital incisions, or volar incisions that cross the fat pads obliquely in a zigzag fashion. Zigzagging is also preferred for opening the palm or wrist. Damage to neurovascular (see Figure 16-1).

Movement of digits within 3 weeks after flexor tenorrhaphy, if permitted at all, must be done very guardedly. After 3 weeks, active motion may progress in a graded fashion.

B. PROGNOSIS. Excursion after tenorrhaphy or tenolysis depends on the mobility of joints, the remodeling of scar tissue so that it yields to the glide of tendons, adequate strength of muscles, and perseverance by the patient. It often takes many months—even up to a year—to regain maximal tendon excursion and joint motion and for the collagen of scar tissue to attenuate and adapt. The patient must be encouraged to persevere and must be made aware of the difficulty and sometimes impossibility of recovering completely normal excursion. Progress may be gauged by serial records of active and passive range of motion of the joints. Additional surgery for tenolysis and/or capsulotomy may improve motion.

V. NERVE INJURIES

The interruption of nerve conduction following injury may be merely physiologic (i.e., neurapraxia) or it may be anatomic if the neuropraxia is transient. The distinction can be made by repeated examination in the first few hours after an open injury and before any anesthetic is administered.

The median, ulnar, and radial nerves are vital to the function of the hand. They are all mixed (sensory and motor) at the elbow, and the median and ulnar nerves are mixed up to the heel of the hand. A knowledge of innervation is essential to determine the level of an injury (see Figures 16-7 and 16-8). Pain and failure to cooperate may lead to a false diagnosis of motor paralysis, whereas absence of sweating over the distribution of an injured nerve objectively identifies sensory paralysis. Two-point discrimination more than 4 to 5 mm apart also signifies impaired sensory function.

Bleeding should be initially controlled by compressing and not by clamping. "Blind" clamping of bleeding points leads to iatrogenic nerve injury and must be avoided. Before clamping or ligating, the vessel must be clearly distinguished from a nearby nerve by accurate dissection under tourniquet control (arm blood pressure cuff at 100 mm Hg above systolic pressure), making blood leak from the vessel by squeezing the extremity, and using loupe magnification and ideal facilities. The patient should be supine.

When blood prevents meticulous exploration, the dissection should extend to normal tissue and then reverse into the zone of injury.

Motor and sensory nerve conduction studies occasionally help to clarify difficult diagnostic problems in chronic cases.

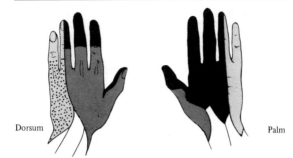

Dorsum   Palm

FIGURE 16-7. Sensory distribution in the hand. Dotted area, ulnar nerve (light dots show distribution of the volar nerves at the wrist, heavy dots show the dorsal nerves at the wrist); diagonal area, radial nerve; darker area, median nerve.(From Way LE, (ed): *Current surgical diagnosis and treatment.* Lange.)

A. TREATMENT

1. Neurapraxia is treated expectantly. How long to defer the exploration of a nerve depends on the mechanism of injury and the surgeon's estimate of its physical impact on the nerve. If there is no sign of regeneration (i.e., return of muscle function and advancement of Tinel's sign) in 4 to 6 months, surgical measures (if applicable) should no longer be deferred. Surgical measures (singly or in combination) may consist of neurolysis, resection of scarred nerve and neurorrhaphy, nerve graft, tendon transfer, tenodesis, arthrodesis, and neurovascular island pedicle flaps.

2. The sooner a divided nerve is repaired, the better. Nerve regenerate at a rate of up to 1 mm per day. After 2 months the motor end plates of the small intrinsic muscles become increasingly resistant to recovery. Neurorrhaphy more than a year after injury gives generally poor return of sensory function. Peripheral neurorrhaphy is highly specialized surgery that can be done properly only by the experienced hand surgeon. Fresh cases being referred should have a surgical skin preparation and the extremity should be immobilized and elevated with or without temporary wound closure and prophylactic antibiotics.

Wrist drop in radial
nerve injury

Forceful extension of
thumb tip is lost in
radial nerve injury

Radial nerve

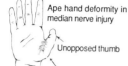

Ape hand deformity in
median nerve injury

Unopposed thumb

Thenar atrophy (especially
the abductor pollicis brevis
which is the thenar muscle
closest to the metacarpal) **Median nerve**

Forceful flexion of tip
of thumb and index is
lost in high median
nerve injury

Thumb web atrophy
and clawing of ring and
little fingers

Loss of abduction and adduction
and inability to cross fingers in
ulnar nerve injury

Ulnar nerve

FIGURE 16-8. Motor loss findings in nerve injuries.

3. Technic of nerve suture. (See Figure 16-9.) All peripheral nerve surgery requires loupe or microscopic magnification as well as microsurgical instruments and suture material (i.e., 8-0 to 12-0 atraumatic nylon).

Freshly incised nerves should be approximated with min-

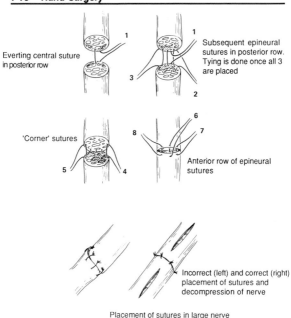

Everting central suture in posterior row

Subsequent epineural sutures in posterior row. Tying is done once all 3 are placed

'Corner' sutures

Anterior row of epineural sutures

Incorrect (left) and correct (right) placement of sutures and decompression of nerve

Placement of sutures in large nerve

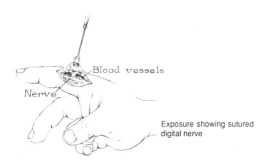

Blood vessels

Nerve

Exposure showing sutured digital nerve

FIGURE 16-9. Methods of neurorrhaphy.

imal section of the stumps. Macerated and scarred nerves require razor blade section across normal nerve tissue before approximation.

Anatomic matching of fascicles and epineural vessels in proximal and distal nerve stumps is essential. Sutures should be atraumatic, fine caliber, as few as possible, and placed into the epineurium or perineurium in such a way as to accurately approximate fascicular stumps without overlap, telescoping, furling, and protrusion from the connective tissue sleeve. Tension must be avoided; if it cannot be overcome by the positioning of joints, a nerve graft should be considered.

Tension on the suture line must be avoided for 3 to 4 weeks postoperatively. This usually requires plaster immobilization. Thereafter the patient should be started on a protocol of progressive range of motion under the direction of the surgeon and hand therapist.

B. PROGNOSIS. A nerve that has been reunited can never regain normal innervation completely. Compensatory factors may substitute adequately for the deficit so that function may be nearly normal. The principal factors that restrict quantitative and qualitative reinnervation are as follows: (1) Inability to reunite and match all divided axons. (2) Distortion due to bleeding, edema, and scar formation. (3) Impairment of circulation and the lack of soft tissue about the injured nerve. (4) Delay in neurorrhaphy. (5) Inexperience in hand surgery. (6) Age of the patient. (7) Motivation of the patient.

VI. BURNS OF THE HANDS

Hand burns occur in the following order of decreasing incidence: thermal, friction, electrical, chemical, and radiation. The impact on function may be catastrophic. The overall economic loss due to deep second- and third-degree thermal burns of the hand is a staggering burden. Preventive safety measures and proper primary therapy can reduce this toll.

While instituting lifesaving measures in the severely burned patient, the upper extremity must simultaneously receive urgent attention. Swelling and the loss of the functional arches of the hand must be avoided as much as possible by elevation, by dermatomy and fasciotomy if brawny edema develops, and by immobilization and positioning (wrist in extension, metacarpophalangeal joints flexed, and, proximal interphalangeal joints in extension). A swollen hand is a claw hand in disguise. Therefore, swelling must be controlled and "fixed" clawing avoided. High-voltage electrical current in contact with the hand spreads deep tissue destruction by coagulation as it passes to its point of exit. The "entry" wound may be far removed from the "exit" burn. The elbow must not be allowed to become fixed in extension and the shoulder in adduction. Whenever possible (and as soon as possible), all joints must be moved actively—often before the burn wound is reepithelialized.

A. TREATMENT. The objective in care of the burned hand is to restore healthy skin cover and joint and tendon motion as early as possible. Burns that do not need debridement and grafting (e.g., first- and second-degree burns) may be treated initially with an ice-water bath and analgesics followed by a soothing cream (e.g., Bacitracin or 1% silver Sulfadiazene). If the burn is deep second degree, is infected, or is already granulating but not healthy and "clean" enough to graft, it should be dressed twice a day with 1% silver sulfadiazine cream or Sulfamylon. Chemical burns are treated initially by copious and sometime prolonged (e.g., 12 to 24 hours) irrigation with tapwater or weak acid (alkali burns) or alkaline (acid burns) solutions. Hydrofluoric acid burns may be neutralized by the local injection of small amount of 10% calcium gluconate.

The chief objective of therapy of deep or extensive burns is to restore effective skin cover to maintain the integrity of deep tissue as rapidly as possible without infection, so that muscle and joint use may be started early and maximal function spared. There is no one rule or one method of accomplishing this, but delay and neglect in the implementation of these principles may lead to permanent disability.

As long as swelling does not prevent active motion and there is no sign of infection, debridement and grafting are not urgent. However, the converse is equally true, and in urgent cases it makes little difference if, during debridement, a small amount of equivocally viable skin is removed in continuity with unequivocally lifeless eschar.

Debridement should be followed by a biologic dressing (autograft, heterograft, or synthetic biologic cover) as soon as hemostasis is adequate to prevent the development of dead space under the graft. Grafting may be immediate or may require waiting for 12 to 24 hours. Immobilization and protection of the hand for 24 to 48 hours is essential so that there will be no shift of the graft on its bed. Sutures or staples may or may not be needed to hold the graft in place.

The thinner (i.e., 0.002 mm) and smaller (i.e., 4 to 10 mm square) the grafts are, the surer they are to take. "Mesh" grafts are suitable for postage stamp grafts, but they must be sutured or stapled in place. Sheets of skin are favored for "clean" wounds with good hemostasis. If the margins lie along lines of stretch, they should be zigzagged with skin darts.

B. FUNCTIONAL DISABILITIES DUE TO HAND BURNS.
Scar leads to a host of characteristic digital deformities (e.g., clawing, buttonhole, swan neck, mallet), adduction contracture of the thumb, and a multitude of other extension and flexion joint contractures. Proper splinting may prevent these deformities and the need for subsequent reconstructive surgery.

VII. FRACTURES, DISLOCATIONS, AND LIGAMENT INJURIES

A. GENERAL PRINCIPLES
1. The history of the degree of force and the mechanism of injury to the hand is essential to the evaluation of these injuries. Radiographs in the anteroposterior, lateral, and oblique planes as well as comparative views of the opposite hand are often indispensable. Pain, distortion, or abnormality of motion (hypermobility or reduced mobility) are usually but not always present. Swelling may mask distortion, and distortion may be mistaken for swelling. To diagnose unexplained continuing skeletal pain one must obtain follow-up radiographs at intervals of 7 to 10 days initially, then monthly.

2. Treatment should be directed at restoration of proper alignment, painless movement, and stability with forceful use of the involved parts. Ultimate function of the whole hand, not radiologic perfection, is what is most important, and functional considerations must dictate the timing and choice of treatment. For example, irreversible and disabling stiffness may be the price of a "perfect" reduction and union of a fracture that has been manipulated too much and immobilized too long. For this reason, in selected cases, it is best to start guarded movements early, particularly in "heavy handed" and older individuals. Instead of using any force to effect a needed reduction it is often best to do an open reduction or settle for imperfect alignment.

3. Initial immobilization should assume the position of maximal function in order to minimize the impact of stiffness. The test of adequate immobilization is freedom from pain. With few exceptions, if one finger needs immobilization, one or more adjacent fingers should also be splinted as well as the wrist. Cast padding, soft gauze, or a spongy cushion such as Reston, and plaster are generally far better for making a custom-fitting splint than boards, sticks, or metal or plastic material. The surgeon must avoid splinting all joints of a digit in extension for fear of stiffness and rotational deformities, and must guard against the hazards of traction technics, which can lead to stiffness and pressure necrosis.

Internal fixation (e.g., Kirschner wires, screws, circlage wire, tension bands, compression plates) should be considered when there is marked instability and when one wishes to allow motion of neighboring tendons and joints. The method of fixation depends on many factors, including the stability of the fracture, the amount of comminution, and the condition of the soft tissue envelope.

4. Open bone and joint injuries should be treated with prophylactic local or systemic antibiotics (or both). When skin and fat cover is lost, it should be replaced by free grafts or pedicle transfer of local or distant tissue.

5. Fracture treatment generally takes precedence over tendon repair, but this does not mean that easily accessible tendon ends should not be reapproximated as a primary procedure.

B. FRACTURES

1. Wrist fractures. Every apparent sprain of the wrist should be considered a fracture until shown to be otherwise by total subsidence of pain or negative follow-up radiographs in 8 to 10 days. The three most common fractures of the wrist are the result of sudden forceful hyperextension or radial deviation.

a. Colles' fracture. The deformity consists of dorsal displacement of the joint surface of the radius, recession of the radial styloid, and fracture of the ulnar styloid. Watch for compression of the median nerve with numbness over its distribution in the hand. Reduction requires anesthesia and should be gentle. The reduction may be lost in the early post-injury period. Therefore, serial radiographs are recommended. The wrist should generally be in the neutral position, not flexed. Immobilization in a long arm cast for 4 weeks, followed by a forearm cast for 2 additional weeks, is frequently adequate. External fixators (e.g., Hoffman, EBI, or Agee) may be required to hold the reduction. Open reduction with internal fixation is needed in unstable fractures. Digital motion with full amplitude of metacarpophalangeal joint and thumb web should be started immediately. Temporary disability commonly persists for 4 to 6 months or more. Residual traumatic arthritis may be unavoidable and require surgery (e.g., ulnar styloidectomy or wrist fusion). Check continuously for the development of compression of the median or ulnar nerves, which may need urgent decompression.

b. Scaphoid fracture. Special radiographic views are essential to rule out these fractures. Pain is maximal in the anatomic snuff box and on radial deviation of the wrist. Reduction is seldom necessary. Immobilization is usually maintained by means of a long arm cast that includes the metacarpophalangeal joint of the thumb for 4 weeks and a short arm cast for an additional 2 weeks. Many patients are then ready to return to work. When there is no radiographic evidence of union, months of immobilization may be necessary, coupled with electromagnetic stimulation. If union does not occur or if avascular necrosis develops, surgery must be considered and may consist of bone grafting, limited wrist fusion, or other procedures. Such cases may have traumatic arthritis and 6 to 12 months of disability.

c. Triquetral fracture. Fracture of the triquetrum is usually a small chip dorsal fracture seen only on the lateral radiographic view. Pain and tenderness are localized to the dorsal-ulnar aspect of the carpus and are often of short duration, requiring only a forearm cast for 1 to 3 weeks.

2. Metacarpal fractures are often nondisplaced. When displacement does occur, the distal segment is usually pulled volarward so that the fracture is bowed to the dorsum (see Figure 16-10). Manipulation and reduction are often difficult. Rotation at the fracture site must be prevented to avoid scissoring of the fingers with flexion after healing has occurred. Open reduction and internal fixation are advocated for unstable fractures. Rigid internal fixation of fracture fragments leads to direct bone healing with reduction of callus formation. This facilitates early range of motion and leads to less tendon adherence in bone, callus, and scar. If splinted, the metacarpophalangeal joints must be splinted in flexion to avoid

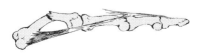

FIGURE 16-10. Dorsal bowing of metacarpal fracture.

disabling stiffness. **Bennett's fracture and Rolando's fracture** occur at the base of the thumb metacarpal.

3. Proximal and middle phalangeal fractures. The most common distortion of these fractures is opposite to that of metacarpal fractures. Here the distal segments are pulled dorsally, causing a volar bowing of the fracture site (see Figure 16-11). Extension of the wrist and flexion of the metacarpophalangeal joint give the relaxation needed for reduction. This, together with side-to-side splinting to the adjacent finger and forearm casting for 3 weeks, usually gives sufficient immobilization. Internal fixation with Kirschner wires—and even open reduction—may be necessary for accuracy of reduction and for very unstable fractures and intraarticular fractures. It is particularly useful in making early motion possible to reduce the likelihood of disabling stiffness of the proximal interphalangeal joint. If joint integrity cannot be reestablished in articular fractures, positioning for a "spontaneous" functional fusion is required or, occasionally, silicone implant joint-spacer arthroplasty is undertaken. Very small chip fractures are treated only for the pain they cause. Intraarticular fracture fragments involving less than a third of the articular surface are sometimes resected.

4. Distal phalangeal fractures present the least hazard to function once pain has subsided (usually 3 to 4 weeks). They are often comminuted and open. Intramedullary fixation with a No. 18 or 19 hypodermic needle or small Kirschner wire is sometimes necessary for displaced shaft and intraarticular fractures, but some cases require only external splinting. This may be achieved by forearm-to-fingertip casting for several days, followed by a digital guard. Open "bursting" type injuries are often too tense to tolerate sutures and should be simply "molded" with nonadherent gauze, and casted.

C. DISLOCATIONS. Most dislocations occur as a result of hyperextension injuries and can be reduced by a combination of

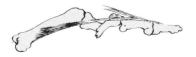

FIGURE 16-11. Volar bowing of phalangeal fracture.

traction and hyperextension and by manipulating the displaced parts back into position. If reduction is impossible without force, open reduction is required.

1. Dislocation of the wrist. Severe injuries of the wrist may cause dislocations about scaphoid and lunate bones. The inexperienced eye may easily fail to notice the abnormality in the radiograph unless it is compared with exactly the same view of the opposite wrist. The scaphoid is often fractured as well as dislocated, whereas the lunate is simply dislocated volarward, where it tends to compress the median nerve and cause dysesthesia. Primary closed reduction under anesthesia is usually successful, but open reduction must be resorted to if this fails. Immobilization is generally for 4 to 6 weeks in a long arm cast.

2. Finger dislocations may occur at any joint and usually involve the dorsal displacement of the distal bone on the proximal one. The proximal interphalangeal joint is most commonly dislocated. The patient often reduces it immediately himself. An unsatisfactory reduction is usually associated with some restrained active or passive motion and imperfect digital stance. When closed reduction is not possible in a fresh case, it means that the head of the more proximal bone has become trapped in a noose formed by displaced tendons, ligaments, and even bands of fascia. The volar plate occasionally fails to clear the joint during reduction and blocks flexion. In other instances, the volar plate has been avulsed so that the phalanx of its origin tends to redislocate. All such difficulties can only be managed surgically. Simple dislocations that are easily reduced and do not tend to redislocate (as verified by radiography) need very little or no splinting beyond the patient's own tendency to favor the part.

D. LIGAMENTOUS INJURIES (SPRAINS AND RUPTURES). Any ligament may be sprained or torn. However, before confirming a diagnosis of a sprain of the wrist, fractures must be ruled out by repeated radiography 1 week after injury. Desmitis (inflammation of a ligament) is a common cause of wrist pain and responds well to rest and trigger-point lidocaine and triamcinolone injections. Ligamentous injuries can be diagnosed with MRI scanning, triple compartment wrist arthrography, or wrist arthroscopy. Abduction force to the metacarpophalangeal joints and abduction or adduction force to the proximal interphalangeal joints are the most common sources of such injuries. Local pain and evidence of relaxation by clinical and radiographic examination under stress are diagnostic.

A small piece of bone is sometimes avulsed. If large, it may require reduction or removal.

Most of these injuries are treated by splinting. An injured finger may be "buddy taped" to the adjacent normal one. Prolonged immobilization invites stiffness, however, which itself is a cause of pain.

Total avulsions of collateral ligaments of metacarpophalangeal joints of the thumb (gamekeeper's thumb) should be repaired if fresh; reconstructed if old.

VIII. AMPUTATIONS

Loss of all or part of a digit is always a shocking experience for the patient, who often brings in the amputated part in the hope that it can be replanted. Replantation may be considered by the experienced hand surgeon when the injury is tidy, the patient young, multiple digits and/or thumb are involved, and the injury is proximal to the distal interphalangeal joint. Any amputation composed of more than just skin requires anastomosis of an artery and vein if it is to survive. The amputated part should be washed with water, covered with a dry gauze and placed in a container or zip lock bag on a bed of ice when a patient is referred to a hand surgeon for possible replantation.

The functional impact of an amputation depends on the digits involved and the plane and extent of the loss. Thus, volar-radial fingertip loss and volar-ulnar thumb tip loss (the surfaces that oppose for pinch) are often disabling amputations. The concepts of (1) hand breadth for stability of grasp, and (2) digital length (especially of the thumb) for effectiveness of pinch must always be considered in planning salvage and reconstruction. Above all, the amputation stump must be rendered pain-free and have durable skin cover. Fingers that are intractably stiff, anesthetic, painful, or too short are often amputated by the surgeon if that will enhance overall function of the hand. Custom-molded prosthetic devices that provide a hook or enhance pinch may be used in selected cases. Other prostheses worn for their cosmetic value have no functional usefulness and are generally discarded by the patient after a time.

A. STUMP CLOSURE. Clots and nonviable tissue should be debrided, but any part or tissue of reconstructive value should be saved. Closure should never be under tension. Bleeding vessels should be meticulously distinguished and separated from nerves by the use of loupe magnification and tourniquet control. Ligatures should be of nonreactive material such as fine nylon. Protruding bone should either be covered with a pedicle flap or rongeured back. Nerve stumps must be recessed or transferred (preferably into a bed of muscle or into the medullary canal of bone) well away from bone stumps or pressure points. Tendons should not be sutured over amputation stumps. Local and systemic antibiotics should be used freely.

The **loss of a fingertip** is the most common amputation. One method of closure of such wounds is by means of a thin (0.002 mm) split thickness onlay graft.* Grafting can be done primarily. The donor site is most often the volar-ulnar aspect of the proximal forearm, which is regionally anesthetized and then stretched tightly as the graft is taken with a razor blade. Anesthesia is required for the digit only if it must be debrided of clots and other debris. The procedure is done using loupe magnification and tourniquet control (blood pressure cuff at 250 mm Hg). The graft may be held in place with narrow strips of fine mesh gauze which is covered with wet gauze carefully tailored to the size of the grafted wound. Dead space is closed by applying two narrow strips of plastic foam (e.g., Reston) at right angles to one another across the digit tip and down the sides and held in place with tubular gauze (Tubegauz). The digit is then immobilized—alone if it is the thumb, or with an adjacent finger—by a well-padded forearm circumferential cast which is worn for 3 to 4 days. Constrictive dressings and garments are avoided, and the extremity is kept elevated. Such grafts survive more often than full thickness skin grafts and invariably take on a satisfactory recipient bed. In time they shrink 50% or more so as to draw normal skin over the defect for satisfactory function. Thinness of the graft precludes cosmetic defect at donor site.

The experienced hand surgeon may selectively employ other grafting techniques consisting of local or distant pedicle flaps. When amputation stumps remain sensitive, the pain may subside with fingertip percussion. If not, surgical revision may be necessary.

---

*The graft should be so thin that writing on the blade can be easily read through it.

IX. INFECTIONS

The most common hand infections are caused by gram-positive cocci and develop out of ignorance or neglect of the pathogenic factors. Tissues and structures whose blood supply is limited or easily impaired (e.g., nail folds, digital fat pads, bones, joints, and tendon sheaths) have the least resistance to infection. Constricting fascia, garments, and jewelry, wounds closed under tension, and dependent position of the hand all favor congestion and the formation of dead space (i.e., seroma and hematoma), which greatly enhances the likelihood of infection of any wound.

Most hand infections can be avoided if proper early treatment is given. The most important preventive measures in the case of hand injuries are (1) Preservation of circulation by elevation and immobilization and the avoidance of tension by sutures, dressings, garments, or swelling. (2) Facilitation of drainage of potential dead space or contaminated wounds by drains or wet dressings. (3) Judicious use of local and systemic antibiotics, along with tetanus prophylaxis. (4) Debridement of clots, foreign bodies, and dead tissue.

Rapid onset of an infection, marked swelling, or unrelenting, throbbing pain often requires bedrest with the trunk flat so the extremity can be continually at rest and propped up on pillows above heart level.

Penicillin, cephalosporin, nafcillin, and vancomycin are currently effective systemic antibiotics for staphylococcal and streptococcal infections. Tobramycin, gentamicin, or a third-generation cephalosporin is effective for gram-negative organisms. Ciprofloxacin is effective for both gram-positive or negative and resistant organisms and can achieve high drug levels in bone.

Incision for drainage should be done over the point of maximum tenderness or fluctuance and parallel to structures of vital functional importance so they are not damaged. This requires anesthesia and tourniquet ischemia.

A. FURUNCLE AND CARBUNCLE. These are common around hair follicles and often require incision and drainage.

B. GRANULATING WOUNDS (THIRD-DEGREE BURNS, ABRASIONS, AVULSIONS) should be debrided and grafted as quickly as possible. Silver sulfadiazine or wet-to-dry dressings are useful for wound care.

C. CELLULITIS is characterized by throbbing pain, local heat, redness, swelling, and tenderness. Elevation, immobilization, empirical antibiotic treatment, and frequent observation are the crucial elements of care. Surgical release of tension on skin and fascia must be done before brawny induration occurs.

Lymphangitis and **lymphadenitis** are treated the same way as cellulitis.

D. PYOGENIC GRANULOMA. Granulation tissue that forms on wounds should be scraped off flush with the skin and compressed to control bleeding for 12 to 24 hours. It is then left exposed to the air to dry up if it is <6 mm in diameter or grafted with a thin shaving of skin if larger. No sutures are needed.

E. PYODERMA is pus-filled blister that often has a central sinus to a collar-button abscess. Treatment consists of unroofing the abscess with adequate drainage of loculated pus, followed by wet-to-dry dressing changes.

F. EPONYCHIA, PARONYCHIA, AND SUBEPONYCHIAL ABSCESS. Incipient cases may respond to rest, elevation, and antibiotics. Surgical drainage of the nailfold can usually be done with a No. 11 pointed scalpel placed flat against the surface of the nail and advanced slowly in a scratching fashion into the point of maximum fluctuance and tenderness. If this is done properly, it is not painful and no blood is drawn—only pus (see Figure 16-12). When the base of the nail floats in pus or the nail is corrugated from chronic pain and recurrent discharge, it is best to undermine and avulse the nailplate with a straight hemostat. The eponychial space should be maintained by placing a small piece of nonadherent gauze in the eponychial fold.

G. SPACE INFECTIONS include infections of the pulp (e.g., felon) and web and of the thenar, hypothenar, midpalmar, dor-

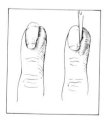

FIGURE 16-12. Incision and drainage of paronychia.

sal subcutaneous, dorsal subaponeurotic, and quadrilateral (Parona) spaces. It also includes infections of the sheaths of the flexor tendons (digital, radial, and ulnar bursae) and the extensor tendons (six compartments at the wrist). If pain, tissue tension, and tenderness are minimal or slight, incision and drainage may not be necessary and there may be a rapid response to rest, elevation, and antibiotics. The chief function of incision is the release of tension. If pus is drained and if there is involvement over a significantly broad or long space (e.g., tendon sheath), catheter-drip administration of local antibiotics (e.g., bacitracin, 50,000 units in 500 ml of Ringer's lactate) should be considered.

1. Felon (see Figure 16-13). The best drainage of a felon is through a midline longitudinal incision, often only 1 to 2 cm long. The vertical strands of fascia (septae) should not be divided. This technique spares the important blood and nerve supply to the digital tip, which may be iatrogenically damaged by the traditional fishmouth and lateral incisions.

2. Flexor tenosynovitis. Kanavel's four signs of flexor tenosynovitis are (1) a finger held in slight flexion, (2) fusiform swelling of the digit, (3) tenderness to palpation along the flexor tendon sheath, and (4) pain with passive extension. The diagnosis is established if pain can be elicited by making the tendon move actively or passively within its sheath. The examiner may passively do this by handling (picking up) only the fingernail as he or she extends the distal digital joint. If this can be done painlessly, then the site of infection rests in the skin or subcutaneous fat and spares the sheath.

Most cases of tenosynovitis that require incision and drainage need only a short volar longitudinal incision in the midline of the middle phalanx of the finger (proximal phalanx

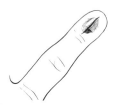

FIGURE 16-13. Incision of felon.

of the thumb) that does not cross the skin flexion creases, with a similarly directed counterincision in the palm. A fine catheter for antibiotic drip (3 to 5 ml/hour) is placed into the distal wound and brought out the proximal wound (see Figure 16-14). This is usually removed in 24 to 48 hours.

Phlegmonous tenosynovitis often destroys digital function unless the flexor sheath is widely opened. This is done through a lateral midaxial incision.

H. BONE AND JOINT INFECTIONS. These structures have particularly low resistance to infection because circulation is limited. All open wounds of bone and joint must be treated as if infection were present, that is, with local and systemic antibiotics, immobilization, and elevation.

I. HUMAN AND ANIMAL BITE INJURIES. Many of these are into joints or flexor sheaths and are considered emergencies for prophylactic treatment (immobilization of the whole hand in bulky dressing, elevation, antibiotics, and close daily followup). When infections become established, they require surgical drainage and are apt to be disabling. Wounds of the soft tissues should be drained and never fully closed.

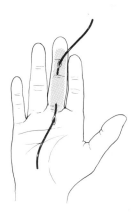

FIGURE 16-14. Drainage and irrigation for septic tenosynovitis.

J. MISCELLANEOUS INFECTIONS

1. Streptococcal gangrene requires prompt fasciotomy, aggressive debridement, and antibiotic treatment.

2. Tuberculosis is an indolent process that most often involves the synovial tissues of joints and tendons. Cultures may take months to be diagnostic. Good response follows synovectomy and antituberculosis drug therapy.

3. Fungal infections involve primarily the nail area. The response to antifungal agents may be good, e.g., griseofulvin systemically. Local ointments usually are not effective for cure.

4. Herpes simplex presents anywhere but most often about the distal phalanx mimicking a felon or paronychia. Pain is out of proportion to any swelling or induration, and is followed in time by the appearance of vesicles which may become purulent and may coalesce into a pyoderma. It may need no treatment since it is self-limiting in about 3 weeks. Acyclovir (Zovirax) a specific antiviral agent, may be useful.

5. Other infections. Gas gangrene, syphilis, deep fungal infections (coccdiodomycosis blastomycosis, actinomycosis, sporotrichosis), tularemia, yaws, and glanders are rare infections diagnosed by history, chronicity, and identification of stigmas and pathogens.

Leprosy is not so much an infection of the hand as it is a motor and sensory paralyzer requiring prophylactic education against trophic ulceration and sometimes reconstructive surgery, including tendon transfers.

X. MISCELLANEOUS DISORDERS

A. DESMITIS, TENDONITIS, MYOSITIS, AND CONSTRICTIVE STATES. Inflammation of ligaments, tendons, or muscles may cause pain and tenderness in many areas of the elbow, forearm, wrist, and hand. Examples of this are **lateral** (tennis elbow) and **medial epicondylitis** and **myositis crepitans.** Repetitive or excessively vigorous effort often initiates the process, but in some cases no cause can be identified. Treatment includes local slow injection of a mixture of lidocaine and triamcinolone, systemic antiinflammatory agents, rest, and, in acute severe cases, temporary immobilization. If longacting steroid is injected, the patient should be warned that it may cause depigmentation and local tissue atrophy that may or may not be reversible.

Constrictive conditions commonly impair nerve and tendon function. **Carpal tunnel syndrome** is characterized by pain and numbness in the hand radiating along the median nerve and even up to the shoulder due to its compression in the carpal tunnel at the wrist. The cause is most commonly nonspecific and consists of an anatomic predilection combined with factors of aging or a shift in the water content of tendons and ligaments. However, it may also result from swelling and space consumption by repetitive effort, trauma, rheumatoid disease, or tumor. A similar state may affect the ulnar nerve in its tunnel at the elbow (**cubital tunnel syndrome**) or the carpal level (Guyon's canal).

Constriction of tendons occurs for similar reasons where they are most snugly tethered by the sheath-pulley systems. The most common stenosing tenosynovitis occurs at the level of the proximal pulleys of the digital flexors in the distal palm as a **trigger finger or thumb,** and about the radial styloid as **DeQuervain's tenosynovitis,** involving the first dorsal compartment of extensor tendons, (the abductor pollicis longus and extensor pollicis brevis).

Initial treatment for most of these conditions is local injection of a mixture of lidocaine and triamcinolone (1:1) into the affected space but not into a nerve. Failure to clear the symptoms after two or three injections combined with appropriate rest of the part (e.g., splinting) justifies surgical release of the constriction.

B. GOUT AND ARTHRITIS. Pain, limitation of motion, and deformity are the complaints that lead to treatment of these conditions. Gout is most often controlled by colchicine or allopurinol (Zyloprim). Tophi are sometimes resectable. The pain of osteoarthritis can be helped by local triamcinolone and systemic antiinflammatory agents. Intractable pain or stiffness can often be corrected by surgery (e.g., joint fusion or implant arthroplasty).

C. RHEUMATOID HAND DISORDERS. This autoimmune disease affects the hand in many ways. The hand surgeon is able to improve its appearance and function, and, in many instances, can forestall disabilities by excisional, incisional, and reconstructive techniques. These include the resection of nodules, synovectomy, tenovaginotomy, and a host of tenoplasty and arthroplasty procedures to correct such deformities as ulnar drift, swan neck, or boutonniere.

D. DUPUYTREN'S CONTRACTURE is a thickening of the palmar fascia of unknown cause. It is commonly mistaken for a callus or tendon problem. It may involve any portion of the fascia and may develop insidiously over years or rapidly in weeks. It may be tender, but the most common complaint is of a lump in the palm or inability to extend the involved digits (usually the ring and little fingers). Treatment is surgical and for the most part consists of excision of the involved fascia. Skill is important to avoid neurovascular injury and postoperative stiffness (e.g., a frozen hand). Occasionally, one may prefer a subcutaneous fasciotomy of a discrete longitudinal band if the skin around it is soft and pliable. Recurrences are not uncommon.

E. TUMORS. Malignancies in the hand are rare. The most common one is squamous carcinoma of the dorsal skin in Caucasians with chronic exposure to sunlight. It can generally be cured with local excision.

Warts (verruca vulgaris), ganglions, inclusion cysts, soft tissue giant cell tumors (xanthomas), and enchondromas of bone are the most common tumors. All may recur if inadequately treated. Warts may be electrodesiccated or treated with a 40% salicylic acid pad. Ganglions may be decompressed by needle aspiration. Surgery for these conditions should be meticulously done under tourniquet and magnification in the operating room.

F. FOREIGN BODIES. The necessity to remove a foreign body depends on its size, depth, location, and the symptoms and signs. Unless superficial and easily seen or felt, it is often best to splint the hand and give antibiotics and tetanus prophylaxis and wait several days or weeks for the stain of blood that hides the foreign body to be absorbed. This makes the need for removal a certainty, and the cystic pocket that often forms around it helps greatly in finding it by dissection with tourniquet control, magnification, and fluoroscopic guidance.

17

Neurosurgery

Lawrence H. Pitts

I. GENERAL PRINCIPLES

A. EVALUATION OF THE NEUROSURGICAL PATIENT.
Neurosurgical diagnosis is based upon a detailed history and a careful physical examination. Headache, visual disturbance, altered consciousness, memory impairment, weakness, paresthesia, incoordination, and speech difficulty are symptoms suggesting disease of the CNS. The physical examination should include specific assessment of mentation, sensory and motor testing, and a thorough cranial nerve examination, including optic fundoscopy. These steps detect clinical signs that permit accurate anatomic localization of the lesion. For patients with nervous system disorders, an accurate history need be taken once, but the physical examination must be repeated and recorded often to gauge the course of the illness and to judge the urgency of other diagnostic steps to be taken before treatment can be given.

1. Plain and tomographic radiographs
a. Plain skull radiographs are useful when bony changes may be present, such as bone erosion or hyperostoses secondary to tumors, or skull fractures may have occurred. CT and MRI have largely replaced skull radiographs and tomograms in evaluating brain and spinal canal disorders.

b. Radiographs of the cervical, thoracic, and/or lumbosacral spine are ordered if clinical assessment indicates disease or injury in these areas. AP, lateral, and right and left oblique views should be obtained. Spine injury is occasionally overlooked, particularly when it is associated with head injury, and tumors of the spine (especially metastatic) are frequently missed also. If one spine lesion exists, suspect another. CT scans of the spine with appropriate image reconstruction by computer technics provide much greater detail of bone and soft tissue than do spine tomograms. MRI is the optimal imaging technic for visualizing spinal cord or canal lesions.

c. Films of the chest, pelvis, and long bones may clarify the neurosurgical problem. For example, long bone fractures may suggest that a child's subdural hematoma is the result of abuse; a mass in the lung may explain hemiparesis and aphasia on a metastatic basis; or the cause of a peripheral nerve lesion may become obvious with findings on radiographs of that extremity.

2. LP is indicated whenever analysis of CSF constituents is likely to help in the diagnosis and treatment. LP is **contraindicated** when an intracranial mass may be or is present because of the risk of tentorial or foraminal herniation in patients with elevated intracranial pressure. LP is contraindicated in the diagnosis of head injury unless meningitis is strongly suspected. If a spinal cord tumor is believed present, LP should be done at the time of myelography; LP done earlier may reduce the accuracy of the myelogram and may worsen the neurologic deficits by altering intraspinal CSF pressure around the tumor.

During the spinal tap, the initial pressure should be measured accurately and the appearance of the fluid recorded. Normal CSF is clear and colorless; yellow staining (xanthochromia) suggests recent subarachnoid hemorrhage (jaundice also causes xanthochromia). Because several hours must elapse before erythrocytes lyse and xanthochromia appears, the absence of xanthochromia in the presence of red-tinged fluid usually reflects very recent subarachnoid hemorrhage or bleeding from the puncture site ("traumatic tap"). Evidence that the tap was traumatic is obtained if the erythrocyte count decreases as more fluid is collected; i.e., compare the first tube of CSF with the third or fourth. CSF content should be analyzed for cell count and type, protein, glucose, and bacterial content. If meningitis is suspected, CSF should be sent for appropriate cultures.

3. CT scan. This noninvasive and safe test is particularly useful for visualizing acute hemorrhage or hydrocephalus and often can demonstrate tumors, abscesses, or infarctions.

4. MRI is the preferred imaging technic for most intracranial or intraspinal lesions. It is more sensitive for many lesions than CT. MR angiography is noninvasive and can visualize some vascular lesions but is not as sensitive or accurate as angiography.

5. Angiography. Cerebral angiography can be done with minimal risk (1%) of a neurologic complication. Radiopaque contrast is injected into the carotid or vertebral arteries, usually by a transfemoral route, and radiographs of the head are taken in rapid sequence as the contrast passes through the brain.

Arterial, capillary, and venous phases (usually within 8 seconds of injection) can be seen. Vascular lesions (aneurysms, arteriovenous malformations, vascular tumors) are readily identified.

B. SPECIAL CONSIDERATIONS IN NEUROSURGERY

1. Seizures are important clinical signs, because the aura, onset, type of seizure, and the postictal state may provide clues to the location of a lesion. Seizures are particularly common in patients with neoplasms, abscesses, and cortical injuries.

Repetitive or continuous seizures (status epilepticus) should be treated vigorously. Phenytoin (Dilantin) is the drug of choice, 750-1000 mg may be given IV over 1 hour as a loading dose. Supplemental doses are usually 100 mg three or four times per day. Phenobarbital is also useful (32-65 mg, three or four times per day) but larger doses may depress consciousness. Diazepam (Valium) given IV (10-50 mg) is highly effective in temporarily controlling status epilepticus, but it must be used with other anticonvulsants.

2. Raised ICP. Almost any space-occupying intracranial lesion can raise the ICP. Clinical indications of elevated ICP are headache, stupor, diplopia, nausea, vomiting, and neck stiffness. Altered blood pressure and heart rate are late signs; typically, the BP is increased and the heart rate is slowed. Apnea may occur if ICP is very high. Raised ICP may be prevented and treated by the following:

a. Hyperventilation. The $PaCO_2$ should be monitored and maintained at 25-35 mm Hg. A good airway is obviously essential.

b. Hypothermia. Because fever causes the brain to swell, the temperature should be controlled by alcohol sponging, antipyretics (aspirin or Tylenol), and hypothermia blankets. Thorazine (5 mg IV every 3-4 hours) minimizes shivering during these maneuvers.

c. Osmotic diuretics. Mannitol (1-3 g/kg/24 hours) causes shrinkage of the brain and reduction of the ICP. Its beneficial effect is transient, and the drug can severely alter serum electrolytes and osmolarity.

d. Steroids. Dexamethasone (Decadron 4-6 mg every 4 hours, IV or orally) or methylprednisolone (Solu-Medrol 125-250 mg IM or IV twice daily) reduces vasogenic brain edema, probably by stabilizing "leaky" sites in the blood-brain barrier. Steroids are most effective when substantial vasogenic edema is present, as with glial or metastatic malignant brain tumors or brain abscess. Steroids do not improve ICP or outcome in patients with head injury.

e. Barbiturates have been used for intracranial hypertension caused by Reye's syndrome and head injury. They may be helpful in lowering ICP resistant to other therapy but are difficult to use because they can cause hypotension.

f. Systemic arterial pressure must be maintained by intravenous infusions of crystalloid or colloid solutions or by the use of pressor agents (norepinephrine or dopamine) to maintain cerebral perfusion pressure (CPP = SAP − ICP) above 70 mm Hg.

3. Infectious CNS processes include meningitis, subdural empyema, brain abscess, and epidural abscess. If focal signs (aphasia, hemiparesis, visual field defects) are present, a CT scan should preclude a mass lesion before LP is done; otherwise, LP should be done to document the specific infecting agent. Broad-spectrum antibiotic coverage (cephotaxime or ceftriaxone, 2 g every 6 hours) should be given until an organism is identified and sensitivities are determined; then a specific antibiotic is chosen which crosses the blood-brain barrier.

4. Fluid balance. Neurosurgical patients should have normal intake and output of fluids (1500-2000 m/24 hours for an adult). Free water (D_5W) should be avoided because it may cause brain swelling. The preferred solution is Ringer's lactate, normal saline, or 5% dextrose in 0.5 normal saline with potassium supplements (40 mEq/day). Fluid balance should be monitored by daily weights and periodic measurements of serum electrolytes and osmolality. Feedings by gastric or enteral lavage may be started early (2-3 days after injury or operation), provided that GI function is normal.

Some neurosurgical patients have profound disturbances of fluid balance. Inappropriate ADH secretion, which most commonly occurs after head trauma, causes retention of free water resulting in low serum Na, high urinary Na, low serum osmolarity, and high urinary specific gravity. Seizures and coma may be the first clinical signs of inappropriate ADH. Treatment includes fluids restriction or use of hypertonic saline.

Diabetes insipidus is seen in patients with pituitary lesions. Urine volume is high and specific gravity is low; serum Na and osmolarity are high. Seizures and stupor may appear. The condition is treated by administration of IV or oral fluids.

Subcutaneous injections of 2-5 mg aqueous vasopressin or 5-15 mg intranasal arginine vasopressin also may be useful when the diagnosis of diabetes insipidus is certain.

Patients who receive steroids, osmotic diuretics, anticonvulsants, and tube feedings (typical neurosurgical patient!) are prone to develop a hyperosmolar state, sometimes leading to nonketotic coma. Consequently, careful monitoring of the fluid and electrolyte status of the neurologic patient is essential.

C. COMA is loss of consciousness from which the patient cannot be aroused by any stimulus. **Stupor** implies that the patient can be partially aroused by loud commands or painful stimuli but promptly lapses into unconsciousness again when the stimulus is withdrawn.

1. Diagnosis of coma consists of determining the specific cause. This requires a careful history (generally from friends or relatives) and a complete physical examination with specific attention to the neurologic examination. Laboratory and radiologic tests of value include serum electolytes, blood glucose, blood urea nitrogen, CT scanning, and, if meningitis is suspected, CSF examination (LP). Medical consultation should be sought promptly.

Coma may be caused by poisoning (e.g., alcohol, barbiturates, narcotics); cerebral lesions (e.g., trauma, vascular accidents, tumors, infections, epilepsy); metabolic disorders (e.g., diabetic coma, hypoglycemia, Addison's disease, uremia, hepatic coma, eclampsia); and other disorders such as severe infection, shock, asphyxia, heat stroke, and hypoxia.

Diagnostic features of common types of coma are listed below:

a. Acute alcoholic intoxication. A history of drinking, alcoholic breath, flushed face, slow and stertorous respirations, diminished reflexes, and a blood alcohol level of above 0.5% point to this diagnosis. **Caution:** Always search for other causes of coma, particularly head injury, in the intoxicated patient.

b. Narcotic poisoning. Even small doses of narcotics may cause respiratory depression and coma in patients with liver insufficiency, myxedema, emphysema, or head injuries and in debilitated or elderly patients.

Findings include cold, clammy, cyanotic skin; pinpoint pupils; respiratory depression (breathing slow and irregular, sometimes Cheyne-Stokes); and a feeble and often irregular pulse.

Acute toxicity due to an overdose of a self-administered narcotic occurs commonly in some localities. Type and purity of the drug are difficult to determine, although a companion or acquaintance may know the patient's drug habits. The examiner should look for needle marks in arms and wrists. Laboratory tests are of value in determining barbiturate, alcohol, or narcotic levels.

c. Diabetic coma. Coma may be precipitated in a diabetic patient by infection or by failure to regulate insulin dosage. Diagnostic features include history of diabetes, gradual onset with blurred vision and thirst, air hunger or Kussmaul breathing, dehydration, acetone breath ("fruity" odor), glycosuria, acetonuria, hyperglycemia, ketonemia, and low plasma bicarbonate.

d. Hypoglycemia. Hypoglycemic reactions in diabetics who take insulin may be precipitated by failure to eat or by vigorous exercise. Mental confusion and bizarre behavior precede coma and convulsions. Tachycardia, perspiration, tremor, and vomiting are other manifestations. The diagnosis is confirmed by finding a low blood glucose level. If hypoglycemia is suspected, glucose should be given after blood is drawn for a glucose determination.

2. Treatment

a. Emergency measures. (1) Identify and treat any life-threatening condition immediately. (2) Establish and maintain an **airway** to provide oxygenation. An endotracheal tube should be inserted if the respiratory rate is <10/minute, or if the PaO_2 is <70 mm Hg, or if the $Paco_2$ is >50 mm Hg with the patient breathing oxygen through a mask. Arterial blood gases should be monitored frequently. (3) Treat shock. (4) When no cause for coma is apparent, obtain blood for glucose determination and toxicologic analysis and immediately administer each of the following: 50 ml of 50% dextrose in water for possible hypoglycemia; 1 ml (0.4 mg) naloxone for possible narcotic overdose; 100 mg thiamine IV for possible Wernicke's (alcoholic) encephalitis.

b. General measures. (1) Observe the patient frequently, record neurologic and vital signs at regular intervals, and change the patient's position every 30-60 minutes to avoid hypostatic pneumonitis and decubiti. A lateral and slightly head-down position is best for patients who are likely to vomit, but endotracheal intubation gives the best airway protection. Have a suction machine and an alert attendant near the bedside. (2) Maintain ventilation. (3) Monitor urinary output through an indwelling catheter. (4) Maintain fluid, electrolyte, and caloric intake. Tube feeding should be started if coma lasts more than 2-3 days. (5) Avoid narcotics, sedatives, and other medications until the diagnosis is established; restlessness can then be treated best by administration of parenteral diazepam (2-5 mg every 2 hours) or morphine sulfate (1-3 mg every hour), as needed.

II. TRAUMA

A. HEAD INJURIES: GENERAL PRINCIPLES. The extent of brain damage is the primary determinant of treatment for patients with head injuries. The prognosis is related to the type and degree of brain damage and to the number and kinds of injuries to other parts of the body.

Injury to the brain results from rapid deceleration, acceleration, and/or the shearing-rotational effects of a blow to the head. These mechanisms may produce **concussion,** a temporary loss of consciousness with no permanent organic brain damage; **contusion,** bruising of the brain; or **laceration,** frank disruption of brain substance. The three types of brain injury can occur singly, but more commonly they are seen in varying combinations.

Contusion may be local, causing focal signs and symptoms (e.g., hemiparesis or aphasia), or it may be generalized, with widespread damage to the brain. Increased vascular permeability in contused brain produces cerebral edema. Decreased respiratory exchange in severely injured patients leads to anoxia and hypercapnia; the resulting cerebral vasodilation contributes still further to cerebral swelling.

1. Emergency management. (1) Establish and maintain adequate ventilation. (2) Control hemorrhage. (3) Treat shock. (4) Examine the patient quickly but thoroughly to ascertain the type and degree of **all** injuries. (5) Splint long-bone fractures. (6) Evaluate the nervous system injury (see below). (7) Do **not** move the patient for any reason (e.g., to obtain radiographs or to transport to another hospital or to another room) until the extent of all injuries is known and the immediate threats to life (e.g., respiratory embarrassment, hemorrhage) have been controlled. (8) If the patient is comatose, assume that the cervical spine is unstable; immobilize the patient in the supine position with sandbags supporting both sides of the head until radiographs exclude a cervical fracture.

2. Evaluation of the nervous system. Every head injury is potentially serious. A thorough neurologic examination should be performed as soon as possible, and a record should be made of the following features: (1) Direct inspection of the head for abrasions, swelling, laceration, blood behind the tympanic membranes, or CSF in the nose or ears. (2) Level of consciousness (Table 17-1). (3) Size of pupils and response to light. (4) Motor response in all 4 extremities (normal, weakness, abnormal flexion, abnormal extension, no movement). (5) Eye movements (spontaneous gaze preference or palsy, response to icewater instillation into the external ear canal if the tympanic membrane is intact and free of obstruction). (6) Corneal response. (7) Cough and gag responses. (8) Breathing pattern. (9) Tendon and plantar reflexes. (10) Ophthalmoscopic examination. **Never artificially dilate the pupils in head injury.** (11) Cervical spine radiographs if there is evidence of injury to that area of if the patient is unconscious on admission. (12) Lumbar puncture should **not** be done unless meningitis is strongly suspected and an intracranial mass lesion has been excluded. (13) CT scan should be done immediately in comatose or deteriorating patients.

Accurate records of the initial physical examination are

Table 17-1. Evaluation of level of consciousness by responses to graded stimuli*

Eye opening	Spontaneous
	To voice command
	With painful stimulus
	None
Motor response	Follows commands
	Localizes painful stimulus
	Complex movement with painful stimulus
	Abnormal flexion in response to pain
	Abnormal extension
	None
Verbal response	Oriented
	Confused
	Speaks only words
	Makes only sounds
	None

*The **best** response is recorded in each of the three categories.

essential, because decisions to repeat diagnostic studies or to operate depend to a great extent upon later variations from the baseline. Repeated examination at frequent intervals is imperative. The most sensitive signs of improvement or deterioration are changes in the level of responsiveness (Table 17-1) or the size of the pupils.

3. Postoperative management. Hypoxia and hypercapnia must be prevented, because they cause cell injury and intracranial vascular dilatation and add to cerebral swelling. Respiratory care, therefore, is very important (see Chapter 2). Measures to maintain normal body temperatures should be used (see page 458). IV hyperosmotic solutions (mannitol 150-300 ml of 20% solution) also help reduce ICP, but they should not be used unless steps are in progress to identify and treat intracranial hematoma by CT scan or diagnostic burr holes.

B. SCALP INJURIES. The scalp is an extremely vascular structure, and injury may cause serious hemorrhage. Bleeding usually is controlled with a simple pressure dressing of several 4 × 4 gauze sponges placed over the wound and held firmly in place by a circumferential dressing. Arterial bleeding can be controlled by firm finger pressure along the edges of the wound or by a hemostat that is attached to the galea and allowed to hang down over the skin edge to pull the galea firmly against the skin and compress the bleeding vessel.

All scalp wounds should be closed as soon as possible, unless they overlie a depressed fracture or a penetrating wound of the skull which requires debridement in the operating room.

1. Scalp lacerations. Shave and wash a **generous area.** If the laceration is large, a 4 × 4 gauze sponge in the wound prevents debris from entering. Cleanse the wound thoroughly with repeated irrigations of saline or Ringer's solution. Infiltrate the circumference of the wound with local anesthetic about 1 inch away from the edges. Remove foreign bodies, which may lead to infection or leave unsightly tattoos. All devitalized tissue should be debrided, taking care not to cut away normal tissue.

The wound is closed with multiple interrupted vertical mattress sutures of monofilament nylon, or the galea and skin may be closed in separate layers. Meticulous technic should be used. Loss of scalp wider than 1 cm often requires treatment in the operating room.

2. Avulsions of the scalp usually include all layers of the scalp down to the periosteum. These injuries should be treated only by experienced surgeons with complete operating room facilities. The surrounding area should be shaved and thoroughly irrigated. If the avulsion is small, the ragged edges can be sparingly trimmed; closure can often be accomplished by tripod extension or modified Z-plasty. If the denuded area is large, the wound is covered with a single layer of fine mesh gauze. A large dressing is placed on top of the gauze, and a firm circumferential dressing is applied to exert even pressure over the area. Delayed closure (using plastic surgical technics) can be performed 8-10 days later.

C. SKULL FRACTURES are no more serious than fractures of any other bone if the brain is not injured; the extent of brain damage determines the prognosis. Skull fractures can be classified according to (1) whether the skin overlying the fracture is intact (closed) or open (compound); (2) whether there is a single fracture line (linear), several fractures radiating from a central point (stellate), or fragmentation of bone (comminuted); (3) whether the edges of the fracture line have been driven below the level of the surrounding bone (depressed) or not (nondepressed).

1. Simple skull fracture (linear, stellate, or comminuted nondepressed). These fractures can be serious if they cross major vascular channels in the skull, such as the groove of the middle meningeal artery or the major dural venous sinuses. If the vessels are torn, epidural or subdural hematomas may form. Patients with these types of fractures should be kept under close observation until it is certain that no such bleeding is occurring. A fracture that extends into the accessory nasal sinuses or the mastoid air cells is considered to be open, because it is in communication with an external surface of the body.

2. Depressed skull fractures. Depressed stellate or comminuted fractures require a surgical procedure to elevate the depressed bone. If there are no untoward neurologic signs and the fracture is closed, operation may be delayed until a convenient time.

3. Open skull fractures. As soon as the patient's general condition permits, a **depressed open skull fracture** should be elevated, debrided, and closed. Until that can be done, the wound is covered with a sterile compression dressing. The scalp wound should not be closed, and no attempt should be made to remove any foreign body protruding from the wound until the patient is in the operating room and all preparations have been made for craniotomy.

Linear or stellate, **nondepressed, open fractures** can be treated by simple closure of the skin wound after thorough cleansing. Open fractures with severe comminution of underlying bone should be treated in the operating room, where proper debridement can be carried out. If possible, the dura should be inspected to make certain that no laceration has been overlooked.

4. Basilar skull fractures may cause rhinorrhea or otorrhea if the dura and arachnoid are torn; they may also cause bleeding from the nose or ears if mucous membranes or skin are lacerated. It is often difficult to tell if blood is mixed with CSF. A drop of the bloody discharge can be placed on a cleansing tissue; if CSF is present, there will be a spreading yellowish-orange ring around the central red stain of blood. There is no evidence that antibiotics improve outcome after basal skull fractures with or without CSF leak. If antibiotics are elected, penicillin (50,000 units/kg) or ampicillin (25 mg/kg) should be given IV every 6 hours. The patient's head should remain elevated to 30 degrees, and fluid intake is restricted to 1200 ml/day. The patient is cautioned against blowing the nose, a maneuver that could contaminate the intracranial space. If a CSF leak persists for longer than 4 days, spinal drainage and acetazolamide (250 mg orally three times per day) can be used to reduce CSF production and lower intracranial pressure. Craniotomy may be required for leaks that continue for more than 2 weeks. Few patients with CSF leaks require surgical repair.

D. TRAUMA TO THE MENINGES. Skull fracture may cause tears in the vascular channels coursing through the meninges and can lead to serious intracranial hemorrhage. Tears in the dura should be repaired to lessen the chances of infection.

E. EPIDURAL HEMATOMA. Hemorrhage between the inner table of the skull and the dura mater most commonly arises from a tear of the middle meningeal artery caused by a skull fracture across the arterial groove in the temporal region. Arterial bleeding strips the dura from the undersurface of the bone and produces still more bleeding because the small bridging veins from the dura to bone are torn. The hematoma rapidly increases in size and compresses the cerebral cortex. If sufficient hemispheric compression occurs, the medial portion of the temporal lobe (uncus and hippocampal gyrus) is forced through the incisura tentorii; this causes pressure on the third cranial nerve and dilatation of the pupil on the same side. Hemispheric compression shifts the brain stem toward the opposite side of the tentorial notch; if it shifts too far, venous hemorrhages into the brain stem lead to irreparable neurologic deficits or death.

An epidural hematoma may arise from torn venous channels in the bone at a point of fracture or from lacerated major dural venous sinuses. Because venous pressure is low, epidural venous hematomas usually form only when a skull fracture has stripped the dura from the bone and left a space in which the hematoma can develop.

Epidural hematoma classically follows a blow to the head that causes unconsciousness for a brief period. After the patient regains consciousness, there may be a "lucid interval" during which there are no abnormal neurologic symptoms or signs. As the hematoma enlarges sufficiently to compress the cerebral hemisphere, there is gradual deterioration of consciousness which progresses to coma and death if the hematoma is not evacuated. As the level of consciousness deteriorates, the pupil on the side of the lesion dilates and hemiparesis occurs.

Even though an epidural hematoma is a curable lesion, the mortality rate is significant because patients are not seen by a physician, or the gravity of injury is not recognized by a physician. A patient may be seen during the lucid interval and discharged. At home, the patient is assumed to be asleep when, actually, the hematoma has increased in size and caused coma instead of sleep. Considering this danger, any patient with a history of a blow to the head leading to even a brief period of unconsciousness should have a thorough neurologic examination and skull radiography. If radiographs show a fracture, the patient should be hospitalized and the conscious level checked at least every hour. If no fracture is demonstrated, the patient may be discharged, but a reliable relative should be instructed to **awaken the patient at least hourly** to make certain that he or she is arousable and not comatose.

Impairment of sensorium is the first indication that operation may be urgently necessary. This is a **true emergency**; if operation is delayed until brain stem hemorrhages occur, the patient is likely to remain comatose even thought the epidural clot is evacuated.

F. SUBDURAL HEMATOMA occurs most commonly when the veins bridging from the cortex to the superior sagittal sinus near the midline are torn, or when an intracerebral hematoma communicates with the subdural space. Bleeding occurs between the arachnoid and the dura; because the arachnoid is attached loosely to the dura, these hematomas can attain tremendous size, even though the bleeding is of venous (low pressure) origin.

1. Acute subdural hematomas are associated with severe head injuries. They arise from a combination of torn bridging veins and frank lacerations of the pia and arachnoid of the cortex. The hematoma is readily demonstrated by CT scanning. Evacuation of the clot may result in significant improvement, but often a major neurologic deficit remains owing to the concomitant cerebral contusion and/or laceration.

2. Subacute subdural hematomas become apparent 1-15 days after injury and are associated with progressive lethargy, confusion, hemiparesis, or other hemispheric deficits. Removal of the hematoma usually produces striking improvement.

3. Chronic subdural hematomas are most common in infants and in adults older than 60 years. They arise from tears in bridging veins after a minor head injury. The hematoma is small initially; it becomes encased in a fibrous membrane, liquefies, and gradually enlarges. The history is usually one of progressive mental or personality changes, with or without focal symptoms (e.g., progressive hemiplegia, aphasia). Papilledema may be present. These findings often suggest a diagnosis of brain tumor, and the hematoma may be discovered unexpectedly during CT or MRI scanning.

Treatment consists of drainage through multiple burr holes. If fluid reaccumulates, craniotomy for removal of the encasing membranes may be necessary.

4. Subdural hygromas are collections of clear or yellow-stained fluid in the subdural space. They probably form through a tear in the arachnoid that allows CSF to escape into the subdural space, producing the same symptoms as a chronic subdural hematoma. If symptoms require, this condition is treated by draining the fluid through multiple burr holes.

G. BRAIN INJURY. Contusions and lacerations of the brain generally cannot be treated surgically, but some neurosurgeons believe that resection of the most severely contused portions of cerebrum may be indicated in selected cases. Intracerebral hematomas are usually associated with lacerations; if the hematoma is large, surgical evacuation is indicated.

H. INJURIES TO THE SPINAL CORD AND NERVE ROOTS.* Laceration, disruption, or dissolution of part or all

---

*See Chapter 16 for peripheral nerve injuries.

of the spinal cord or nerve roots is usually caused by penetrating wounds or severe fracture-dislocations of the bony spine. Concussion of the spinal cord produces temporary interruption of function without anatomically demonstrable changes. Contusion of the cord usually occurs at the site of a fracture-dislocation or a penetrating wound.

1. Diagnosis. Neurologic deficits resulting from trauma to the spinal cord may be partial or complete, and transient or permanent. The diagnosis usually is not difficult, **but spinal cord injury may be overlooked** in comatose patients. It is imperative that cervical spin radiographs be obtained in all patients with severe head injuries; about 6% of such patients have injuries to the spine as well.

a. Symptoms and signs. (1) Weakness or paralysis of the extremities, and diminished reflexes below the level of the injury as a consequence of "spinal shock," which may persist for hours or days. (2) Partial or complete loss of any modalities of sensation below the level of the lesion. (3) Marked weakness and numbness of hands and arms with variable sparing of lower extremity function. (4) Urinary retention. (5) Paralytic ileus with abdominal distention. (6) Respiratory difficulty which frequently accompanies cervical lesions because the intercostal muscles are paralyzed and breathing is purely diaphragmatic. (7) Loss of sweating below the level of the lesion. (8) Point tenderness over the fracture site, with or without gibbus or crepitus.

b. Radiographs may be negative, or they may demonstrate simple fracture or complete fracture-dislocation with marked comminution.

2. Emergency management. A thorough neurologic examination must be performed as soon as possible to establish the level and degree of functional loss. Examine for associated injuries. Spinal cord injury should be assumed present until there is definite proof that none has occurred. Do not move the patient until the full extent of the injury is known, because the spinal cord may be further damaged by improper movement.

Obtain a detailed description of the accident, because management may depend upon whether the injury was caused by hyperflexion, hyperextension, or a direct blow.

If cervical fracture is suspected, place sandbags at both sides of the head as an emergency splinting measure to prevent motion. Several person are required to lift the patient onto bed or x-ray table. One person directs the move; the spine should be kept aligned by applying traction on the chin and occiput.

If patient cannot void, connect an indwelling catheter to gravity drainage.

As soon as the patient's general condition warrants, obtain radiographs of the spine. The physician should accompany the patient to the x-ray department and remain there until satisfactory lateral, anteroposterior, and oblique views have been obtained without rotating the patient's head.

3. Treatment. If cervical fracture or fracture-dislocation is found on radiography, skeletal traction should be instituted using halo or tong devices. If traction does not reduce the fracture within 4-6 hours, closed manipulation by an experienced surgeon, using an image intensifier in the operating room, should be considered. If manipulation is unsuccessful, open surgical reduction should be done.

Decompression of the spinal cord by an appropriate anterior or posterior approach should be done in the following circumstances: (a) progressive neurologic loss; (b) partial neurologic injury with major canal compromise, as shown by MRI or CT scan with intrathecal metrizamide instillation; (c) a potentially infected foreign body in the spinal canal. If decompression is decided on, it should be carried out as soon as the patient's condition is stable and immediately after life-threatening associated injuries have been dealt with. If injury is cervical, skeletal tong traction should be instituted immediately and maintained during the operation. Stabilization of the spine is a necessary part of surgery.

III. CONGENITAL LESIONS

Evaluation of congenital lesions of the CNS requires an understanding of embryology. The formation of the neural groove begins at the midposition of the neural plate, and closure progresses rostrally and caudally. The neural tube gradually separates from the ectoderm and comes to lie within the mesoderm early in embryologic development. Therefore, malformations of the nervous system are frequently associated with malformations of mesodermal and ectodermal elements.

A. CRANIOSYNOSTOSIS (CRANIOSTENOSIS) is premature bony fusion of cranial sutures. Normally, bones of the skull are separated at birth and become joined in a fibrous union at the suture lines after 6 months of age. In craniosynostosis, closure of the sutures begins in utero and progresses after birth.

Early recognition of this condition is important because brain weight doubles in the first year of life. If two more of the sutures fuse prematurely, skull malformation is marked.

1. Diagnosis. The principal clinical feature of craniosynostosis is deformity of the cranial contour; the type of deformity depends upon the suture or sutures involved. Typical patterns of involvement include sagittal suture alone; coronal suture alone; all sutures.

2. Treatment and prognosis. The only treatment is surgical. Operation consists of removing a linear strip of bone, following the line of and including the involved suture. Silastic film is sutured over the edge of the bone to delay regrowth. Major skull reconstruction is now possible for premature closure of skull or facial sutures, including moving the orbits for hypo- or hypertelorism.

B. ENCEPHALOCELES are protrusions of meninges and neural tissue from their normal intracranial location. About 75% of all encephaloceles are in the occipital area. Most protrude extracranially in the midline, but they may project into the nasopharynx, nasal cavity, or orbit.

The sac may be large with a narrow stalk, but more commonly it is sessile in shape. It is often difficult to determine by examination if the mass contains neural structures, CSF, or both. Transillumination with a bright light in a darkened room may show neural tissue as a shadow against the homogeneous red glow of the fluid.

At operation, the neck of the mass and the cranial defect are exposed, the sac is opened, neural contents are replaced within the cranial cavity if possible, and the dura is closed. The bony defect may be repaired later if it persists.

C. DERMAL SINUS tracts are due to incomplete embryonal separation of the neural tube from overlying ectoderm, creating a persistent connection between the skin and the CNS or its investing membranes or bone. Because closure and separation of the neural tube proceed caudally and rostrally from about the midpoint of embryo, dermal sinuses occur most often at either end of the neural tube. Midline cutaneous defects are common in the sacral area; most of these are of no significance because they penetrate no deeper than the sacral fascia. If they extend into the subarachnoid space through a bony defect (spina bifida), the tract may serve as a pathway of infection.

The diagnosis is usually suggested by the cutaneous defect (e.g. dimple, port wine stain, hair tuft) and there may be a history of recurrent meningitis.

The sinus should be excised surgically to prevent meningitis.

D. HYDROCEPHALUS is enlargement of the ventricles of the brain due to a decrease in CSF absorption; an increase in CSF production; or obstruction of CSF flow by a lesion in the normal pathway of CSF circulation. Common sites of obstruction are the foramina of Monro, the aqueduct of Silvius, the foramina of Luschka and Magendie, and the basilar cisterns.

E. HYDROCEPHALUS IN INFANTS

    1. Diagnosis. There is abnormal, progressive enlargement of the head that can be shown by comparison with standard charts. The fontanel is usually wide, tense, and nonpulsating. The fontanel bosses are prominent, and sclerae may be visible above the iris ("sunset sign"). Symptoms of increased intracranial pressure may include irritability, vomiting, and somnolence.

    2. Differential diagnosis. In **obstructive hydrocephalus,** no communication exists between the ventricular system and the subarachnoid absorptive bed. In **communicating hydrocephalus,** the ventricles communicate freely with the subarachnoid space. The following diagnostic steps should be taken to determine the type and cause of hydrocephalus: (1) If the child is moribund, subdural taps should be done bilaterally to exclude a subdural hematoma. A 20-ga short-beveled spinal needle is inserted into the subdural space through the lateral angle of the anterior fontanel or the coronal suture well away from the midline. Fluid emerging spontaneously after the stylet is withdrawn is diagnostic of a subdural hematoma, hygroma, or empyema. Specimens should be obtained for cells, protein, and culture. Fluid should not be aspirated, but it should be allowed to flow until the fontanel becomes soft. (2) A CT brain scan, with and without contrast, should follow the subdural taps. CT scanning or MRI may be done first if the child is stable. Ventricular size and the presence of hematomas, neoplasms, abscesses, etc. can be recognized easily and safely. General anesthesia or sedation (Demerol 1 mg/kg plus Phenergan 1 mg/kg IM) may help to obtain a good study without motion artifact. (3) Lumbar puncture should be done only after an intracranial mass has been excluded.

    3. Treatment. Occasionally the hydrocephalus arrests spontaneously. After ventricular hemorrhage in premature infants, secondary hydrocephalus (from blocked subarachnoid CSF pathways) may arrest after early treatment with spinal taps (to drain bloody CSF) and Diamox (to reduce the CSF formation). Repeated LPs (in communicating hydrocephalus) or ventricular taps (in obstructive hydrocephalus) may be used until definitive treatment can be given.

Several shunting procedures are available to direct the CSF to an absorptive bed. The choice of procedure depends on the type of hydrocephalus. In obstructive hydrocephalus, the fluid must be shunted directly from the ventricular system; in communicating hydrocephalus, the fluid can be shunted from the lumbar subarachnoid space. In both instances, the fluid is shunted into either the peritoneal cavity or the right atrium.

F. HYDROCEPHALUS AFTER INFANCY

1. Diagnosis. In patients over 3 years of age the skull expands poorly to accommodate rising CSF pressure and expanding ventricles. Progressive dementia, headache, somnolence, nausea, vomiting, and occasionally visual impairment are symptoms of hydrocephalus in this group of patients. Urinary incontinence and gait disturbance may appear as the ventricles expand, forming, in association with dementia, the "triad" of occult hydrocephalus. CSF pressure may be normal or only slightly elevated. On the other hand, CSF pressure may be severely elevated, particularly if the ventricles are obstructed, accounting for the appearance of papilledema and visual impairment.

2. Treatment. CSF shunting is the most effective current treatment. Ventriculoperitoneal or ventriculoatrial shunts usually function well for all types of hydrocephalus. Lumbarperitoneal shunts are indicated only if CSF can pass from its ventricular source freely into the lumbar subarachnoid space. Ventriculoperitoneal shunting (Torkildsen procedure) is reserved for patients with obstruction of the aqueduct or the foramina of the fourth ventricle. Drugs to reduce CSF production are usually ineffective, although Diamox (3-4 mg/kg four times per day) may help.

G. PORENCEPHALY is a circumscribed cavity in cerebral tissue that communicates with the ventricle; it is usually caused by a stroke in utero. The most common clinical findings are seizures and, rarely, enlargement of the head. Surgical treatment is indicated only when seizures cannot be controlled by anticonvulsant drug therapy.

H. ARNOLD-CHIARI MALFORMATION consists of elongation and caudal projection of the cerebellar tonsils though the foramen magnum; elongation and kinking of the medulla into the cervical canal so that the fourth ventricle opens into the cervical spinal subarachnoid space; and downward displacement of the cervical spinal cord so that the cervical nerve roots course upward to their respective foramina. Hydrocephalus is often present, as well as congenital anomalies of the cervical vertebrae (e.g., fusion of one or more cervical vertebrae), lower cranial nerve palsies, cerebellar disturbances, and long tract signs.

Hydrocephalus and neural compromise may be relieved by decompression of the posterior fossa and upper cervical laminectomy. If these measures are ineffective, a shunting procedure may be required.

I. PLATYBASIA is a developmental defect characterized by upward displacement of the cervical vertebral column into the base of the skull so that the odontoid process projects into the cranial cavity. Other bony anomalies are frequently associated, such as occipitalization of the atlas, malformation of the foramen magnum, and fusion of the cervical vertebrae.

Symptoms rarely develop before adulthood. Neurologic signs are those of cervical spinal cord compression with weakness, ataxia, sensory loss, and sphincter disturbances. The diagnosis is established by radiography of the skull and cervical spine. Platybasia is present when the odontoid process projects more than 5 mm above a line drawn from the posterior rim of the foramen magnum to the posterior edge of the hard palate (Chamberlain's line).

Transoral removal of the odontoid or decompression of the foramen magnum by suboccipital craniectomy and cervical laminectomy may help. In most cases, arrest of progressive deficits is all that can be accomplished; occasionally excellent functional recovery is seen.

J. SYRINGOMYELIA (AND SYRINGOBULBIA). A syrinx is a central cavitation of the spinal cord (syringomyelia) and/or the brain stem (syringobulbia). Syringomyelia usually occurs in the cervical and upper thoracic cord.

Examination shows dissociated loss of pain and temperature sensation involving the upper extremities, shoulder girdle, and upper thorax, with relative preservation of touch perception. This is produced when the cavity disrupts the decussating pain fibers in the commissures around the central canal. Associated findings are weakness of the muscles of the upper extremities, particularly the intrinsic muscles of the hand, with atrophy and fasciculations. Long tract signs (hyperreflexia, spasticity, extensor plantar responses) are often present in the lower extremities. MRI clearly demonstrates these cystic cavities.

Laminectomy (with or without drainage of the cystic area), myelotomy, or permanent drainage of the cavity into the subarachnoid space or peritoneal cavity have mixed success, and the prognosis is guarded.

K. SPINA BIFIDA OCCULTA is a defect in the laminar arch, most often in the lumbosacral area. Associated anomalies are common in the skin overlying the bifida spine, and the lower extremities may be malformed. It is usually asymptomatic, but urinary incontinence, weakness, atrophy, and sensory loss in the lower lumbar area and along the distribution of the sacral nerve roots may be noted. MRI may demonstrate an intraspinal mass, which is usually a lipoma.

Treatment is indicated only when there are progressive neurologic deficits. The operation consists of laminectomy with removal of any intraspinal mass (lipoma, dermoid).

L. MENINGOCELE AND MYELOMENINGOCELE. A meningocele is a protusion of meninges containing CSF through a defective neural arch. If neural elements are present, it is a myelomeningocele. The lesion usually is in the lumbosacral area, but it may occur at any level. Occasionally it protrudes anteriorly into the pelvic, abdominal, or thoracic cavities. Neurologic deficits (sensory, motor, and sphincter disturbances) suggest that the lesion contains neural tissue. The objective of surgery is cosmetic removal of the mass and prevention of infection and further neurologic deficits. The lesion should be removed if technically feasible. A meningocele or myelomeningocele that has ruptured and is leaking CSF should be repaired emergently if the neurologic deficits are not severe. If there is no CSF leak, operation can be delayed until there is sufficient skin covering to ensure a satisfactory closure. Progressive hydrocephalus is usually treated before removal of the meningocele; increased CSF pressure may threaten the repair.

Prognosis depends upon the extent of associated neurologic deficits and the severity of associated anomalies.

IV. NEOPLASMS OF THE CENTRAL NERVOUS SYSTEM

A. INTRACRANIAL NEOPLASMS. Brain tumors occur in all age groups with approximately equal distribution up to the age of 70 years. Two-thirds of brain tumors in children arise in the subtentorial space (posterior fossa). About 45% of brain tumors are gliomas, 15% meningiomas, 10% pituitary tumors, 5% tumors of nerve sheaths, 5% blood vessel tumors, 5% congenital, and 10% metastatic. Miscellaneous tumors account for the remainder.

Symptoms and signs are produced by the mass effect and neural involvement of the tumor and by secondary effects, such as brain edema or CSF obstruction. Brain tumors almost never metastasize outside the CNS.

1. Local effects

a. Frontal lobe. Personality change (inappropriate behavior, loss of social inhibitions) and mental changes may occur. If ICP is elevated, there may be headache, nausea, vomiting, and papilledema.

If the posterior portions of the frontal lobe are involved, the patient may show forced grasping; if the motor areas of the cortex or subcortical areas are involved, varying degrees of hemiparesis on the contralateral side, increased deep tendon reflexes, and a positive Babinski reflex occur.

Tumor in the dominant frontal lobe may cause expressive aphasia. If convulsions occur, they are frequently of the adversive type (head and eyes turned away from the side of the lesion). Tumors arising beneath the frontal lobes may cause anosmia or visual loss.

b. Parietal lobe. Contralateral weakness is accompanied by defects in the appreciation of the weight, texture, size, and shape of objects. Ability to perceive on the side of the body opposite the lesion may be impaired (astereognosis). Parasagittal tumors (involving the paracentral area) may cause spastic paralysis of the contralateral leg or paraplegia and urinary incontinence. Tumors low in the parietal area may produce visual field defects. If the dominant hemisphere is involved, global aphasia may be present.

c. Occipital lobe. A visual field defect is the major neurologic sign and tends to be more congruous than a visual field defect produced by a lesion in the temporal lobe. Complete homonymous hemianopsia has no localizing value, because it can be produced by a lesion anywhere from the chiasm to the occipital lobe. Isolated visual hallucinations may occur, or they may appear as part of a generalized seizure.

d. Middle fossa. "Temporal lobe seizures" are a common manifestation. Uncinate fits are accompanied by unpleasant olfactory sensations, often with lip-smacking and loss of contact with surroundings. A generalized seizure may follow. The seizure may take the form of momentary episodes of staring, a feeling of unreality, and extreme familiarity (déja vu) or unfamiliarity with surroundings at the time of the attack. Distorted perceptions of sounds, objects, sizes, or shapes may be noted. Visual field defects are common and tend to be incongruous. If the dominant temporal lobe is involved, receptive aphasia or auditory agnosia may occur.

e. Posterior fossa. Early symptoms are produced by involvement of the cerebellum, brain stem, and cranial nerves, and often by obstruction of the flow of CSF. A tumor arising in a hemisphere of the cerebellum causes ataxia of gait and incoordination of the ipsilateral arm and leg. Nystagmus is common. The principal manifestation of a tumor in the midline of the cerebellum is ataxia of the trunk and legs with unsteadiness and falling even while sitting; incoordination of the arms is less frequent. Cranial nerve palsies, particularly of those nerves supplying the extraocular muscles, also occur.

f. Brain stem. Multiple cranial nerve palsies, nystagmus, and incoordination and paresis of extremities. ICP increases and hydrocephalus are uncommon.

g. Cerebellopontine angle tumors are situated in the angle formed by the petrous ridge, tentorium, cerebellum, and brain stem. The vast majority are nerve sheath tumors arising from the vestibular portion of the eighth cranial nerve. Symptoms begin with tinnitus on the involved side followed by nerve deafness. Involvement of the seventh cranial nerve produces facial palsy; involvement of the fifth cranial nerve may cause numbness or paresthesia in the face and loss of the corneal reflex. Involvement of the cerebellum causes ataxia, dysmetria, and nystagmus.

h. Midbrain. Usually involved secondarily by tumors arising from nearby structures. Tumors in the pineal region frequently press on the roof structures of the midbrain causing difficulty in upward gaze (Parinaud's syndrome) and impairment of the pupillary light reflex. Involvement of the red nucleus area produces ataxia, incoordination, and intention tremor.

i. Pituitary gland. Hyperfunction of portions of the gland (acromegaly, Cushing's disease, galactorrhea) or, more commonly, hypofunction leading to amenorrhea, loss of libido, and pubic and axillary hair, and so on. As sellar tumors enlarge, they encroach on the optic chiasm and produce a characteristic bitemporal heminaopsia. Hemorrhage into a pituitary tumor can cause sudden visual loss.

2. General or secondary effects. Increased ICP produced by any space-occupying intracranial mass leads to the classic triad of headache (commonly located in the vertex, worse in the morning after prolonged recumbency, and frequently relieved by standing up); nausea and vomiting; and papilledema. Increased ICP may also cause personality changes, convulsions, cranial nerve palsies, and even homonymous hemianopsia as the posterior cerebral artery passing over the edge of the tentorium is compressed by the tense brain.

3. Diagnosis. Focal symptoms and signs of a brain tumor depend on its location, whether it is situated on the surface or in the deeper tissues, cell type, rapidity of growth, and so on. It is imperative to determine if there is progression. Progression of symptoms justifies the suspicion of brain tumor and the studies outlined below should be obtained.

a. MRI is the preferred initial study and can demonstrate most tumors better than CT scans.

b. CT brain scan usually localizes the tumor accurately.

c. Arteriography is used to localize the tumor either by indicating a tumor "blush," or indirectly by distortion of arteries or veins from their normal position.

4. Treatment of brain tumors. In general, the treatment of brain tumors is surgical exploration and excision through a craniotomy. The tumor should be completely removed without producing a serious neurologic deficit if possible. If the tumor cannot be excised completely, radical subtotal removal should be done to decompress the surrounding brain. If the tumor blocks the flow of CSF, shunting is indicated. Postoperative radiation therapy has considerable value in some tumors but not in other. Chemotherapy of primary and metastatic brain tumors may also help.

B. INTRACRANIAL GLIOMAS. All tumors that arise from the interstitial cells of the CNS are included in this category.

1. Glioblastoma multiforme comprises about 25% of gliomas and is the most malignant primary tumor of the brain. It arises, in the white matter, grows rapidly, and has a strong tendency to cross to the opposite hemisphere. This tumor is highly cellular and pleomorphic, and has many mitoses. The most common sites of occurrence are the frontal, parietal, and temporal lobes, and the highest incidence is in the age group of 40-60 years. Glioblastoma multiforme cannot be completely removed and is resistant to radiation therapy. Most patients die within one 1 year after diagnosis.

2. Astrocytomas account for about 35% of gliomas. They grow relatively slowly and frequently blend diffusely into the surrounding brain. In adults, they arise most often in the frontal, parietal, and temporal lobes and are impossible to remove completely because they extend into deep structures. Astrocytomas are only partially radiosensitive, and survival is usually 3-6 years. Survival may be extended by reoperation. In children, they occur predominately in the cerebellar hemisphere and are often cystic; cystic or solid cerebellar astrocytomas can be completely excised in many cases and recurrence is uncommon.

3. Medulloblastomas (about 10% of gliomas) occur predominantly in children 4-8 years of age, usually boys (3:1). They arise from the lateral wall or roof of the fourth ventricle and frequently seed to other parts of the nervous system. Complete surgical removal is not possible. These tumors are radiosensitive and respond to chemotherapy. Five-year median survival is about 30% for poor-risk tumors and about 70% for more favorable tumors.

4. Ependymomas arising from the lateral ventricles or fourth ventricle may be totally removable. Often, however, they arise from the ventricular walls, rendering them difficult to remove totally. Ependymomas usually respond to radiation therapy.

5. Oligodendrogliomas (5% of gliomas) usually occur in the cerebral hemisphere in adults. Total removal is often impossible, and the cells are relatively radioresistant. Tumors with anaplastic features lead to median survival of about 4 years; other oligodendrogliomas have medial survival of about 10 years.

6. Pinealomas (2%-3% of gliomas) occur in young adults and block flow of CSF early. Some of them can be removed surgically. Alternate treatment is CSF shunting followed by radiation therapy. Prognosis for survival is 3-10 years in malignant tumors.

C. MENINGIOMAS are benign tumors that arise from cells of the pia, arachnoid, and dura. They occur predominantly in the 40-60 age group. Because meningiomas involve the cerebral cortex early in their growth, convulsive seizures often herald their presence. Characteristic locations, in descending order of frequency, are as follows:

1. Parasagittal. Anterior parasagittal meningiomas produce headache and personality changes. Midparasagittal meningiomas cause paresis of the contralateral foot, with or without cortical sensory change, incontinence of urine, and seizures beginning in the contralateral foot. Posterior parasagittal meningiomas produce headache and visual field defects.

2. Convexity of the cerebral hemisphere. In general, these tumors are situated anteriorly and produce mental changes and motor weakness. Tumors in the midparietal area cause motor and sensory loss, and tumors situated posteriorly lead to sensory and visual field losses.

3. Sphenoid ridge. Meningiomas along the inner third of the sphenoid ridge cause extraocular muscle palsies and visual loss with optic atrophy. Meningiomas along the middle third of the ridge usually attain a large size before significant symptoms are produced. Ultimately, encroachment on the temporal lobe causes psychomotor fits, and involvement of the frontal lobe produces mental changes. Meningioma along the outer third of the ridge often grows as a flat plate of tumor (en plaque); progressive exophthalmos from tumor growth into the orbit and a palpable mass in the temporal region are the consequences.

4. Olfactory groove. These usually become quite large before clinical manifestations appear (anosmia and personality changes).

5. Less common locations are suprasellar, in the posterior fossa, and in the region of the gasserian ganglion.

6. Treatment. Surgical removal is indicated in all cases, and complete removal is often possible. Even with subtotal removal, the prognosis is good and is improved with irradiation of the residual tumor.

D. TUMORS OF THE CRANIAL NERVES. The great majority of cranial nerve tumors arise from the sheath of the eighth nerve at the internal auditory meatus (so-called acoustic tumor or vestibular schwannoma). Most can be removed completely. Where total removal is not possible because the capsule is intimately adherent to the brain stem, the prognosis with subtotal removal may still be good. Some of these tumors grow very slowly, and reoperation can be done when symptoms recur.

E. TUMORS OF THE INTRACRANIAL BLOOD VESSELS

1. Hemangiomas are actually malformations with no neoplastic elements. They usually occur in the pons and are often clinically silent, although occasionally they may produce symptoms if the malformation ruptures or obstructs the flow of CSF.

2. Hemangioblastomas are true neoplasms formed by proliferation of angioblasts. They are usually found in the cerebellum of adults where they produce symptoms. If there is associated hemangioblastoma of the retina, the disorder is called **von Hippel-Lindau disease.** Hemangioblastomas in the cerebellum frequently form a large cyst filled with thick yellow fluid. The tumor lies within the wall of the cyst (mural nodule), and surgical removal of the mural nodule is curative. Solid tumors are difficult to excise completely, and the prognosis is less favorable.

F. CONGENITAL INTRACRANIAL TUMORS

1. Craniopharyngiomas are the most common congenital brain tumors (3%-4% of all brain tumors). They arise from epithelial cell rests in the region of the infundibular stalk and consist of squamous epithelium or epithelium of the type seen in developing tooth buds (so-called adamantinomas). The cysts may become quite large. Deposits of calcium above the sella turcica can often be seen by radiography. Symptoms are produced by compression of neighboring structures and consist of endocrine disorders, visual field defects, optic atrophy, and obstruction of CSF flow.

Treatment is surgical removal, although often total removal is impossible because the capsule is adherent to the hypothalamus or the carotid artery. Aspiration of the cyst and subtotal removal of the capsule carries a low operative mortality, and, when coupled with postoperative radiation therapy, often leads to long-term improvement.

2. Epidermoid cysts (pearly tumors, cholesteatomas) arise from embryonic epidermal cells. Symptoms are usually delayed until adulthood. Treatment is surgical removal. If the wall is adherent to vital structures, complete surgical removal is not possible, but long-term survivals have been reported even with incomplete removals.

3. Dermoids resemble epidermoids but contain dermal structures, such as sebaceous glands and hair follicles. Treatment is surgical.

4. Teratomas are derived from the three germinal layers and may attain huge size. Symptoms usually occur in childhood. The prognosis is good if the tumor is removed completely.

5. Chordomas. These slow-growing neoplasms arise from remnants of primitive notochord along the clivus beneath the pons, and they extend into the middle fossa and cerebellopontine angle. They produce multiple cranial nerve palsies combined with long tract signs from pressure on the pons. Marked erosion of the base of the skull is usually visible on basilar radiographs. Total removal is rarely possible, and the prognosis is poor.

6. Colloid cyst of the third ventricle. These cystic lesions in the anterior portion of the third ventricle cause symptoms by intermittent blockage of the CSF flow through the foramen of Monro. Because the cyst hangs from the roof of the ventricle by a stalk, changes in body position may produce, or relieve, sudden violent headache. The lesion should be removed; the prognosis is good.

G. PITUITARY TUMORS most often arise from the anterior lobe and are classified by their endocrine activity.

Endocrine-active tumors may secrete growth hormone (acromegaly), adrenocorticotropic hormone (Cushing's disease, Nelson's disease), prolactin (galactorrhea-amenorrhea), thyrotropic stimulating hormone (hyperthyroidism), or gonadotropic hormones, or they may be mixed secreting tumors. Their symptoms are related to the body's response to an excess of stimulating hormones; consequently, they become clinically manifest before reaching a large size. Endocrine-inactive tumors become clinically important when they become large enough to cause pressure on nerve or brain in the suprasellar region that leads to visual disturbance, extraocular palsies, and headache.

The endocrine-active tumors are often microadenomas and may or may not cause minor changes visible by radiography in the sella turcica. Larger tumors usually cause sellar enlargement and erosion. MRI scanning with the enhancing agent gadolinium can demonstrate pituitary adenomas as small as 3-5 mm and is the diagnostic procedure of choice.

Treatment of pituitary tumors is surgical removal, by the transsphenoidal route for tumors of small or moderate size and by the transfrontal route for tumors with extensive subfrontal or parasellar extension. Some prolactin-secreting tumors can be successfully treated temporarily with bromocriptine, although long-term success is uncertain. Radiation therapy should follow incomplete surgical resection of nonsecreting tumors.

H. INTRASPINAL NEOPLASMS occur at any level of the cord from the foramen magnum to the sacral canal; the greatest number are in the thoracic area. They may arise from the spinal cord, spinal nerves, bone, cartilage, fat, blood vessels, or fibrous tissue, or they may be metastatic. They are rare before age 10 years.

These tumors may be grouped as follows: (1) those arising within the spinal canal, extending extraspinally through a vertebral foramen (dumbbell tumors); (2) those arising within the spinal canal but not invading the dura or cord (intraspinal extradural tumors); (3) those arising within the dura but not invading the spinal cord (intradural extramedullary tumors); and (4) those arising entirely within the substance of the cord (intramedullary tumors).

Most intraspinal tumors are benign, but early diagnosis and treatment are essential to avoid irreversible spinal cord damage.

1. Diagnosis
a. Symptoms and signs. A history of pain in the back with radiation into dermatomal patterns, accompanied by sensory and/or motor root signs, and the appearance of long tract deficits suggest a spinal cord tumor. It is imperative to establish (1) whether symptoms began abruptly and have not changed significantly since onset, in which case an intraspinal tumor is unlikely; (2) whether symptoms began abruptly but remitted and recurred, as is typical of multiple sclerosis; or (3) whether the onset was vague, but progression since the onset has been steady as one would expect with spinal cord tumor.

One of the earlier symptoms of spinal cord tumor is **radicular pain**—pain produced by pressure or traction on the nerve roots. The pain is often experienced in a peripheral area of the dermatome supplied by the root or roots involved; e.g., tumors of the cervical region may cause pain in the shoulder, arm, or hand. Radicular pain has the following distinct characteristics: often restricted to the involved dermatomes; severe, sharp, stabbing, and superimposed on a background of continuous dull, aching pain; made worse by straining; worse at night after prolonged recumbency and temporarily relieved by physical activity. **Paresthesia** and/or **dysesthesia**, which are variously described as numbness, coldness, and tingling, are also in a radicular pattern.

Sensory loss, if it appears, is of a spinal cord type; i.e., a distinct level of sensory loss, generally with an earlier loss of pain sensation. **Motor involvement** may be of the upper motor neuron type (i.e., spasticity, hyperreflexia, and extensor plantar response), or of the lower motor neuron type if the tumor involves the cauda equina.

Hesitancy in urination is an early sign of pressure on the spinal cord. Incontinence and/or retention of urine are late signs.

b. Radiographs of the spine may show erosion, calcium deposition in the tumor, increase in the interpedicular distances, enlargement of the intervertebral foramina, or collapse of vertebrae. The diagnosis of tumor is confirmed by MRI scanning.

2. Treatment and prognosis. When a symptoms and signs progress rapidly, surgical treatment is urgent. Most benign tumors can be removed completely. The prognosis for return of function depends upon the location of the tumor, whether it can be removed completely or not, and the severity and duration of neurologic deficit before excision. Prognosis for intramedullary tumors is more guarded, because the hazard of increasing the neurologic deficit may preclude complete removal. Postoperative radiation therapy may be beneficial in diminishing the mass effect and preventing further neurologic losses.

I. METASTATIC INTRASPINAL TUMORS. The spinal cord is often compressed by metastases to the bones of the spinal column or to the epidural space. If the primary site of malignancy is known, spinal irradiation and high-dose steroid therapy (dexamethasone 25 mg every 6 hours for 1 week) should be given. Surgical decompression by laminectomy or vertebrectomy is appropriate if the patient is medically stable and when neurologic deterioration is very rapid, when a primary cancer site is unknown, or when the primary tumor is known to be unresponsive to radiation therapy.

J. PERIPHERAL NERVE TUMORS

1. Neurilemmomas are the most common tumors of the peripheral nerves; they arise in the supporting tissues, and are usually solitary, well encapsulated, of variable size, and benign. The diagnosis is suggested by a mass in the course of a peripheral nerve. Symptoms include paresthesia or hypesthesia; with tumors of mixed or pure sensory nerves, percussion over the tumor elicits tingling distally (Tinel's sign). Malignant change (sarcoma) occurs rarely. Treatment is by surgical removal, but in some cases excision is difficult and results in permanent neurologic deficit.

2. Neurofibromas are composed of all the elements of peripheral nerves (axis cylinders, myelin sheaths, and connective tissue). They may appear as solitary lesions, but most commonly they are multiple, occurring as part of von Recklinghausen's neurofibromatosis (cafe-au-lait spots, multiple neurofibromas, and multiple brain tumors of all types). Individual tumors causing disabling symptoms can be excised.

Sarcomatous changes are more frequent in neurofibromas than in neurilemmomas. Neurofibrosarcoma may not be clinically distinguished form its benign counterpart, except for the rapidity of its growth. Surrounding structures are infiltrated, and distant metatases may occur.

V. CEREBROVASCULAR DISEASE

A. CEREBRAL ISCHEMIA. Any area of the brain can become ischemic from arterial occlusion (partial or complete) or embolization. Symptoms may be slow and progressive, or sudden and catastrophic. Extracranial cerebrovascular disease is discussed in Chapter 11; intracranial atheromatous plaques most commonly form at the bifurcation of the internal carotid artery into the middle and anterior cerebral arteries.

1. Symptoms and signs of cerebral ischemia depend upon the vessel that is affected:

a. Internal carotid artery. Occlusion usually produces contralateral weakness of the arm and leg, subjective numbness, blindness, and aphasia (if the dominant hemisphere is involved).

b. Middle cerebral artery. Usually the same as internal carotid occlusion, except that blindness does not occur, and the arm is usually weaker than the leg.

c. Anterior cerebral artery. Weakness and/or subjective numbness of the contralateral leg and occasionally the arm.

d. Posterior cerebral artery. Hemianopsia, scintillating scotomas, and (if lesions are bilateral) temporary or permanent cortical blindness.

e. Basilar artery. Usually bilateral symptoms such as quadriparesis, bilateral paresthesia, ataxia, dysarthria, diplopia, dysphagia, blindness, and frequently unconsciousness.

2. Treatment of extracranial disease is discussed in Chapter 11. Revascularization of the brain after intracranial artery occlusion is now possible in selected cases by extracranial-intracranial arterial microanastomosis.

B. INTRACRANIAL ANEURYSM.

Most intracranial aneurysms are congenital lesions located on the anterior portion of the circle of Willis at points of bifurcation of major arteries. Approximately 10%-15% arise in branches of the basilar artery, including the posterior cerebral arteries. About 20% of patients have multiple aneurysms.

1. Diagnosis

a. Intracranial aneurysms produce symptoms by one or more mechanisms; subarachnoid hemorrhage, or less often, intracerebral or subdural hemorrhage; pressure on adjacent structures leading to cranial nerve palsies (third, fifth, second, fourth, and sixth); ischemia from occulusion of neighboring or parent arteries; distention or pressure on pain-sensitive structures causing headache, usually orbital or supraorbital.

b. Subarachnoid hemorrhage typically is a sudden, catastrophic event in a previously healthy person 20-40 years of age. Severe meningeal irritation (stiff neck, photophobia, headache), nausea, and vomiting may stabilize or progress to coma and death within minutes to days.

c. Intracerebral hemorrhage may be associated with profound neurologic loss (hemiplegia, aphasia), coma, and death.

d. The diagnosis of subarachnoid hemorrhage is established by lumbar puncture or CT scan. CSF pressure is usually increased, the fluid is homogeneously bloody, and the supernatant is xanthochromic. CT scans may show diffuse blood in subarachnoid spaces with larger amounts of blood near the ruptured aneurysm.

e. Arteriograms should be obtained as soon as the patient's condition permits.

2. Treatment

a. General. Bed rest, maintenance of fluid and electrolyte balance, and mild analgesics to control headache and restlessness. Anticonvulsants (phenytoin, 100 mg 3 times a day) and nimodipine (60 mg every 4 hours for 14 days) should be given.

b. Surgical. If operation is indicated, it should be done as soon as the patient's condition permits. **Direct intracra-**

nial approach: The objective is to isolate the aneurysm from the circulation without producing a neurologic deficit. Methods include clipping the neck of the aneurysm, clipping the parent vessel proximally and distally, or reinforcing the aneurysm wall with various materials. **Indirect surgical approach:** Ligation of the carotid artery in the neck lowers the pressure in the aneurysm and may reduce the danger of subsequent hemorrhage. In general, this method of treatment is applicable only to aneurysms arising from the internal carotid artery proximal to the circle of Willis and is not used often. **Interventional radiologic treatment** can occlude some aneurysms by placement of balloons or other hemostatic material within the aneurysm.

3. Prognosis. The mortality rate is 35% with the first episode of subarachnoid hemorrhage from ruptured intracranial aneurysm. The danger of a second hemorrhage is greatest within the first 2 weeks after the initial episode.

C. CEREBRAL ARTERIOVENOUS MALFORMATION.

These are congenital lesions that may cause subarachnoid or intracerebral hemorrhage, although hemorrhage is far less common with arteriovenous malformation than with aneurysm. Other manifestations include recurrent convulsive seizures, loss of function of adjacent brain (hemiparesis, aphasia), or progressive mental deterioration. Neurologic deficits may be caused by hemorrhage with subsequent gliosis and cyst formation, or they may result from shunting of blood directly into the venous system leading to local tissue hypoxia and eventual gliosis.

The diagnosis is suggested by the history, the presence of a bruit over the lesion, and sometimes intracranial calcification on radiographs. Cerebral angiography is diagnostic, and CT or MRI scanning with and without IV contrast material often demonstrates the lesion.

Treatment is by obliteration of the malformation either by surgery or by focused irradiation. The prognosis depends upon the size and location of the lesion.

D. INTRACEREBRAL HEMORRHAGE is the cause of stroke

in many hypertensive patients. Hematomas develop most often in the basal ganglia, subcortical white matter, cerebellum, and brain stem. Catastrophic in onset, the lesion depresses consciousness severely and progressively. Because an intracranial mass and brain deformity result from intracerebral hemorrhage, initial diagnostic steps include CT scanning and MRI. Lumbar puncture is usually contraindicated.

Treatment consists of control of hypertension, life support, and removal of the mass by operation if the lesion is positioned in such a place that its removal will restore the patient to useful life. Deep hemorrhages are usually managed without operation. Prognosis depends upon site and severity of hemorrhage.

VI. INTERVERTEBRAL DISK DISEASE

A. PROTRUSION OF LUMBAR INTERVERTEBRAL DISKS. Ninety percent of protrusions occur at the L4-5 and L5-S1 interspaces.

1. Diagnosis

a. Symptoms usually include back pain, with or without leg pain. The pain characteristically spreads to the gluteal region and then down the posterior or posterolateral aspect of the thigh and calf; it is aggravated by coughing, sneezing, or straining and may be relieved by bed rest. Pain is often accompanied by numbness in parts of the foot or lower leg.

b. Signs include spasm of paravertebral muscles; flattening of the lumbar spine with loss of normal lordosis; limitation of back motion, particularly forward flexions; and tenderness to deep pressure over the back or sacroiliac region.

c. Neurologic findings. Straight leg-raising produces leg pain and frequently back pain which is accentuated by dorsiflexion of the foot (further stretching of the sciatic nerve and roots). The ankle reflex is diminished or absent (more common with protrusion at the L5-S1 interspace impinging on the first sacral nerve root). The knee reflex may be diminished with herniations at the L3-4 interspace. Motor evaluation shows weakness of dorsiflexion and/or plantar flexion; weak inversion or eversion of the foot may be found also with herniations at the lower two lumbar interspaces. Weakness of the quadriceps may be present with L3-4 lesions. Sensory status varies from no loss to complete analgesia in the distribution of the root involved.

d. Radiographs. Plain films may be normal or may show narrowing of the involved interspace, arthritic "lipping" of the adjacent vertebral bodies, and/or arthritic changes around the zygoapophysial joints.

e. Special examinations. MRI is noninvasive and usually demonstrates compression of the thecal sac or nerve roots. CT scanning gives better detail of bone abnormalities and often shows disk herniations. Intrathecal instillation of radiopaque contrast is used occasionally in conjunction with CT or plain radiography when noninvasive technics are not diagnostic. Electromyography can be used to identify the involved nerve root by demonstrating fibrillation potentials in the muscles supplied by the root.

2. Differential diagnosis. Lumbar disk disease must be differentiated from tumors, congenital bony abnormalities (spondylolisthesis, spina bifida), and inflammatory disease (abscess, osteomyelitis, rheumatoid disease).

3. Treatment

a. Supportive treatment includes analgesics, NSAIDs, strict bed rest with boards between springs and mattress to prevent sagging, local heat, and muscle "relaxants" (Valium 10 mg three times per day). The patient is often more comfortable in the modified Fowler's or contour position. One or two weeks of bed rest may be necessary before improvement is noted.

After the acute pain subsides, a progressive physical therapy program should be instituted to strengthen the back, abdominal, and leg muscles and to instruct the patient in the proper way to use the back muscles to prevent straining. Support of the back with a corset or brace may be useful when pain is severe.

b. Surgical. Operation is indicated when pain is intractable or when neurologic signs appear. Excision of a diseased disk usually helps. Education of the patient and a well-directed exercise program are essentials of management, whether medical or surgical.

B. PROTRUSION OF CERVICAL INTERVERTEBRAL DISKS

1. Diagnosis

a. Symptoms. Patients with lateral cervical protrusions have frequent bouts of pain involving the neck, shoulder, and scapular region, accompanied by lancinating pain into the arm or hand, and accentuated by straining. Paresthesias into the fingers are common; into the first and second digits if C-6 is involved, the third digit if C-7, and fourth and fifth digits if C-8 is involved.

b. Signs include restricted neck motion, absence of cervical lordosis, spasm of the neck muscles, hypesthesia in a dermatomal pattern in the arm and hand, and weakness in the muscles supplied by the involved root. There is diminished biceps reflex if C-6 is involved and diminished triceps reflex if C-7 is.

  c. Radiographs may be normal if the protrusion is recent, or they may show a narrowed interspace and/or hypertrophic lipping with narrowing of the root foramina. Myelography reveals a defect of the root sleeve. MRI is very sensitive in showing spinal cord compression. CT scans effectively show osteophytes compromising the spinal canal or neural foramina.

  d. With midline protrusions, there may be no history of root pain; a common presenting complaint is spastic paraparesis with or without urinary hesitancy or incontinence. Signs of pyramidal tract involvement are apparent in the lower extremities. Radiographs reveal interspace narrowing, with or without osteophytic spurring at the posterior edge of the vertebrae. Myelography shows an anterior deformity.

  2. Treatment involves use of analgesics, NSAIDs, and home halter traction (5-10 lb) initially; as symptoms subside, a neck brace may be helpful.

  If symptoms fail to improve and/or neurologic deficits are present, operation to remove the offending disk may be necessary. Myelography or MRI should precede operation in order to localize the lesion precisely. In midline or lateral protrusions, the operation of choice is anterior diskectomy with or without intervertebral fusion. A foraminotomy by a posterior approach is an effective alternative for laterally placed disk fragments. Surgery usually prevents progression of neurologic loss and may partially restore lost function.

VII. INFECTIONS OF SCALP, BONE, AND BRAIN

A. PYOGENIC SCALP INFECTIONS should be treated vigorously, as there are abundant communications from the venous channels of the scalp to the diploic spaces of the calvaria and from these spaces to the underlying dura. Treatment of scalp infections includes appropriate antibiotics, drainage of abscesses, and debridement of necrotic tissue.

B. OSTEOMYELITIS OF THE SKULL occurs most commonly after implantation of bacteria into bone by trauma or by extension of infection in contiguous structures such as scalp or sinuses. Appearance of signs and symptoms of osteomyelitis may be delayed for weeks to months after the initial trauma or neighboring infection. Typical manifestations are headache, local evidence of inflammation (with or without a draining sinus), and tenderness. Systemic effects such as fever, leukocytosis, and cervical or suboccipital lymphadenopathy may not be present. Radiographs may be negative early in the course, but later they reveal a characteristic mottled appearance of the bone.

Vigorous antibiotic therapy should be based on results of cultures and sensitivity tests. If inflammation or drainage persists despite antibiotics and initial debridement, infected bone should be excised. Cranioplasty to repair the defect should be deferred until at least 6-12 months after all evidence of infection has disappeared.

C. EPIDURAL ABSCESS usually develops by direct extension from an adjacent infection, although hematogenous spread of bacteria can give rise to this lesion also. The classic findings in cranial epidural abscess are those of a rapidly enlarging space-occupying lesion in association with the symptoms and signs of systemic infection. Acute or chronic spinal epidural abscesses cause cord compression. Pain is prominent, and bony tenderness is always present.

Epidural abscesses require immediate surgical drainage and antibiotics if neurologic deficits are present. Small epidural abscesses can sometimes be treated with antibiotics alone if the patient is neurologically intact and the organism has been identified. MRI is the most accurate way to follow lesion progression or resolution.

D. SUBDURAL ABSCESS is usually the result of direct extension from an overlying area, but they may occur from rupture of an intracranial abscess into the subdural space. Because there are no limiting structures in the subdural space, these abscesses extend over the entire hemisphere, under the brain, and into the interhemispheral fissure.

The abscess is a rapidly enlarging space-occupying lesion and causes lethargy, obtundation, paresis, coma, and papilledema. The diagnosis is based upon a history of primary infection, MRI, and the findings of subdural pus on exploration. Treatment is essentially the same as for epidural abscess.

E. INTRACEREBRAL ABSCESS. A variety of bacteria and parasites cause intracerebral abscesses. In the past, most abscesses were associated with sinusitis or mastoiditis, but now few arise from these sources. Pulmonary infection accounts for 30%, and the remainder result from head injury or bacteremia due to congenital heart disease, drug addiction, or other systemic infection. Abscesses are multifocal in 10%-15% of cases resulting from hematogenous seeding. About 10% of patients with AIDS have intracerebral infection, usually from toxoplasma parasites, but occasionally viruses. In AIDS, intracerebral lymphomas can produce focal mass lesions.

1. Diagnosis. A history of infection (ear, sinuses, or elsewhere) is important. Convulsions, headache, and paresis with progressive lethargy are the symptoms and signs. In the acute phase, the patient may have fever, leukocytosis, and an elevated CSF cell count. In the chronic phase, as the infection is walled off by formation of a capsule, toxic symptoms are replaced by signs of a mass. Lumbar puncture may be dangerous and should be preceded by other studies if focal neurologic deficits are present.

MRI or CT scans often show a characteristic lucent area surrounded by a dense capsule which enhances with iodinated contrast medium and surrounding edema.

2. Treatment. In the acute phase, broad-spectrum antibiotics must be given until the causative organism has been identified; then specific antibiotics are given. If the patient is lethargic or has focal neurologic findings, dexamethasone (6 mg every 6 hours) usually controls the cerebral edema surrounding the abscess.

Surgical treatment consists of aspiration or total excision of the abscess. The mortality rate varies from 15%-50%; the worst results occur in patients who are comatose before operation.

F. AIDS. About 10% of patients with AIDS present with CNS symptoms, and more than 30% have intracranial lesions at the time of death. Cerebral pathology can be varied and multiple, including HIV infection of the brain, progressive multifocal leukoencephalopathy, and coccidioidomycosis. The most common brain mass lesions are toxoplasma abscesses, which almost always are multiple at the time of diagnosis. Patients can present with seizures or focal deficits. When more than one lesion is demonstrated on MRI, antitoxoplasmosis treatment with sulfadiazine and pyrimethamine is started. The patient is followed clinically and with CT or MRI. If either the clinical or radiologic picture worsens or fails to improve within 2 weeks, stereotaxic biopsy of the lesion should be done to exclude AIDS-related cerebral lymphoma. If lymphoma is diagnosed, urgent radiation therapy should be initiated. Severe dementia is usually due to HIV encephalopathy, for which no therapy currently is available.

VIII. PAIN

The neurosurgeon is frequently called upon to carry out procedures for relief of chronic pain of known or unknown origin. Every effort must be made to determine the cause of the pain, and every patient who complains of chronic pain that has no apparent cause or is atypical must be thoroughly evaluated psychiatrically before operation is considered. The most common pain syndromes requiring surgical intervention are trigeminal neuralgia, glossopharyngeal neuralgia, postherpetic neuralgia, and pain produced by advanced malignancies.

A. TRIGEMINAL NEURALGIA

1. Diagnosis. Trigeminal neuralgia is a disorder characterized by severe lancinating pain occurring without warning in the distribution of any of the major branches of the trigeminal nerve. Each pain is a brief stabbing sensation with frequent paroxysms. There may be periods of remission lasting for many months. Many patients describe a "trigger area" somewhere about the face, mouth, or tongue, where stimulation produces the stabbing pain, and the patient may refuse to eat, shave, or talk, to avoid stimulating the trigger area. There is no pain between attacks and no loss of sensation in the distribution of the trigeminal nerve. If there is loss of sensation, a tumor in or near the gasserian ganglion should be suspected.

2. Treatment. Carbamazepine (Tegretol) relieves the pain in approximately 80% of patients with trigeminal neuralgia. In a few cases, phenytoin (Dilantin) 300 mg daily may be effective.

If the pain persists despite adequate medical therapy or if medications are not tolerated, a variety of **surgical procedures** are available.

a. Arteries that cause trigeminal neuralgia by compressing the nerve can be freed surgically and the disorder cured.

b. Passage of a radiofrequency current through a needle placed in the trigeminal ganglion can be used to destroy portions of the ganglion in a graded fashion. This allows preservation of some facial sensation, particularly the first branch of the trigeminal nerve, which is necessary for corneal protection.

c. The peripheral branch of the trigeminal nerve innervating the trigger area can be surgically excised.

d. Craniotomy, either via the temporal fossa (to section or decompress the ganglion) or through the posterior fossa (to section portions of the nerve between the brain stem and the gasserian ganglion) may be employed.

B. GLOSSOPHARYNGEAL NEURALGIA.

The pain is similar to that of trigeminal neuralgia, but it is located in the distribution of the ninth cranial nerve, i.e., in the tonsillar fossa and deep in the neck at the angle of the jaw on the affected side. The diagnosis is confirmed by application of topical anesthesia to the tonsillar fossa on the affected side; in true glossopharyngeal neuralgia, pain is relieved immediately but returns after the local anesthetic has worn off. Intracranial section of the ninth cranial nerve and the upper two filaments of the tenth through a posterior fossa approach gives permanent relief; in some patients, microvascular decompression of the glossopharyngeal nerve can be curative.

C. POSTHERPETIC NEURALGIA.

In a few cases of herpes zoster, severe burning pain persists in the involved area after the infection has run its course. Chronic inflammatory changes are present in the posterior root ganglion and in ascending pathways of the spinal cord and brain stem carrying pain impulses. A variety of medications has been used. Tricyclic antidepressant medications are very effective in some patients. If these fail, high doses of narcotic analgesics can provide prolonged benefit in some patients. Transcutaneous stimulators have limited success. Laminectomy and removal of the spinal root ganglion may be effective. Radiofrequency electrocoagulation of the dorsal root entry zone of the spinal cord has afforded relief of this severe pain.

D. PAIN PRODUCED BY ADVANCED MALIGNANCIES.

Severe pain becomes a problem as inoperable malignancies invade sensitive structures. The pain is deep, boring, and steady, with sharp stabbing pains at times superimposed. Operations for relief of pain in cancer patients should not be considered a last resort. Large doses of narcotics often produce mental dullness and disinterest in life. As a general rule, if the patient's life expectancy is longer than 3-6 months, a pain-relieving surgical procedure should be carried out as soon as the pain becomes significant.

Relief can be given without loss of vital neurologic function by cutting the fibers responsible for pain transmission at an appropriate level in the peripheral or central nervous system. The operation most frequently used is a cordotomy (spinothalamic tractotomy). The spinothalamic tract in the anterior quadrant of the spinal cord on the side opposite the pain is sectioned at the high thoracic or high cervical level, causing loss of pain and thermal sensation on the contralateral side below the level of the section. For pelvic pain involving the midline or for bilateral pain, bilateral cordotomy is indicated. Thoracic cordotomy can be performed by laminectomy and open section, or cordotomy can be done in the awake patient by passage of radiofrequency current through a small needle placed percutaneously into the spinothalamic tract at the C1-2 level.

Pain involving the face, jaw, neck, or brachial plexus can be relieved by sectioning the pain fibers in the medulla at the level of the obex. An alternative procedure is section of the trigeminal, glossopharyngeal, and upper filaments of the vagus nerves intracranially and the upper 3 or 4 posterior cervical roots on the side of the pain.

E. OTHER MODALITIES IN PAIN RELIEF. **Transcutaneous electrical stimulation** of painful areas is safe and may be beneficial. Instillation of small doses of morphine into the lumbar subarachnoid space via subcutaneous reservoirs and tubing into the lumbar sac can dramatically relieve pelvic pain without altering other sensation. Electrodes placed into thalamic or periaqueductal midbrain nuclei can provide pathways for electrical stimulation of these structures, providing marked relief of pain in selected patients.

18

Orthopedics*

Harry E. Jergesen

I. INJURIES TO THE SPINE

A. GENERAL PRINCIPLES. Depending on the severity and the mechanism of the trauma and the anatomic location of the lesion, these injuries may vary from minor soft tissue strain or contusion to extensive fracture-dislocation with severe neurologic impairment.

Fractures may involve the body, pedicle, lamina, transverse process, or combinations of the above. Pathologic fracture may occur with minimal trauma. Dislocations are described by direction and by magnitude (complete or incomplete) of displacement and by the degree of complexity (unilateral or bilateral). Pathologic fracture may occur without evident episodic trauma.

1. Types of injury
a. Direct
(1) *Closed:* Caused by trauma applied through overlying soft tissues without open wounds communicating with the axial skeleton; frequently involves fracture of spinous or transverse processes and rarely the lamina.
(2) *Open:* Generally due to penetrating injuries such as those inflicted by firearms or knives.

b. Indirect.
When these injuries are extensive, they are usually the result of complex combinations of forces (e.g., compression, flexion, extension, or rotation) rather than a single force.

2. Neurologic injury.
Most skeletal injuries of the spine do not involve the cord or nerves. Damage to the spinal cord may complicate any displacement that even transiently reduces the diameter of the canal. Extensive neurologic deficit may occur without evident osteoarticular disruption and, conversely, marked skeletal derangement may not be associated with neurologic loss.

---

*This revised chapter was originally authored by Floyd H. Jergesen, M.D.

Neurologic injury may be intensified by manipulation during emergency care. When the patient is unable to communicate or is likely to have sustained injury to either the cervical or thoracolumbar regions, the head and trunk should be immobilized until the precise involvement can be critically assessed. Multiple levels of the spine may be injured concomitantly.

3. Associated injury to the appendicular skeleton or to the other organ systems of the conscious patient may mask symptoms that might focus attention on spinal injuries.

4. Diagnosis. Unconsciousness or transitory amnesia may obscure the mechanism and extent of initial injury. Determination of the earliest time of onset of any motor or sensory compromise gives insight of prognostic value.

a. Symptoms and signs. The location and extent of superficial soft tissue lesions should be noted because they may indicate the direction and magnitude of force that was applied indirectly to the spine. Palpation of the entire spinal region without manipulation of the patient may reveal sites of deep tenderness. Altered alignment or abnormal prominence of the spinous processes may suggest the presence of occult lesions.

Careful neurologic assessment is an integral part of the general physical examination. When the anatomic site of skeletal disruption, as demonstrated by radiography, is compared with the most proximal level of total neurologic deficit as indicated by clinical examination, that portion due solely to cord damage may be separated from that caused by root injury. Root lesions are characterized by segmental sensory and motor deficits in peripheral nerve distributions.

During the first 24 hours after injury, a partial spinal cord lesion is manifest minimally by sacral sparing—residual perianal sensation and some voluntary motor activity of the toe flexors. Residual reflex activity during this initial period merely indicates that cord function distal to the interruption is not suppressed by spinal shock which persists, as a rule, no longer than 24 hours. Failure to recover any sensory or active motor function distal to the level of the cord lesion during this period suggests complete and permanent spinal cord damage. Return of the bulbocavernosus reflex indicates recovery from spinal shock and precedes the return of deep tendon reflexes.

b. Radiographs. When the patient is unconscious, a preliminary radiograph or fluoroscopic survey of the spine and appendicular skeleton may aid in establishing a more precise initial diagnosis. After a tentative diagnosis has been made and protective measures have been taken against unintentional injury, more extensive investigation by routine radiography can be undertaken. Preexisting skeletal displacement may not be apparent because of spontaneous reduction.

CT may demonstrate occult bone lesions, especially in the region of the spinal canal.

c. Special tests. (1) Determination of spinal fluid dynamics helps differentiate partial from complete blockage of the canal. (2) Myelography localizes precisely the level of spinal canal compromise and its configuration. (3) MRI may define the extent and location of soft tissue injury and neural compromise.

5. Treatment. The prime objectives of early treatment are to protect the spinal cord and nerves from further damage and to minimize discomfort during transportation of the patient to a hospital. This can be accomplished most simply by removal of the injured on a flat surface in the supine position with the neck immobilized in neutral alignment. As soon as possible stabilization of cervical spine injuries, especially in the presence of neurologic loss, can be enhanced by cranial traction directed axially to the spine with the head in anatomic position.

B. SPRAIN OF THE CERVICAL SPINE. The injuries considered here involve supporting muscles, tendons, and ligaments. Motor vehicle accidents are a common cause, while a smaller number are due to sports injuries. "Whiplash" is a nonspecific term employed by the layman to refer to the varied pattern of symptoms that follow automobile accidents.

1. Diagnosis is established by differentiation from more serious osseoligamentous injury and from traumatic lesions of the brain, spinal cord, and nerve roots.

a. Symptoms and signs. The onset of symptoms may be immediate or delayed. In the absence of other more serious injury, delay of onset is often an indication of less severe neck injury. The principal symptom is pain. It is commonly accentuated by neck movements and relieved somewhat by rest. Physical findings include symmetric restriction of active neck movements and diffuse, poorly localized paracervical muscle tenderness. Muscle spasm may be present and is associated with deep, diffuse tenderness.

b. Radiographic examination of the cervical spine must be thorough. In addition to the standard projections, which include the lateral projections in flexion and extension,

CT and MRI may help to differentiate sprain from fracture or dislocation.

2. Differential diagnosis. Radiation of pain or altered sensation in a dermatomal pattern associated with motor dysfunction in the corresponding myotome should immediately suggest the possibility of a focal lesion of a spinal nerve root. Persistent and severe headache requires search for intracranial sources. Difficulty swallowing associated with pharyngeal edema points to a more serious condition than sprain. If blurring of vision and diplopia do not subside promptly they require ophthalmologic investigation. Complaints of dizziness or tinnitus that are not transient suggest eighth cranial nerve dysfunction. Both hemorrhage in the labyrinth and transient ischemia due to vertebral artery compression have been suggested as causes of posttraumatic vertigo.

3. Treatment of cervical sprain is essentially symptomatic. Pain is likely to be intensified by neck movement. Restriction of movement by any method such as external cervical support by a soft collar or brace, or by recumbency in bed may provide comfort. Light cervical traction (2-3 kg) by head halter may give additional relief. Nonsteroidal antinflammatory drugs, analgesics, and sedatives (for apprehensive patients) relieve mild pain. Local application of heat or cold, depending on the patient's preference, may offer additional comfort.

C. FRACTURES, DISLOCATIONS, AND FRACTURE-DISLOCATIONS OF THE CERVICAL SPINE account for about 15% of all derangements of the spine caused by severe trauma.

Neurologic findings peculiar to injuries of the cervical portion of the spinal cord bear emphasis. The body of the third cervical vertebra marks the approximate level of the fourth cervical segment. A **complete** lesion at this site or more proximally causes death by respiratory paralysis. The most common **partial** lesion involves the central region of the cord, which causes flaccid paralysis of the upper extremities and spasticity distally. A lesion of the anterior cord results in partial paralysis and anesthesia. Loss of deep pain and proprioception indicates a lesion posteriorly. Involvement of a lateral half of the cord results in paralysis of the same side of the body with hypalgesia and absence of temperature perception of the opposite side (Brown-Sequard syndrome).

1. Upper cervical spine
a. Fracture of the atlas (Jefferson's fracture). An axial blow to the top of the head may drive the condyles of the

occiput into the lateral masses of the first cervical vertebra, causing fracture of the arches and displacement of the masses. Routine radiographs may demonstrate displacement of the lateral masses while occult fracture may be revealed only by CT. When the spinal cord has not been injured and the fragments are not markedly displaced, immobilization in a halobrace for 12-16 weeks may be the only treatment that is required. Otherwise, skull traction is generally advisable during initial treatment in recumbency followed by brace immobilization. Persistent unstable fractures need posterior occipito-axial fusion.

 b. Fracture of the axis. The most common fracture of the proximal cervical spine involves the odontoid (which should be differentiated from os odontoideum). Subluxation or dislocation of the atlantoaxial joint may be present. Displacement of the odontoid fragment with the atlas partially protects the cord from injury. When necessary, reduction should be obtained by skull traction and maintained by a halo brace until healing is complete, usually by 12 weeks.

 Fracture of the body of the axis may be manifest as a vertical or oblique cleft that extends into the lateral mass or the lamina. When neurologic injury is not present, a halo brace is adequate because of inherent stability.

 An avulsion fracture of the anteroinferior margin of the body suggests injury due to hyperextension and implies an associated lesion of the disk. It may accompany fracture-dislocation of the second and the third cervical segments.

 c. Occipitoatlantal dislocation. This extremely rare lesion is generally fatal because of spinal cord injury. Because extensive ligamentous disruption causes gross instability, treatment by traction should be avoided.

 d. Atlantoaxial dislocation. Traumatic anterior dislocation of the atlas without fracture of the odontoid is very rare and, because of spinal cord injury, is likely to be fatal. The transverse ligament must rupture to permit dislocation.

 Posterior dislocation of the atlas without fracture of the odontoid is rare. It is caused by displacement of the arch upward over the tip of the odontoid.

 e. Atlantoaxial dislocation in children. Spontaneous forward dislocation of the atlas on the axis may occur in children as a complication of upper respiratory tract infection. Initial treatment is by head halter until painful restriction of active motion is relieved. Cervical support by brace or collar should continue until recovered stability can be demonstrated by radiography.

f. Fracture-dislocation of the axis ("hangman's fracture"). Bilateral fracture through the pedicles with forward displacement of the body of the axis on that of C-3 (traumatic spondylolisthesis) may occur as the result of motor vehicle accidents or legal hanging. Displacement of the segments may be corrected by carefully controlled cranial traction until stabilization occurs. External immobilization by a halo brace should be continued until bony healing occurs—generally after a period of 12-16 weeks.

2. Lower cervical spine

a. Compression fracture of the vertebral body. Isolated compression fractures are less common than in the thoracic spine and are more likely to occur in the lower cervical segments. Injury to the spinal cord or nerve roots is uncommon. Because the posterior ligaments are not disrupted and the fragments are impacted, the lesion is mechanically stable and uncomplicated healing is to be expected. Careful radiographic evaluation with supervised lateral flexion-extension views are necessary to differentiate this lesion from fracture-dislocation.

b. Comminuted fracture of the vertebral body. Comminution results from driving the respective disks of the segments above and below into the affected vertebral body (burst fracture, tear-drop fracture). Posterior ligaments are not disrupted. Bone fragments are not impacted and are likely to be displaced. Neurologic damage frequently results from compression of the cord by posteriorly displaced bone fragments and injury to roots by fragments displaced laterally.

When damage to the spinal cord is not present, sustained cranial traction in the anatomic position is necessary until reliable stabilization is provided by initial healing—usually 2-3 months. When cord damage is evident, early laminectomy is liable to increase instability by disrupting undamaged posterior ligaments. Concomitant posterior fusion is unlikely to provide adequate stability for early mobilization of the patient. Compression of the cord unrelieved by traction may be treated more effectively by combined anterior debridement of offending fragments followed by fusion. Any persisting instability may be treated subsequently by posterior fusion without laminectomy.

c. Fracture of spinous process. Fractures of spinous processes occur more frequently in lower than upper cervical spine and may be isolated or may accompany more serious lesions. Fracture is usually caused by indirect violence, such as avulsion by forced flexion or by impingement on adjacent spines during forced extension. The lesion generally can be identified in the lateral radiographic film, but in the cervicothoracic region oblique views can be helpful. Treatment is symptomatic. Fatigue fracture of a spinous process occurs in the distal cervical or proximal thoracic region ("clay shoveler's disease").

d. Forward bilateral dislocation. Complete bilateral forward dislocation without fracture is more apt to occur in the lower than in the upper cervical spine. Both inferior articular processes of the segment above are displaced anterior to the superior ones of the segment below. This implies disruption of the intervertebral disks and tearing of the apophyseal joint capsules and the longitudinal and posterior ligaments. Damage to the spinal cord and nerves is likely to be present. Locked facets may be demonstrated by conventional radiographs or CT.

When neurologic damage is evident (especially an incomplete spinal cord lesion), prompt reduction is necessary to prevent further injury from pressure. Although locked facets make reduction difficult by skull traction alone, it should be tried with the neck slightly flexed and the patient awake. The course of further treatment is variable because of delayed or incomplete ligamentous healing which may permit redislocation or subluxation even though immobilization is not discontinued prematurely. Anterior or posterior arthrodesis has been advocated early in the course, especially when quadriparesis or quadriplegia occur, to facilitate nursing care and to expedite rehabilitation. When neurologic damage is not a factor, a more conservative treatment program is reasonable.

e. Forward unilateral dislocation. Complete unilateral dislocation anteriorly below the level of the axis is characterized by torsional displacement whereby one facet joint remains essentially undisturbed while the other is completely displaced and usually locked. Less extensive disk and ligamentous damage is probable than that of the bilateral lesion. When present, neurologic findings may be asymmetric and involve predominantly the side of displacement. Routine anteroposterior radiographs demonstrate the spinous process of the dislocated segment above to be displaced toward the side of the more involved facet, and lateral views show the body displaced anteriorly less than half of its diameter. CT studies with reformatted views may provide confirmatory evidence.

Reduction may be accomplished by cranial traction with the patient awake, the head being flexed slightly and tilted to the side opposite the dislocated facet joint. When reduction has been effected, the head is placed in anatomic position which is mechanically stable. Immobilization in a halo brace is continued for 12 weeks. Early open reduction is indicated when closed methods fail and especially when neurologic injury is present.

f. Forward bilateral subluxation (incomplete dislocation) may occur alone or it may complicate compression fracture. Neurologic damage is not likely but when it is evident, other accompanying lesions should be sought. Uncomplicated bilateral subluxation can be treated by gentle manual traction with the patient awake, letting the head extend so that its weight can provide the traction force or by gentle traction with a head halter with 2-3 kg of weight. The neck should be protected by a cervical brace for 2-3 weeks. Resubluxation may occur.

g. Forward unilateral subluxation below the level of the C-2 may be caused by minimal injury; it may occur spontaneously, especially during sleep. Younger persons are affected more commonly than older ones. Pain may be a prominent feature. Tilting of the head away from the side of lesion and rotation of the chin slightly toward the unaffected side are the chief physical signs. The lesion is best demonstrated by lateral radiographs or CT.

Reduction can frequently be accomplished by gentle manual traction or by head halter. After reduction, the neck should be protected by a soft collar until discomfort and any restriction of active movement disappears. Recurrence is possible. Any persistence of symptoms requires search for other likely causes.

h. Extension dislocation. Diagnosis is often difficult and at times must rest on speculation because of the inherent stability of the cervical spine, likelihood of spontaneous reduction, and paucity of evidence from standard radiographic examination. Dislocation without significant fracture implies rupture of the anterior longitudinal ligament and disruption of the disk. Injury to the cord may be caused by infolding of posterior longitudinal ligament and by hypertrophic spurs of posterior body that encroach upon the canal anteriorly. The neurologic pattern of incomplete deficit may conform to that of an acute central cord lesion.

Standard radiographic studies may show only widening of disk space or avulsion of a bit of bone from the body of an adjacent vertebra by the anterior longitudinal ligament.

This lesion is stable when the cervical spine is in slight flexion. Treatment by prolonged bracing is adequate. The major therapeutic challenge is care of any neurologic complication.

i. Fracture-dislocation. Compression fracture of the vertebral body may occur as an isolated lesion (see above), or it may be associated with varying degrees of forward (anterior) dislocation. Compression of the superior plate of the body with disruption of the intervertebral disk, displacement of the facet joints, and tearing of the posterior supporting ligaments, account for the major components of this lesion complex. Even though the facet joints do not displace, fracture of the lateral mass can permit subluxation. Injury to the spinal cord and nerve roots may be present. Because of impaction of the bone fragments, fracture healing usually proceeds uneventfully. Treatment is directed to the accompanying dislocation (see above).

Forces that cause lateral flexion may produce compression fracture of the lateral mass or adjacent segment of the cerebral body. Contralateral facet subluxation by distraction, with or without avulsion of an adjacent transverse process, may be associated. Injury to roots or the brachial plexus on the distracted side may be present. Associated damage to the cord may obscure the root lesion initially. Because of inherent stability of the lesion, treatment by external support alone is apt to be adequate; traction may be harmful.

D. FRACTURES OF THE THORACIC SPINE. The thoracic spine is comparatively stable. Fracture results either from direct violence, which may involve only a spinous process; or indirect violence, which may result in compression of the body of the vertebra.

Compression fractures of the thoracic vertebrae are rare in young children and are caused only by severe trauma in older children. In this age group, therefore, unless there is a positive history of severe trauma, a wedge-shaped deformity in the thoracic spine should suggest pathologic fracture. This must not be confused with Calve's or Scheuermann's disease.

Minimal (frequently unrecognized) trauma may cause compression fracture of the body of the thoracic vertebrae in adults with osteoporosis. Disability is usually self-limited and reduction is not indicated. If rest in bed for 3-4 days does not relieve the pain, a surgical corset with shoulder restraints or a brace (Taylor or Arnold type) may provide comfort and permit early ambulation.

Compression fractures of the thoracic spine caused by severe trauma are characterized by wedge-shaped deformity of the vertebral body. No adequate closed method has been devised for reduction of these injuries. Because of the inherent stability of the thoracic spine, prolonged immobilization is required for relief of pain; a long plaster jacket or brace that includes the iliac crests may be the only adequate method of external support that will provide relief from pain.

Rotational fracture-dislocations near the thoracolumbar junction and shear fractures of the thoracic spine are commonly associated with paraplegia. Rotational fracture-dislocation is inherently unstable because of extensive rupture of supporting ligaments, fracture of the vertebral body in the transverse plane, and disruption of the articular facet joints by fracture or dislocation. These fractures may be unstable, and internal stabilization with fusion may be necessary to minimize injury to the cord and to permit early mobilization.

Shear fracture is fracture-dislocation of the thoracic spine in which dislocation takes place at or near the intervertebral disk with fracture of articular processes or pedicles. Forward displacement takes place in the transverse plane.

E. FRACTURES AND FRACTURE-DISLOCATIONS OF THE LUMBAR SPINE

1. Uncomplicated compression fractures. Compression fractures of vertebral bodies caused by hyperflexion injury are the most common fractures of the lumbar spine and occur most often near the thoracolumbar junction. The widespread use of seat belts in automobiles has been accompanied by an increasing incidence of fractures that occur near the lumbosacral level as the result of accidents. Often more than one vertebral body is involved, but deformity may be greatest in one segment. Acute angulation of the spine caused by compression fracture of the body of a vertebra may be associated with varying degrees of disruption of the facet joints, from sprain to complete dislocation.

In older patients with preexisting degenerative arthritis in which there is mild deformity involving no more than one-fourth of the anterior height of the body of the vertebra, the surgeon may elect merely to place the patient at bed rest for a few days. As soon as acute pain is relieved, the back should be braced and increasing physical activity encouraged within the tolerance of pain. In the more active age group, and when the compression deformity involves more than one half of the anterior height of the body of the vertebra, reduction by hyperextension and immobilization in a plaster jacket or plastic brace may be carried out.

2. Comminuted fractures of the vertebral body are characterized by disruption of the adjacent intervertebral disks and varying degrees of displacement of bone fragments. The endplates of the body are forced into the centrum together with the disk. A large fragment of the body may be displaced anteriorly. Posteriorly displaced fragments are apt to cause compression of the cord or cauda equina; and the facet joints may be fractured or dislocated. Careful physical and radiographic examinations are mandatory before treatment is instituted.

The method of **treatment** may be dictated by extent of bone injury and presence of neurologic complications. When neurologic involvement is absent and comminution is not manifest by extensive fragmentation, reduction may not be necessary. Under these circumstances, immobilization in a plaster jacket or brace may be sufficient. It must be determined whether dislocation has occurred or is likely because of posterior element injury (see below). Mobilization of the patient from recumbency should be controlled by periodic physical and radiographic examinations to determine incipient displacement of fragments which may herald or accompany the onset of neurologic deficit. When the posterior elements are intact and compression of the body has been greater than one fourth to one third its former height, reduction by extension of the spine and immobilization in a brace or a plaster jacket should be considered in young adults. When cauda equina injury has occurred, the location and nature of compression must be accurately confirmed by CT examination so that it can be relieved, generally by operative intervention. Closed reduction is usually carried out, followed by posterior instrumentation and fusion to minimize residual neurologic compromise. Bone healing is likely to be slow, and immobilization should be prolonged until stabilization has occurred.

3. Fracture of the transverse processes may result from direct violence, such as a direct blow, or may be incidental to a more serious fracture of the lumbar spine. It may result also from violent muscle contraction alone. One or more segments may be involved. If displacement is minimal, soft tissue injury is likely to be minor. Extensive displacement of the fragments indicates severe soft tissue tearing and hematoma formation.

Treatment depends upon the presence or absence of associated injuries. If fracture of the transverse process is the sole injury, and if pain is not severe upon guarded motions of the back, strapping and prompt ambulation may be sufficient. If displacement and soft tissue injury are extensive, bed rest for a few days followed by prolonged support in a corset or brace may be necessary and slow symptomatic recovery may be anticipated.

4. Fracture-dislocation of the lumbar spine. Severe compression trauma may cause fracture-dislocation with rupture of one disk or, if comminution occurs, two disks. Varying degrees of injury to the posterior elements occur, including unilateral or bilateral dislocation of the facets or fracture of pedicles or facets. Accompanying fractures of spinous and transverse processes and tearing of the posterior ligaments and adjacent muscles can add to the complexity of this severe lesion. The dislocation of the upper segment may be solely in the anteroposterior plane, or it may be complex, with additional displacement in the coronal plane with torsion around the longitudinal axis of the spine.

Treatment depends upon type of injury. Because these injuries are usually unstable, open reduction and internal fixation with fusion is usually carried out as soon as the general condition of the patient permits. With complete dislocation of one or both facets, such surgery is usually necessary. Rigid fracture fixation permits more rapid mobilization and rehabilitation than does nonoperative treatment. External immobilization by a molded cast or plastic brace may be used to supplement the internal fixation if necessary. If there is no neurologic involvement and dislocation was associated with fracture of pedicles or facets, nonoperative treatment may be an option. Reduction is achieved by cautious extension with traction on the lower extremities under radiographic control without anesthesia. When dislocation has been corrected, immobilization in a plaster body cast with a spica extension to incorporate at least one thigh may be necessary for adequate support. Mobilization of the patient from recumbent position should be accomplished slowly because displacement of fragments can occur and neurologic complications may result. When reasonable doubt exists, it is preferable to continue recumbency for 8-12 weeks until initial healing has provided mechanical stability. If closed reduction is not successful, or if extension causes neurologic symptoms, the attempt should be abandoned at once in favor of open reduction. In complete dislocation of one or both facets, open reduction may be necessary.

F. FRACTURE OF THE SACRUM generally is associated with injuries of the pelvis or lumbar spine. Isolated sacral fracture may be transverse or longitudinal. It may also appear as an isolated lesion as a result of direct violence. Linear transverse fracture of the sacrum without displacement that occurs below the level of the second segment should be treated symptomatically. Strapping of the buttocks of males and wearing a snug girdle by females can provide some comfort during the acutely painful stage. If the fracture extends through a sacral foramen and is associated with displacement, there may be injury to one of the sacral nerves and consequent neurologic deficit. If the sacral fragment is displaced anteriorly, reduction should be attempted by means of bimanual manipulation. Great care should be exercised to prevent injury to the rectal wall by pressure of the palpating finger against a sharp spicule of underlying bone.

Longitudinal fractures involve the lateral mass of the first two segments and may extend into the foramens.

G. FRACTURE OF THE COCCYX is usually the result of a blow on the buttock. No specific treatment is required other than protection. Strapping the buttocks together and avoidance of direct pressure may minimize pain. Warn patients that pain may persist for many weeks. Fracture-dislocation can be reduced by bimanual manipulation, but recurrence of the deformity is likely.

II. INJURIES TO THE SHOULDER GIRDLE

A. FRACTURE OF THE CLAVICLE may occur as a result of direct trauma or indirect force transmitted through the shoulder. Most fractures of the clavicle are seen in the lateral half, commonly at the junction of the middle and lateral thirds. About two thirds of clavicular fractures occur in children. Birth fractures of the clavicle vary from greenstick to complete displacement and must be differentiated from congenital pseudoarthrosis.

Because of relative fixation of the medial fragment and the weight of the upper extremity, the lateral fragment is displaced downward, forward, and toward the midline. Anteroposterior radiographs should always be taken, but oblique projections are occasionally of more value. Although injury to the brachial plexus or subclavian vessels is not common, such complications can usually be demonstrated on physical examination.

1. Treatment

a. Without displacement. Immobilization of greenstick fractures is not required in children, and healing is rapid. Complete fractures should be immobilized for 10-21 days.

b. With displacement. In infants and small children, a figure-of-eight dressing may provide support and decrease pain. Healing usually takes 2-4 weeks. Older children and adolescents may require reduction by closed manipulation and immobilization with a figure-of-eight dressing. Reduction need not be exact, because exuberant callus formation will be partially or completely obliterated by remodeling of bone in the late stage of the fracture repair.

c. With displacement or comminution (in adults)

(1) *Closed reduction.* Comminuted fractures of the clavicle with displacement can usually be managed successfully by closed reduction, although in women greater effort must be made to secure accurate realignment without deformity. Fractured surfaces of displaced fragments which cannot be reduced closed can sometimes be manipulated into apposition by seizing the main fragments percutaneously with large towel clamps. A plaster shoulder spica gives more secure immobilization than the figure-of-eight dressing. Immobilization must be maintained for 6-12 weeks.

(2) *Open reduction* may be justifiable occasionally to prevent delay of healing where there is interposition of soft tissue or severe tension by displaced fragments on overlying skin.

d. Fracture of the outer third of the clavicle distal to the coracoclavicular ligaments is comparable to dislocation of the acromioclavicular joint (see below). If the coracoclavicular ligaments are intact and the fragments are not widely displaced, immobilization in a sling and swathe is adequate. If the coracoclavicular ligaments have been lacerated and extensive displacement of the main medial fragment is present, treatment is similar to that advocated for acromioclavicular dislocation.

B. ACROMIOCLAVICULAR DISLOCATION may be incomplete (types I and II) or complete (type III). The acromial end of the clavicle is displaced upward and backward; the shoulder falls downward and inward. Anteroposterior radiographs should be taken of both shoulders with the patient erect. Displacement is more likely to be demonstrated when the patient holds a 5-8 kg weight in each hand. An axillary projection demonstrates backward displacement of the acromial end of the clavicle.

Incomplete dislocation (subluxation) is associated with only minor tearing of the acromioclavicular ligaments, because complete dislocation requires concomitant rupture of the conoid and trapezoid components of the coracoclavicular ligament. These ligaments may be torn within their substance, or they may be avulsed with adjacent periosteum from the acromial end of the clavicle.

1. Treatment

a. Incomplete dislocation. When displacement is minimal initial treatment may be by sling until acute pain from movement and the weight of the upper extremity has been relieved.

b. Complete dislocation. Treatment of complete acromioclavicular dislocations is controversial. It is difficult to maintain reduction and adequate immobilization of complete acromioclavicular dislocations by closed methods. Open operation performed within the first 3 weeks after complete acromioclavicular dislocation offers the best hope of restoring anatomic alignment. If it is deferred longer, the ligaments will have partially healed with elongation, and the deformity can be expected to recur when immobilization is discontinued unless the ligaments have been reconstructed.

Many orthopedists advocate nonoperative treatment for all but the most severely displaced acromioclavicular dislocations. They cite the rapid return of pain-free motion and excellent long-term functional results in patients treated without reduction.

C. STERNOCLAVICULAR DISLOCATION.

Displacement of the sternal end of the clavicle may occur superiorly, anteriorly, or, less commonly, inferiorly. Retrosternal displacement is rare and may be complicated by injury to the great vessels. Complete dislocation can be diagnosed by physical examination. Anteroposterior and oblique radiographs confirm the diagnosis. CT may also be helpful.

For incomplete dislocation, a sling or figure-of-eight dressing usually is adequate. Open reduction with repair of the torn sternoclavicular and costoclavicular ligaments, with or without internal fixation, is normally required to maintain adequate reduction of complete dislocations. However, chronic or recurrent anterior dislocations usually are asymptomatic and are therefore left untreated.

D. FRACTURE OF THE SCAPULA. Fracture of the neck of the scapula is most often caused by a blow on the shoulder or by a fall on the outstretched arm. The degree of fragmentation may vary. The main glenoid fragment may be impacted into the body fragment. The treatment of impacted or undisplaced fractures in patients 40 years or older should be directed toward preservation of shoulder joint function, because stiffness may cause prolonged disability. Open reduction is rarely required even for major displaced fragments except for those involving the articular surface when associated with dislocation of the humeral head. These fractures are likely to involve only a segment of the articular surface and may be impacted. Such fracture occasionally complicates anterior dislocation of the shoulder joint.

Fracture of acromion or spine of scapula requires reduction only when the displaced fragment is apt to cause interference with abduction of the shoulder. Persistence of an acromial apophysis should not be confused with fracture.

Fracture of the coracoid process may result from violent muscular contractions or, rarely, may be associated with anterior dislocation of shoulder joint.

When fracture of the body of the scapula is caused by direct violence, fractures of underlying ribs and pulmonary injury may be associated. Treatment of uncomplicated fracture should be directed toward the comfort of the patient and the preservation of shoulder joint function.

E. FRACTURE OF THE PROXIMAL HUMERUS occurs most frequently during the sixth decade. The classification of proximal humeral fractures is based on the presence or absence of displacement of the articular surface of the humeral head, greater tuberosity, lesser tuberosity, and shaft.

1. Undisplaced fractures of the proximal humerus or minimally displaced fractures of the proximal humerus—with the exception of those of the anatomic neck—require little treatment beyond immobilization of the shoulder in a sling until discomfort subsides. Following this initial period of immobilization, progressive range of motion exercises are started.

2. Single fractures of the proximal humerus
a. Fracture of the anatomic neck. Isolated fracture of anatomic neck of the humerus is uncommon and may be followed by avascular necrosis of the articular fragment even in the absence of displacement. Malhealing of displaced fractures may cause limitation of shoulder motion. When displacement is the determinant of open operation, primary humeral

prosthetic arthroplasty is likely to provide a more satisfactory long-term result than anatomic replacement of the devascularized articular fragment.

b. Fracture of the surgical neck. The main fracture cleft is distal to the tuberosities. Minor comminution of the proximal segment can be disregarded when displacement of those fragments does not occur. Some angulation is likely to accompany any displacement in the transverse plane of the humerus. When angulation >45 degrees occurs in the active person, it should be corrected to avoid subsequent restriction of abduction and elevation. Lesser degrees of deformity require no manipulation, especially in elderly persons. Impacted and minimally angulated fractures can be treated by means of a sling.

Although they do occur, neurovascular injuries are not common complications. Closed manipulation is justifiable, but because persistent instability is a frequent complication, impaction or locking of the fragments is desirable. If reduction is stable, a Velpeau type dressing provides reliable immobilization after correction of anterior angulation. Redisplacement may occur when reduction is not stable or when the arm is immobilized in abduction. When comminution is not extensive, the fracture that has been adequately reduced by closed methods may be stabilized by one or two heavy Kirschner wires introduced percutaneously and obliquely in the deltoid region through the distal fragment into the head of the humerus. With the fragments fixed, the arm is then brought to the side and immobilized either by a sling and swathe or by a plaster Velpeau dressing. Open reduction and internal fixation of uncomplicated fractures of surgical neck are not commonly required.

c. Fracture of greater tuberosity generally is a component of a complex injury, either comminuted fracture of the proximal humerus or anterior dislocation of the shoulder joint. Fracture of the greater tuberosity with no associated injury is apt to be undisplaced. When isolated and displaced fracture does occur, it is likely to be associated with persistent or spontaneously reduced anterior dislocation of the humeral head and longitudinal tear of the capsulotendinous cuff.

When accurate repositioning of the greater tuberosity fragment does not occur following closed reduction of the dislocated humeral head, open operation is desirable to fix anatomically the avulsed fragment and to repair any capsulotendinous tear.

d. Fracture of the lesser tuberosity is generally a part of comminuted fracture of the proximal humerus. Isolated fracture is rare and is due to avulsion by the subscapularis muscle. Because of the broad insertion of that muscle which extends to the adjacent humeral shaft inferiorly, displacement of the bony fragment is unlikely to be marked.

Treatment consists of immobilization in a sling for about 4 weeks.

3. Combined and displaced fracture of the proximal humerus

a. Fracture of the surgical neck and greater tuberosity. Combined and displaced fractures involving the surgical neck and greater tuberosity are unique because the persistently active subscapularis muscle attached to the intact lesser tuberosity causes the proximal articular fragment to be rotated internally in relation to the shaft. It is difficult to correct this torsional displacement by closed methods. It may be accomplished with the aid of the image intensifier by initially inserting, percutaneously and transversely, a small Steinmann pin into the proximal segment which is used to derotate that fragment and to stabilize it while completing the reduction. The two major fragments are then fixed percutaneously as described for unstable fractures of the surgical neck. If reduction of displacement at both fracture sites is not adequate, open reduction and internal fixation of the bone fragments and repair of any rotator cuff tear are indicated. This combined lesion may be complicated by anterior dislocation of the proximal head fragment from the glenoid.

b. Fracture of the surgical neck and lesser tuberosity. Combined and displaced fracture of the surgical neck and lesser tuberosity are significant because the external rotators cause the proximal fragment to be externally rotated with reference to the shaft so that the cartilaginous surface of the humeral head is directed anteriorly. Correction of torsional displacement and adequate reduction are difficult by closed methods but may be achieved by appropriate modification of the technic described for combined fracture of the surgical neck and greater tuberosity. If satisfactory reduction cannot be attained, open reduction with fixation of the bone fragments and repair of any coexisting tear of the rotator cuff is appropriate. Posterior dislocation of the head fragment from the glenoid may complicate this combined lesion.

c. Fracture of surgical neck and both tuberosities is an uncommon but serious lesion generally complicated by displacement of one or all of the component fragments. Displacement of the tuberosities and of the shaft provide a mechanism for subluxation or dislocation of the main articular fragment which may be anterior, posterior, lateral, or inferior. Shattering of the articular segment may permit multidirectional displacement of component fragments. Tear of the rotator cuff may occur as part of the total lesion.

With comminution and displacement of component fragments of the proximal segment, satisfactory functional results are unlikely and delay of bone healing is probable after any type of closed treatment. Avascular necrosis of the articular fragment is an anticipated sequel because of its end-arterial blood supply. Open operation offers the best chance for preservation of some function with tolerable discomfort. Removal of the articular segment and repair of the remaining structures are not as successful in the early treatment of this injury as hemiarthroplasty with fixation of tuberosities to the distal shaft fragment.

A late complication of intraarticular fractures of the proximal humerus is secondary glenohumeral osteoarthritis.

d. Separation of the epiphysis of the head of the humerus. When this injury occurs as a result of birth trauma, it is difficult to recognize because of the absence of a bony nucleus in the capital epiphysis. Even though radiographic examination is negative, the injury should be suspected when there is swelling of the shoulder region and limitation of active movements of the arm. Fracture through the physis may be encountered in older children. Principles of treatment are as for fracture of surgical neck of the humerus. Open reduction is rarely desirable; every effort should be made to reduce by manipulation or traction.

F. DISLOCATION OF THE SHOULDER JOINT. Over 95% of all cases of shoulder joint dislocation are anterior or subcoracoid. Subglenoid and posterior dislocations comprise the remainder.

1. Anterior dislocation presents the clinical appearance of flattening of the deltoid region, anterior fullness, and restriction of motion due to pain. Both anteroposterior and transscapular lateral radiographs are necessary to determine the site of the head and presence or absence of complicating fracture involving either the head of the humerus or the glenoid. Anterior dislocation may be complicated by (1) injury to major nerves arising from the brachial plexus; (2) fracture of the upper extremity of the humerus, especially the head or greater tuberosity; (3) compression or avulsion of the anterior glenoid; and (4) tears of the rotator cuff. The most common sequel, especially in younger patients, is recurrent dislocation. Before manipulation, careful examination is necessary to determine the presence or absence of complicating nerve or vascular injury. Closed reduction of the first dislocation generally requires sedation or anesthesia to provide adequate muscle relaxation.

After closed reduction of an initial dislocation the extremity is immobilized in a sling and swathe for 3-6 weeks before active motion is begun. If a second episode is the result of minor trauma, the lesion is considered permanent and treated accordingly.

2. Subcoracoid dislocation. Uncomplicated subcoracoid dislocation can almost always be reduced by closed manipulation. With associated fracture, or when the dislocation is old, open reduction may be necessary. Even when the dislocation is old, however, closed reduction by skeletal traction may be tried before open reduction is elected.

3. Posterior dislocation is characterized by fullness beneath the spine of the scapula and by restriction of motion in external rotation. A transscapular lateral radiographic view demonstrates the position of the head of the humerus in relationship to the glenoid. This uncommon lesion may be reduced by the same combination of coaxial and transverse traction as described for anterior dislocation. Immobilization following an initial episode should be accomplished by plaster spica or brace with the arm in approximately 30 degree external rotation and elbow flexed at a right angle.

4. Recurrent dislocation of the shoulder is almost always anterior and occurs most often in younger patients, i.e., those who have sustained their initial dislocation at age 30 or less. Various factors can influence recurrent dislocation. Avulsion of the anterior and inferior glenoid labrum or tears in the anterior capsule remove the natural buttress that gives stability to the arm with abduction and external rotation. Other lesions which impair the stability of the shoulder joint are fractures of the posterior and superior surface of the head of the humerus (or of greater tuberosity) and longitudinal tears of the rotator cuff between the supraspinatus and subscapularis. Reduction of the acute recurrent dislocation is by closed manipulation. Immobilization does not prevent subsequent dislocation, and it should be discontinued as soon as acute symptoms subside, usually within a few days.

Adequate curative treatment of recurrent dislocation of the shoulder, so that unrestricted normal use of the joint is possible, almost always requires operative repair of the anterior capsulotendinous cuff.

III. FRACTURES OF THE SHAFT OF THE HUMERUS

Fracture of the shaft of the humerus is more common in adults than in children. Direct violence is accountable for the majority of such fractures, although spiral fracture of the middle third of the shaft may result from violent muscular activity such as throwing a ball. Radiographs in two planes are necessary to determine the configuration of the fracture and the direction of displacement of the fragments. Documentation of torsional displacement about the longitudinal axis of the shaft of transverse and comminuted fractures requires inclusion of the shoulder and elbow in the anteroposterior view. Before initiating definitive treatment, a careful neurologic examination should be done (and recorded) to determine the status of the radial nerve. Injury to the brachial vessels is not common.

A. FRACTURE OF THE UPPER THIRD. Fracture through the metaphysis proximal to the insertion of the pectoralis major is classified as fracture of the surgical neck of the humerus.

Fractures between the insertions of the pectoralis major and the deltoid commonly demonstrate medial displacement of the distal end of the proximal fragment, with lateral and proximal displacement of the distal fragment. Medial displacement of the proximal end of the distal fragment occurs with fracture distal to the insertion of the deltoid in the middle third of the shaft.

Treatment depends upon the presence or absence of complicating neurovascular injury, the site and configuration of the fracture, and the magnitude of displacement.

In infants, skin traction for 1-2 weeks permits sufficient callus to form so that immobilization can be maintained by a sling and swathe or a Velpeau dressing. Open reduction for the sole purpose of accurate positioning of the fragments is rarely justified in children and adolescents, because slight shortening and <15° of angulation will be compensated for during growth. Torsional displacement, however, will not be compensated for and must be corrected initially.

In adults, an effort should be made to reduce completely displaced transverse or slightly oblique fractures by manipulation. To prevent recurrence of medial convex angulation and maintain proper alignment, it may be necessary to bring the distal fragment into alignment with the proximal by bringing the arm across the chest and immobilizing it with a plaster Velpeau dressing. If ends of fragments cannot be approximated by manipulative methods, treatment by skeletal traction may be used for children or open reduction for adults.

B. FRACTURE OF THE MIDDLE AND LOWER THIRDS.

Spiral, oblique, and comminuted fractures of the shaft below the insertion of the pectoralis major may be treated by a hanging cast from the axilla to the wrist with the elbow in 90° of flexion and the forearm in midposition. The cast is suspended from a bandage around the neck by means of a ring at the wrist. Traction is afforded by the weight of the plaster. The patient is instructed to sleep in the semireclining position. As soon as clinical examination demonstrates stabilization (about 6-8 weeks), the plaster may be discarded and a sling and swathe substituted.

When fracture of shaft of humerus is associated with other injuries which require confinement to bed, initial treatment may be by skeletal traction.

Fractures of shaft of humerus—especially transverse fractures—may heal slowly. If stabilization has not taken place after 6-8 weeks of traction, more secure immobilization, such as with a plaster shoulder spica, should be considered. It may be necessary to continue immobilization for 6 months or more.

When complete loss of radial nerve function becomes apparent immediately after injury or after attempts at closed reduction, open operation is indicated to determine the type of nerve lesion or to remove impinging bone fragments. Internal fixation of the fragments can be accomplished at the same time. If partial function of the radial nerve is retained, exploration can be deferred because spontaneous recovery may occur and may be complete by the time the fracture has healed. Open reduction of closed fractures is indicated in the presence of arterial injury or (in adults) if adequate apposition of major fragments cannot be obtained by closed methods, as is likely the case with transverse fractures near middle third of shaft.

IV. INJURIES TO THE ELBOW REGION

A. FRACTURE OF THE DISTAL HUMERUS is most often
caused by indirect violence. Therefore, configuration of the fracture cleft and the direction of displacement of the fragments frequently indicate the mechanism of the injury. Injuries of major vessels and nerves and elbow joint dislocation are apt to be present.

Examination for peripheral nerve and vascular injury must be made and all findings carefully recorded before treatment is instituted.

1. Supracondylar fracture of the humerus occurs proximal to the olecranon fossa; transcondylar fracture occurs more distally and extends into the olecranon fossa. Neither fracture extends to the articular surface of the humerus. Treatment is the same for both types.

Supracondylar fractures are observed more commonly in children and adolescents, and they may extend into the physes of the capitellum and trochlea. Transcondylar fracture is very rare in children.

The direction of displacement of the distal fragment from the midcoronal plane of the arm serves to differentiate the "extension" from the less common "flexion" type. This differentiation has important implications for treatment.

a. Extension-type fracture. The majority of supracondylar fractures are of this type and usually result from hyperextension of the elbow during falls. The usual direction of displacement of the main distal fragment is posterior and proximal. The distal fragment may also be displaced laterally and, less frequently, medially. The direction of these displacements is identified easily on biplane radiographic films. Internal torsional displacement is more difficult to recognize; and unless torsional displacement is reduced, relative cubitus varus with loss of carrying angle will persist.

Displaced supracondylar fractures are surgical emergencies. Immediate treatment is required to avoid occlusion of the brachial artery and to prevent or to avoid further peripheral nerve injury. If hemorrhage and edema prevent complete reduction of the fracture at the first attempt, a second manipulation is required after swelling has regressed.

(1) *Manipulative reduction.* Minor angular displacement (tilting) may be reduced by gentle forced flexion of the elbow under local or general anesthesia, followed by immobilization in a posterior plaster splint in 45 degrees or more of flexion. If displacement is marked but the presence of a radial pulse indicates arterial circulation is not impaired, closed manipulation under general anesthesia should be done immediately. If radial pulses are absent or weak on initial examination and do not improve with manipulation, arteriography and/or surgical exploration of the brachial artery is indicated. Capillary flush in nail beds cannot be relied on as the sole indication of competency of deep circulation. After reduction and casting, the patient should be placed at bedrest, preferably in a hospital, with elbow elevated on a pillow and dressing arranged so

that the radial pulse is accessible for frequent observation. Swelling can be expected to increase for 24-72 hours. During this critical period, continued observation is necessary so that any circulatory embarrassment which may lead to Volkmann's ischemic contracture can be identified at once. The circular bandage must be adjusted frequently to compensate for initial increase and subsequent decrease of swelling. If during manipulation it was necessary to extend the elbow beyond 45 degrees to restore the radial pulse, the joint should be flexed to the optimal angle as swelling subsides to prevent loss of the reduction. If reduction cannot be maintained by closed means, percutaneous K-wire fixation of the fracture fragments allows the elbow to be positioned in more extension.

In children, initial healing takes place in 4-5 weeks, after which time the plaster splint may be discarded and a sling worn for another 2 weeks before active motion is permitted. In adults, the healing period is less rapid, usually 10-12 weeks.

(2) *Traction and immobilization.* In certain instances, supracondylar fractures of the humerus with posterior displacement of the distal fragment should be treated by traction: (a) If comminution is marked and stability cannot be obtained by flexion of the elbow, traction is indicated until the fragments have stabilized. (b) If two or three attempts at manipulative reduction have been unsuccessful, continuous traction under radiographic control for 1-2 days is justifiable before further manipulation. (c) If the radial pulse is absent or weak when the patient is examined initially and does not improve with manipulation, immediate surgical exploration of the antecubital vessels may be necessary. During the early phase of treatment by continuous traction, flexion of the elbow beyond 90 degrees should be avoided because this may jeopardize circulation.

(3) *Operative treatment.* Primary open reduction and internal fixation are indicated when there is associated vascular injury, when adequate closed reduction is not obtained, and when other fractures are present in the same extremity.

b. *Flexion-type fracture of the humerus* is characterized by anterior and sometimes also torsional and lateral displacement of the main distal fragment. Treatment is by closed manipulation. A posterior plaster splint is then applied from the axillary elbow in full extension. Elevation is advisable for at least 24 hours or until soft tissue swelling has reached the maximum, after which time the patient may be ambulatory. When satisfactory reduction cannot be accomplished by closed manipulation, treatment should be by traction with the elbow in full extension until the fragments become stabilized.

2. Separation of the distal humeral epiphyses is an uncommon variation of supracondylar fracture, with or without appreciable displacement. Sprains of the elbow do not commonly occur in children; injury more often involves the distal humeral epiphyses. Radiographic comparison of the injured elbow with the uninjured elbow may show no deviation, but careful physical examination may demonstrate posterior tenderness over the lower epiphyses and also swelling. This combination of swelling and tenderness should suggest epiphyseal separation and warrants protection from further injury by means of a long-arm cast worn for about 3 weeks.

The direction of displacement is determined by careful clinical and radiographic examinations. Depending upon the direction of angulation of the osseous nuclei of the capitellum and trochlea (as demonstrated in the lateral radiograph), immobilization is as described for supracondylar fractures.

3. Intercondylar fracture of the humerus is classically described as being of the T or Y type, according to the configuration of the fracture cleft observed on the antero-posterior radiograph. This fracture is usually seen in adults. Open fracture and other injuries to the soft tissues are frequently present. The fracture often extends into the trochlear surface of the elbow joint, and unless the articular surfaces of the distal humerus can be accurately repositioned, restriction of joint motion, pain, instability, and deformity can be expected.

a. Closed reduction. If the fragments are not widely displaced, closed reduction may be successful. Because comminution is always present, stabilization is difficult to achieve and maintain by manipulation and external immobilization.

(1) *Anterior displacement* may be treated first by a combination of continuous traction with the elbow in full extension and closed manipulation of the main fragments. If adequate positioning can be achieved in this manner, olecranon pin traction is continued until stabilization occurs. The extremity may then be immobilized in a plaster cast.

(2) *Significant posterior displacement* requires overhead skeletal traction through the olecranon. It may be neces-

sary to apply a swathe around the arm or body for simultaneous transverse traction.

b. Open reduction may be indicated if adequate positioning cannot be obtained by closed methods. A requirement for acceptable results of open reduction and internal fixation is that the fragments be sufficiently large so that they can be fixed to one another. Usually, screw and K-wire fixation is combined with the use of low-profile plates bent to conform to the contour of the supracondylar ridges. Comminution may be so extensive that satisfactory stabilization cannot be accomplished by current technics of internal fixation. Under such circumstances, it is better to abandon open operation and to accept the imperfect results of closed treatment. If the proximal radius and ulna are intact, subsequent total elbow replacement arthroplasty is an alternative.

4. Fracture of the lateral condyle of the humerus. The three major varieties of this fracture are (a) fracture of a portion of the capitellum in the coronal plane of the humerus, with or without extension into the trochlea (seen only in adults); (b) isolated fracture of the lateral condyle without extension into the trochlea; and (c) separation of the capitellar epiphysis (in children).

a. Fracture of the capitellum is characterized by proximal displacement of the anterior detached fragment and probably occurs as one component of a spontaneously reduced incomplete dislocation of the elbow joint. The lesion is most clearly demonstrated on lateral radiographs. Closed reduction should be attempted by forcing the elbow into acute flexion. After reduction, the extremity is immobilized in a posterior plaster splint with the elbow in flexion to prevent displacement of the small distal fragment.

When accurate reduction cannot be accomplished by closed technics, open operation may be desirable to avoid or minimize subsequent restriction of elbow movement. If the small distal fragment retains sufficient soft tissue attachment to assure adequate blood supply, it may be temporarily fixed to the main fragment in anatomic position by a K-wire. If the articular fragment lacks significant soft-tissue attachment, avascular necrosis is likely, and removal is indicated.

b. Isolated complete fracture of the lateral condyle without extension into the trochlea is uncommon and is not usually associated with major displacement of the detached fragment. Fracture which involves the entire capitellum and extends into the trochlea is discussed below.

c. Separation of the capitellar epiphysis. Fracture of the lateral condyle of the humerus in children is essentially separation of the capitellar epiphysis, even though the fracture may extend into the metaphysis and the trochlear epiphysis. If the center of ossification of the capitellum is small, minor displacement may be missed on initial examination; further displacement then results from unguarded use. The fact that a part of the extensor muscles originate on the fragment is an important factor in displacement.

(1) *Closed reduction.* Minor displacement may be treated by manipulative reduction and external immobilization in a posterior plaster splint. Careful monitoring of the fracture by radiography is necessary to ensure that reduction is maintained.

(2) *Open reduction.* Because anatomic reduction of displaced fractures is difficult to obtain and maintain by purely closed means, most orthopedists advocate either closed reduction and percutaneous pinning or open reduction and internal fixation under direct vision.

d. Avulsion of the medial epicondylar apophysis in children is rare and may occur without or with dislocation of the elbow. Minor displacement causing localized tenderness and swelling over the medial aspect of the elbow can be treated by immobilization in a sling and swathe for a few days. More extensive injury should be suspected if tenderness and swelling are diffuse. When separation is greater than 1-2 mm, open reduction with K-wire fixation is indicated.

B. FRACTURE OF THE PROXIMAL ULNA. Common fractures of the proximal ulna include fracture of the olecranon and fracture of the coronoid process. Fracture of the coronoid process is a complication of posterior dislocation of the elbow joint, and is discussed below.

Fracture of the olecranon which occurs as the result of indirect violence (e.g., forced flexion of the forearm against the actively contracted triceps muscle) is typically transverse or slightly oblique. Fracture due to direct violence is usually comminuted and associated with other fracture or anterior dislocation of the joint. Because the major fracture cleft extends into the elbow joint, treatment should be directed toward restoration of anatomic position to afford maximal recovery of range of motion and functional competency of the triceps.

The method of **treatment** depends upon the degree of displacement and the extent of comminution. Minimal displacement (1-2 mm) can be treated by closed manipulation with the elbow in full extension and immobilization in a volar plaster splint. Immobilization must be continued for at least 6 weeks before active flexion exercises are begun.

Open reduction and internal fixation are indicated in displaced fractures. Excision of comminuted fragments with repair of the triceps tendon insertion is warranted if the majority of the joint surface is intact.

C. FRACTURE OF THE PROXIMAL RADIUS

1. Fracture of the head and neck of the radius may occur in adults as an isolated injury uncomplicated by dislocation of elbow or the proximal radioulnar joint. This fracture is caused by indirect violence, such as a fall on the outstretched hand, when the radial head is driven against the capitellum. Care must be taken to obtain true anteroposterior and lateral radiographs of the proximal radius as well as of the elbow joint, because small fractures may be obscured by a change from midposition to full supination during exposure of the films.

a. Conservative measures. Nondisplaced fractures and those with minimal displacement may be treated symptomatically with aspiration of tense hemarthrosis to minimize pain. The extremity may be supported by a sling or immobilized in a posterior plaster splint with the elbow in 90 degrees of flexion.

b. Surgical treatment. When the fracture involves more than a third of the articular surface and is comminuted, or when displacement is >1-2 mm, excision of the entire head of the radius is generally recommended. On rare occasions, large displaced single fragments may be amenable to open reduction and internal fixation.

2. Fracture of the proximal epiphysis of the radius in a child is a true epiphyseal separation although the fracture cleft commonly extends into the neck of the bone. Because the articular surface of the proximal fragment remains intact, the prominent features of displacement are angulation and impaction. Wide displacement of the minor proximal fragment may mean that the elbow joint was dislocated but had reduced spontaneously since the injury.

a. Closed reduction. Every effort should be made to reduce these fractures by closed manipulation. Several radiographs taken with the forearm in various degrees of rotation should be examined so that the position can be selected which is best suited for digital pressure on the proximal fragment. Anteroposterior and lateral radiographs with the elbow in flexion are then taken; if angulation has been reduced to <45 degrees, the end result is likely to be satisfactory.

b. Open reduction. If closed reduction is not successful, open reduction and repositioning under direct vision are indicated even in the child.

D. SUBLUXATION AND DISLOCATION OF THE ELBOW JOINT

1. Subluxation of the head of the radius occurs most frequently in infants between the ages of 18 months and 4 years, usually when the child is suddenly lifted by the hand with the forearm in pronation. Because of comparative laxity of the interosseous membrane and other supporting ligamentous structures, the direction of displacement of the radial head is distal in the direction of the longitudinal axis of the shaft. It has been suggested that this permits the proximal part of the annular ligament to become infolded between the radial head and the capitellum. In unreduced subluxations, in addition to tenderness about the radial head and restriction of supination, swelling and tenderness may be present in the region of the ulnar head at the level of the inferior radioulnar joint. The infant holds the forearm semiflexed and pronated. If spontaneous reduction has occurred, diagnosis is dependent upon finding slightly restricted supination associated with discomfort. Radiographs are generally not helpful, but in the older child the distance between the radial head and the capitellum may be increased in comparison with the uninjured side.

Reduction by forced supination of the forearm can usually be accomplished easily without anesthesia. The extremity should be protected in a sling for 1 week. Rarely, in an older child, closed manipulation may be unsuccessful, and open release of the annular ligament may be necessary.

2. Dislocation of the head of the radius. Isolated dislocation of the radius at the elbow is a rare lesion which implies dislocation of the proximal radioulnar and radiohumeral joints without fracture. This lesion, which occurs in children older than 5 years or occasionally in adults, should be differentiated from subluxation of the head of the radius. The direction of displacement of the radial head is usually anterior or lateral, but it may be posterior.

Reduction can usually be accomplished by forced supination of the forearm under anesthesia. The extremity should be immobilized for 3-4 weeks with the elbow in flexion and the forearm in supination.

3. Dislocation of the elbow joint without fracture is almost always posterior. It may be encountered at any age but is most common in children. Complete backward dislocation of the ulna and radius implies extensive tearing of the capsuloligamentous structures and injury to the region of insertion of the brachialis muscle. The coronoid process of the ulna is usually displaced posteriorly and proximally into the olecranon fossa, but it may be simultaneously displaced laterally or medially.

Peripheral nerve function must be carefully assessed before definitive treatment is instituted. The ulnar nerve is most likely to be injured.

In recent dislocations, closed reduction can be achieved (under general anesthesia) by axial traction on the forearm with the elbow in the position of deformity. Hyperextension is not necessary. Lateral or medial dislocation can be corrected during traction. The elbow should be brought into 90° of flexion and a posterior plaster splint applied. Active motion is permitted after 3 weeks.

E. FRACTURE-DISLOCATION OF THE ELBOW JOINT.
Dislocation of the elbow is frequently associated with fracture. Some fractures are insignificant and require no specific treatment; others demand specialized care.

1. Fracture of the coronoid process of the ulna is the most frequent complication of posterior dislocation of the elbow joint. Treatment is the same as for uncomplicated posterior dislocation of the elbow joint (see above).

2. Fracture of the head of the radius with posterior dislocation of the elbow joint. This injury is treated as two separate lesions. The severity of comminution and the magnitude of displacement of the radial head fragments are first determined by radiography. If comminution has occurred or the fragments are widely displaced, the dislocation is reduced by closed manipulation; the head of the radius is then excised. If fracture of the head of the radius is not comminuted and the fragments are not widely displaced, treatment is as for uncomplicated posterior dislocation of the elbow joint.

3. Fracture of the olecranon with anterior dislocation of the elbow joint. This very unstable injury usually occurs from a blow on the dorsum of the flexed forearm. Fracture through the olecranon permits the distal fragment of the ulna and the proximal radius to be displaced anterior to the humerus and may cause extensive tearing of the capsuloligamentous structures around the elbow joint. The dislocation can be reduced by bringing the elbow into full extension, but anatomic reduction of the olecranon fracture by closed manipulation is not likely to be successful and immediate open reduction and internal fixation are usually indicated. Recovery of function is likely to be delayed and incomplete.

4. Fracture of the medial epicondylar apophysis with dislocation of the elbow joint.

Dislocation of the elbow joint in children may be complicated by avulsion of the medial epicondylar apophysis. The direction of dislocation may have been lateral, posterior, or posterolateral. Physical and radiographic examination may not demonstrate the extent of displacement at the time of injury because partial reduction may have occurred spontaneously. Radiographs of the uninjured elbow in similar projections are desirable to compare the exact locations of the two apophyses. The free fragment is normally displaced downward by the action of the flexor muscles. If partial spontaneous reduction of the elbow dislocation has occurred, the detached apophysis may be found incarcerated within the elbow joint between the articular surfaces of the trochlea and the olecranon. This may happen also during manual reduction. Ulnar nerve function must be evaluated before definitive treatment is given.

Dislocation of the elbow joint may be reduced by closed manipulation, but accurate repositioning of a widely separated apophysis cannot be achieved by closed methods. Opinion differs concerning the necessity for anatomic reduction of the apophysis if it is not incarcerated within the elbow joint. Some authorities maintain that fibrous healing of the apophysis causes no disability; others anticipate weakness of grasp or subsequent pain as the result of development of a pseudoarthrosis between the apophysis and the medial condyle. Exuberant bone formation around the apophysis may cause tardy ulnar paralysis. If it is elected not to reduce displacement of an apophysis outside the elbow joint, the extremity should be immobilized at a right angle for 3 weeks in a plaster splint before active motion is permitted.

If the ulnar nerve has been injured, or if the apophysis cannot be displaced from the elbow joint by closed manipulation, open reduction is indicated.

5. Fracture of the lateral condyle with lateral dislocation of the elbow joint

must be differentiated from fracture of the lateral condyle with or without posterior dislocation of the joint (see below). Neither lesion is common. A complicating feature of fracture of the lateral condyle with lateral dislocation is inclusion not only of the entire capitellum but also extension of the fracture cleft into the trochlea. This creates an unstable mechanism which cannot be reliably immobilized in either flexion or extension even though closed reduction has been successful. Open reduction and internal fixation are indicated.

6. Fracture of the lateral condyle with posterior dislocation of the elbow joint. Treatment of this uncommon injury should be divided into two phases. The dislocation should be reduced first by closed manipulation. This maneuver may also simultaneously accomplish adequate reduction of the condylar fracture. If the condylar fragment cannot be adequately repositioned by closed manipulation, open reduction and internal fixation are justifiable to assure anatomic restoration of the articular surfaces.

V. FRACTURES OF THE SHAFTS OF THE RADIUS AND ULNA

A. GENERAL CONSIDERATIONS

1. Causative injury. Spiral and oblique fractures are likely to be caused by indirect injury. Greenstick, transverse, and comminuted fractures are commonly the result of direct injury.

2. Radiography

a. In addition to anteroposterior and lateral films of the entire forearm, including the elbow and wrist joints, oblique views are often desirable.

b. The lateral projection is usually taken with the forearm in neutral position (between complete pronation and supination).

c. For the anteroposterior projection, care must be taken to prevent any change in relative supination of the radius; if this happens, the distal radius is the same in both views, and the fracture may not be demonstrated.

d. Especially in children, films of the uninjured forearm are desirable for comparison of epiphyses and for future reference if growth is impaired.

3. Anatomic peculiarities. Both the radius and the ulna have biplane curves which permit 180 degrees of rotation in the forearm. If the curves are not preserved by reduction, full rotatory motion of the forearm may not be recovered or derangement of the radioulnar joints may follow.

Torsional displacement by muscle activity has important implications for manipulative treatment of certain fractures of the radial shaft. The direction of torsional displacement of the distal fragment following fracture of the shafts is influenced by the location of the lesion in reference to muscle insertion. If the fracture is in the upper third (above the insertion of the pronator teres), the proximal fragment is drawn into relative supination by the biceps and supinator and the distal fragment into pronation by the pronator teres and pronator quadratus. The relative position in torsion of the proximal fragment may be determined by comparing the position of the bicipital tubercle on an anteroposterior film with similar projections of the uninjured arm taken in varying degrees of forearm rotation. In fractures below the middle of the radius (below the insertion of the pronator teres), the proximal fragment characteristically remains in midposition owing to the antagonistic action of the pronator teres on the biceps and supinator; the distal fragment is pronated by the pronator quadratus.

4. Closed reduction and splinting. With fracture and displacement of the shaft of either the radius or the ulna, injury of the proximal or distal radioulnar joints should always be suspected. Swelling and tenderness around the joint may help localize an occult injury when radiographs are not helpful.

In both adults and children, closed reduction of uncomplicated fractures of the radius and ulna should be attempted. The type of manipulative maneuver depends upon the configuration and location of the fracture and the age of the patient. The position of immobilization of the elbow, forearm, and wrist depends upon the location of the fracture and its inherent stability.

B. FRACTURE OF THE SHAFT OF THE ULNA. Isolated fracture of the shaft of the proximal third of the ulna (above the insertion of the pronator teres) with displacement is often associated with dislocation of the head of the radius (Monteggia fracture). If closed reduction cannot be achieved or maintained, open reduction and internal fixation of the ulnar fracture should be carried out.

Fracture of the shaft of the ulna distal to the insertion of the pronator teres is apt to be complicated by angulation. The proximal end of the distal fragment is displaced toward the radius by the pronator quadratus muscle.

An oblique fracture cleft creates an unstable mechanism with a tendency toward displacement, and immobilization in a plaster cast is not reliable. Open reduction and rigid internal fixation are indicated.

Open reduction of uncomplicated fracture of the ulna in children is rarely justifiable because accurate reduction is not imperative; in children under 12 an angular deformity as great as 15 degrees may be corrected by growth. Torsional displacement of uncomplicated fractures of shaft is not likely to occur. Deformity caused by transverse displacement will be corrected by growth and remodeling.

C. FRACTURE OF THE SHAFT OF THE RADIUS. Isolated fracture of the shaft of the radius can be caused by direct or indirect violence; open fracture usually results from penetrating injury. Closed fracture with displacement is usually associated with other injury (e.g., fracture of the ulna or dislocation of the distal radioulnar joint). Radiographs may not reveal dislocation, but localized tenderness and swelling suggest injury to the distal radioulnar joint.

If the fracture is *proximal to the insertion of the pronator teres,* closed reduction is indicated. The extremity should then be immobilized in a plaster cast which extends from the axilla to the metacarpophalangeal joints, with the elbow at a right angle and the forearm in full supination.

If the fracture is *distal to the insertion of the pronator teres,* the forearm should be in midrotation rather than full supination. Because injury to the distal radioulnar joint is apt to be associated with fracture of the radial shaft below the insertion of the pronator teres, weekly anteroposterior and lateral radiographs should be taken during the first month.

If the configuration of the fracture cleft is *transverse rather than oblique,* displacement is less apt to take place following anatomic reduction. In the adult, if stability cannot be achieved or if reduction is not close to anatomic, open reduction and internal fixation are recommended because deformity due to malunion is likely to cause limitation of forearm and hand movements. Open reduction with rigid internal fixation has the added advantage of permitting early range of motion exercises for the elbow and wrist. Children <12 years are likely to recover function provided that torsional displacement has been corrected and angulation does not exceed 15 degrees. Especially if it is convex anteriorly, angulation >15 degrees should be corrected in children even if open reduction is required.

D. FRACTURE OF THE SHAFTS OF BOTH BONES. The management of fractures of the shafts of both bones of the forearm is essentially a combination of those technics which have been described for the individual bones. If both bones are fractured at the same time, dislocation of either radioulnar joint is not likely to occur. If the configuration of the fracture cleft is approximately transverse, stability can be attained by closed methods provided reduction is anatomic or nearly so. Oblique or comminuted fractures are unstable.

Treatment depends in part upon the degree of displacement, the severity of comminution, and the age of the patient.

1. Without displacement. In adults, fracture of the shaft of the radius and ulna without displacement can be treated by immobilization in a tubular plaster cast extending from the axilla to the metacarpophalangeal joints with the elbow at a right angle and the forearm in supination (fractures of the upper third) or midposition (fractures of the mid and lower thirds).

2. Greenstick fractures of both bones of the forearm are common in children. With fractures of the lower third in children <12, if angulation is >15 degrees or if the apex is directed anteriorly, deformity should be corrected.

Angulated greenstick fractures of both bones proximal to the distal third of the shaft have a tendency toward increased deformity if not adequately reduced. Complete the fracture by reversing the direction of angulation until a palpable "give" occurs, indicating that intact bone on the convex surface has been ruptured.

3. With displacement. It is not always possible to anatomically correct displaced fractures of both bones of the forearm by closed methods, but an attempt should be made in adults and children if radiographic studies show a configuration whereby stabilization can be accomplished without operation. Manipulative reduction is recommended if the patient is treated soon after injury and overriding is >1 cm. It is essential that good apposition of the fragments of each bone be obtained.

If treatment is delayed until hemorrhage and swelling have caused induration of the soft tissues, or if overriding is >1 cm, sustained traction may be necessary to overcome shortening. Because prolonged traction on the skin with countertraction on soft tissues is hazardous owing to the possibility of decubiti or vascular injury, skeletal traction may be indicated. When correction of the overriding is demonstrated by radiography, the fragments are manipulated into position under local or general anesthesia.

Persistent overriding without angulation in young children

is not a problem because 0.5 cm of shortening may be corrected by growth. In adolescents and adults, if accurate apposition of fragments or stability cannot be achieved in fractures of both bones, open reduction and internal fixation are recommended. Persistent displacement, particularly excessive rotational or angulatory malalignment, of one or both bones may be associated with delay of healing, restriction of forearm movements, derangement of the radioulnar joints, and deformity.

E. FRACTURE-DISLOCATIONS OF THE RADIUS AND ULNA

1. Fracture of ulna with dislocation of radial head (Monteggia's fracture). Fracture of the ulna, especially when it occurs near the junction of the middle and upper thirds of the shaft, may be complicated by dislocation of the radial head. This unstable fracture-dislocation is categorized commonly under three types. When the radial head is dislocated anteriorly, angulation at the ulnar fracture site is convex in the same direction (type I). In type II, posterior dislocation of the radial head is accompanied by posterior convex angulation at the fracture site of the ulna. The type III lesion—lateral dislocation of the radial head with fracture of the ulna in its proximal third, distal to the coronoid process—is rare. All three types occur in both children and adults.

a. Anterior dislocation of the head of the radius can be caused by direct violence upon the dorsum of the forearm, and it may also be caused by forced pronation. The annular ligament may be torn, or the head may be displaced distally from beneath the annular ligament without causing a significant tear. The injured ligament may be interposed between the articular surface of the head of the radius and the capitellum of the humerus or the adjacent ulna.

Adequate reduction can usually be achieved by closed manipulation in children and sometimes in adults. A posterior plaster splint is applied from the axillary fold to the heads of the metacarpals with the elbow at 110-130 degrees of flexion and the forearm either in midrotation or slight supination. If reduction is satisfactory, the extremity is elevated and observed frequently for signs of circulatory embarrassment for at least 72 hours. Bandages must be adjusted at appropriate intervals to accommodate for changes of soft-tissue swelling which may embarrass circulation soon after reduction and later may cause displacement of the splint and loss of reduction. In children, immobilization is usually carried out for a period of 4-6 weeks.

b. Posterior dislocation of the head of the radius.
This lesion is caused by direct violence to the volar surface of
the forearm. Treatment is by closed reduction. A tubular plaster cast or stout posterior splint is applied from the metacarpal
heads to the axilla with the elbow in full extension and the forearm in midposition. Careful postreduction observation is essential.

c. Open reduction. In children if accurate reduction of
the fracture and the dislocation cannot be achieved and maintained by closed methods, open reduction and internal fixation
with plaster immobilization are indicated until bone healing is
well under way. In adults, open reduction and internal fixation
of the ulnar fracture are usually carried out. Open reduction of
the radial head dislocation is performed only if closed reduction fails, usually owing to interposition of the annular ligament.

**2. Fracture of the shaft of the radius with dislocation
of the ulnar head.** In fracture of the shaft of the radius near
the junction of the middle and lower thirds with dislocation of
the head of the ulna (Galeazzi's fracture), the apex of major
angulation is usually directed anteriorly while the ulnar head
lies volar to the distal end of the radius. (Convex dorsal angulation with the ulnar head posterior to the lower end of the radius is rare.)

a. Closed reduction. Anatomic alignment is difficult to
obtain by closed manipulation and difficult to maintain in plaster, but these technics should be tried before open reduction is
used. Immobilization is carried out in a long-arm cast with the
forearm in supination.

b. Open reduction. If anatomic reduction cannot be
achieved by closed methods, open reduction and internal fixation are recommended.

VI. INJURIES OF THE WRIST REGION

A. SPRAINS OF THE WRIST. Isolated severe sprain of the
ligaments of the wrist joint is not common, and the diagnosis
of wrist sprain should not be made until other lesions, e.g.,
injury to the lower radial epiphysis (in children), complete tears
of carpal ligaments, and carpal fractures and dislocations (in
adults), have been ruled out. If symptoms persist for more than
2 weeks, especially if pain and swelling are present, repeat radiographic examination should be carried out.

Treatment of a simple sprain may be by immobilization with a volar splint extending from the palmar flexion crease to the proximal forearm. The splint should be attached with elastic bandages so that it can be removed several times daily for gentle active exercises and warm soaks.

B. COLLES' FRACTURE encompasses a variety of complete fractures of the distal radius characterized by convex volar angulation and by varying degrees of dorsal displacement of the distal fragment. The fracture cleft may be transverse or oblique; it may be comminuted, and may extend into the radiocarpal joint. Displacement is often minimal, with dorsal impaction and volar convex angulation. As displacement becomes more marked, dorsal and radial tilt of the distal fragment causes increased angulation and rotational displacement in supination of the distal fragment. The normal volar and ulnar inclination of the carpal articular surface of the radius is reduced or reversed.

Avulsion of the styloid process is the usual injury to the distal ulna. Extension of the fracture cleft into the ulnar notch may injure the distal radioulnar articulation. The carpus is displaced with the distal fragment of the radius. Marked displacement at the fracture site causes dislocation of the distal radioulnar and ulnocarpal articulations, and tearing of the triangular fibrocartilage, both radioulnar ligaments, and the volar ulnocarpal ligament. If the ulnar styloid is not fractured, the collateral ulnar fragment may be torn. The head of the ulna lies anterior to the distal fragment of the radius.

1. Symptoms and signs. Clinical findings vary according to magnitude of injury, degree of displacement of fragments, and interval since injury.

2. Complications. Derangement of the distal radioulnar joint is the most common complicating injury. Direct injury to the median nerve by bone spicules is not common. Compression of the nerve by hemorrhage and edema or by displaced bone fragments is frequent and may cause all gradations of sensory and motor paralysis. Initial treatment of the fracture by immobilization of the wrist in acute flexion can be a significant factor in aggravation of compression. Persistent compression of the nerve creates classic symptoms of carpal tunnel syndrome. Other complicating injuries are fractures involving the scaphoid, the head of the radius, or the capitellum.

3. Treatment. Complete recovery of function and a pleasing cosmetic result are goals which cannot always be achieved. Patient's age, sex, and occupation, presence of complicating injury or disease, severity of comminution, and the configuration of the fracture cleft govern the selection of treatment.

Open reduction of recent closed Colles' fracture is rarely indicated. Many technics of closed reduction and external immobilization have been advocated; the experience and preference of the surgeon determine the choice.

a. Minor displacement. Colles' fracture with minimal displacement is characterized by absence of comminution and slight dorsal impaction. Deformity is barely perceptible or may not be visible even to the trained observer. In the elderly patient, treatment is directed toward early recovery of function. In young patients, prevention of further displacement is the first consideration.

Reduction is not necessary. The wrist is immobilized for 3-5 days in a volar plaster splint extending from the distal palmar flexion crease to the elbow. Thereafter the splint may be removed periodically (several times daily) to permit active exercise of the wrist.

b. Marked displacement. Early reduction and immobilization are indicated. When reduction has been delayed until preliminary healing is advanced, open reduction may be elected or correction of the deformity can be deferred until healing is sound. Malunion is corrected by osteotomy and bone grafting.

In the elderly with complicating arthritis, when impaction causes stability, the mild deformity may be accepted in favor of early restoration of function.

(1) *Stable fractures.* Colles' fracture is characterized by comminution of the dorsal cortex. Correction of the deformity creates a wedge-shaped area of fragmented and impacted cancellous bone. Base of the wedge is directed dorsally, and there is no buttress to prevent recurrence of displacement. Stability is partly attained by bringing the volar cortices of fragments into anatomic apposition.

A lightly padded tubular cast extending above the elbow or a "sugar tong" splint is preferred. The plaster should extend distally only to the palmar flexion crease, with the forearm in midposition and the wrist in slight volar flexion and ulnar deviation. In obese patients, immobilization is more reliable if the elbow is included in the plaster.

(2) *Unstable fractures.* If radiographs show extensive comminution with intraarticular extension and involvement of the volar cortex, the fracture is likely to be un-

stable and skeletal distraction is probably indicated. Partially threaded or smooth pins are placed distal to the fracture through the metacarpals and proximal to it through the radius or ulna. These pins may be incorporated in a long-arm plaster cast or, alternatively, they may be fastened to an external fixator. The wires are left in place for 6-8 weeks. Following removal of the pins, the fracture is protected for an additional 2-4 weeks by a short-arm cast or a "sugar tong" splint.

4. Complications and sequelae. Joint stiffness is the most disabling sequel of Colles' fracture. Derangement of the distal radioulnar joint may be caused by the original injury and perpetuated by incomplete reduction; it is characterized by restriction of forearm movements and pain. Late rupture of the extensor policis longus tendon is relatively uncommon. Symptoms of median nerve injury due to compression caused by acute swelling alone usually do not persist more than 6 months. Failure to perform shoulder and elbow joint exercises several times daily can result in disabling stiffness.

C. SMITH'S FRACTURE (REVERSED COLLES'). The fracture site of the radius is 1-2.5 cm above the wrist joint in this lesion. The normal volar concavity of the lower radius is accentuated because the apex of angulation at the fracture site is posterior. The ulnar head is prominent dorsally, and there may be derangement of the inferior radioulnar joint. This lesion should be differentiated from Barton's fracture-dislocation.

The fracture can be reduced by closed manipulation and immobilized with the wrist in neutral position. Unstable fractures may require initial skeletal distraction (see unstable Colles' fracture above). Fractures which cannot be reduced adequately by closed methods may require open reduction and bone plating.

D. FRACTURE OF THE RADIAL STYLOID. Forced radial deviation of the hand at the wrist joint can fracture the radial styloid. A large fragment of the styloid is usually displaced by impingement against the carpal navicular. Avulsion of the tip of the styloid by the radial collateral ligament may occur as well, and may be associated with scapholunate dissociation. If the fragment is large, it can be displaced farther by brachioradialis muscle which inserts into it.

Because the fracture is intraarticular, reduction of large fragments should be anatomic. If the styloid fragment is not displaced, immobilization in a short-arm cast for 3 weeks is sufficient. If the fragment is displaced, manipulative reduction should be tried. If the distal, smaller fragment tends to displace but can be apposed by digital pressure, percutaneous fixation can be achieved by a medium Kirschner wire inserted through the proximal anatomic snuffbox so as to transfix both fragments. The wrist is then immobilized in a snugly molded short-arm cast for 6 weeks.

If closed methods fail, open reduction is indicated because persistent displacement is likely to cause posttraumatic degenerative arthritis.

E. FRACTURE OF THE DISTAL RADIAL EPIPHYSIS. Fracture through the distal radial physis in children is the counterpart of Colles' fracture in the adult. Wrist sprain is rare in childhood and should be differentiated as early as possible from fracture of the distal epiphysis. Such an injury is usually caused by indirect violence due to a fall on the outstretched hand. The magnitude of displacement of the epiphyseal fragment varies.

In some cases, separation and displacement of the epiphysis cannot be demonstrated by radiologic studies and may be quite difficult to identify on clinical examination. The patient may complain of pain in the region of the wrist joint, and slight swelling may be present. Pressure with a blunt object, e.g., the eraser of a pencil, may demonstrate maximal tenderness at the physis instead of at the wrist joint. Buckling of adjacent metaphyseal cortex manifests greater displacement. Displacement is posterior and to the radial side. Marked displacement may be accompanied by crushing of the physis, tear of the triangular fibrocartilage of the distal radioulnar articulation, displacement of the distal ulnar epiphysis, or avulsion of the ulnar styloid.

Both wrists should be radiographed if injury to distal radial physis is suspected. Severe injury, crushing physeal cartilage and fracturing the epiphysis, is likely to impede growth and may even lead to early physeal fusion; continued growth at the distal ulnar physis produces derangement of distal radioulnar joint.

Open reduction is rarely necessary. The trauma of the operation superimposed on the injury is likely to cause early arrest of physeal growth. Closed reduction by manipulation is usually successful if it can be done within the week following injury. A long-arm cast is used for immobilization.

F. FRACTURE-DISLOCATIONS OF THE RADIOCARPAL JOINT. Dislocation of the radiocarpal joint without fracture is rare. Fracture-dislocation of the wrist joint most commonly involves the posterior or anterior margin of the articular surface of the radius. Dislocation without injury to one of the carpal bones is usually associated with fracture of the anterior surface of the radius or the ulna. Comminuted fractures of the distal radius may involve either the anterior or posterior cortex and extends into the wrist joint. Subluxation of the carpus may occur at the same time.

1. Anterior fracture-dislocation of the radiocarpal joint (Barton's fracture) is characterized by fracture of the volar margin of the carpal articular surface of the radius. The fracture cleft extends proximally in the coronal plane in an oblique direction, so that the free fragment has a wedge-shaped configuration. The carpus is displaced volar and proximally with the articular fragment. This uncommon injury should be differentiated from Smith's fracture by radiography.

Treatment by closed reduction may be successful, especially in cases in which the free fragment of the radius does not involve a large portion of the articular surface. Immobilization is with a long-arm cast with the wrist in volar flexion and the elbow at a right angle.

2. Posterior fracture-dislocation of the radiocarpal joint should be differentiated from Colles' fracture by radiography. In most cases the marginal fragment is smaller than in anterior injury and often involves the medial aspect where the extensor pollicis longus crosses the distal radius. If reduction is not anatomic, fraying of the tendon at this level may lead to late rupture. Occasionally, this injury may involve fracture of the radial styloid.

Treatment is by manipulative reduction as for Colles' fracture and immobilization in a snug short-arm cast with the wrist in neutral position.

G. DISLOCATION OF THE DISTAL RADIOULNAR JOINT.

The triangular fibrocartilage is the most important structure in preventing dislocation of the distal radioulnar joint. The accessory ligaments and pronator quadratus muscles play a secondary role. Complete anterior or posterior dislocation implies both a tear of the triangular fibrocartilage and disruption of accessory joint ligaments. Tearing of the triangular fibrocartilage in the absence of major injury to the supporting capsular ligaments causes subluxation or abnormal laxity of the joint. Because the ulnar attachment of the triangular fibrocartilage is at the base of the styloid process, radiographs may demonstrate associated fracture. Diastasis of the radius and ulna is demonstrated by widening of the distal radioulnar joint by radiography compared with the opposite side.

Complete anterior or posterior dislocation of the distal radioulnar joint is rare. Medial dislocation is associated with fracture of the radius. The direction of dislocation is indicated by the location of the ulnar head in relation to the distal end of the radius.

H. FRACTURES AND DISLOCATIONS OF THE CARPUS.
Injury to the carpal bones and ligaments occurs predominantly in men during the most active period of life. Because it is difficult to differentiate these injuries by clinical examination, it is imperative to obtain radiographs of the best possible quality. Anteroposterior views in neutral and in maximum radial and ulnar deviation are necessary as well as lateral views in neutral position. Special views may be necessary such as anteroposterior views in midsupination to demonstrate the pisiform. Carpal tunnel views for the hamate may be necessary.

1. Fracture of the scaphoid is the most common injury to the carpus and should be suspected in any injury to the wrist in an adult male unless a specific diagnosis of another type of injury is obvious. If tenderness on the radial aspect of the wrist in the anatomic snuffbox is present and fracture cannot be demonstrated, initial treatment should be the same as if fracture were present (see below) and should be continued for at least 2-3 weeks. Repeat radiographic examination after this period may demonstrate an occult fracture.

Three types of fracture are distinguished:

a. Fracture of the tubercle is generally not widely displaced, and healing is generally prompt if immobilization in a thumb spica cast is maintained for 4-6 weeks.

b. Fracture through the waist is most common. Blood supply to the proximal fragment is usually not disturbed, and healing takes place if reduction is adequate and treatment is instituted early. If the nutrient artery to the proximal third is injured, ischemic necrosis of that portion of bone may occur.

Radiographic examination in multiple projections is necessary to determine the direction of the fracture cleft and displacement of the proximal fragment. If the proximal fragment is displaced, it can be reduced under local anesthesia by forced dorsiflexion and radial deviation of the wrist. Immobilization in a cast gauntlet with the wrist in slight dorsiflexion is necessary. The cast should extend distally to the palmar flexion crease in the hand and to the base of the thumbnail. Many authorities emphasize that a long-arm cast provides more secure immobilization by restricting forearm pronation and supination. If reduction has been anatomic and blood supply to the proximal fragment has not been jeopardized, adequate bone healing can be expected in 10-12 weeks. Such healing must be demonstrated by the disappearance of the fracture cleft and restoration of the trabecular pattern between the two main fragments. Radiodensity of the proximal fragment in relation to adjacent bone is indicative of osteonecrosis.

c. Fracture through the proximal third of the scaphoid is likely to be associated with ischemic necrosis of the minor fragment. If the diagnosis is made soon after injury, reduction and immobilization in a thumb spica cast promote healing. Radiographs should be taken monthly to determine the progress of bone healing; it may be necessary to prolong immobilization for 4-6 months. The same criteria of radiographic examination as are used for healing of fractures through the waist are used in fractures of the proximal third.

If evidence of healing is not apparent after immobilization for 6 months, further immobilization probably will not be effective. This is especially true if radiographs show that the fracture cleft has widened and if sclerosis is noted adjacent to the cleft. If the interval between time of injury and establishment of a diagnosis is 3 months or more, a trial of immobilization for 2-3 months may be elected. If obliteration of the fracture cleft and evidence of bone continuity are not visible in radiographs after this trial period, some form of operative treatment such as bone grafting is necessary to initiate healing.

If ischemic necrosis had occurred in the proximal fragment, bone grafting is less likely to be successful. Although excision of the avascular fragment may relieve painful symptoms for a time, the patient usually notes weakness of grasp and discomfort after prolonged use.

Prolonged failure of bone healing predisposes to posttraumatic arthritis. Bone grafting operations or other procedures to promote union may be successful, but arthritis causes continued disability. Arthrodesis of the wrist gives the best assurance of relief of pain and a functionally competent extremity.

2. Fracture of the lunate may be manifested by minor avulsion fractures of the posterior or anterior horn. Careful multiplane radiographic examination is necessary to establish the diagnosis. Either of these lesions may be treated by the use of a volar splint for 3 weeks.

Fracture of the body may be manifested by a crack, by comminution, or by impaction. A fissure fracture can be treated by immobilization in a cast.

Complications include persistent pain in the wrist, slight

restriction of motion, and tenderness over the lunate. Radiographic examination may demonstrate areas of sclerosis and rarefaction. Impaction or collapse can be accompanied by arthritic changes surrounding the lunate. This radiographic appearance is referred to as Kienböck's disease, osteochondrosis of the lunate, or ischemic necrosis.

3. Fracture of the hamate may occur through the body and is shown on radiographs as a fissure or compression. Fracture of the base of the hamulus is less common and more difficult to diagnose; special projections are necessary to demonstrate the cleft. Direct trauma involved in specific activities such as swinging a baseball bat typically causes this injury. If the hamulus is displaced, closed manipulation is not effective. Prolonged painful symptoms or evidence of irritation of the ulnar nerve may require excision of the loose fragment.

4. Fracture of the triquetrum is caused commonly by direct violence and is often associated with fracture of other carpal bones. Treatment is by immobilization in a plaster cast.

5. Ligamentous injuries of the carpus. Forced dorsiflexion of the wrist may result in dislocation of the lunate, either alone or in combination with the proximal pole of the scaphoid (perilunate dislocation). These injuries must be differentiated from simple wrist sprain because, when unrecognized, they may result in chronic wrist joint instability and pain. Occasionally, such ligamentous injuries are associated with fractures, most notably of the scaphoid (transscaphoid perilunate dislocation). Radiographs demonstrate soft tissue swelling, abnormal relationships between individual carpal bones, and associated fractures (particularly of the radial styloid, capitate, or scaphoid). Anteroposterior views of the carpus, particularly with the fist clenched, may demonstrate increased distance between the scaphoid and lunate, revealing scapholunate dissociation. Most authorities agree that early recognition of these injuries and prompt, accurate reduction of the dislocated or fractured carpal bones yield the best long-term results. If proper reduction cannot be obtained or maintained, surgical treatment is indicated.

VII. FRACTURES OF THE PELVIS

Fractures of the pelvis may vary in severity from relatively low-energy, stable injuries to those resulting from high-energy forces. The latter injuries are frequently unstable and may be associated with damage to the blood vessels and abdominal viscera. For this reason, management of complex, high-energy pelvic fractures is best carried out by a team of surgical specialists who are able to coordinate the care of the various injuries.

Fractures of the pelvis associated with central dislocation of the hip are discussed in the following section. There is great variability in pattern in the other pelvic fractures; some of the most common fracture patterns are discussed below.

A. AVULSION FRACTURES OF THE PELVIS include those involving the anterior superior and anterior inferior iliac spines, a portion of the iliac crest apophysis anteriorly, and the apophysis of the ischium. The ischial apophysis may be avulsed indirectly. If displacement is minimal, prompt healing without disability is to be expected. If displacement is marked (i.e., >1 cm), reattachment by open operation is justifiable.

B. FRACTURE OF THE WING OF THE ILIUM. Isolated fracture without involvement of the hip or sacroiliac joints most often occurs as a result of direct trauma. With minor displacement of the free fragment, soft-tissue injury is usually minimal and treatment is symptomatic. Wide displacement of the free fragment may be associated with extensive soft-tissue injury and hematoma formation. Healing may be accompanied by ossification of the hematoma with exuberant new bone formation.

C. ISOLATED FRACTURE OF THE OBTURATOR RING involving either pubis or ischium with minimal displacement is associated with little or no injury to sacroiliac joints. This is also true of minor subluxation of the symphysis pubis. Initial treatment consists of bedrest for a few days followed by ambulation on crutches. A sacroiliac belt or pelvic binder may give additional comfort. When discomfort disappears, unsupported weight-bearing may be permitted.

D. COMPLEX FRACTURES OF THE PELVIC RING are due either to direct violence or to force transmitted indirectly through the lower extremities. They are characterized by disruption of the pelvic ring at two points: (1) anteriorly, near the symphysis pubis, manifested either by dislocation of that joint or by fracture through the body of the pubis, by unilateral or bilateral fracture through the obturator ring, or by fracture through the acetabulum; and (2) disruption of the pelvic ring through or in the vicinity of the sacroiliac joint. The disruption can extend partially through the sacroiliac joint as a dislocation and extend into sacrum or adjacent ilium as a fracture. Magnitude of displacement injuries is often associated with extensive hemorrhage into the soft tissues or injury to the bladder, urethra, or intraabdominal organs. When anterior and posterior disruptions are ipsilateral, the entire involved hemipelvis and extremity may be displaced proximally. Anterior disruption may occur on one side and posterior disruption on the opposite side with wide opening of the pelvic ring.

When severe and complex fractures of the pelvic ring are suspected, the extent of associated injuries must be determined at once by physical and radiographic examination. Shock due to blood loss may be present. Treatment of the fracture by reduction should not be instituted until the extent of associated injuries has been determined. Treatment of some of those injuries may be more urgent than that of the fracture lesion. A careful search must be made for possible injury to bowel, bladder, ureters, and major blood vessels.

If displacement and soft tissue injury are minimal, a pelvic sling to facilitate nursing care may be all that is required. When the hemipelvis has been displaced proximally, skeletal traction on the distal end of the femur on the affected side with suspension of the extremity may permit reduction.

If the sacroiliac joint has been dislocated and the ilium is rotated posterior to the sacrum, with opening of the anterior fracture, closed reduction can be attempted. Postmanipulation maintenance of reduction is accomplished by a pelvic sling, a short bilateral thigh spica, or an external fixature. Orthopedic traumatologists advocate surgical fixation of unstable pelvic fractures in multiply injured patients to permit more rapid mobilization, thus avoiding the complications of prolonged bedrest.

VIII. INJURIES OF THE HIP REGION

A. BIRTH FRACTURE OF THE UPPER FEMORAL PHYSES is rare, and diagnosis by physical examination alone is difficult because the skeletal structures involved are deeply situated. Swelling of upper thigh and pseudoparalysis of the extremity following a difficult delivery suggest injury. Radiography may demonstrate proximal and lateral displacement of shaft of femur. Formation of new bone in the region of metaphysis may be demonstrated in 7-10 days. If displacement has occurred, treatment for 2-3 weeks by Bryant's traction is recommended. Alternatively protection by perineal pillow splint for 2-3 weeks may be adequate.

B. DISPLACEMENT AND SEPARATION OF THE CAPITAL FEMORAL EPIPHYSES. Displacement of the capital femoral epiphysis due to trauma in the normal child should be differentiated from idiopathic slipped epiphysis (epiphysiolysis, adolescent coxa vara). However, between the ages of 10 and 16 years, differentiation may be impossible. Mild injury may cause sudden separation and displacement because of weakening of the physis by antecedent disturbance of cartilage growth.

Traumatic separation of the capital femoral epiphysis is rare in normal children, but it may occur as a result of a single episode of severe trauma that otherwise might cause fracture of the femoral neck. Direction of displacement is likely to be the same as in adolescent coxa vara. Although anatomic reduction can be obtained by closed manipulation, immobilization in a plaster spica should not be trusted because redisplacement is possible; internal fixation is more reliable. Traumatic separation of the capital physis associated with dislocation of the hip joint (epiphysis and proximal femur) is a rare lesion with an unfavorable prognosis. Ischemic necrosis of the epiphysis is almost certain.

C. FRACTURE OF THE FEMORAL NECK occurs most commonly in patients over the age of 50. Weakening of bone due to senile osteoporosis or, less commonly, to metastatic disease may predispose to fracture. In contrast, femoral neck fractures in the young result from high-energy trauma and may involve extensive disruption of the blood supply to the femoral head. If displacement has occurred, the extremity usually is externally rotated, adducted, and slightly shortened. Movement of the hip joint causes pain. If the fragments are not displaced and the fracture is stable, pain at the extremes of passive hip motion may be the only significant finding. The fact that the patient can actively move the extremity often interferes with prompt diagnosis.

Before treatment is instituted, anteroposterior and lateral films of excellent quality must be obtained. Gentle traction and internal rotation of the extremity while the anteroposterior film is exposed may demonstrate more clearly the direction of the fracture cleft. When femoral neck fracture is suspected but not clearly demonstrated on radiography, other studies such as CT scan, bone scan, or MRI may provide the diagnosis.

Fractures of the femoral neck may be classified either according to the orientation of the fracture or to the degree of displacement as abduction or adduction.

1. Valgus impacted fracture of the femoral neck. Valgus describes the relationship between the neck and shaft fragment and the head. These fractures occur most often in the proximal femoral neck adjacent to the head. Displacement is apt to be minimal, and impaction is often present. The direction of the fracture cleft approaches the transverse plane of the body, and the angle is 30 degrees or less. The anteroposterior radiograph may show a wedge-shaped area of increased density. A good lateral film demonstrates both the anterior and posterior cortices of the femoral neck. In this plane the neck and shaft fragment may be angulated slightly, so that only the posterior cortex appears to be impacted and the anterior cortices of the fragments appear to be separated.

Impaction is precarious and undependable as a fixation mechanism; if internal fixation is not used, loss of position may occur before healing is sound. If firm impaction can be demonstrated in both the anterior and posterior radiographs, some surgeons recommend conservative treatment, i.e., bedrest followed by non–weight-bearing ambulation. Full weight-bearing is not permitted until complete healing can be demonstrated by radiography (usually 4-12 months after injury). Other surgeons prefer internal fixation because it prevents displacement and permits the patient to be out of bed soon after the operation; however, even unsupported weight-bearing is not permitted any sooner than after nonoperative treatment.

2. Displaced fractures of the femoral neck are characterized by coxa vara deformity. The fracture may be at any level of the neck. A vertical configuration of the fracture line favors proximal displacement of the distal fragment. The fracture should be considered unstable if the angle between the fracture cleft and the transverse plane of the body is >30 degrees. Marked displacement almost always involves comminution of the posterior neck with varying degrees of impaction and loss of bone volume.

This can be a life-endangering injury, especially when it occurs in elderly persons. Treatment is directed toward the preservation of life and restoration of function to the hip joint. In most cases, when the life expectancy of the patient is more than a few weeks, surgery is the treatment of choice. Immobilization of this unstable fracture requires prolonged recumbency with constant nursing care and is associated with more numerous complications than early mobilization. Some surgeons believe that immediate operative treatment is required after fracture; others believe that 1-2 days of evaluation of the general health status of the patient leads to a lower mortality rate. Operative treatment usually consists of either closed reduction and internal fixation or primary prosthetic arthroplasty.

a. Internal fixation. The goal is to preserve the head fragment by attaining stable bony contact and thus to promote healing. A major objective is to allow the patient as much general physical activity during healing as is compatible with the mechanics of fixation. In order to permit necessary preoperative medical evaluation of the patient when internal fixation is elected, initial treatment may be by balanced suspension, skeletal traction, and prompt closed reduction of the fracture. Persistent displacement may cause further compromise of the retinacular blood supply to the articular fragment.

Anatomic or near anatomic reduction and firm fixation are desirable to provide optimal circumstances for bone healing. Comminution at the fracture site, injury to the retinacular blood supply of the capital fragment, excessive stressing of the fracture site by early weight-bearing, and insecure fixation are some of the factors that lead to failure.

The variety of surgical technics and the many fixation appliances available testify to the multiplicity of problems that can be encountered and the variability of opinion concerning treatment. When the fragments are undisplaced or minimally displaced, closed reduction is unnecessary. When displacement occurs, reduction may be obtained by closed means as a preliminary step to fixation or can be accomplished by surgical exposure of the fracture site. Fixation apparatus may consist of multiple pins applied percutaneously or of larger implants that require more exposure. After operation, the patient may be free in bed and mobilized at an early date. To salvage the operative effort if fixation is precarious, traction in balanced suspension or immobilization in a plaster spica for 1-4 months may be necessary until preliminary healing gives additional stability.

Depending upon the relative security of fixation, the extent of weight-bearing must be regulated until bone continuity is restored to the point where displacement of fragments is unlikely. The agile and cooperative patient may be ambulatory on crutches (but within the limitations of acceptable weight-bearing) within a few days after operative treatment. Crutch walking is hazardous in elderly patients because inadvertent loading may disrupt the fracture site.

b. Primary arthroplasty. In selecting primary arthroplasty, the surgeon elects to sacrifice the head fragment either because of extensive injury to the blood supply or because of extensively diseased bone as in pathologic fractures. In some cases, the goal is to permit early unrestricted weight-bearing. When the acetabulum is undamaged or is not the site of preexisting disease, the commonly accepted technic is cemented hemiarthroplasty. In the rare circumstance when there is pre-existing degenerative change in the acetabulum, total joint replacement may be justified.

The most common complications of femoral neck fracture are loss of reduction after reduction and internal fixation, nonunion, and ischemic osteonecrosis of the head fragment. Secondary osteoarthritis (posttraumatic arthritis) may appear later with or without the sequelae mentioned above.

3. Femoral neck fracture in childhood (rare) must be differentiated from congenital coxa vara. Traumatic fracture is usually caused by severe injury. Anatomic reduction should be obtained either by closed or open means. Internal fixation with pins or screws prevents displacement and permits increased mobility. Osteonecrosis of capital epiphysis is a frequent sequela.

D. TROCHANTERIC FRACTURES

1. Fracture of lesser trochanter is quite rare as an isolated injury but may result from the avulsion force of the iliopsoas muscle. It occurs most commonly as a component of intertrochanteric fracture.

2. Fracture of greater trochanter may be caused by direct injury, or indirectly as an avulsion by forceful contraction of the gluteus medius and minimus muscles. It occurs most commonly not in isolation but rather as a component of intertrochanteric fracture.

If displacement is <1 cm and there is no tendency to further displacement (determined by repeated radiographic examinations), treatment may be by bedrest until acute pain subsides. As rapidly as symptoms permit, activity is increased gradually to partial weight-bearing with crutches. Full weight-bearing is permitted as soon as healing is apparent, usually in 6-8 weeks. If displacement is >1 cm and increases on adduction of the thigh, extensive tearing of surrounding soft tissues may be assumed and open reduction and internal fixation are indicated.

3. Intertrochanteric fractures occur most commonly among the elderly. The cleft of an intertrochanteric fracture extends upward and outward from the medial region of the junction of the neck and lesser trochanter toward the summit of the greater trochanter. Comminution, when present, typically involves the lesser and greater trochanters.

It is important both to determine whether comminution has occurred and to assess the magnitude of displacement. These fractures may vary from a simple two-part fracture without significant displacement to ones with severe comminution. Severely comminuted fractures are composed of four major fragments: head-neck, greater trochanter, lesser trochanter, and shaft. Displacement may be so marked that the head-neck fragment forms a right angle with the shaft fragment and the distal fragment is rotated externally 90 degrees.

Non-union in intertrochanteric fractures is unlikely. The factors that may adversely affect healing are osteopenia, comminution, incomplete reduction, and inadequate immobilization. Malunion (varus and external rotation) is abetted by major forces that cause displacement (gravity and muscle activity).

Initial treatment of the fracture in the hospital can be by balanced suspension and, when indicated, by the addition of traction. The selection of definitive treatment depends in part upon the general condition of the patient. Because intertrochanteric fracture is most likely to occur in the elderly, significant concurrent medical problems may have a great effect on the outcome of fracture treatment. Some surgeons believe that delay in open treatment is hazardous to the life of the patient, and they prefer to operate promptly. Others believe that a thorough evaluation of the general health status of the patient should be made and that preliminary treatment of the fracture—reduction by closed technics—can proceed simultaneously.

Although most surgeons favor operative treatment of intertrochanteric fractures whenever feasible, undisplaced fractures can be treated in selected cases by balanced suspension of the lower extremity until the fragments are stabilized by preliminary bone healing. These fractures can also be treated initially by immobilization in a plaster spica. Sufficient healing generally occurs within 2-3 months to permit the patient to progress from a bed and wheelchair regimen to partial weight-bearing with crutches. Unsupported weight-bearing should not be resumed until the fracture cleft has filled with callus.

If comminution is present and displacement is significant, early reduction and immobilization can be provided by skeletal traction prior to operation. If reduction of the fracture has not been accomplished by preliminary traction, it is carried out at the time of surgery. Some surgeons prefer not to anatomically reduce unstable fractures caused by comminution of the medial femoral cortex (calcar). They maintain that medial displacement of the upper end of the main distal fragment enhances mechanical stability and permits earlier weight-bearing and more prompt healing. The chief intent of open operation is to provide sufficient fixation of the fragments by a metallic surgical implant so that the patient need not be confined to bed during the healing process.

Intertrochanteric fracture during childhood can be treated by skeletal traction with a Kirschner wire inserted through the lower femur above the physis or by closed reduction and internal fixation. Varus deformity should be avoided.

E. SUBTROCHANTERIC FRACTURE due to severe trauma below the level of lesser trochanter at the junction of cancellous and cortical bone is most common in men during active years of life. Soft tissue damage is extensive. The direction of the fracture cleft may be transverse or oblique. Comminution occurs and the fracture may extend proximally into the intertrochanteric region or distally into the shaft.

Closed reduction should be attempted by continuous traction to bring the distal fragment into alignment with the proximal fragment. If comminution is not extensive and the lesser trochanter is not detached, the proximal fragment is often drawn into relative flexion, external rotation, and abduction by the predominant activity of the iliopsoas, and gluteus medius and minimus muscles.

Interposition of soft tissue between the major fragments may prevent adequate reduction by closed technics. In adults, subtrochanteric fractures are usually treated by operative means. Open or closed reduction of the fracture is followed by internal fixation, either with a plate and screw device or, alternatively, with an intramedullary rod adapted to provide rotatory control of the fracture fragments. Activity and weight-bearing are restricted according to the degree of fracture comminution, the rigidity of the internal fixation, and the compliance of the patient. Healing is usually complete by 12-16 weeks.

In skeletally immature patients or occasionally in young adults, skeletal traction by means of a Kirschner wire inserted through the supracondylar region of the femur (with the hip and knee flexed to a right angle) is utilized. Repeat radiographs are carried out periodically until reduction is accomplished. If soft tissue interposition is not a factor, reduction can usually be achieved in 48 hours. Thereafter, the extremity is left in this position with an appropriate amount of traction until stabilization occurs (8-12 weeks). The angle of flexion is then reduced by gradually bringing the hip and knee into extension. After 2-3 months of continuous traction, the extremity can be immobilized in a plaster spica if stabilization of fracture has occurred. Full weight-bearing must not be resumed until radiographs show that bone healing obliterates the fracture cleft.

F. TRAUMATIC DISLOCATIONS OF THE HIP JOINT may occur with or without fracture of the acetabulum or of the proximal femur. This injury is most common during the active years of life and is usually the result of severe trauma unless there is preexisting disease of the femoral head, acetabulum, or neuromuscular system. The head of the femur cannot be completely displaced from the normal acetabulum unless the ligamentum teres is ruptured or deficient because of some unrelated cause. Traumatic dislocations can be classified according to direction of displacement of the femoral head from the acetabulum.

1. Posterior hip dislocation. The head of the femur is usually dislocated posterior to the acetabulum while the thigh is flexed, e.g., as may occur in a head-on automobile collision when the passenger's knee is driven violently against the dashboard. The significant clinical findings are shortening, adduction, and internal rotation of the extremity. Anteroposterior, transpelvic lateral, and, if fracture of the acetabulum is demonstrated, oblique projections are required (CT scan may be helpful). Common complications are fracture of the acetabulum, injury to the sciatic nerve, and fracture of the head or shaft of the femur.

If the acetabulum is not fractured or if the fragment is small, reduction by closed manipulation either by Bigelow's or Stimson's method is indicated.

The success of reduction is determined immediately by anteroposterior and lateral radiographs. Interposition of capsule substance is manifest by widening of the joint space. If reduction is adequate, the hip is stable with the extremity in extension and slight external rotation. If a posterior acetabular rim fracture is present, a CT scan after reduction may be used both to assess fracture alignment and to determine whether free bone fragments are present in the joint space.

Postreduction treatment may be by immobilization in a plaster spica or by balanced suspension. Because this is primarily a soft tissue injury, sound healing should take place in 4 weeks. Opinion differs on when unsupported weight-bearing should be resumed. Some believe that disability caused by ischemic osteonecrosis of the femoral head is less likely when complete weight-bearing is deferred for 6 months after injury; others think early loading is not harmful.

If the posterior or superior acetabulum is fractured, dislocation of the hip must be assumed to have occurred even though displacement is not present at time of examination. Undisplaced fissure fractures may be treated initially by bedrest and avoidance of full weight-bearing for 2 months. Frequent examination is necessary to make certain that the head of the femur has not become displaced from the acetabulum.

Minor fragments of the posterior margin of the acetabulum may be disregarded unless they are in the hip joint cavity. Larger displaced fragments often cannot be reduced adequately by closed methods. If the fragment is large and the hip is unstable following closed manipulation, open operation is indicated. If the sciatic nerve has been injured it should be exposed and carefully protected when the posterior hip joint is exposed. The fragment is then placed in anatomic position and fixed. After the operation the extremity is placed in suspension. If fixation of the acetabular fragment is precarious, supplemental skeletal traction may be necessary to prevent redisplacement of the bone fragment and the femoral head.

2. Anterior hip dislocation. Anterior dislocation of the femoral head is far less common than posterior dislocation. In this injury the head of the femur may lie medially on the obturator membrane, beneath the obturator externus muscle, or, in a somewhat more superior position, beneath the iliopsoas muscle and in contact with the superior ramus of the pubis. The thigh is classically in flexion, abduction, and external rotation, and the head of the femur is palpable anteriorly and distal to the inguinal flexion creases. Anteroposterior and lateral films are required.

Closed manipulation with general anesthesia is usually adequate. Postreduction treatment may be by balanced suspension or by immobilization in a plaster spica with the hip in extension and the extremity in neutral rotation. Active hip motion is permitted after 3 weeks.

3. Central dislocation of the hip with fracture of the pelvis. Central dislocation of the head of the femur with fracture of the acetabulum may be caused by crushing injury or by an axial force transmitted through the abducted extremity to the acetabulum. Comminution is commonly present. There are usually two fragments; superiorly, the ilium with the roof of the acetabulum; inferiorly and medially, the remainder of the acetabulum and the obturator ring. Fracture occurs near the roof of the acetabulum, and components of obturator ring are displaced inward with the head of femur. Extensive soft tissue injury and massive pelvic bleeding are likely. Intraabdominal injury must not be overlooked.

In the absence of, or immediately after, complicating injury has received priority attention, closed treatment of the fracture-dislocation by skeletal traction should be tried. Open reduction is difficult and should be carried out only by those who are familiar with the demanding technics of reduction and internal fixation of pelvic fractures. Bidirectional traction is likely to achieve the most satisfactory results in all but the exceptional case. For the average adult, approximately 10 kg of force is applied axially to the shaft of the femur, in neither abduction nor adduction, through a Kirschner wire placed preferably in the supracondylar region. Lateral traction can be applied to a large cancellous bone screw inserted in the midcoronal plane of the femur, at about the level of the lesser trochanter. Force is applied at a right angle to the direction of axial traction and the magnitude is the same. The extremity is placed in balanced suspension. Progress of reduction is observed by portable radiographs made three times per day until adequate positioning is manifested by relocation of the head of the femur beneath the roof of the acetabulum. Bidirectional traction is maintained for 4-6 weeks. Thereafter, the transverse traction component is gradually diminished under appropriate radiographic control until it can be discontinued. Axial traction is maintained until stabilization of the fracture fragments by early bone healing has occurred, usually about 8 weeks after injury. In the next 4-6 weeks, while balanced suspension is continued, gentle, active exercises of knee and hip are encouraged. After discontinuation of balanced suspension, more elaborate exercises to aid recovery of maximal hip function are performed frequently. Full and unprotected weight-bearing is not advised before 6 months. Recently developed open operative technics of reduction and internal fixation of pelvic fractures avoid malposition of fracture fragments and hasten rehabilitation. The most likely long-term sequelae of central fracture-dislocation are osteonecrosis of the femoral head and secondary osteoarthritis.

IX. FRACTURE OF THE SHAFT OF THE FEMUR

A. IN ADULTS, fracture usually occurs as a result of severe direct trauma. Indirect violence, especially torsional stress, is likely to cause spiral fractures that extend proximally, or, more commonly, distally into the metaphyseal regions. These fractures are likely to be encountered in bone that has become osteopenic as a result of disuse or age. Most are closed fractures;

open fracture is often the result of compounding from within. Extensive soft tissue injury, bleeding, and shock are commonly present.

If the fracture is through the upper third of the shaft, the proximal fragment is apt to be in flexion, external rotation, and abduction, with proximal displacement or overriding of the distal fragment. In mid-shaft fracture direction of displacement is not constant, but the distal fragment is almost always displaced proximally if the fracture is unstable; and angulation is commonly present with the apex directed anterolaterally. In complete fracture of the lower third of the shaft the distal fragment is often displaced proximally; upper end of the distal fragment may be displaced posteriorly to the distal end of the upper fragment.

1. Diagnosis. Hemorrhagic shock is likely to be present. Careful x-ray examination in at least two planes is necessary to determine the exact site and configuration of the fracture line. Emergency splints should be removed either by the surgeon or by a qualified assistant so that manipulation does not cause further damage. The hip and knee should be examined for associated injury.

Injuries to the sciatic nerve and to the superficial femoral artery and vein are not common but must be recognized promptly.

2. Treatment depends on age of patient and the site and configuration of the fracture. Displaced, oblique, spiral, and comminuted fractures are unstable and can rarely be treated successfully by closed manipulation and external plaster fixation. Reduction of the fracture with closed or open intramedullary rodding is usually preferred over closed treatment with skeletal traction.

After preliminary traction, biplane radiographs are made to determine the progress of correction of overriding. If alignment and apposition of fragments are not satisfactory, closed manipulation, preferably under general anesthesia, should be carried out while traction is continued.

If soft tissue interposition prevents reduction by closed methods, open reduction should be carried out in adults to avoid delay of bone healing and deformity.

a. Fracture of the upper third. Treatment of subtrochanteric fracture is discussed above. If a comminuted subtrochanteric fracture extends into the upper third of the femoral shaft, skeletal traction through the supracondylar region of the femur may be used to align the bone fragments, and, in some cases, to provide definitive treatment. The extremity is positioned with the hip and knee at a right angle. In some cases, skeletal traction can be through either the lower femur or the tibial tuberosity in balanced suspension. Russell's traction can be used if the patient is small and muscular development is not great. External rotation and abduction of the extremity are usually required to bring the lower fragment into alignment with the proximal fragment.

In adults, operative treatment is usually carried out in order to permit early mobilization, especially when other injuries are present. Rigid internal fixation devices such as interlocked intramedullary rods are used to maintain length and rotatory alignment.

b. Fracture of the middle third. The deformity caused by fracture at this level is not constant. Angulation is commonly present with the apex directed anterolaterally. Initial treatment to achieve alignment and stabilization is by skeletal traction through the tibial tuberosity or the lower end of the femur. Traction in the transverse plane by a swathe around the thigh may be necessary to correct angulation.

c. Fracture of the lower third. In transverse and comminuted fractures, the proximal end of the distal fragment is likely to be displaced posterior to the distal end of the proximal fragment. The same displacement is likely to be encountered in supracondylar fracture. Russell's traction should not be used for comminuted or widely displaced fractures because it may injure the femoral or popliteal vessels.

Closed treatment of distal femoral fractures is usually carried out only if operative treatment is not possible. If closed treatment is chosen, rigorous attention to detail is necessary. After reduction has been accomplished by traction, biplane radiographic examination should be repeated at least weekly to determine maintenance of reduction and progress of healing. When sufficient callus has formed to assure stabilization of the fragments, generally after 12 weeks or more, further immobilization can be given by a 1½ plaster spica or fracture brace. Prior to application of the spica or brace, there should be a period of observation in balanced suspension without traction to determine whether displacement of the fracture fragments by overriding will occur. Angulation can generally be corrected by appropriate wedging.

Elective indications for open reduction and internal fixation may be based on the desire to avoid prolonged recumbency in bed and hospitalization. Some mandatory indications include inability to obtain adequate reduction by closed technics and delay of bone healing. The purpose of open reduction is generally to provide anatomic reposition and rigid fixation that permits the patient to be ambulatory without such external supportive apparatus as casts, splints, or braces. Unprotected weight-bearing without crutches before restoration of bone continuity should not be a goal of open operation of most fractures.

B. INFANTS AND CHILDREN. Femoral fracture at birth occurs most often in the middle third. Comminution is usually not present. Skin traction and plaster immobilization are adequate, although skeletal traction may be necessary in older children. Open reduction is rarely necessary.

Fracture of proximal or middle third of the femur in a child under 2 years of age can be treated with Bryant's traction. Circulatory adequacy must be observed carefully and another method substituted if swelling, cyanosis, or pallor of the foot or obliteration of pedal pulsations cannot be managed by adjustment of dressings. As a rule, sufficient callus is present at the fracture site after 3-4 weeks so that traction can be discontinued. If callus formation is adequate, infants who have not yet begun to walk need no further protection; walking infants may require protection by a plaster hip spica for an extra few weeks.

Preliminary treatment of unstable fracture of the femur in children over 5 years of age can be done by Russell's traction. If the child is uncooperative or if adequate correction cannot be obtained, it may also be necessary to place the sound extremity in traction. Traction is continued until the fracture is stabilized; if it is discontinued before the callus is sufficiently mature, the deformity (especially angulation) may recur even though the extremity is protected by a plaster spica. Correction of angulation and torsional displacement around the long axis of the femur is mandatory. Slight shortening (1-2 cm) can be compensated by growth. Close apposition of fragments is not necessary, because healing will take place in spite of minimal soft tissue interposition. It is usually necessary to continue traction for 3-6 weeks or until sufficient callus is formed to prevent recurrence. Immobilization should be maintained for another 2 months. Weight-bearing must not be resumed until radiographs show that healing is sound.

X. INJURIES OF THE KNEE REGION

A. FRACTURES OF THE DISTAL FEMUR

1. Supracondylar fracture of the femur. This comparatively uncommon fracture (at the junction of cortical and cancellous bone) may be transverse, oblique, or comminuted. The distal end of the proximal fragment is apt to perforate the overlying vastus intermedius, vastus medialis, or rectus femoris muscles and may penetrate the suprapatellar pouch of knee joint to cause hemarthrosis. The proximal end of the distal fragment is usually displaced posteriorly and slightly laterally.

Because the distal fragment may impinge upon the popliteal vessels, circulatory adequacy distal to the fracture site should be verified as soon as possible. Absence of pedal pulsations is an indication for immediate investigation of a possible vascular injury even though prompt closed reduction is judged adequate. Peroneal or tibial nerve injury is a less frequent complication.

If the fracture is transverse or nearly so, closed manipulation under general anesthesia is occasionally successful. Stable fractures with minimal displacement can be treated in a single plaster hip spica with the hip and knee in about 30 degrees of flexion or in a fracture brace. Frequent radiographic examination is necessary to make certain that displacement has not occurred.

Stable or unstable uncomplicated supracondylar fracture may be treated nonoperatively with biplane skeletal traction if soft tissue interposition does not interfere with reduction. If adequate reduction cannot be obtained, it may be necessary to manipulate the fragments under general anesthesia, using skeletal traction to control the distal fragment. If adequate closed reduction cannot be obtained, open reduction and internal fixation are indicated.

When closed treatment is undertaken, traction must be continued for about 6 weeks or until stabilization occurs. The wires can then be removed and the extremity immobilized in a single plaster spica or fracture brace for an additional 2-3 months.

Open reduction and rigid internal fixation of supracondylar fractures have been increasingly used because they permit more rapid mobilization, better fracture alignment, and earlier supervised exercises for knee motion. Regardless of treatment, supracondylar fracture is likely to be followed by restriction of knee motion due to scarring and adhesion formation in adjacent soft tissues.

2. Intercondylar fracture of the femur. This uncommon comminuted fracture, which occurs in older patients, is described as T or Y according to the radiographic configuration of the fragments. Closed reduction is difficult when the proximal shaft fragment is interposed between the two main distal fragments. Maximal recovery of function of the knee joint requires anatomic reduction of the articular components. If alignment is satisfactory and displacement minimal, immobilization for 3-4 months in a plaster spica or fracture brace is sufficient. If displacement is marked, skeletal traction through tibial tuberosity (with knee in flexion) is required. Manual molding of distal fragments may be necessary. Open reduction and bolt fixation of distal fragments may be indicated to restore articular congruity. Occasionally, primary total knee replacement may be indicated, especially if there is severe comminution or preexisting severe degenerative arthritis of the knee. Further treatment is as described for supracondylar fracture.

3. Condylar fracture of the femur. Isolated fracture of lateral or medial condyle of femur is a rare consequence of severe trauma. Occasionally only the posterior portion of the condyle is separated in the coronal plane. Cruciate ligaments or collateral ligament and joint capsule of the opposite side of knee are often injured.

The objective of treatment is restoration of anatomic intraarticular relationships. If displacement is minimal, the knee can be manipulated into varus or valgus (opposite the position of deformity). If anatomic reduction cannot be obtained by closed manipulation, open reduction and fixation of the minor fragment with two to three bone screws is recommended. The ligaments must be explored, and, if found to be injured, repaired primarily if possible.

4. Separation of the distal femoral epiphysis. Traumatic separation of distal femoral epiphysis in children is the counterpart of supracondylar fracture in the adult. Direction of displacement of the epiphyseal fragment is most commonly anterior. Torsional displacement around the long axis of the femur may be present.

Reduction of anterior displacement can be achieved by closed manipulation. After reduction is complete, the knee is flexed to a right angle and a long-leg plaster cast is applied. If the thigh is obese, the plaster should be extended proximally to include the pelvis in a single hip spica.

Peripheral circulation must be observed carefully. After 4 weeks plaster is changed and flexion of the knee reduced to 45 degrees. At the end of the second month, exercises should be introduced to regain complete knee extension.

B. FRACTURE OF THE PATELLA

1. Transverse fracture of the patella is the result of indirect violence, usually with the knee partially flexed. The extent of associated tearing of the patella retinacula depends on the degree of force of the initiating injury.

Swelling of the anterior knee is caused by hemarthrosis. If displacement is present, defect in patella can be palpated and active extension of the knee is lost.

Open reduction is indicated if the fragments are separated more than 2-3 mm. The fragments must be accurately repositioned to prevent early posttraumatic arthritis of the patellofemoral joint. If the minor fragment is small (no more than 1 cm in length), it may be excised. If the fragments are approximately the same size, repair by wire cerclage is preferred.

2. Comminuted fracture of the patella is caused only by direct violence. Severe injury may cause comminution of the articular cartilages of both the patella and the opposing femur. If comminution is not severe and displacement is insignificant, plaster immobilization for 8 weeks in a cylinder extending from the groin to the supramalleolar region is sufficient.

Severe comminution requires excision of the patella.

C. TEAR OF THE QUADRICEPS TENDON occurs most often in patients over 40 years of age. Preexisting attritional disease of the tendon is apt to be present, and the causative injury may be minor. The patient is unable to extend the knee completely. Radiographs may show avulsion of a bit of bone from the superior patella. Operative repair is required for a complete tear.

D. DISLOCATION OF THE PATELLA. Traumatic dislocation of the patellofemoral joint may be associated with dislocation of the knee joint. When this injury occurs alone it may be due to direct violence or muscle activity of the quadriceps, and the direction of dislocation of the patella is lateral. Spontaneous reduction is apt to occur if the knee joint is extended; if so, clinical findings may consist merely of hemarthrosis and localized tenderness over the medial patellar retinaculum. Gross instability of the patella, which can be demonstrated by physical examination, indicates that the injury to the soft tissues of the medial aspect of the knee has been extensive. Recurrent episodes require operative repair for effective treatment.

E. DISLOCATION OF THE KNEE JOINT is uncommon in adults and extremely rare in children. It is caused by severe trauma. Displacement may be transverse or torsional. Complete dislocation can occur only after extensive tearing of the supporting ligaments and joint capsule.

Signs of neurovascular injury below the site of dislocation are an absolute indication for prompt reduction. If pedal pulses do not return promptly, consultation with a vascular surgeon should be sought immediately. A complicating muscle compartment syndrome requires prompt fascial release.

Anatomic reduction of uncomplicated dislocation should be attempted. If impinging soft tissues cannot be removed by closed manipulation, arthrotomy is indicated. After reduction, the extremity is immobilized in a tubular plaster cast extending from inguinal region to toes with the knee in slight flexion. (In the obese patient, a single hip spica should be applied.) A window should be cut in the plaster over dorsum of foot to allow frequent determination of dorsalis pedis pulsation. After 6-8 weeks' immobilization, the knee can be protected by a long leg brace. Intensive quadriceps exercises are necessary to minimize functional loss.

F. DERANGEMENTS OF KNEE JOINT may be caused by trauma or attritional disease. Although ligamentous and cartilagenous injuries are discussed separately, they commonly occur as combined lesions. Arthroscopy, arthrography using single or double contrast media, and MRI can be valuable adjuncts for a precise diagnosis when the usual methods are inconclusive.

1. Injury to the menisci. Injury to the medial meniscus is the most frequent internal derangement of the knee joint.

The significant clinical findings after acute injury are mild swelling and varying degrees of restriction of flexion or extension. Motion may cause pain. Tenderness can often be elicited at the point of pain. If symptoms have persisted for 2-3 weeks, weakness and atrophy of the quadriceps femoris may be present.

Injury to the lateral meniscus less often causes mechanical blockage of joint motion. Pain and tenderness may be present over the lateral joint line. Pain can be elicited by forcible rotation of leg with knee flexed maximally.

Injury to the anterior cruciate ligament should be ruled out by thorough, repeated physical examination. If an isolated meniscus tear is suspected, initial treatment is conservative. Pain caused by tense effusion can be relieved by aspiration. If a hemarthrosis is present, an anterior cruciate ligament tear is likely. If pain is severe, the extremity should be immobilized in a splint with the knee in slight flexion. Younger patients usually prefer to be ambulatory on crutches, but immediate weight-bearing should be restricted. Unrestricted activity must not be resumed until complete motion is recovered and symptoms have subsided. If symptoms continue, abnormal physical findings persist, and diagnostic studies reveal a meniscus tear, operative arthroscopy is the preferred method of treatment.

2. Injury to the collateral ligaments. The collateral ligaments are at risk when excessive varus or valgus force is applied to the knee. Extensive injury to these ligaments may be accompanied by tears of the menisci and the joint capsule.

a. Medial collateral ligament. Forced abduction of the leg at the knee, which is frequently associated with torsional strain, causes injury varying from tear of a few fibers to complete rupture of the ligament. Pain is present over the medial aspect of the knee joint. Tenderness can be elicited at the site of lesion. When only an isolated ligamentous tear is present, radiographic examination may not be helpful unless made while valgus stress is applied to the slightly flexed knee.

Treatment of incomplete tear consists of protection from further injury while healing progresses. Painful hemarthrosis should be relieved by aspiration. The knee may be immobilized temporarily in a splint or a brace. Incomplete rupture of the medial collateral ligament is usually treated with restricted weight-bearing and a brace that permits a free range of knee motion. Complete ruptures, traditionally treated with surgical repair, are increasingly managed with nonsurgical techniques. An initial period of rigid immobilization and restricted weight-bearing is followed by bracing, motion exercises, and progressive weight-bearing.

b. Lateral collateral ligament. Tear of the fibular ligament is often associated with injury to surrounding structures (e.g., the joint capsule, the popliteus muscle tendon, and the iliotibial band). Avulsion of the apex of the fibular head may occur, and the peroneal nerve may be injured.

Pain and tenderness are present over the lateral aspect of the knee joint, and hemarthrosis may be present. Radiographs may show a bit of bone avulsed from the fibular head. If severe injury is suspected, radiographic examination under stress, using local or general anesthesia, is required. A firm, padded, nonopaque object about 20-30 cm in diameter is placed between the partially flexed knees and the legs are forcibly adducted while an anteroposterior exposure is made. Widening of the lateral joint cleft indicates severe injury.

Treatment of partial tear is similar to that described for partial tear of the medial collateral ligament. If complete tear is suspected, and especially if the peroneal nerve has been injured, exploration is indicated. The extremity is protected for 6-8 weeks in a long-leg cast or in a brace with limited motion at the knee.

3. Injury to the cruciate ligaments

a. Anterior cruciate ligament injury is usually accompanied by injury to the menisci or medial collateral ligament. The cruciate ligament may be avulsed with a part of the medial tibial tubercle, or at the femoral attachment, or may rupture within the substance of its fibers. This diagnosis should be suspected when the force applied to the knee results in a "pop," the patient is unable to resume sport or ambulation immediately after the injury, and hemarthrosis is noted on joint aspiration.

A characteristic physical finding is a positive "drawer" sign or a Lachman sign whereby manually applied stress causes excessive anterior excursion of the tibial plateau compared with the uninjured normal knee joint. Anterolateral rotatory instability, elicited by various maneuvers, is virtually always present.

Complete recent rupture of the anterior cruciate ligament within its substance cannot be repaired adequately by suture alone. Primary repair with reinforcement by one of the hamstring tendons is advocated by some. When manifest by avulsed tibial bone, attachment of the fragment in anatomic position by arthrotomy is necessary. Old tears may require reconstructive procedures.

b. Posterior cruciate ligament tear may occur within its substance or at its femoral attachment, or may be manifest by avulsion of a fragment of bone or variable size at its tibial attachment. A posterior "sag" of the proximal tibia may be visible with the patient lying supine and the knees flexed 90 degrees. The diagnosis is made by the "drawer" sign: The knee is flexed at a right angle and the upper tibia is pushed backward; if excessive posterior excursion of the proximal tibia can be noted, tear of the posterior ligament is likely.

Treatment is directed primarily at the associated injuries and maintenance of the competency of the quadriceps musculature. Primary repair of tears within the fibers is difficult and of dubious value. Open reduction and fixation of a fragment of tibia with the attached ligament is feasible and is likely to restore functional competency of the ligament. Late reconstruction is indicated only if symptoms persist despite adequate muscle rehabilitation.

G. FRACTURES OF THE PROXIMAL TIBIA

1. Fracture of the lateral tibial condyle is commonly caused by a blow on the lateral aspect of the knee with the foot in fixed position, producing a valgus strain. Hemarthrosis is always present, as the fracture cleft involves the knee joint. Soft tissue injuries are likely to be present also. The medial collateral and anterior cruciate ligaments may be torn. The lateral meniscus may be torn. If displacement is marked, fracture of the proximal fibula may be present also.

The objective of treatment is to restore the articular surface and normal anatomic relationships. In cases of minimal displacement (less than 4-5 mm) where ligaments have not been extensively damaged, treatment may be by immobilization for 6 weeks in a long-leg cast with the knee in slight flexion. Reduction of marked displacement can be achieved by closed manipulation unless comminution is severe. After radiographic verification of reduction, the extremity can be immobilized in a long-leg cast, preferably with knee in full extension. Many fractures of the lateral condyle of the tibia, especially comminuted fractures, cannot be reduced adequately by closed methods. Open reduction, internal fixation, and supplemental bone grafting are required.

2. Fracture of the medial tibial condyle is caused by the varus strain produced by a blow against the medial aspect of the knee with the foot in fixed position. The medial meniscus, the lateral collateral ligament, and the lateral joint capsule may be torn. Severe comminution is not usually present, and there is only one major free fragment.

Treatment is by closed reduction to restore the articular surface of the tibia to prevent functional elongation of the tibial collateral ligament. The extremity is immobilized for 10-12 weeks in a long-leg cast. During the latter part of this period of immobilization, a brace may be used to allow knee motion exercises. Full weight-bearing is deferred for at least 3 months.

3. Fracture of both tibial condyles. Axial force, such as may result from falling on the foot or sudden deceleration with the knee in full extension (during an automobile accident) can cause simultaneous fracture of both condyles of the tibia. Comminution is apt to be severe. Deformity is either genu varum or genu valgum. Radiographic examination should include oblique projections.

Severe comminution makes anatomic reduction difficult to achieve by closed means and difficult to maintain following closed manipulation alone. If closed treatment is elected, sustained skeletal traction is usually necessary. When stability has been achieved, the extremity can be immobilized for another 4-5 weeks in a long-leg cast with the knee in full extension. Unassisted weight-bearing is not permitted before the end of the third or fourth month.

If closed methods are not effective in achieving and maintaining adequate reduction, surgical treatment is indicated. Some believe open reduction and internal fixation are appropriate in selected cases where comminution is minimal.

Instability and restriction of knee motion are common sequelae. If reduction of the articular surfaces is not adequate, posttraumatic arthritis will appear early.

4. Fracture of the tibial tuberosity. Violent contraction of the quadriceps muscle may cause avulsion of the tibial tuberosity. Avulsion of the anterior portion of the upper tibial epiphysis, uncommon in childhood, must be differentiated from Osgood-Schlatter disease (osteochondrosis of tibial tuberosity).

If displacement is minimal, treatment is by immobilization in a cylinder cast with knee in full extension. Immobilization is maintained for 8 weeks or until healing is apparent.

A fragment displaced >0.5 cm is treated by either closed reduction and percutaneous fixation, plaster immobilization, or open reduction.

5. Fracture of the tibial tubercle usually occurs in association with comminuted fracture of the condyle. The medial intercondylar eminence may be avulsed with adjacent bone attached to the anterior cruciate ligament. In this fracture, anatomic reduction is necessary to restore anterior knee stability.

6. Separation of the proximal tibial epiphysis. Complete displacement is rare; partial separation due to forceful hyperextension of the knee is more common. The distal metaphyseal fragment is displaced anteriorly. If no circulatory or neurologic deficit is present, immediate treatment by closed manipulation is indicated. Reduction can be accomplished by forced flexion of the knee. Initial immobilization by an anterior plaster splint from the upper thigh to the ankle permits frequent observation of the peripheral circulation. After 3 weeks the knee may be extended further and immobilization in a long-leg cast continued for another 3-4 weeks. Partial weight-bearing should be avoided until healing is evident.

Injury to the proximal tibial physis as a result of a blow on the lateral aspect of the knee causes compression but only minor displacement. This lesion, analogous to fracture of lateral condyle in adults, may either retard or arrest the growth of the lateral aspect of the tibia and thus cause tibia valga or knock-knee.

H. FRACTURE OF THE PROXIMAL FIBULA. Isolated fracture of the proximal fibula is uncommon; this fracture is usually associated with fracture of the femur or of the tibia or fracture-dislocation of the ankle joint. The apex of the fibular head may be avulsed by the activity of the biceps femoris muscle or detached with the fibular collateral ligament by a varus strain of the knee.

The fracture usually requires no treatment, but avulsion of the apex of the head may necessitate operative repair of the ligament or tendon. Fracture in this region may be associated with paralysis of the common peroneal nerve.

I. DISLOCATION OF THE PROXIMAL TIBIOFIBULAR JOINT. This extremely rare lesion is caused by the activity of the biceps femoris muscle. Displacement is posterior and can be reduced by digital pressure over the head of the fibula in the opposite direction.

XI. FRACTURES OF THE SHAFTS OF THE TIBIA AND FIBULA

This fracture occurs at any age by is most common during youth and early adulthood. In general, open, transverse, comminuted, and segmental fractures are caused by direct violence. Fracture of the middle third of the shaft (especially if comminuted) is apt to be complicated by delay of bone healing.

If fracture is complete and displacement is present, clinical diagnosis is not difficult. However, critical local examination is of utmost importance in planning treatment. The nature of the skin wounds which may communicate with the fracture site often suggests the mechanism of compounding, whether it has occurred from within or without. Extensive swelling due to hemorrhage in closed fascial compartments may prevent complete reduction immediately. Neurovascular integrity below the level of the fracture must be verified before definitive treatment is instituted. Radiographs in the anteroposterior and lateral projection of the entire leg, including both knee and ankle joints, are always necessary, and oblique projections are often desirable.

A. FRACTURE OF SHAFT OF THE FIBULA. Isolated fracture is uncommon and is usually caused by direct trauma. It is usually associated with other injury of the leg, e.g., fracture of tibia or fracture-dislocation of ankle joint.

B. FRACTURE OF SHAFT OF THE TIBIA. Isolated fracture is likely to be caused by indirect injury, such as torsional stress. Because of mechanical stability provided by the intact fibula, marked displacement is not apt to occur.

If the fragments are not displaced, reliable treatment may be given by immobilization in a long-leg cast or fracture brace.

If fragments are displaced, manipulation under anesthesia may be necessary. Fractures with a transverse orientation tend to be stable after reduction. Oblique and spiral fractures tend to displace unless fragments are locked.

C. FRACTURE OF THE SHAFTS OF TIBIA AND FIBULA IN ADULTS. Simultaneous fracture of the shafts of both bones are unstable lesions which tend to become displaced following reduction. Treatment is directed toward reduction and stabilization of the tibial fracture until healing takes place. For adequate reduction, the fragments must be apposed almost completely, and angulation and torsional displacement of the tibial fracture must be corrected.

If reduction by closed manipulation is anatomic, transverse fractures tend to be stable. Repeated radiographs are necessary to determine whether displacement has recurred. The plaster must remain snug at all times. Recurrent angular displacement can be corrected by wedging the cast in the appropriate direction. If reduction is lost, another type of treatment must be substituted.

If oblique and spiral fractures are unstable following manipulation and immobilization, internal fixation or immobilization in an external fixatur is usually required.

A rarely selected alternative method of treatment of unstable fractures is continuous skeletal traction, which must be continued for about 6 weeks or until preliminary healing causes stabilization. The extremity is then immobilized in a cast or brace for another 8-12 weeks until bone continuity has been restored.

If adequate apposition and correction of the deformity cannot be achieved by closed methods, open reduction and internal fixation are required. The blood supply to intermediate fragments is likely to be disturbed in comminuted and segmental fractures. These unstable closed fractures can usually be treated successfully by closed reduction and external immobilization. However, newer techniques such as unreamed intramedullary rodding with or without interlocking screws may permit more rapid mobilization, more secure fracture fixation, and easier maintenance of knee and ankle motion.

D. FRACTURE OF SHAFTS OF TIBIA AND FIBULA IN CHILDREN. Open reduction and internal fixation of closed fractures in children are rarely necessary. In transverse or short oblique tibial fractures or in the presence of an intact fibula, closed reduction of axial displacement (overriding) is desirable; angular and torsional displacement must be corrected also. If proper alignment is secured, 1 cm of overriding is acceptable.

Comminuted or oblique tibial fractures with displacement of both bones may be treated by skeletal traction with a Kirschner wire inserted across the calcaneus until early bone healing stabilizes the fragments. Further immobilization in a cast is necessary until healing has progressed far enough to permit weight-bearing.

XII. INJURIES OF THE ANKLE REGION

A. ANKLE SPRAIN during childhood is rare. In the adult, it is most often caused by forced inversion and internal torsion of the foot while in plantar flexion. Pain is usually maximal over the anterolateral aspect of the joint; greatest tenderness is apt to be found in the region of the anterior talofibular and calcaneofibular ligaments. Eversion sprain is less common; maximal tenderness and swelling are usually found over the deltoid ligament.

Sprain is differentiated from partial or complete ligamentous tears. Routine radiographic studies are negative. Stress studies with anesthesia, arthrography, or dye injections into the peroneal tendon sheath differentiate ligamentous strain from frank tears. If swelling is marked, elevation of the extremity, application of an elastic wrap, and avoidance of weight-bearing for a few days are advisable. Whereas minor injuries may be treated by an ankle brace or elastic bandage support, major tears require cast immobilization, followed by supervised exercise and rehabilitation.

B. FRACTURES AND DISLOCATIONS OF THE ANKLE JOINT may be caused by direct injury, in which case they may be comminuted and open; or by indirect violence, which often causes typical lesions (see below).

Pain and swelling are the prominent clinical findings. Deformity may or may not be present. Radiographs of excellent technical quality must be obtained in anteroposterior, lateral, and mortise projections to demonstrate the extent and configuration of all major fragments. Special oblique projections and stress examinations may be required. Arthrography may identify capsuloligamentous tears. Many classification schemes for fractures of the ankle have been devised. For the sake of brevity and clarity, these injuries are discussed according to their anatomic location.

1. Fracture of the medial malleolus may occur as an isolated lesion of any part of the malleolus (including the tip) or may be associated with (1) fracture of the lateral malleolus with medial or lateral dislocation of the talus, and (2) dislocation of the inferior tibiofibular joint with or without fracture of the fibula. Isolated fracture does not usually cause instability of the ankle joint.

Undisplaced isolated fracture of the medial malleolus should be treated by immobilization in a short-leg cast with the ankle flexed to a right angle and the foot slightly inverted to relax the tension on the deltoid ligament. Immobilization is continued for 8-10 weeks or until bone healing is sound.

Displaced isolated fracture of the medial malleolus may be reduced by closed manipulation. If anatomic reduction cannot be obtained and maintained by closed methods, open reduction and internal fixation are required.

2. Fracture of the lateral malleolus may occur as an isolated lesion or may be associated with fracture of the medial malleolus, tear of the deltoid ligament, or avulsion of the posterior tibial tubercle. If the medial aspect of the ankle is injured, lateral dislocation of the talus is apt to be present. The tip of the lateral malleolus may be avulsed by the calcaneofibular and anterior talofibular ligaments. Transverse or oblique fracture may occur. Oblique fractures commonly begin anteriorly and inferiorly and extend in the coronal plane in a posterior and superior direction.

If swelling and pain are not marked, isolated undisplaced fracture of the lateral malleolus may be treated by an ankle brace. Otherwise, a short-leg cast should be applied for 6 weeks and an elastic bandage worn thereafter until full joint motion is recovered and the calf muscles are functioning normally.

Isolated displaced fracture of the lateral malleolus should be treated by closed reduction and cast immobilization for 8-12 weeks. If anatomic reduction cannot be achieved by closed methods, open reduction and internal fixation are required.

3. Combined fracture of the medial and lateral malleoli. Bimalleolar fractures are commonly accompanied by displacement of the talus, usually in a medial or lateral direction. In conjunction with dislocation in the coronal plane, concurrent displacement may take place in the sagittal plane, either anteriorly or posteriorly, or in torsion about the longitudinal axis of the tibia.

Bimalleolar fracture may be treated by closed manipulation. A long-leg cast is then applied with the knee in about 45 degrees of flexion and the foot in neutral position. Immediate open reduction must be done if radiographs show that perfect anatomic reduction has not been achieved.

4. Fractures of the distal tibia

a. Fracture of the posterior margin Fracture of the posterior articular margin may involve part or all of the entire posterior aspect and is apt to be accompanied by fracture of either malleolus and posterior dislocation of the talus. It must be differentiated from fracture of the posterior tibial tubercle, which is usually caused by avulsion with the attached posterior lateral malleolar ligament.

Anatomic reduction by closed manipulation is required if the fracture involves >25% of the articular surface. If reduction by closed manipulation is unsuccessful, open reduction is required. Frequent radiographic examination is necessary to make certain that redisplacement does not occur.

b. Fracture of the anterior margin of the tibia (rare) is likely to be caused by forced dorsiflexion of the foot. If displacement is marked and talus is dislocated, tear of the collateral ligaments or fractures of the malleoli are likely to be present. Closed reduction by forced plantar flexion is frequently unsuccessful, resulting in significant residual joint incongruity.

c. Comminuted fractures. Extensive comminution of the distal tibia (pilon fracture) presents a difficult problem of management. The congruity of articular surfaces cannot be restored by closed manipulation, and satisfactory anatomic restoration is usually not possible even by open operation. The best initial treatment for extremely comminuted and widely displaced fractures is closed manipulation and skeletal traction. After traction has been applied and impaction of fragments has been disrupted, displacement may be sufficiently corrected to permit immobilization in a long-leg cast with knee in 10-15 degrees of flexion and foot in neutral position. With the extremity immobilized in plaster, continuous skeletal traction is maintained until stabilization by early bone healing occurs. An alternative is distraction with a wire or pin in the calcaneus and one or two wires or pins in the shaft of the tibia. If reduction by calcaneal pin traction is not adequate, open reduction with limited internal fixation of major fracture fragments may restore tibial length and joint alignment.

Healing is likely to be slow. If the articular surfaces of the ankle joint have not been properly realigned, disabling posttraumatic arthritis is likely to occur early. Early arthrodesis is indicated to shorten the period of disability.

5. Complete dislocation of ankle joint. The talus cannot be completely dislocated from ankle joint without fracture unless all ligaments are torn.

6. Incomplete dislocation of the ankle joint. Major ligamentous injuries in the region of the ankle joint are usually associated with fracture.

a. Tear of the deltoid ligament. Pain, tenderness, swelling, and ecchymosis in the region of the medial malleolus without fracture suggest partial or complete tear of the deltoid ligament. If fracture of the lateral malleolus or dislocation of the tibiofibular syndesmosis is present, the cleft between the medial malleolus and talus is likely to be widened. If widening is not apparent, radiographic examination under stress is necessary to demonstrate instability.

Interposition of the deltoid ligament between the talus and the medial malleolus often cannot be corrected by closed manipulation. If widening persists after closed manipulation, surgical exploration is indicated so that the torn ligament can be removed from the joint space and repaired.

b. Tear of anterior talofibular ligament with the adjacent joint capsule is caused by forced inversion and internal torsion of the foot in plantar flexion. Stress examination demonstrates anterior subluxation of talus in relation to tibia.

Rupture of the anterior talofibular ligament may be associated with tear of the calcaneofibular ligament. Stress examination by forced inversion of the foot demonstrates tilting of the talus greater than similar examination of the opposite normal joint. Tear of both ligaments may be associated with fracture of the medial malleolus and medial subluxation of the talus.

Instability of the ankle joint characterized by a history of recurrent sprains may result from unrecognized tears of the supporting ligaments.

Recent isolated tear of the anterior talofibular ligament or combined tear of the calcaneofibular ligament should be treated by immobilization for 4-6 weeks in a plaster boot. Some surgeons advise early operative repair. Associated fracture of the medial malleolus creates an unstable mechanism. Unless anatomic reduction can be achieved and maintained by closed methods, open reduction and internal fixation of the malleolar fragment are indicated.

7. Dislocation of the tibiofibular syndesmosis. Both the anterior and posterior tibiofibular ligaments must be torn before the distal tibiofibular joint can be dislocated. Lateral dislocation of the talus is also an essential feature, and this cannot occur unless the medial malleolus is fractured or the deltoid ligament is torn. The distal fibula is commonly fractured, but it may remain intact, and dislocation may be caused by a tear of the interosseous membrane; less commonly the fibula may fracture proximally (Maisonneuve fracture).

Anatomic reduction by closed manipulation is difficult to achieve, but should be tried. If immediate and repeated radiographic examinations do not demonstrate that anatomic reduction has been achieved and maintained, open reduction and internal fixation with a syndesmotic screw should be performed as soon as possible.

8. Separation of distal tibial and fibular epiphyses. The most common injury of the ankle region of children is traumatic separation of distal tibial and fibular physes. Sprain is rare in children. Separation of the distal fibular physis may occur as an isolated injury, or it may be associated with separation of the tibial physis. If epiphyseal displacement has occurred, treatment is by closed manipulation and plaster immobilization. Open reduction is indicated if anatomic reduction has not been obtained. Special care should be exercised in identifying physeal injuries that extend into the articular cartilage. If injury has been severe or if reduction is inadequate, disturbance of growth is likely to follow.

XIII. INJURIES OF THE FOOT

A. FRACTURE AND DISLOCATION OF THE TALUS
1. Dislocation of the subtalar and talonavicular joints without fracture occasionally occurs. The ankle joint is not in-

jured. Displacement of the foot can be either in varus or valgus. Reduction by closed manipulation is usually not difficult. Incarceration of the posterior tibial tendon in the talonavicular joint may prevent reduction by closed manipulation. After reduction, the extremity should be immobilized in a short-leg cast for 4 weeks.

2. Fracture of the talus. Major fracture commonly occurs through the body or the neck; the uncommon fracture of the head involves a portion of the neck with extension into the head. Indirect injury usually causes closed fracture as well as most open fractures; severe comminution is infrequent. The proximal or distal fragments may be dislocated. Flattening of the articular surface either may result from compression fracture at the time of the initial injury or may occur later in association with complicating avascular necrosis.

a. Fracture of the neck. Forced dorsiflexion of the foot may cause this injury. Undisplaced fracture of the neck can be treated adequately by a non–weight-bearing short-leg cast for 8-12 weeks. Dislocation of the body or distal neck fragment with the foot may complicate this injury. Fracture of the neck with anterior and frequently medial dislocation of the distal fragment and foot can usually be reduced by closed manipulation. Subsequent treatment is the same as that of undisplaced fracture.

Dislocation of the proximal body fragment may occur separately or may be associated with dislocation of the distal fragment. If dislocation of the body fragment is complete, reduction by closed manipulation may not be possible. In this event, open reduction should be done promptly to prevent or minimize extent of avascular necrosis. Bone healing is likely to be retarded because some degree of ischemic necrosis is probable.

Complete dislocation of the neck fragment from the talonavicular and subtalar joints is rare; but if it does happen, avascular necrosis of the fragment is to be expected even though anatomic reduction is promptly accomplished. If satisfactory reduction by closed manipulation is not possible, immediate open operation with reduction of the fragment or its removal is advisable, because delay may cause necrosis of overlying soft tissues.

b. Fracture of the body. Closed uncomminuted fracture of the body of the talus with minimal displacement of fragments is not likely to cause disability if immobilization is continued until healing occurs. If significant displacement occurs, the proximal fragment is apt to be dislocated from the subtalar and ankle joints. Even though prompt adequate reduction is obtained by either closed manipulation or open operation, extensive displacement of the proximal body fragment is likely to be followed by avascular necrosis. If reduction is not anatomic, delayed healing of the fracture may follow.

c. Compression fracture of the superior surface of the trochlea of the talus from the initial injury (which is likely to have been violent) cannot be reduced. When this lesion occurs as a separate entity or in combination with other major fractures of the body, prolonged protection from weight-bearing is the major means of preventing further collapse that is likely to occur.

Osteochondral fracture of a portion of the articular surface may occur with relatively mild ankle injuries.

B. FRACTURE OF THE CALCANEUS is commonly caused by direct trauma. Because this is likely to occur as a result of a fall from a height, fracture of the spine may also be present. Comminution and impaction are general characteristics. Minor impactions and fissure fractures are easy to miss so radiographs must be prepared in multiple projections. In some instances, minor impactions of articular surfaces are evident only by CT imaging.

Various classifications have been advocated. Fractures that are generally comminuted and disrupt the subtalar and calcaneocuboid articulations should be distinguished from those that do not; this differentiation has important implications for treatment and prognosis.

1. Fracture of the tuberosity. Isolated fracture is not common. It may occur in a vertical or a horizontal direction.

a. Horizontal fracture may be limited to the superior portion of the region of the former apophysis and represents an avulsion by the Achilles tendon. Where the superior minor fragment is widely displaced proximally with the tendon, open reduction and fixation may be necessary to obtain the most satisfactory functional result.

Further extension of the fracture cleft toward the subtalar joint in the substance of the tuberosity creates the "beak" fracture. The minor fragment may be displaced proximally by the action of the triceps surae. If displacement is significant, reduction can be achieved by skeletal traction applied to the proximal fragment with the foot in equinus. Immobilization is obtained by incorporation of the traction pin or wire in full extremity plaster with the knee flexed 30 degrees and the foot in plantar flexion. If adequate reduction cannot be accomplished in this way, open reduction is advised.

b. Vertical fracture occurs somewhat medially in the sagittal plane. Because the minor medial fragment normally is not widely displaced, plaster immobilization is not required. Comfort can be enhanced by limitation of weight-bearing with the aid of crutches. The cleft of a vertical fracture may occur superiorly near the coronal plane of the body and represent an osseous avulsion of the insertion of the triceps surae.

2. Fracture of the sustentaculum. Isolated fracture is a rare lesion which may be caused by forced eversion of the foot. Where displacement of the larger body fragment occurs, it is lateral. Incarceration of the tendon of the flexor hallucis longus in the fracture cleft has been reported. Generally this fracture occurs in association with comminution of the body.

3. Fracture of the anterior process is caused by forced inversion of the foot. It must be differentiated from midtarsal and ankle joint sprains. The firmly attached bifurcate ligament (calcaneonavicular and calcaneocuboid components) avulses a bit of bone. Maximum tenderness and slight swelling occur midway between the tip of the lateral malleolus and the base of the fifth metatarsal. The lateral radiographic view projected obliquely is the most satisfactory to demonstrate the fracture cleft. Treatment is by a non–weight-bearing short-leg cast for 4 weeks with the foot in neutral position.

4. Fracture of the body may occur posterior to the articular surfaces, in a general vertical but somewhat oblique plane, without disruption of the subtalar joint. Most severe fractures of the calcaneal body are comminuted and extend into the subtalar and frequently the calcaneocuboid joints. Fissure fractures without significant displacement cause minor disability and can be treated simply by protection from weight-bearing, either by crutches alone or in combination with a short-leg cast until bone healing is sufficiently sound to justify graded increments of loading.

a. Nonarticular fracture. Where fracture of the body with comminution occurs posterior to the articular surface, the direction of displacement of the fragment attached to the tuberosity is proximal, causing diminution of the tuber joint angle. Because the subtalar joint is not disrupted symptomatic posttraumatic degenerative arthritis is not usual even though some joint stiffness persists permanently. Marked displacement should be corrected by skeletal traction applied to the main posterior fragment to obtain an optimal cosmetic result. Success of reduction can be judged by the adequacy of restoration of the tuber joint angle.

   b. Articular fractures are of three general types:

(1) *Fracture of the body without communication* may involve the posterior talar articular surface. Where displacement of posterior fragment of the tuberosity occurs, the direction is lateral. Fractures of this category with more than minimal displacement should be treated by the method advocated for nonarticular fracture of the body.

(2) *In fractures with minor comminution,* the main cleft occurs vertically, in a somewhat oblique lateral deviation from the sagittal plane. From emergence on the medial surface posterior to the sustentaculum it is directed forward and rather obliquely laterally through the posterior articular facet. The sustentaculum and medial portion of posterior articular surface remain undisplaced with relation to the talus. The body below the remaining lateral portion of posterior articular surface with the tuberosity are impacted into the lateral portion of the posterior articular facet. Some authorities have recommended open reduction and bone grafting. Lack of precise reduction, determined in part by restoration of the normal tuber joint angle, causes derangement of the subtalar joint, and symptomatic posttraumatic arthritis is a frequent sequel.

(3) *Fracture with extensive comminution* extending into the subtalar joint may involve the entire posterior articular surface with impaction into the substance of the underlying body. There are many variants; the clefts may extend across the calcaneal groove into the medial and anterior articular surface, and detachment of the peroneal tubercle may be a feature. This serious injury may cause major disability in spite of the best treatment, because the bursting nature of the injury defies anatomic restoration.

   Some surgeons advise nonintervention. Displacement of fragments is disregarded. Initially, a compression dressing is applied and the extremity is elevated for a week or so. Warm soaks and active exercises are then started, but weight-bearing is avoided until early bone healing has taken place. In spite of residual deformity in the region of the subtalar joint (which may be intensified by weight-bearing) acceptable functional results may be obtained by those willing to put up with the discomforts involved.

   Other surgeons advocate early closed manipulation which can partially restore the external anatomic configuration of the heel region, a cosmetic goal particularly desirable for women.

Persistent and disabling painful symptoms originating in the deranged subtalar joint may require arthrodesis for adequate relief. Concomitant involvement of the calcaneocuboid joint is an indication of the more extensive triple arthrodesis.

C. FRACTURE OF THE TARSAL NAVICULAR.

Minor avulsion fractures may occur as a feature of severe midtarsal sprain and require neither reduction nor elaborate treatment. Avulsion fracture of the tuberosity near the insertion of the posterior tibial muscle is uncommon and must be differentiated from a persistent, ununited apophysis (accessory navicular) and from the supernumerary sesamoid bone, the os tibiale externum.

Major fracture occurs either through the middle in a horizontal plane, or more rarely, in the vertical plane, or is characterized by impaction of its substance. Fatigue fractures of the tarsal navicular occur rarely in long distance runners and may be difficult to diagnose by radiography. Only noncomminuted fractures with displacement of the dorsal fragment can be reduced. Closed manipulation by strong traction on the forefoot and simultaneous digital pressure over the displaced fragment can restore it to its normal position. If a tendency to redisplacement is apparent, this can be counteracted by temporary fixation with a percutaneously inserted Kirschner wire. Comminuted and impacted fractures cannot be anatomically reduced. Some authorities offer a pessimistic prognosis for comminuted or impacted fractures. They contend that even though partial reduction has been achieved, posttraumatic arthritis supervenes, and that arthrodesis of the talonavicular and cuneonavicular joints will be ultimately necessary to relieve painful symptoms.

D. FRACTURE OF THE CUNEIFORM AND CUBOID BONES.

Because of their relatively protected position in the midtarsus, isolated fractures of the cuboid and cuneiform bones are rarely encountered. Minor avulsion fractures occur as a component of severe midtarsal sprains. Extensive fracture usually occurs in association with other injuries of the foot and often is caused by severe crushing. Simple classification is impractical because of the complex character and the varied manifestations of the whole injury.

E. MIDTARSAL DISLOCATIONS

through the cuneonavicular and the calcaneocuboid joints or, more proximally, through the talocalcaneonavicular and the calcaneocuboid joints may occur as a result of twisting injury to the forefoot. Fractures of varying extent of adjacent bones are frequent complications. When treatment is given soon after the accident, closed reduction by traction on the forefoot and manipulation is generally effective. If reduction is unstable and displacement tends to recur upon release of traction, stabilization for 4 weeks by percutaneously inserted Kirschner wires is recommended.

F. FRACTURES AND DISLOCATIONS OF THE METATARSALS

are likely to be caused by direct crushing or indirect twisting injury to the forefoot. Besides osseous and articular injury, complicating soft tissue lesions are often present. Tense subfascial hematoma of the dorsum of the forefoot, if not relieved, may cause necrosis of overlying skin or may even lead to gangrene of the toes by interruption of the arterial supply.

1. Tarsometatarsal dislocations. Possibly because of strong ligamentous support and relative size, dislocation of the first metatarsal at its base occurs less frequently than similar involvement of the lesser bones. With tarsometatarsal dislocation involving the lesser metatarsals, associated fractures are common. Dislocation is more commonly caused by direct injury but may be the result of stress applied indirectly through the forefoot. Direction of displacement is ordinarily dorsal, lateral, or a combination of both.

Closed reduction should be carried out as soon as possible. Skeletal traction applied to the involved bone by a Kirschner wire or a stout towel clamp can be a valuable aid to manipulation. Even though persistent dislocation may not cause significant disability, the resulting deformity can make shoe fitting difficult for men and the cosmetic effect undesirable for women. Open reduction with evacuation of dorsal subfascial hematoma and Kirschner wire stabilization is a preferred alternative to unsuccessful closed treatment. When effective treatment has been deferred 4 weeks or even longer, early healing prevents satisfactory reduction of persisting displacement by closed technics. Under such circumstances, it is better to defer open operation and to direct treatment toward recovery of function. Extensive operative procedures and continued immobilization can increase joint stiffness. Reconstructive operation can be planned more suitably after residual disability becomes established.

2. Fractures of the shafts. Undisplaced fractures of the metatarsal shafts cause no permanent disability unless nonunion occurs. Displacement is rarely significant where fracture of the middle metatarsals is oblique and the first and fifth are uninjured, because they act as splints. Incomplete fractures should be treated by stiff-soled shoe (with partial weight-bearing) or, if pain is marked, by a short-leg walking cast.

Great care should be taken in displaced fractures to correct angulation in the longitudinal axis of the shaft. Persistent convex dorsal angulation causes prominence of the head of the involved metatarsal on the plantar aspect with the implication of concentrated local pressure and production of painful skin callosities. Deformity of the shaft of the first metatarsal due to convex plantar angulation can transfer weight-bearing stress to the region of the head of the third metatarsal. After correction of angular displacement, the cast should be molded well to the plantar aspect of the foot to minimize recurrence of deformity and to support the longitudinal and transverse arches.

If reduction is not reasonably accurate, fractures through the shafts near the heads (the "neck") may cause great discomfort from concentrated pressure over the plantar surface, resulting in reactive keratosis formation. Every effort should be made to correct convex dorsal angulation by appropriate reduction. If adequate reduction of unstable metatarsal fractures cannot be obtained, open reduction and percutaneous Kirschner wire fixation should be carried out without delay.

3. Fatigue fracture of the shafts of the metatarsals has been described by various terms, e.g., march, stress, and insufficiency fracture. Its varied clinical manifestations may delay precise diagnosis, even to the point of confusion with osteogenic sarcoma. Commonly, it occurs in active young adults, such as military recruits, who are unaccustomed to vigorous and excessive walking. A history of a single significant injury is lacking. Incipient pain of varying intensity in the forefoot which is accentuated by walking, swelling, and localized tenderness of the involved metatarsal are cardinal manifestations. Depending upon the stage of progress, radiographs may not demonstrate the fracture cleft, and callus formation may ultimately be the only clue. More obvious findings may vary from an incomplete fissure to a clear transverse cleft. Persistent unprotected weight-bearing may arrest bone healing and even result in displacement of the distal fragment. The second and third metatarsals are most frequently involved near the junction of the middle and distal thirds. The lesion can occur more proximally and in other lesser metatarsals. Because weight-bearing may prolong and aggravate symptoms, protection in either a short-leg walking cast or a heavy shoe with a reinforced sole is recommended. Weight-bearing should be restricted until painful symptoms subside and healing is demonstrated by radiography.

4. Fracture of the tuberosity of the fifth metatarsal. Forced adduction of the forefoot may cause avulsion fracture of the tuberosity of the fifth metatarsal and, where supporting soft tissues have been torn, activity of the peroneus brevis muscle may increase displacement of the avulsed proximal fragment. If displacement of the minor fragment is minimal, adhesive strapping or a stiff-soled shoe is adequate treatment. If displacement is significant, treatment should be by a walking boot until bone healing occurs. Nonunion is rare. It is important to recognize that fractures more proximal in the fifth metatarsal—those through the proximal diaphysis—have a tendency to progress to delayed union or nonunion. These fractures should be immobilized in a cast; some authors have even recommended primary internal fixation. In the adolescent, fracture in the tuberosity should be differentiated from a separate ossific center of the tuberosity and in the adult, from the supernumerary os vesalianum pedis.

G. FRACTURES AND DISLOCATIONS OF PHALANGES OF TOES. Fractures of the phalanges of toes are caused most commonly by direct violence (crushing or stubbing). Spiral or oblique fracture of the shafts of the proximal phalanges of the lesser toes may occur as a result of indirect twisting injury.

Comminuted fracture of the proximal phalanx of the great toe, alone or in combination with fracture of the distal phalanx, is the most disabling injury. Because wide displacement of fragments is not likely, correction of angulation and support by an adhesive dressing and splint usually suffice. A weight-bearing plaster boot may be useful for relief of symptoms arising from soft tissue injury. Spiral or oblique fracture of proximal phalanges of the lesser toes can be treated adequately by binding the involved toes to the adjacent uninjured toe. Comminuted fracture of the distal phalanx is treated as a soft tissue injury.

Traumatic dislocation of the metatarsophalangeal joints usually can be reduced by closed manipulation. These dislocations are rarely isolated and usually occur in combination with other injuries to the forefoot.

H. FRACTURE OF THE SESAMOIDS OF THE GREAT TOE is rare, but it may occur as a result of crushing injury. It must be differentiated from partite developmental lesions. Undisplaced fracture requires no treatment other than a foot support or a metatarsal bar. Displaced fracture may require immobilization in a walking plaster boot with the toe strapped in flexion. Persistent delay of bone healing may cause disabling pain arising from arthritis of the articulation between sesamoid and head of the first metatarsal. If a foot support and metatarsal bar do not provide adequate relief, excision of sesamoid may be necessary.

XIV. INFECTIONS OF BONES AND JOINTS

A. OSTEOMYELITIS is an infection of bone and is classified according to origin as primary or secondary, according to microbial flora, and according to course as acute, subacute, or chronic.

Primary osteomyelitis is caused by direct implantation of microorganisms into bone and is usually localized to that site. Open (compound) fractures, penetrating wounds (especially those due to firearms), and surgical operations on bone are the most common causes. Operative treatment is usually necessary; treatment with antimicrobial drugs is adjunctive.

Secondary (acute hematogenous) osteomyelitis is usually due to spread through the blood stream. It may result from direct extension of infection in contiguous soft tissues or from septic arthritis in an adjacent joint.

1. Acute pyogenic osteomyelitis (secondary or hematogenous). About 95% of acute secondary osteomyelitis cases are caused by pyogenic organisms, usually a single strain. Secondary contamination during treatment may produce a mixed infection.

Acute hematogenous osteomyelitis occurs predominantly during the period of skeletal growth, with peak incidence during childhood. About 75% of cases in children are due to staphylococci; group A streptococci and *Haemophilus influenzae* are the next most common pathogens; and the remainder of cases are caused by a wide variety of organisms. Preexisting infection of another organ system is present in about half of cases. The tibia and femur are the most commonly involved of the long bones. The initial lesion may become progressive or chronic, or the infection may resolve with or without treatment.

If the initial lesion is not controlled, spread of infection causes bony destruction that differs in infancy, childhood, and adulthood owing to the vascular supply of bone. During infancy, terminal ramifications of the nutrient artery perforate the growth plate and end in the cartilaginous precursor of the epiphysis. This may explain both the frequency of complicating septic arthritis during infancy and subsequent disturbances of growth. Infection may spread rapidly throughout the entire length of the bone, but involucrum formation is not characteristic.

In children, initial localization of infection in calcellous bone is rapidly followed by edema which causes increased intraosseous pressure. Suppuration follows edema, and the escape of exudate beneath the periosteum causes elevation with disruption of vascular channels. The inflamed periosteum starts to produce a shell-like layer of new bone which can be identified by radiography. Disturbance of blood supply to the inner surface of the cortex from thrombosed branches of nutrient vessels leads to necrosis of compact bone and sequestration. Because the epiphysis is separated from the metaphysis by the growth plate, it is protected from direct involvement.

In adulthood, metaphyseal and epiphyseal vessels communicate across the scar of the previous growth plate, and microorganisms can enter the epiphysis through the nutrient artery. This permits organisms to reach subchondral bone of joints and precipitate a complicating septic arthritis. Because the periosteum of adults is rather fibrous and adherent, extensive subperiosteal abscess formation is not a prominent feature. However, periosteal inflammation can be identified by demineralization and absorption of the cortex. Involucrum formation and extensive cortical sequestration occur in adulthood. Involvement of the diaphysis, chronic infection of the marrow, and abscesses of the soft tissues surrounding bone are more common sequelae in adults.

a. Diagnosis

(1) *Symptoms and signs.* In infants and children, the onset is often sudden, with marked toxicity; an insidious onset may produce more subtle symptoms. Voluntary movement of the extremity is inhibited. Tenderness followed by swelling and redness are the local manifestations.

Onset in adults is less striking. A history of intravenous drug abuse may suggest a source of the infection. Generalized symptoms of bacteremia may be absent; vague, shifting, or evanescent local pain may be the earliest manifestation. Limitation of joint motion may be marked, especially in patients with spine involvement or when lesions are near joints.

(2) *Laboratory tests.* ESR and white count are often elevated. Identification of the causative organism is often possible by blood culture. Exudates may be recovered for culture by aspiration of extraosseous tissues in areas of

tenderness or directly from the involved bone. In severe infections of more than 2 days' duration, material for culture and smear is usually obtained during open surgical treatment.

(3) *Radiographs.* Significant changes in bone cannot be identified by radiography before 7–10 days after onset in infants and 2–4 weeks after onset in adults, but extraosseous soft tissue swelling adjacent to the infection may appear within 3–5 days after onset of symptoms. Xeroradiography may demonstrate subtle changes in extracortical soft tissues that are not apparent on routine radiographs. CT and MRI may reveal both soft tissue edema and replacement of normal fatty marrow with edema fluid or pus. If antimicrobial therapy was started early, radiographic changes in bone may not appear for 3–5 weeks. Subperiosteal new bone formation is a late manifestation of healing.

b. Differential diagnosis. Acute local infections of bone must be differentiated from the prodromal states of viral illnesses and from traumatic injuries.

Acute hematogenous osteomyelitis must also be differentiated from suppurative arthritis, rheumatic fever, cellulitis, tuberculosis, mycotic infections, and Ewing's sarcoma. The pseudoparalysis associated with acute osteomyelitis in infancy may simulate poliomyelitis. When symptoms are mild, osteomyelitis may initially mimic Legg-Perthes disease.

c. Complications. Delayed diagnosis or inadequate early treatment can lead to chronic osteomyelitis. Other complications include soft tissue abscess formation, septic arthritis, and metastatic infections to other organs. Pathologic fracture may occur at sites of extensive bone destruction.

d. Treatment. Toxic patients require IV administration of fluid and electrolytes. If accompanying anemia is severe, it should be corrected by blood transfusion. Immobilization of the affected extremity by splinting or casting is advisable for relief of pain and protection against pathologic fracture. Although antibiotics are of great benefit, they are not always curative. The mainstay of therapy is surgery. Treatment must be individualized, and only broad guidelines are given here.

(1) *Surgical.* During the first 2–3 days after the onset of acute infection, open surgical treatment can be avoided in many cases, especially in infants and children. If vigorous general care and appropriate antibiotic therapy are instituted promptly, the progress of the local lesion may be

controlled and spread of the infection halted before suppuration and significant tissue destruction have occurred.

If an abscess has formed beneath the periosteum or has extended into soft tissues of infants and children, it should be drained at least once daily by aspiration. Pain and fever that persist longer than 2-3 days after initiating aspiration and antimicrobial therapy suggest spread. Surgical decompression of the medullary cavity by drilling or limited fenestration should be done promptly with the hope of minimizing progression of bone necrosis. Subsequent treatment of the local lesion may be by open or closed technics. Open treatment of the wound by packing requires multiple dressing changes, which are painful and frequently cannot be accomplished except under general anesthesia. Closed wound treatment with intermittent suction drainage provides egress of exudates and minimizes the likelihood of secondary contamination. Antibiotics can also be administered locally through the drainage tube in concentrations that systemically would be toxic.

Radical surgical technics such as extensive guttering and diaphysectomy should be reserved for the treatment of chronic osteomyelitis.

(2) *Antibiotic therapy* is aided by identification of the organism and its antibiotic sensitivities. Because acute infections in children are usually due to staphylococci or β-hemolytic streptococci, appropriate systemic antibiotics for these organisms should be administered without waiting for culture reports. Chemotherapy should be continued for about 2-3 weeks after the patient becomes afebrile or repeated wound cultures fail to show growth.

e. Prognosis. Mortality rate in treated acute osteomyelitis is about 1%, but morbidity continues to be high. If effective treatment is instituted within 48 hours after onset, prompt recovery can be expected in about two thirds of cases. Chronicity and recurrence of infection are likely when treatment is delayed.

2. Chronic pyogenic osteomyelitis may occur as a consequence of acute infection or may appear as an indolent, slowly progressive process with no striking symptom. Recurrent infection is manifested by exacerbation of symptoms with or without drainage after a quiescent period of days, weeks, or years.

a. Diagnosis

(1) *Symptoms* may be so mild and the onset so insidious that there is little or no disability, but recurrent fever,

pain, and swelling are common. There may be a history of injury. The infection may communicate through a sinus to the skin surface with periodic or constant discharge of pus.

(2) *Laboratory tests.* Leukocytosis, anemia, and acceleration of ESR are inconstant. The causative organisms should be cultured and drug sensitivity studies performed. Culture of exudates from sinus orifices may be misleading because skin contaminants are likely to be present. More reliable specimens can be obtained by taking samples of suspected tissue at operation or by deep aspiration at a distance from sinus tracts.

(3) *Radiographs.* Structural alterations of bone depend upon the stage, extent, and rate of progress of disease. Destruction of bone may create diffuse areas of radiolucency. Bone necrosis becomes apparent as areas of increased density and is due in part to osteopenia in surrounding vascularized bone. Involucrum and new bone formation are healing responses which may be identified beneath the periosteum or within the bone. Subperiosteal new bone is seen as a lamellar pattern. Progressive resorption of sclerotic bone and reformation of normal trabecular pattern also suggest healing.

CT may be helpful in identifying deep areas of bone destruction. Sinograms made with contrast media may aid in localization of sequestra or points of persistent infection and demonstrate the course of sinus tracts and soft tissue abscesses. Occasionally, bone scanning with radioisotopes localizes otherwise occult infection.

b. Differential diagnosis. Chronic pyogenic osteomyelitis should be differentiated from benign and malignant tumors; from certain forms of osseous dysplasia; from fatigue fracture; and from specific infections discussed below.

c. Complications. The most common complication is persistence of infection with acute exacerbations. Persistent infection may cause anemia, weight loss, weakness, and amyloidosis. Chronic osteomyelitis may disseminate to other organs. Acute exacerbations can be complicated by serous effusions in adjacent joints or by frank purulent arthritis. Constant erosion and progressive destruction of bone cause structural weakening which can lead to pathologic fracture.

Before epiphyseal closure, osteomyelitis can produce overgrowth of a long bone from chronic hyperemia of the growth plate. Focal destruction of a physeal plate can create asymmetric growth.

Rarely, after years of drainage, pseudoepitheliomatous hyperplasia, squamous cell carcinoma, or a fibrosarcoma arises in persistently infected tissues.

d. Treatment

(1) *General.* During the quiescent phase, no treatment is necessary and patients live essentially normal lives. Minor exacerbations accompanied by drainage may be managed adequately with dressing changes. More acute episodes may require immobilization, bedrest, local heat, and mild analgesics.

(2) *Medical.* Occasionally, when the drug sensitivities of the causative organism are known, systemic antibiotic treatment without surgical intervention is advantageous. This is especially true during the early phase of a recurrence without external drainage or abscess formation.

Copious drainage and clinical and radiographic evidence of progressive bone destruction and sequestration require more aggressive treatment.

(3) *Surgical.* Soft tissue abscesses without sequestration can be treated by operation and open or closed drainage. Similar treatment may also suffice for Brodie's abscess, a rare, walled-off infection of bone. Removal of a sequestrum with drainage of the abscess cavity often permits rapid healing. With the exception of the fibula, metatarsals, and possibly metacarpals, diaphysectomy should be avoided in adults, if possible, because the resected shaft does not regenerate. More extensive and long-standing infections may require more radical surgery (diaphysectomy or amputation). Recently introduced technics such as distraction osteogenesis may be used to reconstitute extensive bone defects.

e. Prognosis.
Even after vigorous treatment, recurrence of infection is likely. This is usually due to incomplete removal of all areas of infected soft tissue scar or necrotic bone.

B. MYCOTIC INFECTIONS OF BONES AND JOINTS. Fungal infections of the skeletal system are usually secondary to a primary infection in another organ system, frequently the lower respiratory tract. Although skeletal lesions have a predilection for the cancellous extremities of long bones and the bodies of vertebrae, the predominant lesion (a granuloma with varying degrees of necrosis and abscess formation) doesn't produce a characteristic clinical picture.

The main mycotic infections of skeletal system are **coccidioidomycosis,** which is usually secondary to a primary pulmonary infection; **histoplasmosis,** which usually represents dissemination from a primary focus in the lungs; **cryptococcosis** (torulosis or European blastomycosis), an uncommon chronic granulomatous pulmonary disease that may be disseminated to the nervous system and rarely to the skeletal system; and North American blastomycosis, which may be disseminated to skeletal structures from the lungs or, less commonly, from cutaneous lesions. Treatment is with amphotericin B (Fungizone). Surgical debridement and in some cases saucerization are often required.

C. SYPHILIS OF BONES AND JOINTS. Syphilitic arthritis or
osteitis may occur during any stage of congenital or acquired infection. Neurotrophic arthropathy (Charcot's joints) can be caused indirectly by syphilitic disease of the spinal cord. In infancy, congenital syphilis typically causes epiphysitis and metaphysitis. Radiologically, a zone of sclerosis appears adjacent to the growth plate but is separated from another similar zone by one of rarefaction. Partial replacement of the rarefied bone by inflammatory tissue precedes suppuration, which may allow epiphyseal displacement because of structural weakening.

Congenital syphilis causes periostitis and osteoperiostitis in childhood and adolescence. Bone involvement is frequently symmetric, and periosteal proliferation along the tibial crest causes the classic "saber shin." A painless bilateral effusion of the knees (Clutton's joints) is a rare manifestation.

In adults, gumma formation is a tertiary manifestation. This granulomatous process is characterized by localized destruction of bone accompanied by surrounding areas of sclerosis. Extensive destruction with accompanying rarefaction may cause pathologic fracture. Periostitis in the adult is likely to occur in the bones of the thorax and in the shafts of long bones. The radiographic picture of syphilitic osteitis in the adult is not diagnostic, but bone production is generally more pronounced than bone destruction.

Osteoarticular lesions due to other causes must be differentiated from syphilis. Serologic studies usually provide confirmatory evidence. Biopsy is not necessary to establish a direct diagnosis, but it may differentiate a gumma from other lesions. A favorable response to penicillin supports the diagnosis.

The only local treatment necessary is immobilization to provide comfort or protection from fracture if the bone is seriously weakened. Lesions of bones and joints respond promptly to adequate chemotherapy.

D. TUBERCULOSIS OF BONES AND JOINTS. Infection of the musculoskeletal system with *M. tuberculosis* is usually caused by hematogenous spread from the respiratory or GI tract. Tuberculosis of the thoracic or lumbar spine may be associated with an active lesion of the genitourinary tract.

1. Diagnosis

a. Symptoms and signs. Onset of symptoms is generally insidious. Pain in an involved joint may be mild and accompanied by a sensation of stiffness. It is commonly accentuated at night. Limping and restriction of joint motion are seen. As disease progresses, the joint becomes fixed by muscle contractures, organic destruction of the joint, and healing in soft tissues and bone.

Local findings during the early stages may be limited to tenderness, soft tissue swelling, joint effusion, and increase in skin temperature about the involved area. As the disease progresses without treatment, muscle atrophy and deformity become apparent. Spontaneous external drainage of abscess leads to sinus formation. Progressive destruction of bone in the spine, especially in the thoracolumbar region, may cause a gibbus.

b. Laboratory tests. Diagnosis rests upon recovery of acid-fast bacilli from joint fluid, tissue exudates, or tissue specimens. Biopsy of the lesion or of a regional joint lymph node may demonstrate the characteristic histologic picture but does not differentiate tuberculosis from other mycobacterial lesions.

c. Radiography. The earliest changes of tuberculous arthritis are soft tissue swelling and distention of the capsule by effusion. Subsequently, bone atrophy causes thinning of trabecular pattern, narrowing of the cortex, and enlargement of the medullary canal. As joint disease progresses, destruction of cartilage causes narrowing of the joint space and focal erosion of the articular surface, especially at the margins. Extensive destruction of joint surfaces causes deformity. As healing takes place, osteosclerosis becomes apparent around areas of necrosis and sequestration. Where the lesion is limited to bone, especially in the cancellous portion of metaphysis, the radiographic picture may be that of single or multilocar cysts surrounded by sclerotic bone. As intraosseous foci expand toward the limiting cortex and erode it, subperiosteal new bone formation takes place.

2. Differential diagnosis. Tuberculosis of the musculoskeletal system must be differentiated from other subacute and chronic infections, rheumatoid arthritis, gout, and occasionally

from osseous dysplasia. Infections caused by nontuberculous atypical mycobacteria can be differentiated only by culture.

3. Complications. Destruction of bones or joints may occur in a few weeks or months if adequate treatment is not provided. Deformity due to joint destruction, abscess formation with spread into adjacent soft tissues, and sinus formation are common. Paraplegia is the most serious complication of spinal tuberculosis. As healing of severe joint lesions takes place, spontaneous fibrous or bony ankylosis follows.

4. Treatment

a. General. In acute infections where synovitis is the predominant feature, treatment can be conservative, at least initially; immobilization, aspiration, and antibiotic therapy may suffice. A similar approach is used for infections of large joints of the lower extremities in children during an early stage. It may also be used in adults either as definitive treatment of mild infections or before operation.

b. Surgical. Various types of operative treatment are necessary for chronic or advanced tuberculosis of bones and joints. The advent of effective drug treatment has broadened the indications for synovectomy and debridement at the expense of more radical surgical procedures such as arthrodesis and amputation. Even though the infection is active and all involved tissue cannot be removed, supplementary chemotherapy may permit healing to occur. In the past, arthrodesis of weight-bearing joints was carried out when function could not be salvaged. Prosthetic replacement in the hip has been used successfully in cases in which the disease has been clinically arrested.

c. Chemotherapy of osteoarticular tuberculosis is based on the systemic administration of drugs to which the strain of pathogen is likely to be susceptible as indicated by in vitro testing. Resistant strains may emerge during administration of single drugs; therefore, combinations of antituberculous agents are recommended (Chapter 4).

E. PYOGENIC ARTHRITIS (suppurative, infectious, or septic arthritis) is an acute or chronic inflammation of joints caused by a variety of microorganisms.

1. Classification can be based on the mechanism of introduction of the pathogen or the microbial etiology.

a. Primary pyogenic arthritis can be the result of direct implantation of microorganisms into joints through penetrating wounds or can complicate percutaneous procedures (e.g., arthrocentesis or intraarticular drug therapy). Joint infections that follow open surgical operations are discussed below.

b. Secondary pyogenic arthritis is generally bloodborne; it can also result from direct extension from an adjacent focus of osteomyelitis or from an extraarticular soft tissue infection.

c. Chronic pyogenic arthritis is usually a sequel to untreated or unsuccessfully treated acute primary or secondary pyogenic arthritis.

2. Acute pyogenic arthritis. Pyogenic cocci (staphylococci, streptococci, pneumococci, and meningococci) are the most frequent pathogens. Enteric gram-negative bacilli, especially *E. coli,* may produce infection in adults. *H. influenzae* is a frequent pathogen in children 6 months to 2 years.

In acute hematogenous arthritis, the larger joints are commonly involved. An acute or chronic infection of nearby bone or soft tissue may secondarily involve a joint. Infections of other organ systems (skin, respiratory, and genitourinary tracts) are possible sources of blood-borne infections. Although a single joint is generally involved in adults, multiple joints may be involved by hematogenous arthritis in children. Antecedent trauma to the area may be misleading.

The initial reaction is an acute synovitis. The intraarticular fluid during this phase may show a few polymorphonuclear leukocytes. Later, the synovial fluid changes to pus; edema and cellular infiltration occur in the subsynovial soft tissues. Destruction of cartilage follows, especially at the point of contact of opposing joint surfaces. Continued infection may produce destruction of synovia and capsular components as well as cartilage and bone. Following successfully treated early infections, there may be no permanent sequelae, but extensive tissue destruction after severe and indolent infections can be only partially repaired, and fibrous or complete bony ankylosis may result.

a. Diagnosis

(1) *Symptoms and signs.* Systemic disease or another serious infection may distract attention from the infected joint. Migratory polyarthralgia or multiple joint symptoms may be misleading. Systemic symptoms include fever, chills, and malaise. Pain is generally progressive and is usually accentuated by active or passive joint motions. The patient tends to limit motion of involved joint. Local tenderness and warmth are present over the joint and are

often accompanied by soft tissue swelling and joint effusion.

(2) *Laboratory tests.* Examination of joint fluid is crucial. During the incipient stage of infection, the fluid may be grossly clear or only slightly turbid, but it tends to become purulent as the infection progresses. The white cell count is likely to be >50,000/ml, with >90% polymorphonuclear neutrophils. The fasting blood glucose level is usually >50 mg/dl above that of the synovial fluid. The mucin clot produced by addition of acetic acid to the synovial fluid tends to fragment or form a flocculent precipitate (in comparison to its normal ropy consistency), which suggests an inflammatory cause of the effusion. ESR is almost invariably accelerated.

Gram stain alone may suggest the appropriate antibiotic. Culture of the blood and synovial fluid establishes a definitive diagnosis and provides specific information on antibiotic sensitivities.

(3) *Radiographs.* Findings depend in part on the virulence of the infection. Radiographic changes lag behind the clinical and pathologic process. During the first 2 weeks, the joint capsule can be seen on radiography to be distended by effusion. As the inflammatory reaction spreads, demarcation between capsule and fat becomes obliterated. Increase in intraarticular pressure from effusion may cause widening of the joint cleft in hip infections, especially in infants, where subluxation can occur. Comparative radiographs of the opposite normal joint can aid in the identification of subtle changes. With persistent hyperemia and disuse, demineralization of subchondral bone occurs adjacent to the joint space and extends centrifugally. Trabecular detail is progressively lost and the compact subchondral bone appears accentuated. Destruction of cartilage is reflected by narrowing of the width of the joint space until subchondral bone is in apposition.

b. Complications. Joint infections can disseminate to other sites either via the blood stream or directly.

c. Differential diagnosis. Acute pyogenic arthritis must be differentiated from other acute arthropathies (rheumatic fever, rheumatoid arthritis, gout and pseudogout, and gonococcal arthritis). Hematogenous osteomyelitis, rheumatic fever, and epiphyseal trauma may mimic acute septic arthritis in childhood.

Acute pyogenic arthritis may complicate other types of preexisting joint disease, notably rheumatoid arthritis or neurotrophic arthropathy. Concomitant or recent systemic treatment with corticosteroids may cloud the diagnosis, especially during the prodromal stage, by modification of physical signs. Polyarthralgia may occur in systemic viral infections or allergic reactions, but other features of pyogenic arthritis are lacking. Acute infections or inflammations of periarticular structures (e.g., septic bursitis and tenosynovitis, osteomyelitis, cellulitis, and acute calcific tendinitis) may be difficult to differentiate. Transient synovitis of the hip in infancy and childhood may be especially difficult to distinguish from bacterial infection, and culture of aspirated joint fluid may be the only method of differentiation.

d. Treatment

(1) *General.* Analgesics and splinting of the involved joint in the position of maximum comfort alleviate pain. Pain caused by increased intraarticular pressure can be relieved by intermittent aspiration or surgical drainage. Bilateral suspension of the lower extremity in abduction with traction may prevent subluxation or dislocation of a septic hip joint, especially in infants and children.

(2) *Specific.* Definitive treatment is based on surgery and antibiotic therapy. The specific operation depends in part upon the infecting agent, the stage of the infection, and the response of the patient.

During the first 48-72 hours after onset, intermittent aspiration relieves intraarticular tension and evacuates exudates. When infection is due to *Staphylococcus aureus,* open or tube drainage is preferable because of the chondrolytic nature of the altered synovial secretions. If infection is not recognized or not treated effectively within the first 72 hours, immediate drainage by open or closed tube methods is advocated. Open drainage implies arthrotomy without closure of the surgical wound, whereas closed drainage indicates closure of the surgical wound with an indwelling tube or percutaneous insertion of a tube via a small trocar into the joint cavity. Arthroscopically assisted drainage and debridement of infected knee joints has been used successfully by some surgeons.

(3) *Antibiotics* should be given based on smear and culture reports.

e. Prognosis.

If effective treatment is instituted within 48-72 hours of onset, prompt response can be expected in an otherwise healthy patient. Defervescence, disappearance of pain, return of uninhibited joint motion, resorption of joint effusion, and a decreasing sedimentation rate are some of the factors that indicate a favorable response to treatment.

Prompt diagnosis and aggressive treatment can prevent the most serious sequel of acute joint infection: loss of function due to bone and soft tissue destruction during the subacute or chronic stage.

3. Gonorrheal arthritis, caused by *N. gonorrhoeae,* is almost always secondary to infection of the genitourinary tract. Joints become infected by hematogenous route, and symptoms appear 2-3 weeks after onset of gonorrhea. Clinical evidence of involvement of multiple joints is often present at the onset, but symptoms are usually transient in all joints but one. Large weight-bearing joints are most often affected. Systemic symptoms may accompany acute arthritis. Initial synovitis with effusion progresses to a purulent exudate with destruction of cartilage which may lead to fibrous or bony alkalosis.

The precise diagnosis is established by recovery of the causative microorganism from the involved joint by culture, which may be successful in only a minority of acute cases. Gonorrheal arthritis must be differentiated from rheumatoid arthritis, pyogenic arthritis caused by other organisms, acute synovitis, Reiter's disease, and gout.

Nonspecific treatment includes immobilization of the joint, bedrest, and analgesics as necessary for pain. If the joint fluid is purulent and recurs rapidly, systemic antibiotic treatment can be supplemented by instillation of the effective antibiotic into the infected joint cavity, repeated once or twice at daily intervals.

The prognosis for preservation of joint function is good if the diagnosis is established promptly and treatment is vigorous.

4. Chronic pyogenic arthritis may follow acute primary or secondary pyogenic arthritis. Pyogenic cocci and enteric gram-negative rods are the most common organisms. The original bacterial strain is sometimes supplanted by another during treatment, or a mixed infection may occur.

The infection can be continuously or intermittently active. Uninterrupted progress from the acute stage is characterized by local pain and swelling, restriction of joint motion, sinus formation, and increasing deformity. Radiographs show progressive destruction of cartilage manifested by narrowing of the joint cleft, erosion of bone, and even infraction or cavitation. Even though the course is indolent, it is that of continued deterioration. Episodic abatement may follow treatment with antibiotics in the recurrent type. Occult infections may be unrecognized for long periods because they do not produce striking clinical findings. They may occur concomitantly with other joint diseases or may complicate surgical operations such as arthroplasty or internal fixation of fractures.

Chronic pyogenic arthritis must be differentiated from chronic nonpyogenic microbial affections of joints, gout, rheumatoid arthritis, and symptomatic degenerative arthritis.

The goal of treatment is eradication of infection and restoration of maximum joint function. Bacterial sensitivity tests provide a basis for selection of antimicrobial drugs. Operative destruction of the joint by arthrodesis or resection is often necessary to eliminate chronic infection.

5. Salmonella osteomyelitis and arthritis. Infection of bones and joints occurs as a complication in <1% of cases with typhoid fever. The precise diagnosis depends upon recovery of *Salmonella typhi* from the osteoarticular focus, and treatment is essentially the same as for other salmonella infections and osteomyelitis in general.

In otherwise healthy patients, the bone lesion of salmonellosis is more likely to be solitary and may exhibit any of the manifestations of acute or chronic pyogenic osteomyelitis. In infants and children, it commonly affects the metaphysis of a major long bone, especially the lower femur, proximal humerus, or distal tibia. In the adult, in addition to the shafts of long bones, the lesion may be found in the metaphyses or epiphyses; other probable locations include the ribs and spine.

Infants and children with sickle cell disease complicated by antecedent episodes of marrow thrombosis and bone infarction can present a somewhat different picture because there is a tendency toward diaphyseal localization multiple foci, and symmetric involvement.

19

Pediatric Surgery

Alfred A. deLorimier
Michael R. Harrison

I. SPECIAL CONSIDERATIONS IN PEDIATRIC MANAGEMENT

Infants and young children have a relatively low tolerance to infection, trauma, blood loss, and nutritional and fluid disturbances. The management of these disorders in infants and children differs somewhat from their treatment in adults, and the margin of safety is narrower. Certain unique aspects of surgical care in infants and young adults deserve emphasis.

A. FLUID AND ELECTROLYTE MANAGEMENT. Parenteral fluids must be adjusted to the size of the patient.

1. Daily maintenance fluid and electrolyte requirements may be calculated according to body weight (Table 19-1). The physiologic limits of water replacement are 30 ml/kg above or below these mean daily requirements. Maintenance electrolyte requirements may be given IV by using such solutions as 5% dextrose and 0.2% saline ($D_5\frac{1}{4}$ NS) with potassium chloride added to a concentration of 20 mEq/L.

Maintenance requirements are higher when there is visible perspiration or abnormally high environmental temperature, fever, or hyperventilation.

2. Previously existing deficits from external fluid losses such as vomiting, diarrhea, and third-space losses into the bowel lumen, peritoneal cavity, or large wounds require rapid blood volume expansion. When a severely contracted blood volume exists, Ringer's lactate should be given rapidly in a volume of 10-20 ml/kg. Rehydration may then be continued with 5% dextrose and 0.45% saline until the clinical status of the baby is improved.

3. Acute blood loss is replaced by transfusion in 10-20 ml/kg increments to maintain vital signs, urine output, and normal hematocrit. Normal blood volume is 85 ml/kg in infants and 75 ml/kg in children. Chronic blood loss is replaced only when hemoglobin drops below 8-9 g/dl.

Table 19-1. Maintenance requirements

Age Size	Premature <2 kg	Infants 2-10 kg	Children 11-20 kg	>20 kg
Water (ml/kg/24 hr)	125-175	125	100	40-60
Sodium (mEq/kg/24 hr)	2-4	2-4	1-3	1-2
Potassium (mEq/kg/24 hr)	1-3	2-4	1-3	1-2
Calories (Cal/kg/24 hr)	125-150	100-125	60-100	30-60
Protein (g/kg/24 hr)	3-4	3-3.5	2.5-3	1-2.5
Urine output (ml/kg/24 hr)	1-3	1-3	1-3	1-3

Newborns of any size require only half normal maintenance for the first 1-2 days.

   4. Continuing losses such as GI secretions, chest tube or bile drainage, and third-space losses require replacement along with maintenance requirements (Table 19-2).
   5. The fluid requirements should be reassessed continuously and the orders should be rewritten at intervals of not more than 8 hours. Placement of a catheter in the right atrium by percutaneous subclavian or internal jugular vein puncture or by a cutdown in the external jugular vein or brachial vein allows monitoring of central venous pressure. Methods for evaluating the response to therapy include assessment of weight, skin turgor, mucous membrane moisture, pulse and central venous pressure response, skin perfusion, urine output and specific gravity, serum and urine osmolarity, hemoglobin, hematocrit, and serum electrolyte changes.

B. NUTRITION An infant requires 100 cal/kg/24 hours and 3 g protein/kg/24 hours to achieve a normal weight gain of 10-15 g/kg/24 hours. These high caloric and protein requirements decline with age but increase with sepsis, stress, and trauma. The catabolic state associated with prolonged starvation and the increased energy expenditures accompanying surgical conditions should be treated by providing adequate calories and protein.
   1. Gastrointestinal feeding. The best means of alimentation is through the GI tract. If the GI tract is functional, standard infant formulas, blenderized meals, or prepared elemen-

Table 19-2. Replacement of abnormal losses of fluids and electrolytes

Type of fluid	Na⁺ (mEq/liter)	K⁺ (mEq/liter)	Cl⁻ (mEq/liter)	HCO₃⁻ (mEq/liter)	Replacement
				Electrolyte content	
Gastric (vomiting)	50 (20–90)	10 (4-15)	90 (50-150)	—	D₅½ NS + K⁺ 20-40 mEq/L
Small bowel (ileostomy)	110 (70-140)	5 (3-10)	100 (70-130)	20 (10-40)	Lactated Ringer's
Diarrhea	80 (10-140)	25 (10-60)	90 (20-120)	40 (30-50)	Lactated Ringer's ± HCO₃
Bile	145 (130-160)	5 (4-7)	100 (80-120)	40 (30-50)	Lactated Ringer's ± HCO₃
Pancreatic	140 (130-150)	5 (4-7)	80 (60-100)	80 (60-110)	Lactated Ringer's ± HCO₃
Sweat					
Normal	20 (10-30)	5 (3-10)	20 (10-40)		
Cystic fibrosis	90 (50-130)	15 (5-25)	90 (60-120)		

tal diets can be given by mouth, through nasogastric or naso-jejunal feeding tubes, or through gastrostomy and jejunostomy tubes placed surgically.

2. Intravenous feeding. When it is necessary to infuse concentrated solutions which thrombose peripheral vessels (>15% glucose), a catheter is placed into the right atrium where the large blood flow dilutes the solution immediately.

The catheter may be placed percutaneously through the subclavian or internal jugular veins, or by cutdown over the external jugular, anterior facial, internal jugular, or brachial veins. This should be performed with strict aseptic technic. The catheter should be of inert material such as Silastic or polyvinyl tubing. The tubing should be sutured to the skin to prevent accidental dislodgement. Dressings should be changed daily and cleansed with iodine solution. If more than 7 days of parenteral nutrition will be required, a Broviac catheter should be used.

Standard IV alimentation solutions containing an amino acid source (2%-5%), glucose (10%-30%), electrolytes, vitamins, and some trace elements are widely available. The electrolyte composition of each solution should be recognized and adjusted if necessary. The solution must be infused at a constant rate to prevent wide fluctuations of blood glucose and amino acid concentrations. This requires the use of an infusion pump. Complications of IV feeding include clotting or accidental dislodgement of the catheter requiring replacement in a new site, sepsis, thromboembolism, acidosis, hyperammonemia, liver damage, and sudden hypoglycemia following abrupt cessation of the infusion.

The risks of a central venous catheter can be avoided by using less concentrated solutions of glucose (<12%), in combination with an emulsified fat solution (Intralipid) given through peripheral veins. Intralipid may not be mixed with other solutions. It may be given alone or concurrently with an amino acid–glucose solution by employing a "Y" tube with the two columns of fluid meeting near the level of the peripheral vein needle. Intralipid 10% (1 g = 10 ml = approximately 10 calories) is given as a continuous infusion at a rate of 10-40 ml/kg/24 hours. The amount of Intralipid should not exceed 4 g/kg/24 hours. Large infusion volumes of the maintenance glucose and fat solutions (100-200 ml/kg/24 hours) may be necessary to provide adequate calories through peripheral vessels. Fluid and electrolytes must be closely monitored.

When properly given, any of these technics can maintain normal growth in infants.

C. TEMPERATURE. Infants lose heat rapidly from their relatively large body surface area. The infant must be kept in an incubator warmed to 32° C or by using an overhead heating element, with temperature monitored continuously. For operation, a warmed room, a warming mattress, and warmed humidified anesthetic gases are required.

D. PREOPERATIVE AND POSTOPERATIVE CARE. All newborns receive 1 mg vitamin K (AquaMephyton) IM. Whole blood or packed red cells are cross-matched. Oxygen and humidity are used as needed. Premedication is not usually necessary. Drugs useful in the surgical care of pediatric patients are listed in Table 19-3.

II. DISORDERS OF THE NECK

A. BRANCHIOGENIC CYSTS AND FISTULAS. During the first month of fetal life, the primitive neck develops four external branchial clefts. Each cleft overlies outpocketings of the foregut, the pharyngeal pouches, so that the external cleft is separated from the internal pouch by only a membrane. The ridges between the clefts, or branchial arches, ultimately form portions of the face and neck. Persistent branchial clefts result in cysts or fistulas lined by squamous or columnar epithelium and surrounded by lymphoid follicles.

1. Diagnosis

a. A persistent first branchial cleft may present as a cyst or fistula in front of or below the ear or below the margin of the mandible. The tract commonly extends to the external auditory canal near the facial nerve.

b. A second branchial cleft remnant may be a cyst or fistula located along the anterior border of the sternocleidomastoid muscle. The tract extends between the internal and external carotid arteries, coursing above the hypoglossal nerve to the tonsillar fossa (see Figure 19-1).

c. A third branchial cleft remnant is a sinus tract extending from the pyriform sinus to the thyroid gland. Almost all of these are on the left side.

d. A cyst produces localized painless swelling unless secondary infection has occurred, in which case erythema and tenderness are present. If a fistula opens into the pharynx, a sour taste may be noted.

e. A fistula produces mucoid material or crusting from a pinpoint skin opening over the middle or lower third of the ster-

Table 19-3. Drugs useful in pediatric surgery

Emergency drugs: single IV dose

Atropine	0.1 mg/kg	Push intracardiac or IV
Epinephrine (Adrenalin)	0.1-1 ml 1:1000	1 mg/dl D_5W, titrate IV drip
Isoproterenol (Isuprel)	0.1-1 mg/kg/min	40 mg/dl D_5W, titrate IV drip
Dopamine (Intropin)	5-40 mg/kg/min	
Lidocaine (Xylocaine)	1 mg/kg	
$NaHCO_3^-$	1 mEq/kg	Slow pushes prn, pH <7.2 or 2 mEq/kg/5 min arrest
Calcium gluconate 10%	10 mg (0.1 ml)/kg	Slow push
Glucose 50%	1 ml/kg	
Furosemide (Lasix)	1 mg/kg	
Mannitol	1 g/kg	
Hydrocortisone (Solu-Cortef)	10-50 mg/kg	
Dexamethasone (Decadron)	2 mg/kg	High dose, short course Rx
Hydralazine (Apresoline)	1 mg/kg	Slow IV to decrease BP
Succinylcholine	1 mg/kg	2 mg/kg IM
Pancuronium or vecuronium	0.1 mg/kg	IV
Ketamine	2 mg/kg	6-10 mg/kg IM

Analgesics and sedatives

Drug	Dose	Route
ASA (aspirin)	5-20 mg/kg	Orally, rectally; every 3-6 hr prn
Acetaminophen (Tylenol)	5-20 mg/kg	Orally, rectally; every 3-6 hr prn
Codeine	0.5-1.5 mg/kg	IM, orally; every 4-6 hr prn
Morphine sulfate	0.1-0.2 mg/kg	IV, IM; every 4-6 hr prn
Meperidine (Demerol)	1-2 mg/kg	IV, IM; orally; every 4-6 hr prn
Naloxone (Narcan)	0.005 mg/kg	IV, IM; every 5 min prn × 3
Nalorphine (Nalline)	0.1 mg/kg	IV, IM; every 15 min prn × 2
Chloral hydrate	10-50 mg/kg	Orally, rectally; every 8 hr prn
Midazolam (Versed)	0.05-0.2 mg/kg	IV, IM, (orally 0.5/Hg; rectally 0.3/ kg)
Secobarbital (Seconal)	1-2 mg/kg	IV, IM, orally; every 6 hr prn
Pentobarbital (Nembutal)	1-2 mg/kg	IV, IM, orally; every 6 hr prn

Gastrointestinal drugs

Drug	Dose	Route
Metoclopramide (Reglan)	0.1 mg/kg	IV, orally; every 6 hr prn
Senna concentrate (Sennekot)	1-2 tsp, bid >1 yr old	
Bisacodyl (Dulcolax)	0.3 mg/kg	Orally, rectally; every 8 hr prn
Cascara	0.2 ml/kg	Orally; every 8 hr prn
Mg hydroxide (Milk of Magnesia)	0.5-1 ml/kg	Orally; every 8 hr prn
Mg citrate	4 ml/kg	Orally; every 8 hr prn
Dioctyl sulfosuccinate (Colace)	2 mg/kg	Orally; every 8 hr prn
Mineral oil	1-2 tsp	Orally; prn
Ferrous sulfate (Fer-in-Sol)	1 mg/kg	Orally; every 8 hr prn

Continued.

Table 19-3. Drugs useful in pediatric surgery—cont'd

Antibiotics		
Aqueous penicillin	50,000-100,000 U/kg/24 hr	IV; every 12 hr (newborn)
	25,000-400,000 U/kg/24 hr	IM, orally; every 4-6 hr
Ampicillin	50-200 mg/kg/24 hr	IM; every 4-8 hr
Methicillin and oxacillin	100-200 mg/kg/24 hr	IM; every 4-6 hr
Gentamicin	3-5 mg/kg/24 hr	IV, IM; every 12 hr (newborn)
Cephalothin	50-100 mg/kg/24 hr	IV, IM; every 4-6 hr
Clindamycin	10-40 mg/kg/24 hr	IV, IM; every 6 hr
Neomycin	50-100 mg/kg/24 hr	Orally; every 6 hr (bowel prep)
Nafcillin	25 mg/kg	IV, IM; every 6 hr
Vancomycin	10 mg/kg	IV; every 6 hr
Cefoxitin	40 mg/kg	IV; every 6 hr

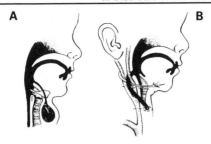

FIGURE 19-1. A, Thyroglossal duct cyst. **B,** Branchial cleft fistula.

nocleidomastoid muscle. Milking the tract from above downward may produce mucoid material at the orifice of the fistula. If the fistula becomes secondarily infected, symptoms of inflammation are present.

f. Branchiogenic cysts and fistulas are bilateral in approximately 10%.

2. Treatment. Surgical excision through a transverse incision is the treatment of choice. If the tract is long, it may be necessary to place a second or third transverse incision above the first for ease of dissection.

B. THYROGLOSSAL DUCT CYSTS, SINUSES, AND FISTULAS. Thyroglossal duct cysts and sinuses may develop from cell rests at any point along the migratory path of the thyroid gland. If the cyst suppurates and drains externally, a fistula results. The cysts contain mucoid material and are lined by squamous or columnar epithelium. Mucous glands occur in 60% of tracts. Scattered islands of thyroid follicles may be present. Sinuses pass a variable distance upward toward the foramen cecum at the base of the tongue. Multiple tracts are common.

1. Diagnosis
a. Thyroglossal duct cysts may be asymptomatic, may be large enough to cause symptoms by pressing on adjacent structures, or, if infected, may be tender and have a discharge. They are found in the midline of the neck anywhere from the submental region to the suprasternal notch, but are most commonly located at the level of the hyoid bone. They vary in size from a barely palpable nodule to a mass 3-4 cm

diameter. Motion of the cyst during protrusion of the tongue is characteristic.

b. Thyroglossal duct fistulas usually develop after a thyroglossal duct abscess has been incised and drained. A deeply placed cord of dense tissue passing upward in the neck with attachment to the hyoid bone suggests the diagnosis.

2. Differential diagnosis. Dermoid cysts may also occur in the midline. Ectopic thyroid tissue is clinically difficult to distinguish from a cyst; a radioactive scintiscan identifies thyroid tissue.

3. Treatment. Cysts and sinuses should be excised because they are apt to become infected. The tracts must be completely removed, including the central portion of the hyoid bone and a block of tissue to the base of the tongue (see Figure 19-2). Infected cysts must be drained, and definitive removal should be delayed until the inflammation has subsided. A sinus or cyst recurs if a branch of the original sinus is overlooked at the first operation.

C. CERVICAL LYMPHADENOPATHY

1. Pyogenic lymphadenitis. Acute inflammation of cervical lymph nodes in the submandibular and anterior cervical triangles usually develops after a respiratory infection. These enlarged nodes ordinarily subside within several weeks. Occasionally, a streptococcal or staphylococcal abscess develops in the nodes and incision and drainage are necessary.

2. Granulomatous lymphadenitis. Typical or atypical tuberculous lymphadenitis develops slowly and may suppurate. The diagnosis is established by appropriate skin tests. These nodes should be excised rather than drained to prevent a chronically draining sinus. Necrotic nodes can be removed by curettement.

3. Lymphoma. Lymphomatous nodes are usually located in the posterior as well as the anterior cervical triangle. These nodes may be solitary, but they are usually multiple, rubbery-hard, matted together, and painless.

4. Metastatic tumor. Metastatic cervical nodes in children are usually due to primary thyroid carcinoma or neuroblastoma.

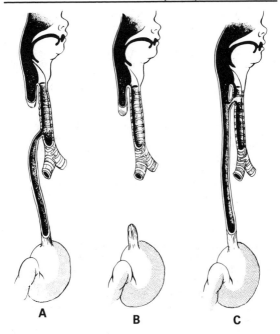

FIGURE 19-2. Esophageal anomalies. **A,** Esophageal atresia; **B,** esophageal atresia without fistula; **C,** H-type tracheoesophageal atresia.

III. RESPIRATORY DISORDERS

A. SURGICAL RESPIRATORY EMERGENCIES

1. Certain aspects of respiration peculiar to infants must be appreciated:

a. Babies are obligate nasal breathers. Mouth breathing is an acquired habit which may not be learned for days or weeks.

b. Infants breathe primarily by diaphragmatic movement. The accessory and intercostal muscles contribute little to ventilation in the newborn.

c. An infant's response to hypoxia is an increase in respiratory rate before an increase in volume. Normal tidal volume is approximately 10 ml/kg.

d. Infants have a flaccid chest wall and mediastinum. Paradoxical motion and increased work in breathing occur with any degree of respiratory distress.

e. Infants have a small, flaccid airway. The tracheal cartilages are readily compressed by slight external pressure. The subglottic area is the narrowest part of the upper airway, measuring about 14 mm^2. If mucosal edema of 1 mm occurs, it reduces the subglottic area to 5 mm^2.

f. Air swallowing develops rapidly during respiratory distress and produces abdominal distention and impaired diaphragmatic excursion.

g. During ventilatory assistance, transpulmonary pressure must be <30 cm of water to prevent alveolar rupture.

2. Symptoms and signs suggestive of respiratory distress in the newborn include (a) Respiratory rate >40/minute. (b) Retraction of the chest wall. (c) Stridor. (d) Cyanosis. (e) Episodes of choking. (f) Episodes of apnea.

3. Differential diagnosis of surgical respiratory emergencies. The diagnosis must be established as soon as possible. Causes of airway obstruction above the thoracic inlet can be identified by physical examination, by attempting to pass a tube through the nasopharynx and esophagus, or by direct laryngoscopy. Intrathoracic lesions must be diagnosed by chest radiography, bronchoscopy, esophagoscopy, CT or MRI.

Surgically treatable causes are choanal atresia, Pierre Robin syndrome; congenital laryngeal obstructions due to webs, cysts, or tumors; compression of the trachea by vascular rings, neck masses, and mediastinal masses; tracheal stenosis, congenital lobar emphysema, and lung cysts; alveolar rupture and pneumothorax; esophageal anomalies; and diaphragmatic hernia. See below.

B. CHOANAL ATRESIA. Complete obstruction at the posterior nares due to choanal atresia may be unilateral and relatively asymptomatic. When it is bilateral, severe respiratory distress is manifest by marked chest wall retractions on inspiration and a normal cry.

1. Diagnosis. There is arching of the head and neck in an effort to breathe, and the baby is unable to eat. The diagnosis is confirmed by inability to pass a tube through the nares to the pharynx. With the baby in a supine position, radiopaque material may be instilled into the nares and lateral radiographs of the head taken to outline the obstruction.

2. Treatment. The emergency treatment of choanal atresia consists of maintaining an oral airway by placing a nipple, with the tip cut off, in the mouth. The membranous (10% of cases) or bony (90%) occlusion may then be perforated by direct transpalatal excision, or it may be punctured and enlarged by using a Hegar's dilator. The newly created opening must be stented with plastic tubing for 5 weeks to prevent stricture.

C. PIERRE ROBIN SYNDROME is characterized by micrognathia, glossoptosis, and cleft palate. The small lower jaw allows the tongue to fall back and occlude the laryngeal airway.

Treatment. The infant should be kept in the prone position during care and feeding; a nasogastric or gastrostomy tube may be necessary. If conservative measures fail, tracheostomy is indicated. The tongue may be sutured forward to the lower jaw, but this frequently breaks down. In time the lower jaw develops normally. These infants eventually learn how to keep the tongue from occluding the airway.

D. CONGENITAL LARYNGEAL OBSTRUCTIONS may be due to intraluminal webs or cysts or to extraluminal tumors such as hemangiomas, cystic hygromas, large congenital goiters, or thyroglossal cysts.

1. Diagnosis. These infants have stridor and chest wall retraction. When the vocal cords are involved the cry is hoarse or aphonic. Examination of the neck and direct laryngoscopy usually identify the cause.

2. Treatment. An airway must be established by placing an endotracheal tube through the larynx or by tracheostomy. Webs and cysts as well as extraluminal tumors must be excised.

E. TRACHEAL OBSTRUCTION BY VASCULAR RINGS AND MEDIASTINAL TUMORS. Vascular rings may compress and encircle the trachea and esophagus, producing respiratory distress and dysphagia. Mediastinal tumors cause respiratory distress by displacement of the lungs or compression of the airways. There are five types of vascular rings: (1) double aortic arch; (2) right aortic arch and persistent left ligamentum arteriosum; (3) anomalous origin of the right subclavian artery; (4)

anomalous origin of the innominate artery; (5) anomalous origin of the right common carotid artery.

Masses causing respiratory distress may involve the anterior, middle, or posterior mediastinum. Examples of such masses include:

Anterior mediastinum—teratoma, lymphangioma, and, in older children, lymphoma, extrathoracic goiter, and thymoma.

Middle mediastinum—pathogenic lymph node enlargement (lymphoma, etc.), aneurysm, bronchogenic cyst.

Posterior mediastinum—neurogenic tumor (neuroblastoma), gastrointestinal duplication (neurenteric cyst), bronchogenic cyst, achalasia or hiatus hernia, mediastinal meningocele.

1. Diagnosis. These infants have a characteristic inspiratory and expiratory wheeze, stridor, or crow. The head is held in an opisthotonic position to prevent compression of the trachea. If the head is forcibly flexed, the stridor is increased and apnea may be produced. There may be hesitation on swallowing with episodes of choking—so called "dysphagia lusoria." Chest radiographs may show compression of the trachea. A-P and lateral esophagograms may show indentation of the esophagus. When there is no esophageal indentation, a tracheogram may be necessary to demonstrate tracheal compression due to an anomalous origin of the innominate or left common carotid artery. An arteriogram is sometimes necessary. Esophagoscopy and bronchoscopy may be helpful in assessing the degree and level of compression.

2. Treatment

a. Vascular rings. The aortic arch anomaly must be completely dissected and evaluated through a left thoracotomy. The smallest component of a double aortic arch must be divided. An anomalous right subclavian artery is divided at its origin. The anomalous innominate or left carotid arteries are pulled forward by placing sutures between their adventitia and the sternum. The accompanying fibrous bands and sheaths constricting the trachea and esophagus must also be divided. However, the attachment between the vessels and the anterior wall of the trachea must be left intact, so that suturing the vessel to the sternum pulls the trachea open. Occasionally, symptoms persist postoperatively because of deformed tracheal cartilage rings. The abnormal area of trachea may require excision.

b. Mediastinal tumors are excised. Lymphomas require chemotherapy.

F. CONGENITAL TRACHEAL STENOSIS

1. Diagnosis. The stenosis may be localized to any segment of the trachea or the entire trachea may be affected. Short segmental stenosis is usually due to submucosal fibrous thickening, while long stenosis is caused by complete tracheal cartilage rings. The symptoms of fixed tracheal narrowing are increased work of breathing on inspiration and expiration. Usually there is an attempt to pass an endotracheal tube and the smallest size tube cannot be placed into the trachea. Chest radiography may outline the narrowing with air-contrast, but bronchoscopy and bronchogram clarify the extent of involvement.

2. Treatment. Median sternostomy is excellent for upper tracheal exposure or posterolateral thoracotomy on the side opposite the aortic arch provides the best surgical access for the lower trachea. For segmental stenosis shorter than one-half the tracheal length, the affected areas should be excised with anastomosis. After transection of the lower end of the trachea, an endotracheal tube can be placed into one or the other bronchus or distal trachea for ventilation, while resection of the proximal area of trachea and the first part of the anastomosis is being developed. For longer lengths of stenosis, usually with complete tracheal rings, the anterior portion of the trachea is incised longitudinally and the appropriate size endotracheal tube is advanced to the carina. The defect in the trachea is covered with a pericardial patch or cartilage taken from a resected rib, placing the attached periosteum on the side of the lumen.

G. CONGENITAL LOBAR EMPHYSEMA may be due to deficient bronchial cartilage, partial obstruction by a redundant or edematous membrane, or compression of the bronchus by an anomalous pulmonary vessel. About one half of the cases are due to formation of an excessive number of alveoli or so-called polyalveolar lobe. Lobar emphysema almost always involves the upper lobes or middle lobe. The emphysematous lobe becomes progressively enlarged, compresses the normal lung, and displaces the mediastinum to the opposite side.

1. Diagnosis. These infants have wheezing, dyspnea, and cyanosis. The chest is hyperresonant, and the breath sounds are decreased over the involved lobe. The diagnosis is established by chest radiography showing the overdistended lobe and compression of the normal lung. The mediastinum may be displaced and the emphysematous lobe may herniate into the opposite chest.

2. Treatment. Occasionally, bronchoscopy and aspiration of mucus or removal of a foreign body are curative. In severely distressed infants, immediate thoracotomy is usually required, and the abnormal lobe must be resected. Relatively asymptomatic patients should be followed closely and may require no treatment.

H. PULMONARY CYSTS AND SEQUESTRATIONS

1. Pulmonary cysts may be congenital or acquired. They may become large enough to be confused with lobar emphysema or pneumothorax and to produce symptoms of severe pulmonary insufficiency.

2. In cystic adenomatoid malformation, usually only one lobe is involved by cysts containing proliferating respiratory epithelium but no cartilage or bronchioles.

3. Pulmonary sequestration may be intralobar or extralobar. An extralobar sequestration presents as a soft, rounded mass lying between the dome of the diaphragm and the lower lobe, usually on the left side. They are usually asymptomatic. Intralobar sequestration has no direct bronchial communication, but becomes infected by collateral ventilation from adjacent lung. Sequestrations are supplied by an artery directly from the aorta, above or below the diaphragm.

4. Treatment. The involved lobe should be removed to relieve the symptoms of respiratory insufficiency and to prevent pulmonary suppuration.

I. ALVEOLAR RUPTURE. Rupture of an alveolus may occur spontaneously or may be caused by excessive intratracheal pressure during resuscitation or mechanical ventilation. Initially, air dissects along the bronchovascular planes, producing pulmonary interstitial emphysema. Further dissection of the air may produce pneumomediastinum or pneumothorax. Mediastinal air does not readily dissect into the tissues of the neck and may markedly compress the trachea. An incision above the clavicles may be necessary to release mediastinal air. Pneumothorax requires tube thoracotomy.

IV. ESOPHAGEAL ANOMALIES

1. Classification. There are three common types of esophageal anomaly:

a. Esophageal atresia in which there is a blind proximal pouch and the distal esophagus communicates with the trachea as a tracheoesophageal fistula (Figure 19-2**A**). This anomaly accounts for 85% of cases.

b. Esophageal atresia with a blind proximal esophageal pouch, no tracheoesophageal fistula, and a rudimentary distal esophagus (Figure 19-2**B**). This accounts for 10% of cases.

c. No esophageal atresia, but an H-type tracheoesophageal fistula (Figure 19-2**C**). This accounts for 4%-5% of esophageal anomalies.

Esophageal stenosis, esophageal web, and esophageal atresia with fistula to the proximal pouch or with multiple fistulas are all rare.

2. Diagnosis

a. Symptoms and signs. The infant appears to have excessive salivation because of inability to swallow. There are repeated episodes of cyanosis, coughing, and gagging. Attempts to feed these babies result in choking and regurgitation. Pneumonia is common owing to aspiration from the blind proximal pouch and/or reflux of gastric contents through the tracheoesophageal fistula. When there is a fistula to the distal esophagus, abdominal distention is common, because air is forced into the bowel during crying.

b. Radiographic findings. A nasogastric tube passed through the nose does not traverse the expected esophageal length. If 1 ml propylidine (Dionosil) or barium is injected into the tube, followed by air, it outlines the blind pouch on anteroposterior and lateral chest radiographs. The contrast material should then be evacuated from the pouch to prevent aspiration. The presence or absence of air in the stomach indicates whether a distal tracheoesophageal fistula is present. The most reliable methods of diagnosing an H-type tracheoesophageal fistula are video-esophagography and endoscopy.

3. Treatment

a. General measures. A sump catheter should be placed in the upper esophageal pouch and connected to continuous suction. The head of the bed should be elevated. The infant should be placed in a humidified incubator and should be turned from side to side every hour and stimulated to cry and cough. Antibiotic therapy is begun immediately: ampicillin 50 mg/kg every 6 hours IV; and gentamicin 2.5 mg/kg every 8 hours.

b. Surgical treatment. Infants with a tracheoesophageal fistula may require gastrostomy to control reflux of gastric juice and to vent air pushed through the tracheoesophageal fistula into the stomach. Full-term infants without severe associated anomalies may then undergo extrapleural thoracotomy for division of the tracheoesophageal fistula and primary esophageal anastomosis as soon as the lungs are clear. Definitive repair may be delayed if there is significant pneumonia or if the infant is premature or has severe associated anomalies.

In most cases of atresia without fistula and in some cases of atresia with fistula, the proximal and distal ends of the esophagus are too far apart for immediate repair. The short proximal pouch may be elongated by daily stretching with a 22-24 Fr bougie over a period of 2-10 weeks. During this time, a sump suction catheter is maintained in the upper pouch and the infant is fed by gastrostomy. It may be necessary to perform a transpleural division of the tracheoesophageal fistula in order to feed the baby by gastrostomy while the pouch is being elongated. In the final stage, extrapleural thoracotomy and anastomosis of the two esophageal segments are usually possible. Extra length can be gained by one or more circumferential incisions through the muscularis of the proximal and distal esophageal segments. If the two esophageal ends cannot be brought together, a conduit between the cervical esophagus and the stomach can be constructed from either colon or greater curvature of the stomach after 1 year of age.

In infants with H-type tracheoesophageal fistula, the fistula may be located above the thoracic inlet in two thirds of cases. These fistulas may be divided through a left transverse cervical incision. Intrathoracic fistulas may be divided by an extrapleural right thoracotomy. A gastrostomy is commonly employed for feeding until the esophageal closure is healed.

V. DIAPHRAGMATIC EVENTRATION AND POSTEROLATERAL (BOCHDALEK) DIAPHRAGMATIC HERNIA

Eventration of the diaphragm may be a congenital defect in which the diaphragm consists of a thin membrane lacking tendon and muscle, or it may be acquired by injury to the brachial plexus during birth; the latter is usually associated with Erb's palsy. The phrenic nerve may be injured during thoracotomy, producing diaphragmatic paralysis.

Posterolateral (Bochdalek) diaphragmatic hernia is a congenital defect in the posterolateral portion of the diaphragm caused by failure of the septum transversum to fuse with the pleuroperitoneal folds during the eighth week of fetal life. The defect occurs on the left side three to five times more frequently than on the right side. During fetal development, the intestinal contents are pushed into the pleural cavity by abdominal muscle tone (Figure 19-3). Varying degrees of pulmonary hypoplasia result, depending on the size of the defect and the amount of intestinal content compressing the lungs.

1. Diagnosis. The onset and severity of symptoms depend upon the degree of pulmonary hypoplasia and the amount of lung compressed by the bowel. These infants have markedly labored respiration and cyanosis. The heart sounds are displaced, and there is apparent dextrocardia with left-sided hernias. The ipsilateral chest is flat to percussion and has diminished breath sounds. The abdomen is characteristically scaphoid. The diagnosis is confirmed by chest radiography showing

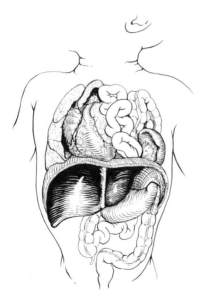

FIGURE 19-3. Congenital posterolateral (Bochdalek) diaphragmatic hernia.

the bowel, spleen, and portions of the liver within the thorax. The lungs, mediastinum, and trachea are displaced to the opposite chest.

2. Treatment

a. General measures. A nasogastric tube should be placed in the stomach to prevent distention of the bowel with air. Oxygen should be given, but ventilation by mask is avoided. For severely distressed infants, an endotracheal tube should be placed and ventilation assisted with transpulmonary pressure <30 cm water. Very rapid shallow breathing with high FiO_2 prevents hypoxia, hypercapnia, and acidosis. A catheter should be inserted into the distal aorta via an umbilical artery (the right radial or temporal artery is an alternative site), and the arterial blood gas and pH levels should be monitored. Metabolic acidosis due to hypoxia requires adjustment in ventilation technic, and bicarbonate should be used only sparingly.

b. Surgical treatment. Infants with eventration may develop severe respiratory distress, and they may require a thoracotomy and plication of the diaphragm to prevent paradoxical motion of the diaphragm and mediastinum.

For infants with a posterolateral diaphragmatic hernia, an abdominal incision is preferred. The bowel is reduced from the pleural space and a hernia sac lining the pleural space should be looked for and excised. A chest tube should be placed in the pleural space and connected to water-seal without suction. The diaphragmatic defect is closed. Large defects require a Teflon or Gortex patch for repair. Forced expansion of the lung must not be attempted lest alveoli be ruptured. A gastrostomy is beneficial. A large ventral hernia may be created by closing the skin, but not the fascia, to accommodate the intestine in the small abdominal cavity.

c. Postoperative care. Ventilatory support is usually necessary. Pulmonary hypertension and heart failure may require vasodilators (tolazoline) and cardiotonic drugs (dopamine).

VI. NEONATAL INTESTINAL OBSTRUCTION

A. GENERAL PRINCIPLES. The cardinal symptoms and signs of neonatal intestinal obstruction are (1) Polyhydramnios in the mother. (2) Vomiting. (3) Abdominal distention. (4) Failure to pass meconium.

1. Polyhydramnios is related to the level of obstruction, occurring in approximately 45% of women who have infants with duodenal atresia and 15% of those who have infants with ileal atresia. When a tube is passed into the stomach of a newborn, a residual >40 ml is diagnostic of obstruction.

2. Vomiting occurs early in upper intestinal obstruction, and it is bilestained if the obstruction is distal to the ampulla of Vater.

3. Abdominal distention is related to the level of obstruction, being most marked in distal obstructions.

4. Meconium is passed in 30%-50% of newborn infants with intestinal obstruction, but the failure to pass meconium within the first 24 hours is distinctly abnormal.

Approximately one fourth of infants with congenital obstructions weigh less than 5.5 lb.

Causes of neonatal intestinal obstruction include intestinal atresia or stenosis, annular pancreas, malrotation with peritoneal bands or volvulus, meconium ileus, Hirschsprung's disease, and imperforate anus.

B. CONGENITAL DUODENAL OBSTRUCTION. Duodenal atresia and stenosis and annular pancreas are frequently associated with other anomalies, and 30% of these patients have Down's syndrome. In 25% of the patients with duodenal atresia, the obstruction is proximal to the ampulla of Vater.

1. Diagnosis. Abdominal radiographs show gastric and duodenal distention (double-bubble sign) when obstruction of the duodenum is almost complete. Total absence of gas distal to the duodenum indicates atresia rather than stenosis. Barium enema (in saline) identifies the presence or absence of malrotation of the colon. The colon is usually very narrow (microcolon).

2. Treatment. A nasogastric tube should be placed and continuous suction applied. Dehydration should be treated preoperatively. Duodenal atresia, stenosis, and annular pancreas should be treated by a side-to-side duodenoduodenostomy between the proximal and distal second part of the duodenum, avoiding the area of obstruction to prevent injury to the ampulla of Vater. The overdistended proximal duodenum frequently fails to function well for many days, and a gastrostomy is helpful for decompression and to check gastric residual during graded feedings. An excessively dilated proximal duodenum requires excision along the antimesenteric wall of the bowel to narrow the lumen.

C. MALROTATION OF THE MIDGUT. During the tenth week of fetal development, the small bowel and colon undergo counterclockwise rotation and fixation to the posterior peritoneum. If bowel rotation fails to occur, intestinal obstruction may be produced by two mechanisms. First, when the cecum is arrested in the upper abdomen, filmy or dense adhesive bands from the right abdomen to the cecum may obstruct the duodenum and other portions of the small bowel. Second, the failure in fixation of the mesentery produces a narrow "universal mesentery" based on the superior mesenteric vessels. This predisposes to volvulus of the intestine, always following clockwise torsion of the bowel and mesentery. The mesenteric blood supply then becomes compromised and may lead to infarction of the entire small and proximal large bowel if the volvulus is not reduced immediately. This is a true emergency, where time counts.

1. Diagnosis. Mesenteric bands usually produce symptoms of duodenal obstruction early in infancy. The abdomen is not distended, and abdominal radiographs show little gas in the small bowel. In contrast, when volvulus occurs, the bowel is usually distended. Bloody stools are a late sign of bowel infarction. A barium enema confirms the abnormal position of the colon and cecum. Because symptoms and abdominal findings may be minimal until bowel infarction is irreversible, emergency barium enema is mandatory if malrotation is suspected.

2. Treatment. The adhesive bands are divided through upper abdominal transverse incision. When a volvulus is present, the torsion is reduced by counterclockwise rotation of the gut. The duodenum is mobilized and placed in the right lower quadrant, and, following appendectomy, the cecum is placed in the left lower quadrant. Frankly necrotic bowel should be resected and continuity established either by primary anastomosis or by Mikulicz enterostomy. After reduction of the volvulus, intestine with questionable viability should be left alone and the abdomen re-explored 12-24 hours later to confirm the viability of the bowel.

D. JEJUNAL, ILEAL, AND COLONIC ATRESIA OR STENOSIS. Small intestinal and colonic atresias probably follow a vascular accident in utero such as volvulus, intussusception, or gangrenous obstruction. Following aseptic necrosis and resorption of the segment of bowel, the atresia may be a membranous occlusion, may produce two blind ends connected by a cord, or there may be a complete separation of the bowel ends. Multiple atresias occur in 10%. Infarction of long lengths of bowel in utero results in abnormally short intestine.

1. Diagnosis. The vomiting, distended infant should have abdominal roentgenograms. Air is sufficient contrast to outline the presence of obstruction, and barium by mouth is not indicated. The colon cannot be distinguished from the small bowel in the newborn, Therefore, a barium enema (in saline) demarcates the colon and determines the presence of colonic obstruction or malrotation. The colon is usually small in caliber (microcolon) because it has been unused, but it is not abnormal. The onset and severity of symptoms from intestinal stenosis depend upon the degree of narrowing of the lumen.

2. Treatment. A transverse upper abdominal incision is used for jejunal atresia, and a tranverse infra-umbilical incision is employed for ileal or colonic atresia. The bulbous dilated proximal blind end of the bowel should be resected. When there is a long length of greatly dilated bowel, the diameter should be reduced by folding in the antimesenteric half of the circumference with a running suture or by resecting the antimesenteric wall of the bowel. End-to-oblique anastomosis is preferred. A gastrostomy is valuable because prolonged postoperative functional obstruction of the dilated proximal bowel frequently occurs.

E. MECONIUM ILEUS. About 15%-20% of infants born with cystic fibrosis have meconium ileus. **Cystic fibrosis** is an inherited disease transmitted as an autosomal recessive trait. The disease affects all the exocrine glands. The secretion from the mucous glands is abnormally viscid and produces varying degrees of obstruction of the bronchi and the pancreatic and bile ducts. Obstruction of the distal small bowel in utero occurs because of the abnormal viscosity of intestinal mucus and not because of pancreatic enzyme deficiency.

1. Diagnosis. Enormous abdominal distention may produce dystocia at birth. Dilated intestinal loops are palpable, and plain abdominal radiographs show dilated loops of bowel of varying diameter. Air-fluid levels are not prominent because of delayed layering of the viscous fluid. Small "soap" bubbles of gas can be seen in the meconium-filled bowel. Calcification in the abdomen may be seen. About 50% of cases are complicated by volvulus and atresia, with or without perforation of the bowel, and meconium peritonitis. The sodium and chloride content of sweat and fingernails is abnormally high (>60 mEq/L).

2. Treatment. A nasogastric tube should be placed into the stomach and connected to suction. Under fluoroscopic control, enemas containing methylglucamine diatrizoate (Gastrografin), which is hygroscopic, or acetylcysteine (Mucomyst), which is mucolytic, may effectively unplug the meconium in uncomplicated cases. Most patients require operation with Mikulicz resection of the most dilated portion of the ileum. Proximal and distal bowel loops may be irrigated with acetylcysteine. Subsequently, the Mikulicz enterostomy is closed.

F. HIRSCHSPRUNG'S DISEASE. Congenital absence of myenteric ganglion cells, extending for a varying distance from the anus, produces functional obstruction of the colon. The normally ganglionic bowel proximal to the aganglionic segment becomes markedly dilated and hypertrophic. The transition zone between aganglionic and ganglionated bowel is at the rectosigmoid in 75% of cases. The entire colon lacks ganglion cells in 10% of cases.

1. Diagnosis. Invariably, constipation begins at birth and may be obstinate enough to cause intestinal obstruction in the neonatal period. Paradoxically, symptoms of abdominal distention and diarrhea in infancy are due to Hirschsprung's disease until proved otherwise. Rectal examination may reveal a tight and narrow anus and rectum. Diagnosis is suspected by barium enema (in saline) showing a normal or small caliber distal intestine and dilatation of the bowel above the transitional zone. No effort should be made to evacuate the contents of the colon before barium enema, so that the transition zone will be retained. The infant is usually unable to evacuate the barium during the next 24 hours. Suction mucosal biopsy of the rectum is safe and simple, but interpretation requires an experienced pathologist. Full-thickness biopsy is definitive in confirming the absence of ganglion cells.

Enterocolitis is a serious and often fatal complication before the first year of life.

2. Treatment. Conservative measures to evacuate colon are inadequate.

For infants less than 1 year old, colostomy should be performed at the transition zone (established by biopsy) in an area of ganglionated bowel.

When the child weighs more than 20 lb, a choice of three abdominoperineal pull-through procedures is available.

a. In the Swenson procedure (Figure 19-4) the overly dilated ganglionated colon and the aganglionic colon

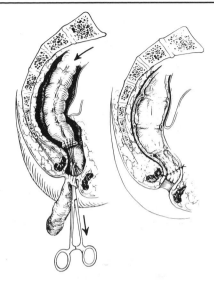

FIGURE 19-4. Swenson abdominoperineal pull-through.

and rectum are excised to a point 1.5 cm anteriorly and 0.5 cm posteriorly from the dentate line. The normally ganglionated bowel is anastomosed to the anal sphincters.

b. The Soave operation (Figure 19-5) consists of dissecting the mucosa out of the residual rectal stump to 1.0 cm above the dentate line. The proximal bowel is pulled through the rectal muscular sleeve and sutured to the distal rectal mucosa.

c. In the Duhamel procedure (Figure 19-6) the overly dilated and aganglionic bowel is removed down to the rectum at the level of pelvic peritoneal reflection. The proximal bowel is brought between the sacrum and rectum and sutured end-to-side to the rectum 1.0 cm above the dentate line. The intervening spur of rectum and bowel is divided to form a side-to-side anastomosis.

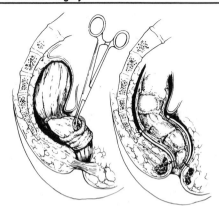

FIGURE 19-5. Soave endorectal pull-through.

G. ANORECTAL ANOMALIES. Two important types of anorectal malformations must be distinguished, depending on whether the distal rectum extends through the levator ani (puborectalis) muscle: the low (translevator) type of imperforate anus or ectopic anus; and the high (supralevator) type of imperforate anus or anorectal agenesis (Figure 19-7).

The low type of imperforate anus may be diagnosed by the presence of an ectopic (and usually stenotic) anal orifice or fistula tract anterior to the normal position. In the male, a fistula tract may extend along the perineal raphe; more rarely,

---

FIGURE 19-6. Duhamel abdominoperineal pull-through. **A,** The rectum has been transected at the peritoneal reflection of the pelvis. The aganglionic and overly distended colon has been resected. The transected normally ganglionated end of the colon is being drawn down behind the rectum. **B,** The end of the proximal colon is anastomosed to an incision made in the posterior wall of the rectum 1.5 cm above the dentate line. **C,** The anterior wall of the colon and the posterior wall of the rectum are divided, and anastomosis is performed with a gastrointestinal stapling device to form a common rectal reservoir.

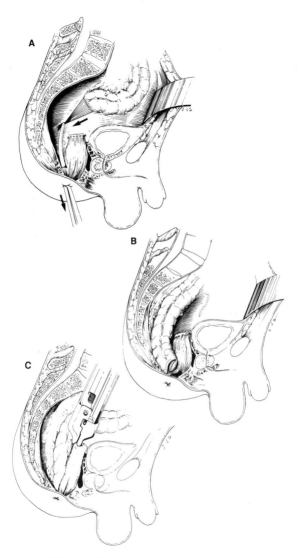

FIGURE 19-6. For legend see opposite page.

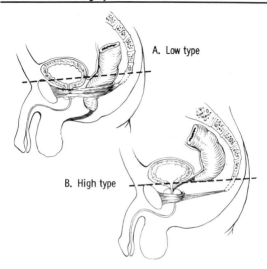

FIGURE 19-7. Imperforate anus. **A,** Low type; **B,** high type.

the fistula is higher and enters the bulbous urethra. In the female, the ectopic orifice may be in the perineum, vestibule, or lower vagina.

In the high type, the distal rectum and anus fail to develop. In the female, there is usually a fistula to the upper vagina or, rarely, to the bladder. In the male there is usually a fistula to the prostatic urethra or bladder.

1. Diagnosis. The most definitive test is careful examination of the perineum for meconium. The presence of a meconium fistula from the bowel to the perineum is the most reliable indicator of a low type anomaly. It is usually safe to wait 12-24 hours to allow meconium to appear.

If a communication between the bowel and perineum cannot be seen, a lateral upside down radiograph of the infant pelvis is sometimes helpful but may be misleading. This should be taken several hours after birth to allow time for swallowed gas to travel to the distal end of the rectum. The baby should be held upside down for several minutes, and the radiograph should be centered over the greater trochanter. Radiographic studies of the spine often reveal vertebral anomalies. IV urograms of renal ultrasonography and voiding cystourethrograms must be done because of the frequency of associated urinary malformations, particularly with anorectal agenesis. MRI scans of the lumbosacral spine identify the presence of a tethered spinal cord, which must be divided to prevent neurologic deficits.

2. Treatment. If a meconium-containing fistula can be demonstrated in the perineum or low vagina, the malformation is a low anomaly and can usually be surgically repaired from a perineal approach with a good prognosis for continence. If a fistula cannot be demonstrated or is high in the vagina, the anomaly is the high type. This malformation requires a sigmoid colostomy in the newborn period. When the infant grows to 20 lb, the anorectal agenesis should be repaired by sacroperineal operation in which the distal colon is brought within the levator-sphincter muscle complex and is sutured to the perineum. In this anomaly, the external anal sphincter and the internal sphincter are deficient. Therefore, continence is dependent upon a functional complex of levator skeletal muscle. The rectum and colon associated with imperforate anus anomalies usually have very poor peristalsis, and constipation is a lifelong problem.

VII. NEONATAL JAUNDICE

The numerous medical causes of direct-reacting hyperbilirubinemia in the newborn include giant cell hepatitis, cytomegalic inclusion disease, herpes simplex, toxoplasmosis, rubella, syphilis, and galactosemia. Antibodies in the baby's serum detect infections causes. Surgically treatable causes of jaundice are biliary atresia and choledochal cyst (see below). During the first months of life, liver function studies cannot identify these various conditions. Microcephaly, chorioretinitis, intracranial calcification, and cytomegalic inclusion bodies in the cells of urinary sediment suggest toxoplasmosis or cytomegalic inclusion disease. Following IV ^{99m}technetium-labeled iminodiacetate compounds (HIDA, PIPIDA, or DISIDA) the appearance of the isotope in the bowel rules out biliary atresia but not choledochal cyst. Needle biopsy of the liver is diagnostic in 60% of cases. Surgical exploration, cholangiography, and open liver biopsy establish the diagnosis in more than 90% of cases. Because results in surgically correctable cases of jaundice are so poor after 90 days of age, surgical exploration is advocated before 3 weeks of age.

A. BILIARY ATRESIA. In extrahepatic atresia, both the major extrahepatic and intrahepatic ducts are obliterated, but numerous proliferating cholangioles and varying grades of cirrhosis may be seen on liver biopsy. The cause of biliary atresia is unknown, but it is probably acquired after birth. The scarred bile ducts and gallbladder are dissected into the porta hepatis and removed. A Roux-en-Y jejunostomy to the porta hepatis may result in satisfactory bile drainage in 50% of cases. Most of the patients develop varying severity of cirrhosis. Long-term survival is 30%.

Intrahepatic biliary atresia is characterized by a total absence of intrahepatic ducts with few cholangioles and little cirrhosis. The extrahepatic bile ducts are patent but narrow. These patients may live for 3-5 years.

B. CHOLEDOCHAL CYST. The three types of choledochal cysts are cystic dilatation of the common bile, diverticulum of the common bile duct, and choledochocele. These cysts commonly have thick fibrous walls which lack an epithelial lining. Commonly there is an anomalous communication of the pancreatic duct to the common bile duct. The onset of symptoms is usually between the age of 3 months and adulthood. Females are affected four times as frequently as males. The symptoms are the triad of jaundice, pain, and abdominal mass.

These cysts should be excised with Roux-en-Y choledochojejunostomy. Associated pancreatic duct anomalies may produce recurrent pancreatitis.

VIII. GI PROBLEMS IN OLDER INFANTS AND CHILDREN

A. HYPERTROPHIC PYLORIC STENOSIS. Progressive hypertrophy of the circular muscle of the pylorus produces narrowing and obstruction of the pyloric canal. The cause is unknown. There is a familial tendency, and males—particularly first-born males—predominate over females 4:1.

This disorder must be differentiated from feeding problems, gastroesophageal reflux, hiatus hernia, pylorospasm, intracranial lesions, uremia, adrenal insufficiency, duodenal stenosis, and malrotation of the bowel.

1. Diagnosis. The symptoms are nonbilious projectile vomiting, failure to gain weight or weight loss, dehydration, and diminished number of stools. The onset of symptoms may occur shortly after birth but is usually delayed until 2-3 weeks after birth. Prominent gastric waves may be seen traversing from the left costal margin across the upper abdomen. A pyloric "tumor" or "olive" 1-2 cm in size is palpable in the upper abdomen in more than 95% of cases. This latter finding is diagnostic, and radiographic studies to show the pyloric "string sign" are usually not necessary. Ultrasound may outline the thickened pyloric muscle.

2. Treatment. A Fredet-Ramstedt pyloromyotomy through a right upper quadrant muscle-splitting incision is curative. This is an elective operation that should be performed only after dehydration and metabolic alkalosis have been treated. Postoperatively, feeding may begin within 6 hours, starting with 1 oz of 10% dextrose solution every 2 hours; increasing amounts of formula are then given every 3-4 hours. There should be no mortality in the treatment of this disease. Complications such as duodenal mucosal perforation, intraabdominal bleeding, and aspiration of vomitus must be carefully watched for in the immediate postoperative period.

B. INTUSSUSCEPTION. Telescoping of a segment of bowel (intussusceptum) into the adjacent segment (intussuscipiens) produces intestinal obstruction, and it may result in gangrene of the intussusceptum. The terminal ileum is usually telescoped into the right colon, producing ileocolic intussusception, but ileo-ileal, ileo-ileocolic, jejuno-jejunal, and colo-colic intussusceptions also occur. In 95% of infants and children the cause is unknown, but this disorder may be related to adenovirus infection. The peak age is in infants 5-9 months old; 65% are less than 1 year old; and 80% are less than 2 years old. Causes such as Meckel's diverticulum, polyps, lymphoma, intramural hematoma (Henoch-Schonlein purpura), and hypertrophic Peyer's patches are reported with increasing frequency in children older than 1 year.

1. Diagnosis. The typical patient is a healthy, robust child who has sudden onset of crying and doubles up his knees on the abdomen because of pain. The ratio of males to females is 3:2. The pain is intermittent, lasts for about 1 minute, and is followed by intervals of apparent well-being. Reflex vomiting is a frequent early sign, and vomiting from bowel obstruction occurs later in the course. Blood and mucus in the rectum produce a "currant jelly" stool. In small infants, colicky pain may not be apparent; these babies become withdrawn, and the most prominent symptom is vomiting. Pallor and sweating during colic are frequent. A mass is usually palpable along the distribution of the colon. A hollow right lower quadrant (Dance's sign) may be noted. Occasionally the intussusception is palpable on rectal examination. The blood count usually shows a polymorphonuclear leukocytosis and hemoconcentration. Barium enema is diagnostic.

2. Treatment. Hypovolemia and dehydration must be corrected. Barium enema reduction may be attempted if there is no evidence of advanced small bowel obstruction or perforation. The patient is sedated, and barium enema is then performed with a surgeon present. The enema bag must not be raised to more than 36 inches above the patient, and under fluoroscopic control the barium enema distends the intussuscipiens and reduces the intussusceptum in 65%-70% of cases.

If enema reduction cannot be accomplished, the patient is anesthetized and the abdomen is explored through a right lower quadrant transverse incision. The intussusception is then reduced by gentle, retrograde compression of the intussuscipiens and not by traction on the proximal bowel. Intestinal resection is indicated if the bowel cannot be reduced or if the bowel is gangrenous. Mikulicz resection may be necessary in critically ill patients. Resection of a Meckel's diverticulum, polypectomy, and incidental appendectomy may be performed. A lymphoma requires removal of the involved bowel and its lymphatic drainage. Intussusception recurs in 1%-2% of cases.

C. GASTROESOPHAGEAL REFLUX. Persistent nonbilious vomiting in infants may be due to gastric outlet obstruction (pyloric stenosis, antral web, or duodenal obstruction proximal to the ampulla of Vater) or malfunction of the gastroesophageal junction at the diaphragmatic hiatus. CNS lesions and sepsis must be excluded. Barium studies often reveal some reflux of gastric contents up the esophagus with or without hiatus hernia and also help rule out congenital esophageal stenosis and achalasia with megaesophagus. In the majority of infants and children with vomiting and reflux, symptoms are controlled by upright feeding and resolve spontaneously when the child begins to sit up and walk. Metoclopramide, 0.1 mg/kg orally every 6 hours, may stop the reflux.

However, some children develop complications of reflux; failure to thrive; abortive sudden death syndrome; aspiration episodes with stridor, bronchitis, or pneumonia; repeated severe vomiting; esophagitis and ulceration with bleeding; anemia; and esophageal structure formation. Acid reflux can be demonstrated with an esophageal pH probe. A Nissen or Thal fundoplication antireflux operation is indicated when sequelae of reflux are documented.

D. OMPHALOMESENTERIC DUCT ANOMALIES. When the entire duct remains intact it is called an **omphalomesenteric fistula.** When the duct is obliterated at the intestinal end but communicates with the umbilicus at the distal end, it is called an **umbilical sinus.** When the epithelial tract persists but both ends are occluded, an **umbilical cyst** or intraabdominal **enterocystoma** may develop. The entire tract may be obliterated but form a band between the ileum and the umbilicus.

The most common remnant of an omphalomesenteric duct is a Meckel's diverticulum, which occurs in 1%-3% of the population. Meckel's diverticulum may be lined in part or totally by small intestinal, colonic, or gastric mucosa, and it may contain aberrant pancreatic tissue. In contrast to duplications and pseudodiverticula, it is located on the antimesenteric border of the ileum 10-90 cm from the ileocecal valve.

1. Diagnosis. Omphalomesenteric remnants may produce symptoms of continuous mucous discharge at the umbilicus, umbilical mass, or abscess. Intestinal obstruction may develop from a persistent band occluding the bowel lumen or by volvulus of the intestine about the band.

Meckel's diverticulum may cause painless, sudden, severe intestinal hemorrhage due to peptic ulceration of the adjacent bowel. The hemorrhage usually occurs in infants less than 2 years old. Peptic ulceration may lead to perforation and generalized peritonitis.

Meckel's diverticulum with a narrow lumen may become occluded and result in diverticulitis, with a clinical picture similar to appendicitis. A Meckel's diverticulum may also become inverted into the bowel lumen and act as a leading edge for an intussusception.

2. Treatment. Umbilical fistulas, sinuses, and cysts should be excised to prevent the development of infection. Meckel's diverticulum should be considered the source of peritonitis or massive GI bleeding when some other cause cannot be identified. Usually the omphalomesenteric remnant can be excised and the communication with the ileum oversewn. Resection of the small intestine is occasionally required.

IX. ABDOMINAL WALL DEFECTS

A. INGUINAL HERNIA AND HYDROCELE. Autopsy studies have shown that the processus vaginalis remains patent in more than 80% of newborn infants. With increasing age, the prevalence of a patent processus diminishes; at 2 years, 40%-50% are open, and in adult autopsy specimens, 25% are open. Actual indirect inguinal hernia develops in 1%-5% of children; 45% occur in the first year of life.

1. Diagnosis of a *hernia* in infancy and childhood can be made only by the demonstration of an inguinal bulge originating from the internal ring. Commonly, the bulge cannot be elicited at will, and signs such as a large external ring, "silk glove" sign, and thickening of the cord are not dependable. Under these circumstances, a reliable history alone may be sufficient. In males, hernias are found on the right side in 60% of cases, on the left side in 25%, and bilaterally in 15%. Bilateral hernias are more frequent in premature infants. The processus may be obliterated at any location proximal to the testes or labia. When the bowel herniates into the scrotum, it is referred to as a complete indirect inguinal hernia; when it extends to a level proximal to the testes in the male or external ring in the female, it is an incomplete inguinal hernia. Direct inguinal and femoral hernias are very rare in infancy and childhood.

Incarcerated inguinal hernia accounts for approximately 10% of childhood hernias, and the greatest incidence is in young infants. In 45% of females with incarcerated hernia, the contents of the sac consist of various combinations of ovary, tube, and uterus. These structures are usually a sliding component of the sac.

Hydroceles almost always represent peritoneal fluid trapped in a patent processus vaginalis; hence, they are commonly called communicating hydroceles. Hydrocele is characteristically an oblong, nontender, soft mass that transilluminates with light. The sudden appearance of fluid confined to the testicular area may represent a noncommunicating hydrocele secondary to torsion of the testes or testicular appendage, or epididymo-orchitis. Rectal examination and palpation of the peritoneal side of the internal ring may distinguish an incarcerated hernia from a hydrocele or other inguinoscrotal mass.

2. Treatment. If expert anesthesia is available, an inguinal hernia in an infant or child should be repaired soon after diagnosis. In premature infants under constant surveillance in the hospital, hernia repair may be deferred until the baby is strong enough to be discharged home. Ordinarily, transfixion suture of the hernia sac at the internal ring, including transversalis fascia, is all that is required. When there is a large internal ring, it may be necessary to narrow the internal ring with multiple sutures placed in the transversalis fascia, but use of abdominal muscles for the repair is unnecessary.

An incarcerated hernia in an infant can usually be reduced initially before operation. This is accomplished by sedation with meperidine (Demerol) 2 mg/kg and secobarbital 2 mg/kg and by elevating the foot of the bed to keep abdominal pressure from being exerted on the inguinal area. When the infant is well-sedated, the hernia may be reduced by gentle pressure over the internal ring in a manner that milks the bowel into the abdominal cavity. During this time, nasogastric suction and IV fluids are used as required for bowel distention and fluid and electrolyte losses. If the bowel is not reduced after a few hours, operation is required. If hernia is reduced, operative repair should be delayed for 24 hours to reduce edema in the tissues. Bloody stools and marked edema or red discoloration of the skin around the groin suggest strangulated hernia, and reduction of the bowel should not be attempted. Emergency repair of incarcerated inguinal hernia is technically difficult because the edematous tissues are friable and tear readily. Gangrenous intestine should be resected, but black, hemorrhagic discoloration of the testis or ovary does not require excision of the gonad.

B. UMBILICAL HERNIA. A fascial defect at the umbilicus is frequent in the newborn, particularly in premature infants. The incidence is higher in blacks. In most children, the umbilical ring progressively diminishes in size and eventually closes. Protrusion of bowel through this defect rarely results in incarceration. Because of these two factors, surgical repair is not indicated unless the intestine becomes incarcerated or unless the fascial defect is >1.5 cm in the diameter after the age of 3 years.

C. OMPHALOCELE occurs once in every 10,000 births. It is a defect in the periumbilical abdominal wall in which the celomic cavity is covered only by peritoneum and amnion. The omphalocele may contain small and large bowel, liver, stomach, spleen, pancreas, and bladder. This defect results from an arrest in mesoblastic infiltration of the ventral body wall. When this mesoblastic arrest takes place in the eighth to tenth week of fetal development, a small defect occurs in which the cord is at the apex of the sac; this is a **fetal omphalocele,** or hernia into the cord. If arrest in mesoblastic infiltration occurs during the third week of fetal development, a large abdominal wall defect is formed and the umbilical cord is located at the edge of the omphalocele. This is **embryonic omphalocele.** Major anomalies are associated with embryonic omphalocele in 50% of cases and involve the CNS, cardiovascular, genito-urinary, and skeletal systems. Malrotation of the midgut is commonly associated with omphalocele. More than half of these babies are born prematurely.

Treatment. The conservative treatment of omphalocele consists of painting the amniotic sac with povidone-iodine every 3 hours to form a sterile eschar which becomes vascularized beneath the membrane. Over a period of time, contraction of the skin and the abdominal wall occurs and the skin grows over the granulating portion of the omphalocele. The disadvantages of this technic are the risk of rupture of the omphalocele, the potential for infection, and the prolonged period of hospitalization required until the defect has healed. It is indicated only for patients with extremely large defects which might not be covered by a surgical approach, or for infants who are critically ill because of prematurity, pulmonary complications, or severe associated malformations.

The fetal type of omphalocele, with a small abdominal defect, can be treated by excising the omphalocele sac and reapproximating the abdominal wall muscles and skin edges.

The large embryonic omphalocele may be treated by staged closure with a "silo" of prosthetic material (usually Silastic-coated Dacron) sutured to the abdominal skin and then removed after the viscera have been progressively reduced into the expanded abdominal cavity. If early closure by this technic is not possible owing to respiratory insufficiency from impaired diaphragmatic excursion, cardiac insufficiency from compression of the inferior vena cava, or vascular insufficiency and infarction of bowel, the omphalocele can be covered with skin and the ventral hernia repaired in stages when the child is older. Teflon or Marlex mesh may be used to bridge the large abdominal defect, and adjacent skin flaps can be mobilized to cover the mesh.

The skin edges can be undermined in the plane between the subcutaneous fat and the abdominal fascia well around the back, inguinal area, and costal margin, and then approximated in the midline to cover the abdominal wall defect. Closure of the abdominal wall without entering the abdominal cavity minimizes distortion of the hepatic veins which would engorge the liver, making abdominal closure more difficult.

D. GASTROSCHISIS. This abdominal wall defect probably follows intrauterine rupture of a fetal omphalocele. It is characterized by a full-thickness defect in the ventral abdominal wall lateral to and usually to the right of a normal insertion of the umbilical cord. There may be a bridge of skin between the defect and the cord. The small and large bowels are herniated through to the abdominal wall defect and, having been bathed in the amniotic fluid, have a very thick, shaggy membrane covering the bowel wall. The loops of intestine are usually matted together, and the length of intestine appears to be abnormally short. Because the bowel has not been contained intraabdominally, the abdominal cavity fails to enlarge and cannot accommodate the protuberant bowel. Over 70% of these infants are premature or small for gestational age. Malrotation of the intestine is almost always present, and other associated anomalies are infrequent.

Treatment. These defects can sometimes be closed primarily.

If the abdominal cavity is not large enough to accept the exteriorized bowel, a tube may be formed from Silastic-covered nylon mesh to encompass the bowel, and the tube is sutured to the abdominal wall defect. When this tube is suspended from the top of an isolette, the intestines can be progressively milked into the expanded abdominal cavity. The fibrogelatinous pseudomembrane surrounding the matted loops of bowel resorbs. Once the bowel is reduced, the Silastic "silo" may be removed and the abdominal wall layers may be reapproximated.

A gastrostomy should be performed for gastrointestinal decompression during the period of ileus, which may be prolonged. Intravenous feeding is essential for postoperative nutrition.

X. NEOPLASMS

A. NEUROBLASTOMA. Of all childhood neoplasms, neuroblastoma is second only to leukemia and brain tumors in frequency. Two thirds of cases occur within the first 5 years of life. This tumor is of neural crest origin and may arise anywhere along the distribution of the sympathetic chain. The tumor is retroperitoneal in 65% of cases, adrenal in 40%, posterior mediastinal in 15%, and cervical or sacral in 5%. Site of origin cannot be determined in 10% of cases.

The biologic behavior of neuroblastoma is frequently different in infants <1 year old compared with older children. The tumor is frequently localized in infants, but distant metastases have developed in >70% of older children at the time of diagnosis. In infants, distant metastases are commonly confined to the liver and subcutaneous tissues, whereas in older children bone and lymph node metastases are most common.

1. Diagnosis. Symptoms in infants are an isolated tumor, hepatomegaly, or subcutaneous nodules. Older children may have an isolated tender mass, but they frequently have pain in the bones and joints and associated malaise, fever, vomiting, and anemia, which may mimic infection or rheumatic fever.

Hypertension occurs in <20% of patients.

Abdominal neuroblastoma may be distinguished from other tumors by the hard, irregular surface of the tumor and the tendency to cross the midline.

Radiographs and CT scan show a soft tissue mass displacing surrounding structures, and calcification is present in 45% of the tumors. For retroperitoneal tumors, an IV pyelogram shows displacement or compression of the adjacent kidney, without distortion of the renal calyces.

Approximately 70% of neuroblastomas produce norepinephrine and its precursors or metabolites. The breakdown products of excess norepinephrine production, most commonly VMA and HVA, should be measured in urine specimens at intervals so that the clinical course of the patient can be followed. An HVA/VMA ratio >1 is associated with a poor prognosis. Serum ferritin level <75 ng/ml is associated with a good prognosis, whereas values >140 ng/ml indicate a poor prognosis. Excised tumor should be analyzed for the oncogene n-*myc;* multiple copies are associated with a poor prognosis and warrant very aggressive treatment.

2. Treatment. A localized neuroblastoma should be excised without irradiation. An unresectable primary tumor and its metastases should be treated by combination chemotherapy. This may produce tumor regression which is sometimes permanent in infants but usually only temporary in older children. Following regression with chemotherapy, residual primary tumor should be excised and total body irradiation with bone marrow transplantation rescue may result in survival in 25%.

The 2-year "cure" rate in infants with distant metastases is 80%.

B. WILMS' TUMOR arises within the capsule of the kidney and consists of a variety of epithelial and sarcomatous cell types such as abortive tubules and glomeruli, smooth and skeletal muscle fibers, spindle cells, cartilage, and bone. Hence the tumor is also called nephroblastoma, embryoma, carcinosarcoma, or mixed tumor of the kidney. About 10% of cases are clear cell, rhabdoid, or anaplastic sarcomatous tumors which have poor prognosis. 80% of patients are under 4 years old. Bilateral tumors occur in 5%-10% of cases. Metastases most commonly occur to the liver and lungs.

    1. Diagnosis. A large, firm, smooth, lateral abdominal mass is always palpable. An IV urogram shows distortion of the calyces and kidney silhouette. Very rarely there is nonfunction of the kidney, in which case the mass must be distinguished from hydronephrosis. Cystoscopy, retrograde urograms, and renal arteriograms are unnecessary. CT scan of abdomen and chest are helpful.

    2. Treatment. The preferred treatment is immediate nephrectomy and excision of all the surrounding tissues within Gerota's fascia, including lymph nodes along the aorta and inferior vena cava. Radiation therapy to the tumor bed is required when regional nodes contain tumor, or if the tumor has broken through the capsule. Very large tumors should be treated with chemotherapy preoperatively to reduce the size of the tumor; nephrectomy should then be performed. The nephrectomy is accomplished through an abdominal or thoracoabdominal incision. Dactinomycin and vincristine should be given postoperatively. Doxorubicin improves the tumor-free survival for more advanced stages of the tumor or for unfavorable histologic clear cell, rhabdoid, and anaplastic tumors.

    Patients with distant metastases are curable. Solitary liver and lung metastases should be resected. Multiple metastases should be treated with irradiation in conjunction with chemotherapy. The cure rate is >85% when this tumor is treated in pediatric oncology centers.

C. TERATOMAS are congenital tumors derived from pluripotential embryonic cells. They are located in the midline or paramedian parts of the body. Teratomas consist of cells representing the three germ layers such as neural tissue, dermal epithelial elements and teeth, intestinal and respiratory epithelium, chorioepithelioma, and mesenchymal tissue such as smooth and striated muscle, connective tissue fat, cartilage, and bone. There are benign and malignant types of teratomas. Metastases usually consist of endodermal sinus (yolk sac carcinoma) tumor. Sites of origin in order of frequency are the ovaries, testes, anterior mediastinum, presacral and coccygeal regions, and retroperitoneum. Most ovarian teratomas are benign "dermoid" tumors. Most testicular teratomas are malignant, and the incidence of malignancy is higher than in the normal population in undescended testis and in pseudohermaphrodites. Most of the mediastinal, retroperitoneal, and coccygeal teratomas are benign. Serum for human chorionic gonadotropin and alphafetoprotein should be drawn to detect a malignant germ cell component to the tumor and as a marker to follow the course of the patient. These tumors should be excised because of their malignant potential and the symptoms produced by their size. Germ cell (yolk sac or endodermal sinus) malignancy is curable with chemotherapy, using a combination of vincristine, bleomycin, actinomycin, cyclophosphamide, and doxorubicin.

D. RHABDOMYOSARCOMAS. The histologic varieties are the embryonal cell, alveolar cell, and pleomorphic types. Sarcoma botryoides is a variant of the embryonal type which is characterized by grape-like masses located in mucosal-lined cavities such as bladder, vagina, bile ducts, middle ear, and sinuses. The embryonal type of tumor occurs primarily in infants and children and arises from the urogenital tract or the skeletal muscles of the head and neck, the extremities, and the trunk. The alveolar cell type occurs in adolescents and young adults and arises from skeletal muscles in the trunk and extremities. The pleomorphic type develops mainly in adults. Metastases spread to regional lymph nodes and to the lungs and liver. Treatment requires radical excision. Radiation therapy and dactinomycin, vincristine, and cyclophosphamide are supplements to surgical excision or are used for disseminated tumor.

E. CYSTIC HYGROMA AND LYMPHANGIOMA. These tumors of lymph vessels occur at the junction of large lymphatic trunks in the neck, axilla, and groin. Cystic hygromas contain large cysts with a well-defined capsule. Lymphangiomas consist of microcystic lymph masses and characteristically invade surrounding structures without respect for tissue planes. Whether these tumors are true neoplasms or whether they represent malformations of the lymphatic system is controversial. Indications for treatment are cosmetic deformity, functional impairment, and prevention of repeated lymphangitis. These lesions do not respond to drugs or injection of sclerosing agents, and they are radioresistant. Excision is the only method of treatment. Every effort should be made to spare normal structures, particularly nerves.

20

Organ Transplantation

John P. Roberts
Chris Freise

I. OVERVIEW

Problems following solid organ transplantation are the result of three factors: (1) the technical aspects of implantation of the graft, (2) the rejection process and concurrent immunosuppression, and (3) the interaction between the first two parts. The problems are related to both the specific organ transplanted and general difficulties that occur in all transplant patients despite the organ they received. For example, renal dysfunction in a cardiac transplant patient has a very similar list of probable causes to renal dysfunction in a liver transplant patient, but these are different from the list in the kidney transplant patient with renal dysfunction.

The occurrence of the complications is very time dependent, and the time after transplant is an important consideration in making a list of probable diagnoses of a symptom complex. For example, a fever in a transplant patient 1 week after transplant has a different probability of being a viral infection than a fever 1 month after transplant. Similarly, the ordering of the differential diagnosis of liver dysfunction following liver transplant is different at 1 month than at 1 year.

The technical aspects of transplantation between different allografts are related primarily to the vascular anastomosis for each organ and for organs that require anastomosis of an epithelialized structure (bile duct, bronchus, ureter, or pancreatic duct). Overall, the incidence of complications is greater for the epithelial anastomosis than for the vascular anastomosis.

The postoperative course following transplantation can be divided into several periods. In the different periods the expected problems reflect the three parts listed above.

A. In the **immediate postoperative course** (first 5 days), most complications are related to bleeding, thrombosis of the vascular anastomosis (frequency of which is inversely proportional to the diameter of the anastomosis), and problems with function of the new organ.

1. Bleeding frequently requires immediate reexploration, if the coagulation status has been normalized. The tolerance for the amount of blood being given prior to reexploration depends somewhat on the organ. Whereas a 6-unit postoperative transfusion requirement may be tolerated in an adult liver recipient, it would not be in a kidney transplant recipient.

2. Vascular thrombosis is rare in thoracic organ transplantation but is more common in renal, pancreatic, and liver transplantation. In patients receiving these organs, although it is theoretically possible to reexplore grafts with thrombosis prior to severe injury, this has generally not been successful. An exception has been the transplanted liver. Because of its dual blood supply (portal vein and hepatic artery), thrombectomy of the artery has been successful, although severe injury to the biliary tree usually results. This is because the hepatocytes can survive on portal blood flow whereas the biliary tree requires arterial blood flow.

3. During this early postoperative period **rejection** is relatively uncommon. Hyperacute rejection is possible but with modern immunologic technics is rare in ABO blood type compatible grafts. The major complications related to the immune system are complications arising from administration of the immunosuppressive agents. These include hyperglycemia and mental status changes due to corticosteroids, renal and neurological dysfunction from cyclosporine, and decreased white blood and platelet counts from antilymphocyte preparations.

B. In the next period of time, **5 to 21 days,** the primary technical concern is the epithelial anastomosis. Leakage at this anastomosis has been of major concern in lung and heart/lung transplantation (bronchus), liver transplant (bile duct), and kidney transplant (ureter). The common cause is probably related to blood supply to the distal aspect of the donor structure. Leakage at these anastomoses is frequently life-threatening and is generally treated by reexploration. Temporization in liver and kidney transplantation can be done by drainage of the bile or urine flow proximal to the leak and percutaneous drainage of associated fluid collections.

1. During this time, **rejection** becomes an important factor in morbidity and mortality. Most acute allograft rejections occur within the first month. There are two major caveats in the diagnosis and treatment of rejection. The first is that rejection is manifest in all organs as graft dysfunction only in its late stages; the second is that rejection is less damaging to the graft and more easily reversed if treated early. For example, if hyperglycemia is used as a marker in pancreas rejection, 90% of the islets are rejected prior to development of hyperglycemia, and treatment of rejection at this point in the clinical course results in graft loss. This has led to the concept of graft surveillance by biopsy in heart, liver, and lung transplantation. The serum creatinine may be an early enough marker of rejection prior to irreversible graft dysfunction to be useful in kidney transplantation. Pancreas transplantation is more successful in combined kidney/pancreas transplantation, probably because the kidney graft serves as a marker of rejection for the pancreas. Similarly, rejection of the lung graft can be demonstrated by heart biopsy and can serve as a marker for rejection of combined heart/lung transplantation.

2. The most common **infections** during the first two periods are of bacterial origin. These infections are primarily pneumonia, wound infection, abscesses, and infections related to indwelling catheters.

C. In the **later posttransplant course** (21 days to 6 months), rejection and infection dominate the clinical course as technical problems become unusual. The most common **technical problems** during this period are stenosis of the epithelial and vacular anastomoses. In general, these are treated (at least temporarily) by balloon dilatation and stenting but may require reoperation.

1. Infections during this period are usually secondary to opportunistic organisms. The primary cause of infectious morbidity is CMV. These CMV infections can range from minimal significance with only asymptomatic viremia or viuria to febrile leukopenic episodes with minimal morbidity to a overwhelming infection with pneumonia, hepatitis, or pancreatitis (with substantial mortality). A CMV infection should be high in the differential diagnosis of febrile transplant patients during this period. Fortunately, it appears that antiviral prophylaxis (acyclovir and gancyclovir) may be effective in preventing or alleviating the disease, and gancyclovir therapy may be effective in treating acute infection. Other infections include pneumocystis pneumonia, which can be eliminated by sulfa prophylaxis, and fungal infections.

2. In the time following 6 months posttransplant, **hepatitis, chronic rejection, hypertension, renal dysfunction,**

and **drug toxicity** dominate the picture. Many of the late complications are specific to each organ, although cyclosporine nephrotoxicity, hypertension, and hypercholesterolemia pertain to all organs.

II. IMMUNOLOGY OF ORGAN TRANSPLANTATION

In order for recognition of a transplantated organ by the host to occur, a difference in cellular proteins between the donor and recipient must exist so that the donor can be recognized as foreign. In human transplantation, the proteins that have been found to be most important in rejection are those derived from a major histocompatibility gene complex. In the human, the gene products from this complex are called the HLA antigens. These gene products are grouped by the different loci (A, B, and DR) and are found on chromosome 6. The antigens found in the A and B loci are called HLA class I antigens, and those found in the DR loci are called class II antigens. The proteins produced by these genes have enormous variability, so each individual human is almost unique.

The basic concerns related to these genes in clinical transplantation have to do with the degree to which the donor and recipient have the same gene products, or are "matched." Identical twins are obviously are identically matched, having received a complete set of identical chromosomes from each parent. Nonidentical siblings could have received the same set of HLA genes by receiving the same chromosome 6 from each parent (HLA-identical or 2-haplotype match), received only one copy that is the same (1-haplotype match), or have received copies that are completely different (0 haplotype). The importance of HLA antigens can be seen in a living related kidney transplant, in which a recipient of an HLA-identical kidney from a sibling has a 5-year graft survival of 90%, whereas recipients of a 0- or 1-haplotype match have a 64% 5-year graft survival, and those patients receiving a transplant from an unrelated cadaveric donor have a 50% 5-year graft survival. The benefit of matching of HLA antigens in cadaver grafts is debated widely. Cadaver grafts that share 6 antigens (two from each loci: A, D, and DR) appear to have improved survival compared with less well matched grafts, and these kidneys are currently shared throughout the United States. The benefit of lesser degrees of HLA matching in graft outcome is unclear. In heart and liver transplantation, extensive matching is precluded by the relatively short preservation times and paucity of donors of these organs. In a retrospective analysis, no benefit was seen for HLA matching of donor and recipients in liver transplantation.

Although the HLA antigens are a major cause of immune rejection in transplantation recipients, they are not the only antigens that can illicit a response, as recipients of kidneys from HLA-identical siblings still require immunosuppression. The identity of these other proteins (*"minor antigens"*) is unclear.

REJECTION. Rejection of the transplanted organ is the bane of the transplant surgeon and physician. Without rejection there would be no need for immunosuppressive drugs, with their systemic toxicity and increased risk of infection. The rejection process is made up of three major processes: (1) the recognition of foreign proteins (antigens), (2) the amplification of the responsive cells, and (3) the attack of the immune system on the transplanted organ. Although these events may occur simultaneously, they can be analyzed separately. The two major types of rejection are antibody mediated (humoral) and that mediated directly by the lymphocyte infiltration and destruction of the graft (cellular rejection). The most common type of solid organ rejection in patients with a negative cross-match (see later discussion) is the cellular type. The components of this cellular rejection are (1) foreign protein, (2) a macrophage (antigen-presenting cell), (3) two classes of lymphocytes—T-helper and T-cytotoxic cells, and (4) chemical signals between cells (primarily interleukin (IL)-1 and IL-2).

In this model of cellular rejection the foreign protein antigen is ingested by the macrophage, and a fragment of the antigen (epitope) is delivered to the T-helper cell in conjunction with secretion of the chemical signal IL-1 by the macrophage. This results in the stimulation of the T-helper cell to proliferation and requires the production by the T-cell of IL-2 and its receptor (IL-2 receptor). The response by the T-helper cell requires stimulation in the presence of both HLA class I and class II. This production of IL-2 also causes the activation and proliferation of cytotoxic T-cells that react to the foreign protein in the presence of class I antigens. These cells cause destruction of the foreign cells by a variety of mechanisms. Although the steps above are a simplification of the cellular rejection process, they represent the target sites for the current immunosuppressive drugs.

III. IMMUNOLOGIC TECHNICS IN TRANSPLANTATION

Prior to transplantation, the immunology laboratory plays an important role in determining the outcome following transplantation. This is because the immune response has some predictable aspects to it that can be determined prior to transplantation, and clinical decisions can be made using this information, such as selecting the appropriate donor-recipient pair or even altering immunosuppression.

A. HLA TISSUE TYPING. Tissue typing is particularly important in living related transplantation of kidneys, as the long-term prognosis for graft survival depends upon the degree of HLA matching. Tissue typing also plays a role in cadaver kidney transplantation, as kidneys with six antigens in common (six-antigen match) with a recipient are shared currently throughout the United States. The clinical uses of matching in other solid organ transplants are controversial, as no direct relationship to graft survival has been documented except for pancreas transplantation, in which matching the graft and recipient at the DR locus appears to improve survival.

The primary method for determining the HLA type of an individual is through **serologic typing.** This is done by taking antibodies to a known HLA antigen and mixing them with the recipient cells and complement; if the cells are killed, the antigen to which the test antibody was directed is known to be on the surface of those cells, and in this way each of the antigens belonging to the A, B, and DR classes is identified. This same procedure can be done on the donor, and the degree of matching between the donor and the recipient can be determined. A six-antigen match occurs when the two antigens from each of the A, B, and DR loci are identical.

B. CROSS-MATCHING. In all the solid organs (except possibly for liver transplantation), the identification of preformed antibodies in the recipient serum directed against the donor cells (positive cross-match) carries a poor prognosis for graft survival secondary to a high incidence of rejection. This can take the form of "hyperacute rejection" when these antibodies react immediately to the proteins in the vessels of the graft and lead to intravascular thrombosis and graft loss within minutes or hours.

Patients acquire these antibodies from previous blood transfusions, previous organ transplants, and, for females, from previous pregnancies. These events represent exposure to foreign antigens to which the patient forms antibodies. These antibodies can represent a significant problem in finding a suitable organ for transplantation. A patient with antibodies in his or her serum to many potential donors is said to be sensitized. To determine the degree of sensitization of a patient, serum from a particular patient is mixed with cells isolated from volunteers who represent the potential donor pool. This test is called the *panel reactive antibody* (PRA) and can be used in the rough sense to decide how long a particular patient may have to wait prior to transplantation. It can be calculated that a patient who has a PRA of 90% would have a high likelihood of being cross-match–positive against a single donor and would require testing against 50 to 100 donors to find one with whom the cross-match is negative. A patient with a 10% PRA would most likely have a negative cross-match with the first available donor.

A cross-match is performed by taking the recipient's serum and mixing it with the donor cells along with complement. If the donor cells are killed, the patient is said to be cross-match–positive. It has been found that transplanting a kidney, heart, or pancreas into a cross-match–positive patient leads to a high incidence of graft loss. The effect of a positive cross-match on survival following liver transplantation is unclear.

C. ABO TYPING. ABO blood typing is done in the usual fashion. Of the four possible blood types, donors of the O type can donate an organ to any recipient, whereas organ patients of the AB blood type can receive organs from donors of any blood type. An ABO-identical transplant is a transplant performed between two patients of the same blood group. An ABO-compatible transplant is performed from an O donor to a recipient of any of the other blood types or transplants to an AB recipient from a non-AB donor. ABO-incompatible transplants are occasionally performed as emergent transplants in liver transplantation, but in general are not performed in kidney or heart transplants without special protocols. ABO-compatible but not identical transplants should in general be performed only in emergency situations, as the use of the donor from one blood type to a recipient of another blood type reduces the potential pool of available organs of the donor blood type. The effect can be seen on patients with O blood type (the universal donor); waiting time for these patients tends to be much longer than for patients of other blood types as organs are transplanted into non–O blood type recipients.

IV. IMMUNOSUPPRESSION*

The development of better regimens for immunosuppression and improved immunosuppressive agents, particularly cyclosporine, have been responsible for a substantial part of the increase in survival. With these current survival rates, the impact of new immunosuppressive agents and immunosuppressive regimens will primarily be in lowering morbidity and thereby the costs of transplantation.

Many of the immunosuppressive regimens and agents currently used in transplantation reflect regimens and agents developed for renal transplantation. The earliest regimen was a combination of azathioprine and prednisone. This regimen in the 1970s yielded the first long-term survival of hepatic and heart allografts. However, graft loss was relatively high; moreover, relatively high doses of prednisone were necessary to maintain immunosuppression in these patients. These high doses of prednisone (>0.1 mg/kg/day) led to significant long-term morbidity.

The introduction of cyclosporine into the immunosuppressive regimen of liver allograft recipients revolutionized immunosuppression. Foremost, the introduction of cyclosporine led to the marked improvement in graft and patient survival that has been seen throughout the 1980s and, importantly, also paved the way for the development of new immunosuppressive strategies, such as synergistic regimens and sequential therapy, which have already contributed to decreased morbidity related to the immunosuppressive regimens.

In the 1990s we will see the introduction of an even greater number of agents. This should allow for the tailoring of immunosuppressive regimens to the individual patient. For example, it is anticipated that while patients may receive relatively potent immunosuppressive regimens during the immediate posttransplant period, when the risk of rejection is highest, patients who do not develop rejection may be switched to alternative regimens that, while providing less immunosuppression, will likewise decrease the long-term morbidity of the immunosuppressive agents. Alternatively, patients who demonstrate a greater number or more severe episodes of rejection will be switched to a more potent agent(s) that, while running

---

*Parts of this section are taken from Lake JR, Roberts JP, and Ascher NL: Maintenance immunosuppression after liver transplantation. Seminars in Liver Disease 12:73-79, 1992.

the risk of greater side effects, will be expected to provide adequate immunosuppression and thereby prevent graft loss.

A. AGENTS

1. Corticosteroids. Corticosteroids (i.e., prednisone and prednisolone) have been used as immunosuppressive agents since the earliest days of transplantation. Even today, almost every regimen includes corticosteroids as a major component. Corticosteroids are used not only for maintenance immunosuppression but also for treatment of established rejection as well. Corticosteroids act at a variety of levels in a cascade of immunologic events leading to rejection. For example, corticosteroids appear to block the production of IL-1. This inhibition of IL-1 production leads to impaired activation of the T-cell and its subsequent production of IL-2, which is important for clonal expansion in response to HLA class II antigens. Corticosteroids also appear to be cytotoxic to activated lymphocytes. In addition, corticosteroids decrease HLA class II antigen expression, inhibit the inflammatory response of other cells (e.g., eosinophils), and prevent the migration of inflammatory cells into damaged tissues. Finally, corticosteroids also inhibit monocyte transformation into macrophages and may inhibit the effects of other antigen-presenting cells as well.

Corticosteroids are often given as a bolus intravenously either immediately prior to transplant surgery, during surgery, or immediately after surgery. Relatively high doses of prednisone or prednisolone are used during the early posttransplant period, and the dose is rapidly tapered to the desired maintenance level. Generally the maintenance dose is 5-10 mg of prednisone per day in adults and 0.1 mg/kg/day in children.

The side effects of corticosteroids are well-known and include fluid retention, hypertension, hyperglycemia, impaired wound healing, myopathy, growth retardation in children, aseptic necrosis of the hip, cataracts, and decreased bone mineralization. These latter long-term side-effects are the most troubling and most disabling side-effects of corticosteroids, and a number of programs have therefore attempted to develop regimens that eventually remove corticosteroids from the patient's immunosuppressive regimen. Other strategies such as the attempt to alleviate bone loss with bisphosphonates (etidronate) or calcitonin are also being tried.

2. Azathioprine. Azathioprine was part of the original regimen used for immunosuppression. More recently, azathioprine has been used largely as part of the so-called triple immunosuppressive regimen in combination with cyclosporine and prednisone. This immunosuppressive regimen likely represents the most common regimen currently used for immunosuppression of the allograft recipient. Azathioprine represents a modification of the parent compound, 6-mercaptopurine (6-MP), and is converted in vivo to 6-MP, which represents the active compound. Azathioprine is an antimetabolite that exerts its immunosuppressive effects through purine metabolism, thereby inhibiting cell division. Consequently, the most rapidly dividing cells in the body are most sensitive to this agent. Currently, azathioprine is used primarily as a steroid- and cyclosporine-sparing agent, in combination with prednisone and cyclosporine. It can be administered either IV or by mouth, and the dosages used are 1-2 mg/kg/day, generally given as a single dose.

The side-effects of this agent are directly related to its effect on cell proliferation, and thus the cells that are most rapidly dividing are most likely to be affected. The major side-effect of azathioprine is bone marrow suppression. In particular, azathioprine has its most significant effects on white blood cells. This effect is dose-related and can be easily reversed either by temporary discontinuation or, more often, by decreasing the dose of azathioprine. Azathioprine also has been shown to produce hepatotoxicity, which, in its earliest stages, resembles histologically an ischemic insult to the liver.

3. Cyclosporine. Cyclosporine represents the major advance in immunosuppression that occurred in the late 1970s and early 1980s. This agent has become a cornerstone of most immunosuppressive regimens currently in use. Cyclosporine is a lipophilic endecapeptide that comes as both an intravenous and an oral preparation, either as an oil-based liquid or in capsule form. When given orally, cyclosporine is absorbed primarily in the small intestine. The oral bioavailability is low, on the order of 10%-30%. Because it is very lipophilic, it requires bile salts for maximal absorption. Cyclosporine absorption is inhibited by a variety of clinical conditions, including biliary diversion (e.g., T-tube drainage), diarrhea, steatorrhea, decreased gastric emptying, and short gut. In pediatric patients, the bioavailability of cyclosporine correlates directly with the length of the bowel in the individual patient. To facilitate the absorption of cyclosporine in a patient with biliary diversion following liver transplantation, bile is refed orally or by an enteral tube. In addition, the T-tube is capped as early as possible following transplantation to reestablish the normal biliary conduit. Cyclosporine is metabolized by a variety of metabolic pathways, including hydroxylation, demethylation, reduction, and carboxylation. To a large extent, cyclosporine metabolism is via the P-450 system, and thus inducers or inhibitors of P-450 can have dramatic effects on cyclosporine metabolism and blood cyclosporine levels. Agents that commonly increase cyclosporine metabolism, resulting in decreased levels, include phenytoin, coumadin, phenobarbital, and rifampin. Conversely, drugs such as ketoconazole and erythromycin can lead to increased levels. Cyclosporine is stored in body fat, so that patients with increased body fat often take longer to achieve adequate cyclosporine blood levels than those with less body fat. Cyclosporine is excreted into bile largely as metabolites, but there is a small enterohepatic circulation of the parent compound as well. Cyclosporine circulates bound to a variety of serum lipoproteins. Approximately half of the cyclosporine in the bloodstream is attached to red blood cells and white blood cells.

The **immunologic effects** of cyclosporine represent a relatively specific effect on T-lymphocytes. Intracellularly, cyclosporine binds to a cytosolic protein and acts to inhibit T-cell proliferation by blocking transcription of IL-2 mRNA, leading to decreased IL-2 production and secretion by T-cells. In the absence of IL-2 production, the proliferation of T-lymphocytes is inhibited. These effects of cyclosporine appear to be relatively specific for T-helper cells. Besides its effect on IL-2 production, cyclosporine also inhibits the secretion of a variety of lymphokines, including gamma interferon.

Cyclosporine is absorbed poorly from the gastrointestinal tract in the early posttransplant period. Thus, many programs administer cyclosporine IV during the immediate posttransplant period at a dose of 2-5 mg/kg/day, often given as a continuous infusion. Oral cyclosporine is begun at a dose of 10-20 mg/kg/day in divided doses once gastrointestinal tract function returns. Subsequent dosing of cyclosporine is adjusted according to blood levels. Currently, two methods exist for cyclosporine blood level determination: HPLC and radioimmunoassay RIA. The older polyclonal RIA assay measured both parent compound and metabolites. However, the newer monoclonal RIA available measures only parent compound and has an advantage over HPLC (which also measures only parent compound) by being technically easier.

The most important side-effect of cyclosporine is **nephrotoxicity.** Acutely, cyclosporine nephrotoxicity is manifested by a fall in urine output, impaired natriuresis, and a fall in GFR. This reflects the acute effects of cyclosporine on intrarenal blood flow and is rapidly reversed by a decrease in cyclosporine dosage. The nephrotoxicity of cyclosporine appears to be worse with IV cyclosporine than with oral cyclosporine at the same blood level. Virtually all patients develop some decrease in GFR associated with cyclosporine administration which can vary from 10%-70%. There is quite a variation in the individual susceptibility to the nephrotoxic effects of cyclosporine. Histologically, one can demonstrate interstitial fibrosis and vascular sclerosis in the kidney with chronic cyclosporine administration. In addition to the decrease in GFR, cyclosporine can also produce marked increases in serum potassium concentrations. This hyperkalemia responds well to mineralocorticoid (Florinef) administration. The concomitant administration of NSAIDs and cyclosporine can cause severe renal dysfunction. This is probably secondary to their inhibition of intrarenal prostaglandins which support the GFR during cyclosporine administration.

Cyclosporine is associated with a number of other side-effects, including hypertension, which is usually easily controlled by medications, hypercholesterolemia, hypertrichosis, gingival hyperplasia, gout, and hepatotoxicity, which is usually manifested by minor increases in serum liver enzymes that respond simply to lowering cyclosporine dose. CNS toxicity is one of the more disabling side-effects of cyclosporine. Neurologic signs and symptoms seen following transplantation include headache, sleep disturbance, psychosis, encephalopathy, seizures, tremors, myoclonus, cortical blindness, hemiplegias, spastic quadrapareses, and coma. The cause of the cyclosporine-associated neurotoxicity is unclear, but patients with decreased serum magnesium concentrations and decreased serum cholesterol levels appear to be at increased risk for this cyclosporine-associated neurotoxicity following liver transplantation. CNS symptoms are often associated with dramatic changes seen by CT or MRI of the brain and vary from minor white matter changes to hemorrhagic infarcts that reverse with time. Although most patients with CSA neurotoxicity recover completely, some are left with residual gait, visual, or speech disturbances.

Cyclosporine administration is also associated with malignancies, in particular B-cell lymphoma. Many of these lymphomas are associated with Epstein-Barr virus infection and may respond to lowering the immunosuppression and intravenous administration of high doses of acyclovir.

4. Antilymphocyte preparations. Currently, there are

two forms of antilymphocyte preparations available in this country: a monoclonal antibody directed against CD3-bearing lymphocytes (OKT3) and polyclonal preparations generated by immunizing animals with various lymphocyte preparations (ATG or MALG). Both of these agents are used for treatment of established rejection. Both of these have been incorporated into maintenance immunosuppression protocols, termed sequential therapy. In these protocols, patients are treated for relatively brief periods of time (<2 weeks) with one of these preparations in the immediate posttransplant period. The rationale for these regimens is discussed later.

Polyclonal preparations suffer by being relatively nonselective for lymphocytes. Thus, they tend to decrease total white blood counts and platelet counts as well. These preparations also require administration through a central venous catheter and have been reported to cause allergic reactions as well as serum sickness. The monoclonal preparation OKT3 is given via peripheral intravenous access. OKT3 is specific in its effects against CD3-bearing T-lymphocytes and thus does not affect total white blood counts or platelet counts. There is, however, a dramatic first-dose reaction that consists of fever, chills, hypotension, and occasionally pulmonary edema and bronchospasm. The severity of this reaction can be decreased by pretreatment with high-dose corticosteroids (10-20 mg/kg of methylprednisolone). These effects lessen with each successful dose and may be related to the release of lymphokines as a result of OKT3 administration. Other side effects of OKT3 include diarrhea and aseptic meningitis, which is typically seen on day 4-5 of OKT3 administration and is manifested by headache and neck stiffness. The use of OKT3 is limited by the development of antimurine antibodies, as OKT3 is a mouse monoclonal. Low titers of antibody can be overcome by increasing the dose of OKT3. Both preparations also have been associated with an increased risk of CMV infections when used as treatment for established rejection episodes. Both have also been associated with an increased risk of B-cell lymphoma.

5. Combination therapy. Every regimen currently used for liver allograft immunosuppression represents a combination of these individual agents. It is difficult to compare the relative efficacy and side-effects of the various regimens because few randomized trials have compared the different regimens directly. The earliest regimen employed was azathioprine and prednisone with or without an antilymphocyte preparation. Although successful, this regimen was associated with a relatively high incidence of graft loss secondary to refractory allograft rejection and also required relatively high doses of prednisone (≥10 mg in adults) with significant long-term corticosteroid toxicity.

Later regimens used cyclosporine and prednisone. With this regimen, there was a decreased incidence of graft loss and improved survival, but still this regimen required relatively high doses of cyclosporine and prednisone with its subsequent long-term toxicity. This led to the development of so-called triple therapy regimens, which included cyclosporine, azathioprine, and prednisone. The theory behind adding azathioprine to prednisone and cyclosporine was that this would allow use of lower doses of each individual drug and, it was hoped, lower long-term side-effects. This regimen also has been associated with a lower incidence of retransplantation and chronic rejection. The arguments against triple therapy include the increased immunosuppression and thus the higher risk of opportunistic infections or malignancies.

Finally, because of the effect of intravenous cyclosporine on urine output and renal function in the early transplant period, sequential protocols have been developed. Patients undergoing transplantation are often very edematous, and patients undergo marked fluid shifts during the immediate posttransplant period. The use of IV cyclosporine impairs the renal elimination of fluid such that the principal advantage of sequential therapy is to avoid the use of IV cyclosporine and to allow initiation of cyclosporine only once renal function has returned to normal. Many programs use quadruple immunosuppression (sequential therapy) as a standard maintenance immunosuppression protocol, and many use such a protocol for patients with impaired renal function prior to transplant. Both MALG and OKT3 have been incorporated into sequential regimens. These regimens appear to delay the onset of rejection by 1-2 weeks but probably do not decrease the overall incidence of rejection. Most sequential regimens delay the administration of cyclosporine until day 5-14 following transplant, depending on renal function. Whether avoidance of intravenous cyclosporine leads to better long-term renal function is unclear. The criticism of the use of antilymphocyte preparations for maintenance immunosuppression has been that this could lead to an increased frequency of posttransplant malignancy and opportunistic infections.

B. NEW AGENTS. A number of immunosuppressive agents are currently undergoing testing in this country. Most are still at the stage of laboratory and animal testing and are not discussed here. Two agents, however, FK-506 and mycophenolate mofetil (RS-61443), are currently in clinical testing, and the preliminary results with these agents are discussed.

1. FK-506. FK-506 is a macrolide produced by a *Streptomyces* species that was discovered in Japan. It appears to have a similar mechanism of immunosuppressive action to cyclosporine. Like cyclosporine, it inhibits IL-2 synthesis by lymphocytes and may decrease the expression of IL-2 receptors on activated lymphocytes as well. Although similar in action to cyclosporine, FK-506 is 50-100 times more potent by weight.

Clinical studies of FK-506 began at the University of Pittsburgh in 1988, and currently more than 1000 patients have been treated at that institution thus far. These results, plus the results of a U.S. multicenter, open-label, randomized trial, indicate that FK-506 is a potent immunosuppressive drug that produces results, in terms of graft and patient survival, comparable to those of cyclosporine.

The initial hope was that FK-506 would be associated with fewer side-effects and, in particular, less nephrotoxicity. However, FK-506 appears to have a similar side-effect profile to cyclosporine. In particular, FK-506 has both acute and probably chronic nephrotoxicity. The acute nephrotoxic effects of FK-506 are very similar to those of cyclosporine in that they are greater with IV administration, are dose-dependent, and are reversible with dose reduction. FK-506 does have a substantially lower incidence of hypertension and does not produce hypertrichosis. It also exhibits neurotoxicity, and a CNS syndrome similar to that with cyclosporine has been seen with FK-506. FK-506 can also lead to glucose intolerance and in high doses causes diarrhea and poor appetite.

Thus far, FK-506 has generally been used in combination with prednisone. However, a number of patients treated at the University of Pittsburgh have now been taken off prednisone and are currently managed with FK-506 as the sole immunosuppressive agent. FK-506 also may be effective as a rescue agent for patients with refractory rejection, as it appears to differ from cyclosporine in that it can be used to treat rejection. This may be the major use of this drug in the future.

2. Mycophenolate mofetil. Mycophenolate mofetil is a prodrug of a compound, mycophenolic acid, which has a mechanism of immunosuppressive action distinct from that of cyclosporine or FK-506. Mycophenolate mofetil is rapidly hydrolyzed following absorption to yield the parent compound.

Mycophenolate mofetil is an inhibitor of purine synthesis. Lymphocytes, unlike most other cell types, possess a single pathway for purine synthesis, and thus inhibition of this pathway leads to a selective inhibition of lymphocyte proliferation. Although inhibition of T- and B-cell proliferation is the primary effect of the drug, the immunologic effects of this agent may be more complex. Mycophenolate mofetil has been used successfully for immunosuppression in a variety of animal allograft models, including heart, pancreatic islets, and renal transplants.

Clinical studies with mycophenolate mofetil as an immunosuppressive agent in transplantation are just beginning in this country. Its use to date has been largely as a rescue agent for patients either intolerant of cyclosporine or with refractory rejection. Primary trials in both kidney and liver allograft recipients are currently underway.

The toxicity of this drug is minor. Despite its similar mechanism of action to azathioprine, mycophenolate mofetil in therapeutic doses does not lead to bone marrow suppression, nor does it exhibit nephrotoxicity or hypertension. The only side-effects noted thus far include skin rash and minor gastrointestinal upset. Long-term follow-up information on the safety of the parent compound, mycophenolic acid, already exists. A cohort of patients with psoriasis has now been treated for almost 20 years with mycophenolic acid with essentially no serious long-term sequelae, although 12% of the patients had uncomplicated episodes of herpes zoster. The incidence of malignancy in that cohort does not appear to be different from the cancer incidence in the United States as a whole.

How this agent will be used as an immunosuppressive agent in maintenance protocols is unclear. It seems logical to replace azathioprine with mycophenolate mofetil in a triple-drug regimen that includes cyclosporine and prednisone. It also offers promise in being able to replace or minimize the amount of cyclosporine or FK-506 necessary to prevent rejection.

V. INFECTIONS AFTER TRANSPLANTATION

Infection in the transplant patient occurs primarily as the result of a technical complication related to the transplant or as a complication of immunosuppressive therapy. Drs. R. Rubin and N. Tolkoff-Rubin have derived important concepts concerning infection in the post-transplant patient, and most of the discussion arises from their concepts. When considering the methods of prophylaxis, diagnosis, and treatment of infections, it is important to realize that different infections occur in different time periods following transplant. The timetable for occurrence in transplant patients is shown in Figure 20-1.

In general, infections occurring in the early posttransplant period are related to **bacterial infection** and arise from the usual sources (i.e., pneumonia, indwelling catheters, and technical complications related to the implantation of the organ). Prevention of infection is related to the use of prophylactic antibiotics, careful hand-washing, and some limitation of patient exposure to potential pathogens. The overuse of antibiotics is to be condemned, as longer prophylactic courses result primarily in the emergence of resistant gram-negative organisms. This is particularly true in patients with indwelling catheters (such as a T-tube) following transplantation. Repeated antibiotic treatment for bacterial colonization of these catheters results in colonization with more resistant organisms and secondary complications of antibiotics, such as *Clostridium difficile* colitis. In general, the use of prophylactic antibiotics in these patients should be limited to the immediate postoperative period. Their use for radiologic studies such as routine cholangiography should be condemned.

The next period following transplant, 1-6 months, is a time when augmentation of immunosuppression is frequently used to treat rejection. During this time, infection by the **herpes family viruses,** primarily herpes simplex virus and CMV, tend to be common. CMV infections arise from one of three different sources: (1) reactivation of a previous infection in the recipient, (2) introduction of the virus via the transplanted organ, or (3) introduction of virus from blood products. The incidence of CMV infections can be quite low in patients who are serologically negative for CMV antibodies prior to transplant, who receive an organ from a serologically negative donor, and who subsequently receive serologically negative blood products. Although this scenario is possible in some situations, the urgency for heart and liver transplantation generally precludes this matching. Therefore, prophylaxis for these viral infections has become paramount.

Whereas the herpes simplex infections tend to be relatively easy to prevent with low doses of oral acyclovir, high doses of oral acyclovir have been found to be necessary to prevent CMV disease in patients following renal transplantation. Although this has not yet been rigorously tested for liver or heart transplantation, most major centers have begun using

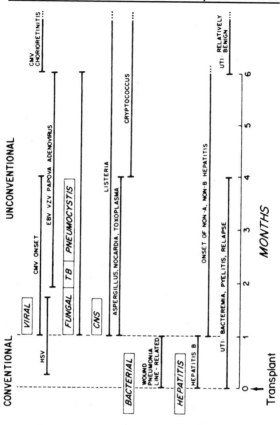

FIGURE 20-1. Timetable for occurrence of infection in the organ transplant recipient. Exceptions to this timetable should initiate a search for an unusual hazard. CMV = cytomegalovirus; HSV = herpes simplex virus; EBV = Epstein-Barr virus; VZV = varicella-zoster virus; CNS = central nervous system; UTI = urinary tract infection. (From Rubin RH, Tolkoff-Rubin NE: *Transplant Proc* 23:4, 2068, 1991.)

some form of acyclovir prophylaxis. The usual dose is 3200 mg daily. The other antiviral that has been applied in transplantation is gancyclovir. A study in heart transplant patients demonstrated a marked reduction in the incidence of CMV disease following 1 month of IV gancyclovir therapy. Current research involving comparison of high-dose oral acyclovir versus IV gancyclovir is now underway. It may well be that a short course of IV gancyclovir, followed by oral acyclovir, is the best protocol in prevention of CMV disease. In general, the oral acyclovir is continued for 3 months following transplant, at which time the incidence of CMV falls dramatically. A controversial point is the use of prophylactic DHPG in patients undergoing antilymphocyte therapy. This therapy appears to decrease the probability of subsequent CMV infections following this time of augmented immunosuppression.

Two other major types of infection appear during this time period. The first is **fungal infections,** both *Candida* infections and potentially fatal *Aspergillus* infections. The oral candidiasis can be prevented with topical antifungal agents. The importance of fluconazole in preventing these infections is unknown. In general, amphotericin is reserved for treatment of serious infections, including *Candida* esophagitis, peritonitis, and complicated urinary tract infections.

An *Aspergillus* infection in the transplant patient is devastating, with few documented survivors. The primary goal in the management of this disease in the transplant patient is prevention. *Aspergillus* is an ubiquitous organism in the environment, and outbreaks in hospitalized patients appear primarily because of poor construction practices. It is extremely important that building management personnel understand the risk of remodeling and construction to the immunosuppressed patient. Even a simple project such as the replacement of a few ceiling tiles can release huge quantities of *Aspergillus* into the air.

Another common infection is *Pneumocystis carinii* pneumonia. In some series, up to 10% of transplant patients have had severe infections with this organism. The use of trimethoprim-sulfamethoxazole (TMP/sulfa) or inhaled pentamidine appears to be effective in preventing these infections. Protocols with TMP/sulfa on an alternate-day schedule appear to be adequate, whereas pentamidine is given once a month. The duration of therapy is unclear. Some centers use TMP/sulfa on a permanent basis in recipients; others cease therapy after 6-12 months. For centers that stop therapy, it may be important to restart therapy if the patient undergoes treatment for rejection.

Another infection in this population is **tuberculosis.** Management of the patient with a positive TB skin test prior to transplant is controversial, but most centers would treat with a 6-month course of standard therapy. Infections in the post-transplant patient are frequently difficult to diagnose and usually present with fever of unknown origin.

VI. ORGAN DONATION

A major contribution to organ transplantation that can be made by all physicians is in providing organs from cadaver donors for transplantation. For organ donation to occur, it is crucial that the physician (1) recognize the potential donor, (2) be cognizant of the principles of medical management of the donor, (3) understand how to approach the family for consent for donation, and (4) understand the referral process for organ donors.

A. THE POTENTIAL DONOR. Currently, a potential donor is a patient who is brain dead but whose heart is beating. Although research is being conducted to determine the feasibility of recovering organs from other patients, such as trauma victims who expire in the emergency room, the technics to rapidly cool and preserve these organs have been used only in animals.

The major causes of death of organ donors are trauma, cerebrovascular accident, and anoxia. In these patients the primary reasons for exclusion from donation are HIV positivity, hepatitis B surface antigen positivity, IV drug abuse, and most malignancies (although brain tumors, nonmelanoma skin cancers, and carcinoma in situ of the cervix may be acceptable). These exclusions exist because conditions pose a substantial risk of disease transmission via the donor organ. Currently there is much debate over the use of organs from hepatitis C antibody–positive individuals. The issues are related primarily to the high false-positive rate of the current hepatitis C screening tests and the relatively slow rate of progression of the disease in the recipient. Currently, most centers refuse hepatitis C–positive donors for renal transplantation, although transplantation into seriously ill heart and liver patients is frequently performed. The use of these organs in hepatitis C–positive recipients is also being studied.

It is difficult to set age criteria for donation, as kidneys and livers have been recovered from donors well past the age of 70 years. The contraindications for potential organ donation have been diminishing as the need for organ donors has grown. It is best always to refer a potential donor if any doubt exists.

B. MEDICAL MANAGEMENT. At the time of recognition of brain death, fluid and electrolyte problems usually require immediate attention. In general, these patients are quite volume depleted secondary to previous attempts to prevent brain swelling. This can be further complicated by the diabetes insipidus that frequently develops in the brain-dead patient. Many of these patients are on pressor agents in order to treat hypotension secondary to the hypovolemia. After brain death is established, aggressive volume expansion is needed. Replacement of water deficits is necessary to reverse the hypernatremia that is common with diabetus insipidus and previous water restriction. Replacement of urine output should be begun with either D_5W or $D_5\frac{1}{4}$ NS. DDAVP should be administered to patients with diabetes insipidus (0.3 µg/kg IV) to prevent excessive urinary losses. Pitressin is a second-line agent because it causes a greater decrease in renal and hepatic blood flow. Other electrolyte disturbances (particularly hypokalemia) should also be treated.

Once adequate volume replacement has been achieved, it is usually possible to decrease the amount of pressor agents to lower levels. Systolic blood pressure should be maintained between 100-120 mm Hg. This is usually achieved with dopamine at a dose of less than 10 µg/kg/min. Many patients with severe head injury, particularly with gunshot wounds, may develop coagulopathy requiring large amounts of FFP, cryoprecipitate, and blood. In general, the coagulopathy associated with these injuries is a consumptive coagulopathy, and the elevated prothrombin time should not exclude liver donation. Temperature regulation should be maintained, as hypothermia can make the donor prone to cardiac arrest.

C. BRAIN DEATH. The procedure for the declaration of brain death varies with the locale. All cerebral and brain stem activity must be absent. All potentially interfering conditions such as hypothermia and drug intoxication should be eliminated. The use of ancillary studies such as EEG, cerebral blood flow studies, and apnea trials depends on local standards. Brain death declaration must be performed by a physician who has no conflict of interest in the donation of the organs.

D. DONATION REFERRAL. When a potential donor is identified, a call should be made to the local organ procurement agency or to the United Network for Organ Sharing (UNOS 1-800-292-9537). This referral provides information about the donation process, and usually a coordinator from the local organ procurement agency comes to the hospital to arrange donation. It is important in this process for brain death to be explained to the family and for the family to accept that the patient is dead prior to the request for organ donation. A study by Garrison found that if the explanation of brain death and the request for organ donation occurred at the same time, only 18% of the families agreed to organ donation. When the discussion of brain death and the family's understanding of brain death took place prior to the request for donation, donation occurred in 57% of the cases.

E. ORGAN SHARING. In October 1987 a nationwide organ-sharing system was instituted. The system is structured such that potential organs are first offered to local programs. If no local recipient is available, the organ is offered to centers within a defined geographic region. If no regional recipient is available, the organ is then offered nationally. The selection of recipient is based upon criteria that take into account the level of care the recipient requires. Patients in the intensive care setting are assigned the highest priority. Patients who are still able to work are assigned the lowest priority.

VII. RENAL TRANSPLANTATION

A. INDICATIONS. The first clinically successful renal transplant was performed in 1946 by Hufnagel, Hume, and Landsteiner. With developments in surgical technic, tissue typing, postoperative management, and immunosuppression over the last 45 years, the indications for renal transplantation have grown to include nearly all causes of end-stage renal disease. In 1990, nearly 10,000 renal transplants were performed, and it is estimated that nearly half of the 20,000 patients who begin chronic dialysis each year are transplant candidates. Successful renal transplantation has been performed from cadaveric donors, living related donors, and living nonrelated donors, with 1-year graft survival greater than 80% at most centers. The main problems following transplantation can be categorized into technical complications, rejection, and complications of immunosuppression.

B. DONOR SELECTION. Approximately 30% of transplanted kidneys are from living donors. Advantages include more favorable results with living donors, immediate organ availability, and an increased chance of immediate graft function. The potential candidate for living kidney donation undergoes a meticulous screening process. This includes a thorough history, physical examination, and blood work to exclude any underlying renal disease or hypertension. Blood group and tissue typing, as well as a leukocyte cross-match and mixed lymphocyte culture, are required to select the best donor candidate on an immunologic basis. Finally, the potential donor requires an IV pyelogram and an arteriogram prior to donation to detect vascular and urinary tract anomalies. In general, the left kidney is used because of the longer renal vein unless a situation such as multiple renal arteries dictates using the right kidney.

If no living donor is available, the recipient is placed on a list with other recipients until a cadaveric donor is available. Eligibility for any particular kidney is based on several factors, including the cross-match results, time waiting on the list, and degree of matching. Kidneys procured from cadaveric donors are usually transplanted within 48 to 72 hours, depending on the method of storage. Kidneys from living related donors are transplanted immediately after donor nephrectomy.

C. SURGICAL TECHNIC. The recipient is usually dialyzed shortly before the transplant to optimize volume status, electrolytes, and acid-base status. The transplanted kidney is typically placed in a retroperitoneal location in the iliac fossa of the recipient. The donor renal artery is anastomosed in an end-to-side fashion to the recipient's external iliac artery. Alternatively, an end-to-end anastomosis to the mobilized internal iliac artery may be performed. The vein is anastomosed end to side to the external iliac vein (Figure 20-2). The donor ureter is attached to the bladder using two common technics. The Politano-Leadbetter technic requires creation of a submucosal tunnel in the bladder with anastomosis of the ureteral mucosa to bladder mucosa through an anterior midline cystostomy. The second technic, an extravesicular uretero-neocystostomy, does not require a large bladder incision and requires a shorter length of ureter, with less risk of an inadequate blood supply to the ureter (Figure 20-3). In patients without an adequate bladder, an ileal loop is constructed 4-6 weeks prior to the time of transplant.

D. POSTOPERATIVE MANAGEMENT. The allograft in the

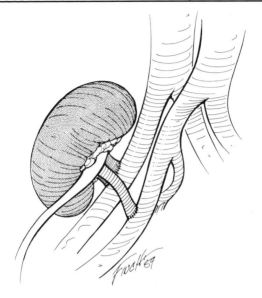

FIGURE 20-2. Anastomosis of renal vessels to external iliac artery and vein. (From Letourneau JG, Day DL, Ascher NL: *Radiology of organ transplantation*, St. Louis, 1991, Mosby–Year Book.)

early postoperative period requires immediate diagnostic and therapeutic intervention. Close monitoring of urine output and fluid status is essential. Adequate replacement of urinary losses is necessary to avoid renal dysfunction secondary to volume depletion. Postoperative anuria occurs in 10-30% of recipients, with the higher incidence of early renal dysfunction secondary to acute tubular necrosis in cadaveric recipients. Usually only 10% of cadaveric recipients require dialysis until renal function is adequate.

The cause of postoperative anuria/oliguria needs to be determined rapidly. In general, anuria is related to a mechanical problem, whereas oliguria is related to allograft dysfunction.

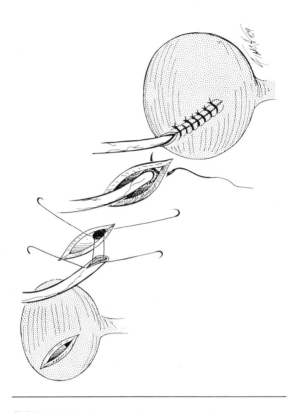

FIGURE 20-3. Extravesicular uretroneocystostomy. Bladder incision; ureteral anastomosis to bladder mucosa; closure of bladder muscle over anastomosis; completed tunneled anastomosis. (From Letourneau JG, Day DL, Ascher NL: *Radiology of organ transplantation,* St. Louis, 1991, Mosby–Year Book.)

Once mechanical obstruction of the indwelling Foley catheter (usually by a clot) has been ruled out by irrigation, the volume status of the patient should be assessed, preferably with a CVP line or pulmonary artery catheter. Fluid replacement to restore intravascular volume should be initiated in the volume-depleted patient. A potential problem is the urine production of the native kidney. Native urine output can be quite high in some patients (particularly patients with polycystic kidney disease) and can mask allograft dysfunction.

Radiologic evaluation using various imaging technics is required if urine output remains low in the face of an adequate volume status. Ultrasonography is helpful to diagnose ureteral obstruction due to technical complications at the anastomosis or fluid collections that may be obstructing the ureter by extrinsic compression. With the addition of duplex and color Doppler imaging, blood flow to the kidney can be evaluated as well. Nuclear medicine technics are valuable for assessing renal function. DTPA and iodine-131 iodohippurate (Hippuran) are the two major radionuclides used in the evaluation of renal allograft function. DTPA renal scans evaluate the vascular flow pattern of the kidney as well as the gross anatomy of the ureter and bladder. Scans are performed over 30 minutes, with uptake of contrast within 6 seconds indicating adequate flow to the graft. Peak activity in the parenchyma should be reached within 2 minutes, followed by a gradual decline in radioactivity in the renal parenchyma and an increase in radioactivity in the urinary collecting system and bladder. Hippuran scans are more sensitive in evaluating renal function. Peak activity is also reached in 2-4 minutes, with gradual decline over the next 30 minutes. In rejection, acute tubular necrosis, and cyclosporine toxicity, the typical findings are poor uptake and poor excretion on a nuclear medicine scan. A urine leak usually appears as an extravasation of tracer outside of the bladder. The cause of oliguria is assumed to be graft dysfunction secondary to ATN or possibly rejection if the above studies do not reveal technical problems.

In the stable renal transplant recipient, Foley catheters are typically left in place 3-7 days, and IV fluids are tapered as the patient begins taking normal amounts of oral fluids. Early removal of nonessential IV lines is important to avoid infectious complications in the immunosuppressed patient.

E. POSTOPERATIVE IMMUNOSUPPRESSION. The protocols currently used by most transplant centers include a combination of corticosteroids, azathioprine, cyclosporine, and antilymphocyte preparations (OKT3, MALG, or ATGAM). Each of these agents decreases recognition and destruction of the allograft by different mechanisms, and each has its own set of complications. However, infection is a complication shared by all of these agents and is the most common adverse side-effect following transplantation.

Sequential therapy with administration of antilymphocyte preparations, prednisone, and azathioprine in the immediate posttransplant period, followed by the addition of cyclosporine when renal function is stabilized, is often used to avoid the nephrotoxicity of cyclosporine in the early transplant period. This protocol is used most often following cadaveric transplantation. Most protocols taper corticosteroids over the first few months after transplant and adjust cyclosporine based on monitoring cyclosporine blood levels. Antilymphocyte preparations are typically used in the early period after transplantation and during rejection episodes when corticosteroid pulses are ineffective or the patient is at high risk for graft loss.

F. RESULTS OF TRANSPLANTATION. With improvements in surgical technic, postoperative management, and immunosuppressive agents, long-term graft and patient survival have increased over the last 3 decades. Living related HLA-identical transplants continue to have the best prognosis for both patient and graft survival, with an overall 91% and 90% 5-year survival rate, respectively, reported in one series. With the addition of cyclosporine to immunosuppressive protocols, the 3-year patient and graft survival exceeds 95% in living related identical transplants. Living related HLA–nonidentical transplants have a 3-year patient and graft survival of 91% and 79%, respectively, in the cyclosporine era. Cadaveric transplants in the cyclosporine era have an 83% and 70% patient and graft 3-year survival. The results of cadaveric transplantation are influenced to some extent by the degree of HLA matching.

G. COMPLICATIONS. The majority of surgical complications are experienced in the immediate postoperative period. The two main types of complications can be classified as **vascular** and **urologic.**

1. Renal artery thrombosis is a rare complication occurring in about 1% of transplants. The risk of this complication is higher with size mismatch of donor renal artery and recipient internal iliac artery when an end-to-end anastomosis is performed, in kidneys with multiple renal arteries, in traumatized kidneys due to rough handling, and in the presence of an unidentified renal artery intimal flap. Sudden loss of urinary output, not due to an obstructed Foley catheter or inadequate vascular volume, should necessitate a work-up with duplex Doppler ultrasonography. Loss of signal is indicative of no flow to the kidney. Alternatively, a nuclear medicine renal scan is informative, with lack of isotope uptake by the kidney indicating no blood flow.

2. Renal artery stenosis occurs in up to 15% of transplanted kidneys. Difficult to control hypertension should suggest the possibility of stenosis. Diagnosis with renal Duplex ultrasonography followed by arteriography to better define the anatomy and degree of stenosis should be done prior to operative repair or angioplasty. Initial success rates for both methods with most lesions are similar (75%-80%), but the restenosis rate following angioplasty is not well-defined. Anastomotic strictures do less well with angioplasty and probably should be repaired by operative intervention.

3. Aneurysms occurring in the renal artery are either pseudoaneurysms at the anastomotic site or mycotic aneurysms secondary to bacterial or fungal infection. A rapidly expanding, tender pulsatile mass in the region of the kidney suggests a mycotic aneurysm. Arteriography is confirmatory for diagnosis. Treatment consists of appropriate antibiotics and removal of the transplanted kidney.

4. Venous complications are less frequent, with thrombosis occurring in 1%-4% of transplants. Causative factors include intimal damage during retrieval, kinking at the iliac vein anastomosis, or pressure secondary to a lymphocele, urinoma, or hematoma. Occasional, severe rejection can result in venous occlusion. Heparin therapy for incomplete occlusion and transplant nephrectomy for complete occlusion are the indicated therapies.

5. Urologic complications include ureteral obstruction, urinary fistula, or bladder leak. These complications generally present with decreased urine output, and mechanical obstruction of the Foley must first be ruled out. Obstruction occurs in 1%-9% of transplants, and diagnosis can be made with ultrasonography demonstrating hydronephrosis. A leak is usually diagnosed by a nuclear medicine renal scan. Intervention for urologic complications usually requires reimplantation of the transplanted ureter or anastomosis to the native ureter. Stabilization of the patient and graft function by preoperative percutaneous nephrostomy are often beneficial.

6. A relatively uncommon postoperative complication is the development of a **lymphocele** in the area of the transplanted kidney. This complication can be minimized by careful ligation of lymphatics during the dissection along the iliac vessels. Urinary tract obstruction with hydronephrosis is the typical clinical finding on presentation, and diagnosis can be confirmed with ultrasonography. Operative drainage into the peritoneal cavity is usually required. A newer treatment option uses the laparoscope for drainage into the peritoneal cavity.

7. Renal allograft rejection occurs in the majority of transplant patients, usually in the early posttransplant period. Episodes can be classified as hyperacute, acute, and chronic rejection, based on time of onset, clinical course, and histologic features.

Evaluation of the rejecting allograft requires a biopsy to confirm the diagnosis. Tissue can be obtained by percutaneous transplant biopsy, which remains the gold standard. Fine-needle aspiration has become more popular recently, especially for serial monitoring of allografts. The addition of flow cytometric technics and immunofluorescence staining has increased the utility of fine-needle aspiration.

a. Hyperacute rejection occurs as the result of pre-formed antibodies, with destruction of the graft in the first 24 hours. Accurate cross-matching prior to transplantation has fortunately made this form of rejection rare.

b. The presenting signs and symptoms of *acute rejection* include fever, decreased urine output, graft tenderness and swelling, and occasionally leukocytosis. Cyclosporine nephrotoxicity and infection must be ruled out, and percutaneous biopsy is typically performed to confirm the diagnosis. Treatment consists of high-dose corticosteroids for 3-4 days, which is effective in the majority of cases. In steroid-resistant rejection episodes, MALG or OKT3 can be used, with a high rate of response, but an associated high rate of viral and bacterial infections.

c. Chronic rejection presents with worsening renal function, usually accompanied by hypertension and proteinuria. Treatment is effective only for short intervals and does not alter the eventual progression of the disease to graft loss. The role of cyclosporine in preventing chronic rejection is under investigation.

8. Cyclosporine is known to alter renal hemodynamics through increased vasoconstriction of vascular smooth muscle. The nephrotoxic potential of cyclosporine requires frequent monitoring of drug levels, and the diagnosis of nephrotoxicity must be differentiated from rejection when an elevated creatinine is measured.

9. Posttransplant hypertension is a significant problem that has increased in frequency with the use of cyclosporine. Other contributing factors include chronic rejection, renal artery stenosis, recurrence of renal disease in the transplanted kidney, and renin production by the native kidneys. Native nephrectomy is helpful in some patients. A bruit over the transplanted kidney may be indicative of renal artery stenosis, and surgical correction or percutaneous transluminal dilatation are possible treatment options. Treatment of cyclosporine-related hypertension requires dosage adjustment and often the addition of antihypertensive agents such as angiotensin-converting enzyme inhibitors or calcium channel blockers.

VIII. HEART TRANSPLANTATION

Human cardiac transplantation was first performed 25 years ago in Cape Town, South Africa, following its perfection in animal models by Norman Shumway. During the early years of this procedure, the operation was almost always technically successful, but complications in the postoperative period limited the 1-year survival rate to 20%. With improvement of the diagnosis and management of rejection, particularly with the use of transvenous endomyocardial biopsy, and the introduction of cyclosporine, the 1-year survival has increased to 80%-90%. Almost 20,000 cardiac transplants have been performed worldwide. The 5-year survival rate is on the order of 70%.

A. INDICATIONS. The primary reason for adult cardiac transplantation is cardiomyopathy, followed by coronary artery disease. In children, congenital heart disease, followed by cardiomyopathy, is the major indication. For patients with congestive heart failure, the 1-year survival without transplant ranges from 50%-70%, which is less than the survival expected from transplantation (80%-90%). A poor outcome can be expected for patients when their ejection fraction falls below 20%. Major contraindications to performing transplantation are pulmonary hypertension and elevated pulmonary vascular resistance, because this may result in acute failure in the transplanted heart. Therefore, catheterization of the right heart is performed prior to transplant, and if pulmonary hypertension or increased vascular resistance is found, consideration should be given to either heart/lung or lung transplantation, heterotopic heart transplant, or transplant with a larger donor organ. In general, patients with other organ system failure should be excluded, although simultaneous heart/kidney transplant has been performed successfully. As with many areas of surgery, it is difficult to come up with absolute age requirements, as physiologic age is probably more important than chronologic age. As in kidney transplantation, a positive cross-match is an absolute contraindication to cardiac transplantation. Exclusion criteria are the same as in any transplant (i.e., patients with active systemic infection, life-limiting cancer, or expected problems with noncompliance of the medical regimen after transplant).

B. DONOR SELECTION. The donor is usually younger than 60 years old, with coronary angiography suggested for donors over 40. A normal ECG and echocardiogram and, at the time of organ recovery, the appearance of good cardiac function are necessary. The heart is generally preserved in a hypothermic crystalloid cardioplegia solution, and the maximum preservation time is currently 4-6 hours.

C. ORTHOTOPIC CARDIAC TRANSPLANTATION. The transplantation of the adult heart is performed by placing the patient on cardiopulmonary bypass and then excising the heart along the atrioventricular groove and transecting the aorta and pulmonary artery. The donor heart is implanted by sewing the donor's left atrium to the recipient's left atrium, and right atrium to right atrium. The pulmonary artery and aorta are then reconstructed by end-to-end anastomoses (Figure 20-4). The graft is then reperfused and the patient warmed. The pericardial and pleural cavities are drained, and temporary pacing wires are placed. Early postoperative care is similar to those patients who undergo other cardiac surgeries. Patients frequently require intropic support for a few days as the myocardium recovers.

D. IMMUNOSUPPRESSION. Triple or quadruple immunosuppression, as outlined previously, is used following cardiac transplantation. Importantly, transvenous myocardial biopsy is performed on a regular basis during the first 3-6 months to look for evidence of rejection. This is done by using a percutaneous approach to introduce the biopsy forceps into the right side of the heart, and taking a septal biopsy, allowing a histologic diagnosis to be made. Treatment of rejection is the same as

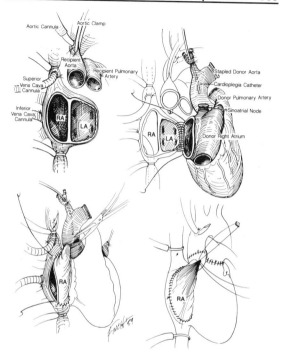

FIGURE 20-4. Cardiac transplantation. (From Letourneau JG, Day DL, Ascher NL: *Radiology of organ transplantation,* St. Louis, 1991, Mosby–Year Book.)

with other organs—high-dose corticosteroids or antilymphocyte preparations. Surveillance with regular biopsies has allowed diagnosis of rejection to be made and treated prior to the development of myocardial dysfunction.

E. LONG-TERM PROBLEMS. The long-term problems with cardiac transplantation are similar to those in all transplant patients—rejection, infection, and drug toxicity. Infection tends to be the primary cause of death, with causes similar to those in recipients of other transplanted organs. The antiviral drugs acyclovir and gancyclovir are important for decreasing the morbidity and mortality from CMV infection following transplant. Coronary artery disease is another major problem that is seen in 30%-40% of post–cardiac transplant patients. The cause of this is unclear, although it is possibly related to rejection or to CMV infection. The ischemia produced by this disease is generally silent, and angiography is recommended in these patients as routine annual follow-up. The disease cannot be treated with bypass grafting or percutaneous transluminal angioplasty. Retransplantation is the only alternative for patients with life-threatening disease. The presentation in these patients is usually congestive heart failure or arrhythmia. This disease is probably one of the leading causes of sudden death following cardiac transplantation.

IX. HEART/LUNG TRANSPLANTATION

The use of heart/lung transplant has been emerging over the last 10 years. Approximately 1000 have been performed, with a 1-year survival of 50%-70%. The primary indications for this operation are primary pulmonary hypertension, Eisenmenger's syndrome, and cystic fibrosis. The merits of heart/lung transplant versus lung transplantation are unclear in patients with a normal heart. These indications should become clear over the next several years, although isolated lung transplant is probably preferred if possible because of the ability to obtain two lungs and one heart from each donor, thereby potentially allowing three different patients to be transplanted.

A. INDICATIONS. Heart/lung transplant indications include pulmonary disease with right ventricular dysfunction, a decreased cardiac output, and oxygen desaturation. Current contraindications are for patients at high risk for postoperative complications, such as those taking steroids and those at significant risk for adhesions between the lung and chest wall (prior thoracotomy, empyema, or pleuritis), as this leads to intra- and postoperative problems with bleeding.

B. DONOR SELECTION. The most common reason for not using the lung has been poor pulmonary function. This is usually related to aspiration, and therefore chest radiography to exclude even minor abnormalities in the pulmonary parenchyma, a recent sputum culture, and Gram stain and bronchosopy at the time of organ recovery are necessary to eliminate the possibility of infection. The other major consideration is the cardiac function of the donor, and the criteria are the same as for cardiac transplantation. Donors are matched by ABO type and size to the recipient. The lungs are recovered by hypothermic flushing of the heart/lung preparation. In general, prostaglandin is used to provide pulmonary arterial dilatation during organ recovery.

C. OPERATIVE TECHNIC. As with cardiac transplantation, the patient is placed on bypass. The donor heart/lung block is implanted with the anastomosis of the trachea, right atrium, and aorta. The bronchial anastomosis is the most problematic, as the blood supply is somewhat tenuous and is usually reinforced with a vascularized patch of pleura or omentum.

D. IMMUNOSUPPRESSION. Steroids are usually given during the operation but are avoided during the immediate postoperative period to allow healing of the tracheal anastomosis. Other immunosuppression is the same as for heart transplant patients. The management of these patients is helped by routine surveillance with transbronchial lung biopsy for pulmonary rejection and endomyocardial biopsy to look for evidence of cardiac rejection. Rejection is treated with steroids or antilymphocyte preparations.

E. LONG-TERM CARE. The complications in heart/lung transplant are similar to those in cardiac transplant. Primary problems are related to lung infections, CMV in particular, and prophylaxis as with cardiac transplants is mandatory. The major technical problem arising in heart/lung transplant is healing of the epithelial anastomosis of the bronchus. This can be complicated by stricture and dehiscence, which are frequently life-threatening. Strictures are best managed with stenting of the anastomosis. Another long-term problem is bronchiolitis obliterans, which is a progressive, obstructive airway disease that is probably related to rejection, occurs in 30%-40% of patients, and is frequently fatal.

X. LUNG TRANSPLANTATION

Over the last several years, there has been a great interest in the use of lung transplantation to treat patients with pulmonary disease who do not have irreversible cardiac disease. This was a change from the use of heart/lung transplantation in this situation. The first successful lung transplantation was performed in 1983, but the number performed has since accelerated so that there have been more than 500 transplants performed to date.

A. INDICATIONS. General indications for lung transplantation are cases of primary pulmonary fibrosis in which the transplanted lung is more compliant and receives most of the ventilation and perfusion. In general, double-lung transplantation is performed in patients with obstructive disease or those having bilateral septic complications of the lung, such as patients with cystic fibrosis, as removing the source of sepsis is considered to be important. The general criteria for choosing a recipient are similar to those for combined heart/lung transplantation. Patients who have right ventricular dysfunction may be considered for single-lung transplantation, as the dysfunction may be reversible when a normal pulmonary vasculature is present.

B. OPERATIVE TECHNIC. The criteria for donor selection are the same as for heart/lung transplantation. The operative technic, in general, has been standardized to a single-lung transplant through a unilateral thoracotomy. A test clamping of the pulmonary artery is performed, and if the artery pressure rises to an unacceptable level, femoral bypass is initiated. The lung is then removed, and the donor left atrial cuff surrounding the pulmonary veins is anastomosed to the recipient's left atrium. This is followed by the bronchial and then pulmonary anastomosis. In general, the bronchial anastomosis has been reinforced with an omental or pleural flap.

C. IMMUNOSUPPRESSION. Immunosuppression is the same as for heart-lung transplantation, with avoidance of steroid administration in the early postoperative period to allow healing of the bronchial anastomosis. The major complications are those of pulmonary transplantation, including problems with the bronchial anastomosis, rejection, and bronchiolitis obliterans.

XI. PANCREAS TRANSPLANTATION

Although insulin provides control of hyperglycemia and ketosis, it appears to do little to prevent complications such as retinopathy, neuropathy, and nephropathy. It has been hoped that pancreas transplantation could, if performed early enough, prevent these complications from developing. The dilemma of pancreas transplantation is that the patient must trade off the use of insulin for the use of immunosuppressive agents with their known complications. This has limited the use of pancreas transplantation, for the most part, to patients with diabetic nephropathy and indications for kidney transplantation. Because these patients would receive immunosuppression for their kidney transplant, they can undergo pancreas transplantation with no additional risk from the immunosuppressive drugs. Although pancreas transplantation has been done without kidney transplantation, the graft survival does not appear to be as good. This is probably because the kidney acts as a harbinger of rejection of the pancreas graft. A rise in creatinine can signify rejection in the kidney and lead to more immunosuppression, whereas an equivalent marker for rejection is not available in pancreas transplantation. The first pancreas transplantations were performed at the University of Minnesota in 1966, but as with most organ transplantation, good survival was not obtained until the early 1980s, when the use of cyclosporine became prevalent. Survival following pancreas transplantation is now quite good, with a patient survival rate of better than 95% at the 1-year date and a graft survival of approximately 70%-80% in patients receiving a pancreas and kidney at the same time. Survival for patients receiving a pancreas by itself is approximately 50%. Whether pancreas transplantation prevents the complications of diabetes is unclear. It does appear to prevent diabetic nephropathy in the transplanted kidney.

A. PATIENT SELECTION. The primary concern in patients considered for simultaneous kidney/pancreas transplantation is the existence of other cardiovascular disease in these diabetic patients. Therefore, evaluation for coronary artery disease and aortoiliac disease is very important.

B. OPERATIVE TECHNIC. The major requirements for the pancreas donor is no history of pancreatitis or diabetes and a normal gland at the time of recovery. The donor operation supplies the pancreas and the duodenum with the portal vein, splenic artery, and superior mesenteric artery. To perform the vascular anastomosis, the splenic artery and superior mesenteric artery are joined by a Y-graft of donor iliac artery.

In general, a midline approach to the abdomen is used. The iliac vessels are isolated and the vessels supplying the pancreas are anastomosed to the iliac vessels. The major technical advance in pancreas transplantation has been drainage of the pancreatic exocrine secretions into the bladder. This is done by anastomosing the duodenum to the bladder (Figure 20-5).

C. IMMUNOSUPPRESSION. In general, immunosuppression is identical to that for kidney transplantation. The serum creatinine is used as the main indicator of rejection, but many programs follow the urinary amylase excretion as a secondary marker of rejection. It has been found that a fall in urinary amylase may be an indication of rejection. Rejection is treated with corticosteroids or antilymphocyte preparations.

D. COMPLICATIONS. Infection and rejection are the major complications of pancreas transplantation. Complications unique to pancreas transplantation include a metabolic acidosis secondary to pancreatic and duodenal excretion of bicar-

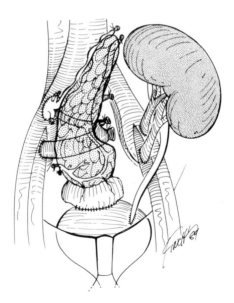

FIGURE 20-5. Combined pancreas/renal transplantation. (From Letourneau JG, Day DL, Ascher NL: *Radiology of organ transplantation*, St. Louis, 1991, Mosby–Year Book.)

bonate into the bladder. This is treated with high doses of oral bicarbonate. In general, this problem disappears after a time for unknown reasons. Other complications include graft pancreatitis, graft thrombosis, and intraabdominal abscess.

XII. LIVER TRANSPLANTATION

Dr. Thomas Starzl performed the first human liver transplant in 1963. Although this sparked worldwide interest in the field, a long-term survivor was not obtained until 1967. Early 1-year survival rates were poor; approximately 30% until 1980 when cyclosporine was introduced as the principal immunosuppressive agent. Cyclosporine (as well as technical advances and improved patient management) ushered in survival rates of 65% in the early 1980s and 1-year survival rates of 80% or better today.

A. PATIENT SELECTION. Careful selection of potential recipients and improved preoperative management have contributed to the improved transplant results. Appropriate indications for liver transplantation can be divided into general indications applicable to most forms of chronic liver disease and specific indications appropriate to one or only a few diseases. Diseases for which liver transplantation is applicable in most cases include ascites refractory to medical management, encephalopathy that significantly impairs lifestyle, variceal hemorrhage that is refractory to sclerotherapy, and the hepatorenal syndrome. Indications that apply to specific liver diseases include refractory pruritus (chronic cholestatic disorders such as primary biliary cirrhosis or extrahepatic biliary atresia), severe metabolic bone diseases with fracture (primary biliary cirrhosis), recurrent cholangitis (primary sclerosing cholangitis [primary biliary cirrhosis] or extrahepatic biliary atresia), neurotoxicity (Wilson's disease), and correction of metabolic diseases related to impaired synthesis of a liver-specific protein (familial hypercholesterolemia, tyrosinemia, α1-antitrypsin deficiency, hereditary oxalosis, Crigler-Najjar type II).

Although these indications for liver transplantation are generally accepted, the decision regarding exact timing of the surgery is made difficult by the variable natural history of the liver disease. Ideally, transplantation should be performed at a time when a patient's general medical condition would minimize operative mortality and morbidity but the liver disease severely jeopardizes 1-year survival. Natural history data suggesting when liver transplantation is appropriate may be helpful in primary biliary cirrhosis, fulminant liver disease, and sclerosing cholangitis. Unfortunately, the natural histories of diseases such as chronic active hepatitis with cirrhosis are much less predictable; consequently, decisions regarding the timing of transplantation are more difficult.

The contraindications to liver transplantation have evolved as the field has developed. Widely accepted contraindications include sepsis, extrahepatic malignancy, and positive HIV serology. Relative contraindications to liver transplantation include HBsAg antigenemia with evidence of active viral replication, advanced age, renal failure, and active infection.

B. DONOR SELECTION. The requirements for the potential liver donor are similar to those for other organs. No test of liver function in the donor is currently predictive of function following transplantation. Some work is being done with the metabolism of lidocaine as a possible test. Until recently the preservation of the donor liver was performed in a hyperosmolar, potassium-rich solution initially used for renal preservation. The mechanism of action of these solutions appears related to the impermeant solutes that maintain a relatively normal state of hydration of the cell during preservation. A new solution with a different set of impermeant substances—hetastarch, raffinose, and lactobionate—may extend the maximum preservation time from 10 to 20 hours.

C. OPERATIVE TECHNIC. Orthotopic liver transplantation remains a surgical tour de force. Much of the improved survival following liver transplantation can be related to improvements in the surgical and anesthetic technics.

1. The **operative challenge** of liver transplantation can be traced to the impaired coagulation mechanisms of liver failure and the chronic portal hypertension. The combination of large nests of vessels to divide and the lack of coagulation factors and platelets to provide hemostasis lead to the possibility of extensive blood loss. The technical problems of recipient hepatectomy are compounded in patients with previous right upper quadrant surgery, and these operations should be deferred to liver transplantation, particularly central portosystemic shunts. Management of variceal hemorrhage by radiologically placed intrahepatic shunts is the preferred method of controlling variceal hemorrhage in the potential liver transplant recipient.

2. The **anesthetic management** is directed toward maintaining adequate intravascular volume and a functioning hemostatic system. This requires supplementation of clotting factors with fresh frozen plasma and cryoprecipitate and correction of thrombocytopenia. The anesthesiologist also must be able to administer large volumes of blood and blood products rapidly. The development of the rapid transfusion device allows for the delivery of warmed blood at a rate >2 L/min. The third anesthetic problem is the maintenance of a normal electrolyte balance. Hypocalcemia from administration of large volumes of citrated blood, acidosis, and hyperkalemia from reperfusion of the donor organ and from the banked blood are common intraoperative events.

D. VENOVENOUS BYPASS. When liver transplantation was first attempted in animals, normal dogs did not tolerate prolonged clamping of the portal vein and inferior vena cava. Hemodynamic instability led to the development of a method of shunting the blood from the portal vein and inferior vena cava to the superior vena cana (venovenous bypass). Later work showed that bypass was not necessary in dogs that had preexisting portal hypertension. Many humans also tolerated vessel clamping without the use of the bypass. In liver transplantation, clamping the portal vein and intrahepatic cava has three undesirable effects: loss of preload from decreased venous return, an increase in vena caval pressure that theoretically can impede renal venous return and compromise renal function, and bowel edema from obstruction of the portal system. Because of these concerns, the Pittsburgh group reinstated the use of the bypass first in heparinized patients (which led to excessive bleeding) and then in a heparinless system. The incidence of renal dysfunction and blood loss was diminished in their patients using the bypass compared with historical controls. Other groups have reported successful liver transplantation without bypass and without an increase in renal dysfunction or blood loss. It is possible to overcome the loss of preload and maintain good urinary output during the anhepatic phase without bypass by use of the rapid transfusion device. Currently, advocates of the bypass describe the benefits as allowing for an extended anhepatic phase when training surgeons or in difficult technical situations. The use of bypass is not without risk. Pulmonary embolism, nerve injury, lymphoceles, and wound infection have all been reported as complications of the bypass. The specific benefits of bypass are unclear and would have to be determined in a randomized trial.

E. BILIARY RECONSTRUCTION. The biliary drainage procedure is responsible for the majority of complications following liver transplantation. Early reports of liver transplantation showed an incidence of 34%-53% and a mortality of 25%-30% from biliary tract complications. Recently, the incidence of biliary complications has decreased to 12%-13%. Improvements have come from standardization of biliary tract reconstruction to either a choledochocholedochostomy (donor bile duct to recipient duct) in recipients with normal bile ducts (Figure 20-6) or a Roux-en-Y choledochojejunostomy in patients with abnormal bile ducts (e.g., patients with extrahepatic biliary atresia or sclerosing cholangitis).

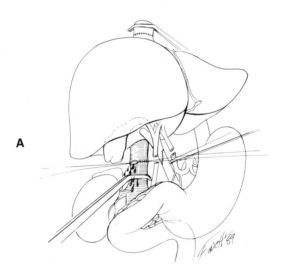

FIGURE 20-6. A, Liver transplantation following completion of vena cava anastomosis and portal vein anastomosis. Portal vein blood is allowed to flow through liver and drain out inferior vena cava to remove preservation solution from the liver. **B,** Completed liver transplant with duct-duct biliary anastomosis done over transhepatic tube. **C,** Completed liver transplantation with biliary anastomosis as done as duct to Roux-en-Y jejunal limb over stent.

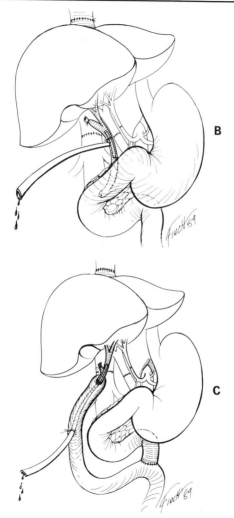

FIGURE 20-6, cont'd. For legend see opposite page.

F. COMPLICATIONS. Biliary complications require immediate intervention with diversion of the bile, usually performed via transhepatic biliary drainage and drainage of any associated bile collection. Whether bile leaks need operation is controversial. Our experience has been that leakage from the transhepatic tube exit site or minor anastomatic leaks can be managed with percutaneous or nasobiliary drainage. Disruption of the anastomosis requires revision, whereas late strictures may be managed by balloon dilation and stenting. Two caveats have been suggested in the setting of biliary complications. The first is that ultrasonography may be unreliable in diagnosing biliary tract dilation in the liver transplant recipient, and the second is that the presence of biliary tract problems should raise suspicion of an hepatic artery thrombosis.

1. Hepatic artery thrombosis. Because liver transplantation interrupts the arterial collaterals to the liver, subsequent thrombosis of the hepatic artery results in total loss of arterial blood flow to hepatic parenchyma and the biliary tree, leading to hepatic necrosis and biliary complications. The biliary tract lesion can resemble sclerosing cholangitis with bile duct strictures and dilation. The incidence of hepatic thrombosis is about 3%-10%, with a higher rate in pediatric patients and in patients with complex vascular reconstructions. Hepatic artery thrombosis occurring immediately after transplant is particularly hazardous because new collaterals have not developed; the mortality in this setting is 50%. Current emphasis has been on early detection by the use of Doppler ultrasonography to test for arterial patency in the postoperative period and the use of aspirin to prevent thrombosis.

Thrombosis in the immediate postoperative period usually requires retransplantation, although it is possible that early recognition, thrombectomy, and anastomotic revision may allow preservation of the liver and biliary tree. Late thrombosis may lead to abscess formation and biliary strictures or follow a more benign course, possibly owing to development of colleterals to the liver.

2. Portal vein thrombosis. Thrombosis of the portal vein occurs in 1.8% of transplants and carries a better prognosis. Liver function may be maintained, but portal hypertension and variceal hemorrhage frequently develop. Angiographic attempts to reopen the portal vein may be successful if performed early. Otherwise, portosystemic shunting procedures may be necessary.

3. Nonsurgical complications in the immediate post-operative period. Renal dysfunction is common in the post-transplant period. Some series report the need for dialysis in 25% of patients after transplantation. Immediate renal dysfunction in liver transplant recipients is often related to the use of cyclosporine. Acute **cyclosporine toxicity** is mediated by reduction of renal blood flow and GFR. The acute nephrotoxicity of cyclosporine can be minimized by the use of low doses. The use of lower doses is possible because of the concomitant use of azathioprine in the postoperative period. Substitution of antilymphocyte preparations for the early use of cyclosporine in a sequential protocol may allow for good renal function in the immediate postoperative period.

4. Rejection. With improvement in the operative technic of liver transplantation and improved care of the critically ill patient, liver transplant rejection has been recognized as a major clinical problem. Percutaneous liver biopsy has defined the incidence of rejection; depending on the criteria used, 20%-80% of patients undergoing transplantation experience rejection at some point in their clinical course. Approximately one half of late mortality is related to rejection.

Laboratory features of rejection are nonspecific and include an elevation in transaminase, bilirubin, and alkaline phosphatase. In prospective studies by Williams and Freese, neither the absolute level nor the change in liver tests could distinguish acute rejection from other causes of graft dysfunction. Moreover, some patients with histologic evidence of acute rejection may have normal or unchanged liver tests. For this reason, liver histology has become the most specific indicator of rejection. Most groups use a combination of clinical, biochemical, and histologic features for diagnosis.

Because of the large number of causes of graft dysfunction and the toxicity of the immunosuppressive agents used to treat rejection, one approach involves weekly biopsies following transplantation to provide the early, specific diagnosis of rejection and treatment based upon these finding. The biopsies are continued until two successive biopsies show no evidence of rejection.

XIII. SUMMARY

Improved survival following liver transplantation in the 1980s was not the result of any one advance. Earlier patient referral and better patient selection have led to recipients who are likely to be long-term survivors while not eliminating those marginal patients who benefit from transplant. Improvements in donor organ recovery have increased the pool of acceptable organs available and therefore have decreased waiting time, allowing transplantation prior to irreversible deterioration of the recipient. Better operative technics have led to fewer complications, and technics of anesthetic management have decreased intraoperative death and postoperative morbidity. Immunosuppression and treatment of rejection have improved, resulting in a decrease of retransplantation and more organs available to other patients while not increasing the complications of immunosuppression. Advances have occurred in an accelerated fashion since 1980. It is believed that a plateau in improvements has not been reached yet and that the 1990s will herald not only improved survival but decreased costs, complication, and hospital stays.

Abbreviations

AAA	Abdominal aortic aneurysms.
ABC	Airway, Breathing, Circulation.
ABG	Arterial blood gas.
ABI	Ankle/brachial index.
AC	Alternating current.
ACD	Acid citrate dextrose.
ACT	Activated coagulation time.
ACTH	Adrenocorticotropic hormone.
ADP	Adenosine diphosphate.
ADH	Antidiuretic hormone.
AFP	Alpha-fetoprotein.
AHF	Antihemophilic factor.
AICD	Automatic implantable cardioverter defibrillator.
AIDS	Acquired immunodeficiency syndrome.
AJCC	American Joint Committee on Cancer.
AMP	Adenosine monophosphate.
AOM	Acute otitis media.
AP	Anteroposterior.
ARA-C	Cytosine arabinoside.
ASA	American Society of Anesthesiologists.
ASD	Atrial septal defect.
ATGAM	Antithymocyte gamma-globulin.
ATN	Acute tubular necrosis.
ATP	Adenosine triphosphate.
AV	Aortic valve.
A-V	Arteriovenous; arterioventricular; atrioventricular.
AVM	Arteriovenous malformation.
BAO	Basal acid output.
BCC	Basal cell carcinoma.
BP	Blood pressure.
BSA	Body surface area.
BUN	Blood urea nitrogen.
CABG	Coronary artery bypass grafting.
CAD	Coronary artery disease.
CAF	Cyclophosphamide, Adriamycin (doxorubicin), [5-] fluorouracil.
Cal	Calories.
CAVH	Continous arteriovenous ultrafiltration.
CBC	Complete blood cell count.
cc	Cubic centimeter.

CEA	Carcinoembryonic antigen.
cGy	Centigray (1 rad).
CHF	Chronic heart failure.
CHOP	Cyclophosphamide, Adriamycin, vincristine, prednisone.
CIN	Cervical intraepithelial neoplasia.
CL	Cleft lip.
CMV	Cytomegalovirus.
CNS	Central nervous system.
CO	Carbon monoxide.
CO_2	Carbon dioxide.
COPD	Chronic obstructive pulmonary disease.
CP	Cleft palate.
CPB	Competitive protein binding.
CPD	Citrate phosphate dextrose.
CPDA	Citrate phosphate dextrose adenine.
CPK	Creatine phosphokinase.
CRF	Corticotropin-releasing factor.
CSA	Cyclosporin A.
CSF	Cerebrospinal fluid.
CSII	Continuous subcutaneous insulin infusion.
CT	Computed tomography.
CVP	Central venous pressure.
CXR	Chest radiograph.
DC	Direct current.
DCIS	Ductal carcinoma in situ.
DDAVP	1-deamino-8-D-arginine vasopressin.
DDT	Dichlorodiphenyltrichloroethane.
DES	Diethylstilbestrol.
DHPG	Dihydroxyphenylglycol; dihydroxyproproxy-methylguanine.
DI	Diabetes insipidus.
DIC	Disseminated intravascular coagulation.
DIT	Diiodotyrosine.
DKA	Diabetic ketoacidosis.
dl	Deciliter.
DNA	Deoxyribonucleic acid.
DPG	Diphosphoglycerate.
DTPA	Diethylenetriaminepenta-acetic acid.
D_5W	5% dextrose in water.
EBA	Extrahepatic biliary atresia.
EBV	Epstein-Barr virus.
ECF	Extracellular fluid.
ECG	Electrocardiogram.
EEG	Electroencephalogram.

EFAD	Essential fatty acid deficiency.
EGD	Esophagogastroduodenoscopy.
Eq	Equivalent.
ER	Estrogen receptor.
ERCP	Endoscopic retrograde cholangiopancreatography.
ESR	Erythrocyte sedimentation rate.
ESWL	Extracorporeal shock wave lithotripsy.
FAP	Familial adenomatous polyposis.
FB	Foreign body.
FDA	Food and Drug Administration.
FIGO	International Federation of Gynecology and Obstetrics.
FFP	Fresh frozen plasma.
FNA	Fine-needle aspiration.
FOAM	5-fluorouracil, vincristine, Adriamycin, and methotrexate.
FTI	Free thyroxine index.
FU	Fluorouracil.
FUDR	Floxiuridine.
G-CSF	Granulocyte colony-stimulating factors.
GFR	Glomerular filtration rate.
GI	Gastrointestinal.
GM-CSF	Granulocyte-macrophage colony-stimulating factors.
GnRh	Gonadotropin-releasing hormone.
G6PD	Glucose-6-phosphate dehydrogenase.
GU	Genitourinary.
H_2O	Water.
HbCO	Carboxyhemoglobin.
HBsAg	Hepatitis B surface antigen.
HCG	Human chorionic gonadotropin.
HgB	Hemoglobin.
HIDA	Hepato-iminodiacetic acid.
HIV	Human immunodeficiency virus.
HL-A	Human leukocyte antigen.
HPLC	High-pressure liquid chromatography.
HPV	Human papilloma virus.
HSV	Herpes simplex virus.
HTLV	Human T-cell leukemia/lyphoma virus.
HUS	Hemolytic-uremic syndrome.
HVA	Homovanillic acid.
ICP	Intracranial pressure.
ICU	Intensive care unit.
IDDM	Insulin-dependent.
IFN	Interferon.

IgA	Immunoglobulin A.
IGF	Insulin-like growth factors.
IgG	Immunoglobulin G.
IHSS	Idiopathic hypertrophic subaortic stenosis.
IL-2	Interleukin-2.
IM	Intramuscular.
INH	Isoniazid.
INR	International normalized ratio.
IPPB	Intermittent positive-pressure breathing.
IQ	Intelligence quotient.
ITP	Idiopathic thrombocytopenic purpura.
IU	In utero; intrauterine international units.
IV	Intravenous.
IVP	Intravenous pyelography.
kg	Kilograms.
17-KS	17-ketosteroid.
JVD	Jugular venous distention.
JVP	Jugular vein pulse; jugular venous pressure.
KOH	Potassium hydroxide.
KUB	Kidney, ureter, and bladder.
LAD	Left anterior descending [coronary artery].
LATS	Long-acting thyroid stimulator.
LDH	Lactic dehydrogenase.
LFT	Liver function test.
LGV	Lymphogranuloma venereum.
LM	Laryngeal mask.
LP	Lumbar puncture.
LV	Left ventricular.
LVH	Left ventricular hypertrophy.
LVOTO	Left ventricular outflow tract obstruction.
MAC	Maximal acid output; minimal aesthetic concentration.
MALG	Minnesota antilymphoblast globulin.
MAO	Monoamine oxidase.
MAP	Mean arterial pressure.
MB	Subunits of isoenzyme of creatine kinase.
MBC	Minimal bactericidal concentration.
MEA	Multiple endocrine adenomatosis.
MEN-I	Multiple endocrine neoplasia-I.
mg	Milligrams.
MI	Myocardial infarction.
MIBG	Methyl isobutyl guanidine.
MIC	Minimal inhibitory concentration.
MIT	Monoiodotyrosine.
ml	Milliliters.

mm	Millimeter.
6-MP	6-mercaptopurine.
MRA	Magnetic resonance angiography.
MRI	Magnetic resonance imaging.
MSH	Melanotropins.
MVO_2	Myocardial oxygen consumption.
Nd/YAG	Neodymium/yttrium-aluminum-garnet [laser].
nmol	Nanomole.
NO	Nitrous oxide.
NPH	Neutral protamine Hagedorn (insulin).
NPO	Nothing by mouth.
NS	Normal saline.
NSAID	Nonsteroidal anti-inflammatory drug.
NYHA	New York Heart Association.
O_2	Oxygen.
OGTT	Oral glucose tolerance test.
OHCS	Hydroxycorticosteroid.
o,p′ DDD	Mitotane.
OR	Operating room.
ORIF	Open reduction with internal fixation.
OS	Opening snap.
osm	Osmole.
P2	Second heart sound.
PA	Posteroanterior.
PABA	Para-amino benzoic acid.
PAsys	Pulmonary artery systolic pressure.
PAmean	Pulmonary artery mean pressure.
PBC	Primary biliary cirrhosis.
PBI	Protein-bound iodine.
PBS	Polybrominated salicylanilide.
PC	Platelet count.
PCA	Patient-controlled analgesia.
PCO_2	Pressure carbon dioxide.
PCWP	Pulmonary capillary web pattern.
PDA	Posterior descending artery; patent ductus arteriosus.
PDS	Polydioxanone sutures.
PEG	Percutaneous endoscopic gastrostomy.
PEEP	Positive end-expiratory pressure.
pg	Picogram.
PGE_1	Prostaglandin E_1.
po	By mouth.
PPF	Plasma protein fraction.
prn	As required.

PS	Physical status.
PSA	Prostate-specific antigen.
PSP	Phenolsulfonphthalein.
PT	Prothrombin time.
PTCA	Percutaneous transluminal coronary artery.
PTFE	Polytetrafluroethylene.
PTH	Para-thyroid hormone.
PTT	Partial thromboplastin time.
PTU	Propylthiouracil.
PV	Peritoneovenous.
Qp/Qs	Increase in pulmonary blood flow.
QRS	Vector loop in ventricular depolarization.
Q-T	Time from beginning of QRS complex to end of T wave.
RBC	Red blood cells.
RCA	Right coronary artery.
RDA	Recommended daily allowance.
RE	Resting energy.
Rh	Rhesus [factor].
RIA	Radioimmunoassay.
RNA	Ribonucleic acid.
RQ	Respiratory quotient.
RVV	Russell's viper venom.
Rx	Drug; therapy; prescription.
S1	First heart sound.
S3	Extradiastolic filling sound.
SAL	Suction-assisted lipectomy.
SAP	Systemic arterial pressure.
SCC	Squamous cell carcinoma.
SFA	Superficial femoral artery.
SGOT	Serum glutamate oxaloacetate transaminase.
SIADH	Inappropriate secretion of antidiuretic hormone.
SLE	Systemic lupus erythematosus.
SOAP	Subjective, Objective, Assessment, Plans.
SMZ	Sulfamethoxazole.
ST	[Segment] of electrocardiogram.
T_3	Triiodothyronine.
T_4	Thyroxine.
TB	Tuberculin; tuberculosis.
TBG	Thyroxine-binding globulin.
TBI	Thyroid-blocking immunoglobulins.
TBPA	Thyroid-binding prealbumin.
TFT	Thyroid function test.
TGA	Transposition of the great arteries.
Tl	Thallium.

TIA	Transient ischemic attacks.
TIPS	Transjugular intrahepatic portosystemic shunts.
TMP	Trimethoprim.
TNF	Tumor necrosis factor.
TNM	Tumor node metastasis.
TOF	Tetralogy of Fallot.
torr	mm HG pressure.
TPN	Total parenteral nutrition.
TRH	Thyrotropin-releasing hormone.
T_3RU	Triiodothyronine resin uptake.
TRU	Transrectal ultrasonography.
TSH	Thyroid-stimulating hormone.
TSI	Thyroid-stimulating immunoglobulins.
TTP	Thrombotic thrombocytopenic purpura.
UNOS	United Network for Organ Sharing.
U/P	Urine to Plasma [ratio].
USP	United States Pharmacopeia.
UTI	Urinary tract infection.
UV	Ultraviolet.
VIP	Vasoactive intestinal polypeptide.
VMA	Vanillylmandelic acid.
VSD	Ventricular septal defect.
vWd	von Willebrand's disease.
VZV	Varicella virus.
WBC	White blood cell.
WDHA	Watery diarrhea, hypokalemia, and achlohydria.
ZE	Zollinger-Ellison.

Index